Disorders of Human Learning, Behavior, and Communication

Ronald L. Taylor and Les Sternberg
Series Editors

H. Carl Haywood David Tzuriel
Editors

Interactive Assessment

With 20 Illustrations

Springer-Verlag
New York Berlin Heidelberg London Paris
Tokyo Hong Kong Barcelona Budapest

H. Carl Haywood, Vanderbilt University, Nashville, TN 37203, USA

David Tzuriel, Bar Ilan University, Ramat-Gan 52 900, Israel

Series Editors: Ronald L. Taylor and Les Sternberg, Exceptional Student Education, Florida Atlantic University, Boca Raton, FL 33431-0991, USA

Library of Congress Cataloging-in-Publication Data
Interactive assessment / [edited by] H. Carl Haywood, David Tzuriel.
p. cm.—(Disorders of human learning, behavior, and communication)
Includes bibliographical references and index.
ISBN 0-387-97587-X (alk. paper)
1. Behavioral assessment. 2. Psychological tests. I. Haywood, H. Carl, 1931–. II. Tzuriel, David. III. Series.
BF176.5.157 1991
153.9′3—dc20 91-21039

Printed on acid-free paper.

Production managed by Ellen Seham; manufacturing supervised by Jacqui Ashri.
Typeset by Best-set Typesetter Ltd., Chai Wan, Hong Kong.
Printed and bound by Edwards Brothers, Inc., Ann Arbor, MI.
Printed in the United States of America.

9 8 7 6 5 4 3 2 1

ISBN 0-387-97587-X Springer-Verlag New York Berlin Heidelberg
ISBN 3-540-97587-X Springer-Verlag Berlin Heidelberg New York

Preface

The terms *interactive* and *dynamic* would never have been associated with psychological and psychoeducational assessment a generation ago. They have currency now because of widespread dissatisfaction with the normative, standardized testing model, criticism of theoretical concepts of intelligence, recognition of abuses of standardized intelligence testing, and frustration with prediction and classification as primary goals of assessment.

It is almost certainly true that public policy concerns propel scientific activity far more often than science propels public policy! In the case of psychological assessment, public policy concerns have arisen in the last 20 years primarily around issues of possible "discrimination" against members of ethnic minorities. At the same time, there has been a resurgence of dedication to "excellence in education" goals. These concerns have led to such extreme measures as prohibition of the use of standardized intelligence tests to determine school placement decisions, especially for minority children. They have led also to a search for alternatives to standardized, normative testing. The chapters in this volume represent a variety of answers to this need.

As happens often with significant social and scientific developments, interactive approaches to psychological assessment have been explored both conceptually and clinically in many places and by many persons at the same time. We have tried in this volume to demonstrate the widespread nature of these developments: a Russian-German tradition, represented in the work of Vygotsky and subsequently the German Lerntest movement; a Swiss-Israeli tradition that has crossed both the Mediterranean and the Atlantic; an American-Canadian-Australian tradition that has strong roots in experimental psychology; a Swiss-French tradition that displays both neo-Piagetian and experimental roots. Our determination to show such a widespread series of developments in interactive approaches to assessment has been intended both to reveal and to encourage diversity in this kind of work. Still in its infancy, interactive assessment will not be recognizable 20 years from now as any single one of the approaches represented in this book. Instead, the healthy diversity that characterizes the field today will have produced methods and materials that are stronger than any of today's programs. Indeed, diversity is the theme of this book: diversity in concepts, geography, materials, programs, and applications.

In any edited book there is a certain amount of discontinuity, difference in general approach, and unevenness with respect to such variables as density of documentation, writing style, and economy. While emphasizing healthy diversity, we have tried to overcome some of the disadvantages of edited books through organization. Each author was invited to contribute to the book for quite specific reasons, usually to achieve "coverage" of the domains that the editors thought important and because each author was doing important work in interactive assessment. We have sequenced the chapters to flow from the most abstract to the most applied, from concerns about theories of human ability to concerns about public policy in education and psychology. Although some of the concepts of interactive assessment are difficult on first reading, readers should be assured that most of them will come up again.

The book is organized in five parts: theory, research, applications, case studies, and policy. Each of the parts is introduced by a brief discussion of its own domain, intended to orient readers to the compelling questions treated in that part. Within parts, diversity is again the emphasis. The book ends with a very brief summary epilogue.

Although we have emphasized diversity in this book, both editors have, and are happy to acknowledge, large conceptual debts to Reuven Feuerstein. In our opinion, Professor Feuerstein has been the most enduring, insistent, consistent, creative, and caring of the many persons who have contributed to the development of interactive assessment. His clinical contributions, through the Learning Potential Assessment Device, will continue to have direct benefits for persons whose intellective potential is underassessed by standardized methods. In one form or another Feuerstein's concepts will be represented in the programs, materials, and techniques of many other innovators in this field.

H. Carl Haywood
David Tzuriel

Contents

Contributors

Adrian F. Ashman, University of Queensland, St. Lucia, Queensland, Australia

John D. Bransford, Vanderbilt University, Nashville, TN, USA

M. Susan Burns, University of Pittsburgh, Pittsburgh, PA, USA

Jerry S. Carlson, University of California, Riverside, Riverside, CA, USA

Robert N. F. Conway, University of Newcastle, CAE Campus, Newcastle, New South Wales, Australia

J. Prasad Das, University of Alberta, Edmonton, Alberta, Canada

Victor R. Delclos, Tulane University, New Orleans, LA, USA

Rogers Elliott, Dartmouth College, Hanover, NH, USA

Joel E. Fagan, Alberta Children's Hospital and The University of Calgary, Calgary, Alberta, Canada

Reuven Feuerstein, Hadassah-WIZO-Canada Research Institute, Jerusalem, Israel

Jürgen Guthke, University of Leipzig, Leipzig, Germany

Ted S. Hasselbring, Vanderbilt University, Nashville, TN, USA

H. Carl Haywood, Vanderbilt University, Nashville, TN, USA

Shlomo Kaniel, Bar Ilan University, Ramat-Gan, Israel

Kevin J. Keane, Lexington School for the Deaf, Jackson Heights, NY, USA

Steve M. Killip, Board of Education for the City of London, London, Ontario, Canada

Pnina S. Klein, Bar Ilan University, Ramat-Gan, Israel

Gary F. Krapf, Chesterfield County Schools, Chesterfield, VA, USA

Carol H. Lamb, The Learning Centre, Calgary, Alberta, Canada

Heather E. MacKenzie, H. E. MacKenzie and Associates, Calgary, Alberta, Canada

John C. Masters, Vanderbilt University, Nashville, TN, USA

Jack A. Naglieri, Ohio State University, Columbus, Ohio, USA

Lorna Oberholtzer, Central Winipeg School Board, Winipeg, Manitoba, Canada

Jean-Louis Paour, University of Provence, Aix-en-Provence, France

Marilyn T. Samuels, The Learning Centre, and The University of Calgary, Calgary, Alberta, Canada

Ian M. Shochet, Charles Sturt University, Bathurst, New South Wales, Australia

Harry Silverman, Ontario Institute for Studies in Education, Toronto, Ontario, Canada

Guylaine Soavi, University of Provence, Aix-en-Provence, France

Abraham J. Tannenbaum, Teachers College, Columbia University, New York, NY, USA

David Tzuriel, Bar Ilan University, Ramat-Gan, Israel

Cheryl A. Utley, Vanderbilt University, Nashville, TN, USA

Susan R. Vaught, Temple University Health Sciences Center, Philadelphia, PA, USA

Nancy J. Vye, Vanderbilt University, Nashville, TN, USA

Mary Waksman, Toronto, Ontario, Canada

Karl Heinz Wiedl, University of Osnabrück, Osnabrück, Germany

Sabine Wingenfeld, University of Arkansas, Fayetteville, AR, USA

Part 1
Theoretical Bases of Interactive Assessment

This first section of the book is designed to provide a conceptual base on which the technology of interactive assessment may rest. In keeping with the theme of diversity that characterizes both this book and the developmental stage of cognitive assessment, these chapters reflect rather different theoretical positions. The editors believe that the theoretical task that confronts psychologists and educators is not to determine which, if any, of these different positions is correct, but instead to enlarge our own perspective by entertaining these diverse points of view.

It is not likely that one can have an actual theory of interactive assessment. Psychological and psychoeducational assessment is a technology that derives benefit from theories about its several components. The most important set of theory concerns the nature, development, and relative modifiability of whatever it is that one hopes to assess—ability, intelligence, learning potential, scholastic aptitude. Each of the four chapters in this section on theory contains a model of the nature of human ability. It is reasonable to expect that each model should demand, or at least be consistent with, a certain set of assessment goals, practices, and interpretation. Readers with especially sharp eyes will look for those models and determine for themselves to what extent the authors have related concepts of ability to assessment models.

Each of these four chapters also has a bit of history in it. In Chapter 1, Tzuriel and Haywood begin with a quite broad orientation, discussing some of the problems with standardized, normative assessment and describing some early work in the testing movement. They then narrow progressively down to a particular emphasis on the dynamic assessment approach that is associated with Feuerstein.

In Chapter 2, Haywood, Tzuriel, and Vaught place interactive assessment within a special conceptual context, a transactional perspective on the nature, development, and modifiability of human ability. In the process, they suggest that some other approaches to assessment are also consistent with a transactional perspective, and they view these approaches (e.g., neuropsychological assessment and curriculum-based assessment) as complementary rather than as competing with dynamic/interactive assessment.

Chapter 3, by Guthke and Wingenfeld, reflects a different history, that of the Lerntest movement in Germany that grew in part from the concepts of Vygotsky. Based more clearly on traditional psychometric approaches, but definitely expanding upon and departing from them, the learning test concept has the concepts of modifiability and of ability-performance discrepancy in common with the other concepts. Contemporary political events in Germany make much of the work presented here, as well as the investigators who have accomplished that work, much more accessible than in the past.

The essential aspect of any interactive assessment approach is transfer of training. In Chapter 4, Das and Conway have emphasized that aspect, generalizing on the concepts of Vygotsky but reflecting also Das's close association with the neuropsychology of A. R. Luria. The cognitive processes that Das and Conway discuss are somehow more narrowly defined than are those of Feuerstein or Guthke, so it would not be surprising to see a greater volume of research on those processes done under a classical experimental psychology model.

Every one of these four theoretical chapters is rooted in empirical research, and to the extent that they are useful they will lead to further research, with each empirical iteration being more sharply focused than its predecessors. The editors have seen these four as representative, but hardly as exhaustive, of the current theoretical approaches to interactive assessment.

1 The Development of Interactive-Dynamic Approaches to Assessment of Learning Potential

David Tzuriel and H. Carl Haywood

Development of Standardized Testing

Traditional methods of assessing mental ability have been intimately related to concepts of intelligence (see Haywood, Tzuriel, & Vaught, Chapter 2 in this volume). Most proponents of conventional testing approaches believe in the existence of "intelligence" as a more-or-less fixed entity. This approach has served as a guide for the design of testing procedures that would justify the concept. A more practical approach has been to devise tests simply for applied purposes, such as classifying children for different educational "tracks" or allocating a school system's resources. A third source of influence on the testing movement has been the pressure of social movements and the particular needs of societies. We focus here on this third aspect, the development of psychological assessment procedures in response to problems and needs posed by social processes such as accelerated urbanization, industrialization, mass production, and attempts at universal education. We try to demonstrate that psychometric practices mirror, to some extent, the social movements and circumstances of their time. Traditional, standardized assessment procedures have grown up in that manner, and the newer approaches described and advocated in this book have developed as well in response to changing societal demands. In later sections, we describe the development of interactive (dynamic) approaches to psychological and psychoeducational assessment, emphasizing approaches that have sprung from conceptual schemes that themselves reflect changes in societal needs and demands.

According to Feuerstein, Rand, Jensen, Kaniel, and Tzuriel (1987), the spread of standardized-psychometric practice has been seen by some as a response to historical events (Cremin, 1964), particularly democratization of the educational system and the inclusion of persons who had previously been considered ineligible for and inaccessible to education. Social scientists as well as educational establishments have responded to social needs by developing complex schemes for assessing a variety of mental functions, diagnostic profiles, classification systems, and labeling categories.

Needs for standardized testing brought about by social processes have been accelerated by historical events that, at first glance, seem to have little to do with psychological testing. The growing dissatisfaction with standardized tests over the last two decades, and consequently the development of alternative interactive-dynamic methods, can also be conceived of as a response to social changes, a point discussed in the following paragraphs.

Interest in testing in the United States was accelerated by the widespread use of standardized testing during World War I for military personnel selection. In less than 2 years the Army Alpha test was given to 1.7 million military recruits in the United States and the data gathered constituted the prime source of various studies of group differences in ability (Tuddenham, 1962). Between the world wars, group testing of both aptitude and achievement in schools became popular. The use of aptitude tests to select candidates for special military training constituted one of the signal successes of psychology in World War II. The launching of the first earth-orbiting satellite by the Soviet Union in 1957 also led, indirectly, to renewed efforts to refine standardized tests. The National Defense Education Act (NDEA) provided financial assistance for school testing programs in order to identify students with outstanding aptitudes and abilities (Haney, 1981). The proliferation of large-scale testing programs was facilitated by the development of automated optical test scoring equipment in the 1950s (Baker, 1971). Minick (1987) stated that the static measures of ability came into wide use because they serve the function of selecting personnel for educational, military or industrial placement in order to maximize the return on a given investment in training or instruction.

S. White (1981) analyzed the success of the testing movement as a social enterprise according to notions of test validity and social values. A crude indicator of the social success of standardized testing in American society is the growth of the various indexing terms in the periodical literature and the gradually increasing size of Buros's compilation of tests. According to White, this growth seems to be due to two factors: (a) need of social institutions to deal with large numbers of persons for such purposes as personnel assignments, college placement, and program evaluation; and (b) a high rate of technical development, including the popular diffusion of statistics and "number consciousness" in society (Boorstein, 1974).

Historians (e.g., Karier, 1976) have suggested that the testing movement grew as a function of its role as an instrument of "order and control in the corporate liberal state." Haney (1981) suggested that testing has succeeded because of its status as an applied science of psychology.

Haney (1981) raised the argument that social attitudes and values influence both the public's view of standardized tests and professional writing about testing. According to Haney, constructs such as aptitude, ability, and achievement seem to have a life of their own, not only because of tradition but also "because they allow 'multi-interpretations' and various sorts of aggrandizement in the business of testing and test interpretation" (p. 1031). As an example Haney cited the contrast in attitudes toward the utility of test information between elementary and secondary versus higher levels of schooling.

In elementary and secondary levels it is widely accepted that when the purpose of testing is classification for educational placement the value of the test is judged in terms of the benefits derived from such special placement (Reschly, 1980). In contrast, the value of tests given in high school is discussed in terms of their ability to predict post–secondary school performance. Astin (1971), who criticized this approach, argued that selective admission based on prediction of future performance in school is perhaps missing the main point of education. Astin suggested instead that the criterion for determining the utility of an admissions policy or an educational program should be whether or not the students acquire skills and knowledge that are of value either to themselves or to society. In an attempt to explain the emphasis on predictive validity of testing at postsecondary levels as opposed to elementary and secondary levels, Haney (1981) suggested that it is related to attitudes about education. In elementary education there is a broad commitment to educating all students to their full potential, but at the postsecondary level the sorting and selection functions of schooling predominate.

Zigler and Seitz (1982) suggested using social competence scales, rather than intelligence tests, as a major indicator of the success or failure of social and educational intervention programs. They argued that intelligence tests have been used to evaluate the success of intervention programs for reasons that are mostly historical: many such programs had IQ gain as a primary goal (e.g., Garber & Heber, 1981; Gray & Klaus, 1965; Ramey, Collier, Sparling, Loda, Campbell, Ingram & Finkelstein, 1976; Skodak & Skeels, 1945; B. L. White, 1975). Other reasons, however, are related to the tests' nature: intelligence tests are available, easy to administer, require little time to administer, and have good measurement characteristics. Their generalizability, as indicated by relation to many aspects of behavior that have theoretical and practical significance (Kohlberg & Zigler, 1967; Mischel, 1968), is another reason for choosing them as evaluation criteria. Because IQ has been found to be the best available predictor of school achievement, and because compensatory education programs have been directed to the prevention and remediation of deficient school achievement, the ability of intelligence tests to sample a broad spectrum of abilities has been a compelling rationale for their use. Another reason that Zigler and Seitz (1982) cited for the popularity of intelligence tests as outcome measures is the ease of demonstrating improvement. Once it became obvious that the most common outcome of any intervention effort was a 10-point increase in IQ (see

Eisenberg & Connors, 1966), researchers used it to show the effectiveness of their programs. Considerable research, however, has suggested that such IQ changes probably result from motivational changes that influence the children's test performance rather than from increases in "intelligence" (e.g., Seitz, Abelson, Levine, & Zigler, 1975; Zigler, Abelson, & Seitz, 1973; Zigler & Butterfield, 1968).

Dissatisfaction with Standard Psychometric Testing

The development of the testing movement has been paralleled, especially in recent years, by dissatisfaction and critical arguments from both professional and lay critics (e.g., Baily & Harbin, 1980; Bronfenbrenner, 1979; Brown & Ferrara, 1985; Feuerstein, Rand, & Hoffman, 1979; Gamlin, 1989; Gould, 1981; Gupta & Coxhead, 1988; Haney, 1981; Haywood, Filler, Shifman, & Chatelanat, 1975; Lidz, 1987b; Mercer, 1975; Minick, 1987; Missiuna & Samuels, 1988; Tzuriel, 1989a; Tzuriel & Klein, 1985; Tzuriel, Samuels, & Feuerstein, 1988; Vernon, 1979; Vygotsky, 1978). The dissatisfaction has been nourished by humanistic trends that have focused on the individual; they emphasize the unique environmental factors that block or facilitate the fulfillment of human potential.

The criticism has been centered on three main points: (a) bias toward minority groups and special education groups as well as selective interpretation of results in those groups (Feuerstein, et al., 1979; Gould, 1981; Gupta & Coxhead, 1988; Haney, 1981; Haywood, Brown, & Wingenfeld, 1990; Kamin, 1974; Mercer, 1975; Messick, 1980; Sewell, 1987; Tzuriel, 1989a; Vygotsky, 1978); (b) lack of consideration of motivational, personality, and social adequacy factors that are crucial for effective human functioning (Feuerstein et al., 1979; Gardner, 1983; Penrose, 1963; Phillips, 1984; Scarr, 1981; Sternberg, 1987; Weaver, 1946; Zigler & Butterfield, 1968; Windle, 1962); and (c) lack of adequate information given by standardized psychometric tests for actual intervention, prescriptive teaching, and remediation processes (Feuerstein et al., 1979; Haywood, 1984; Haywood, Brown, & Wingenfeld, 1990; Vernon, 1979). The criticism has been discussed extensively in the literature cited above and in Chapter 2 by Haywood, Tzuriel, and Vaught (this volume), and is not repeated here.

The Development of An Interactive Assessment Approach

Together with the growing concern over the uses and abuses of standard tests, there have been attempts to modify the testing procedures and suggest novel assessment approaches (Brown & Ferrara, 1985; Budoff,

1967, 1987; Carlson & Wiedl, 1978, 1979; Coxhead & Gupta, 1988; Feuerstein, et al., 1979; Guthke, 1982; Haussermann, 1958; Haywood & Switzky, 1974, 1986; Lidz & Thomas, 1987; Mearig, 1987; Paour 1979; Tzuriel, 1989a; Tzuriel & Klein, 1985, 1986, 1987; Vygotsky, 1929, 1962, 1978). The need for change in assessment procedures can be conceptualized on both molar and molecular levels. On a molar level change has been impelled by two emerging forces: (a) democratization and humanization of the educational system; and (b) the notion that standardized, static testing procedures are not uniformly valid, and thus might "penalize" some subgroups, such as minority ethnic groups and recent immigrants. Efforts to develop interactive-dynamic procedures by Vygotsky, Feuerstein, Budoff, Carlson and Wiedl, Guthke, Campione and Brown, Haywood, Tzuriel, Gamlin, Lidz, Mearig, Stott, and others, have converged in the last decade. Development of interactive-dynamic assessment approaches has constituted a novel response to the growing concern about conventional testing. Ramey and MacPhee (1981) posed the question of whether dynamic assessment can be considered as a new paradigm that is necessary in order to respond to the new needs of assessment. As others have done, they referred to three criteria: (a) dissatisfaction with the existing philosophical-theoretical stance underlying the practice of conventional tests; (b) the existence of demographic, sociological, political, and economic conditions that create pressures to change conventional methods of assessment of large groups of persons; and (c) the emergence of novel theoretical views of the concept of intelligence, its structure, and origins that lead consequently to development of new paradigms. The two key figures who have played leading roles in changing the conventional testing assessment approach have been Vygotsky and Feuerstein, both from outside the dominant psychological mainstream in the United States. Both Vygotsky and Feuerstein have responded to social needs and cultural-historical changes for assessing human cognitive potential rather than assessing only contemporary performance.

Vygotsky's cultural-historical theory emerged at a time when educational backwardness of a large portion of the population was coupled with the social need to assimilate several national groups into the Soviet Union, and to adopt and implement Marxist theory in various spheres of life. What Vygotsky was actually trying to do consciously extended Marx's historical materialism and Engels's anthropolitical views to the ontogenetic plane (Sutton, 1981, 1987). Vygotsky criticized standard testing procedures mainly because they suggested that mental deficits and backwardness of cultural development of nationalities might be associated with a particular sociocultural level. Standard tests were criticized by Vygotsky because they had been constructed in one social context and artificially transplanted to another. A deeper basis for his criticism was that children grow up in a unique cultural-social environment that reflects historical development and a complex system of economic and cultural conditions. Thus, the study of the children within national minorities cannot be isolated from the cultural-social context. Because children are natural products of and inseparable from their particular environment, tests should be adapted to the specific conditions in which the children are developing (Vygotsky, 1929).

Feuerstein's dynamic assessment approach evolved within the historical-social framework of a massive immigration to Israel by hundreds of thousands of Jews from all over the world. Many of the immigrants coming from Asian and North African countries had to go through an accelerated process of adjustment and assimilation to both a new country and a different cultural context. The new immigrants confronted a relatively modern society with demands for a sophisticated level of technology. Social pressures for integration of the newcomers into the mainstream of the developing society posed a challenge to construct new approaches for the assessment of the abilities and potential of persons that would take into account the diverse cultures from which the newcomers arrived and allow fulfillment of the individuals' learning potential, especially those whose performance on conventional psychological tests would ordinarily have placed them outside the mainstream of education and vocational opportunity. Although testing became a necessary tool for selection of people in order to prepare them for roles in a technically advanced society, an emerging need has grown for novel methods of assessment in a multicultural society. The confrontation of immigrants with their new country created a state of disequilibrium in the well-established definitions of intelligence and the specific techniques used to assess individual differences in intellectual development.

Feuerstein's dynamic assessment approach has been used recently with Ethiopian immigrant Jews who came to Israel (Kaniel, Tzuriel, Feuerstein, Ben-Shachar & Eitan, in press). The need to apply this approach with native, black, and Hispanic Americans and Canadians has been discussed recently by Emerson (1987), Haywood (1977, 1988), Sewell (1987), and Williams (1990).

On a molecular level, the interactive-dynamic assessment movement has been motivated mainly by dissatisfaction with the ability of conventional assessment methods to provide information about individuals' learning ability that can be translated directly into practice by educators and members of other helping professions (see, e.g., Meyers, Pfeffer, & Erlbaum, 1985). Educators and clinicians need to know not only the actual manifest performance but also the nature of learning processes, specific deficient functions that impair learning, and mediational strategies that can facilitate learning (e.g., Campione & Brown, 1987; Feuerstein et al., 1979). The dynamic-interactive assessment procedures have brought with them a "fresh" look at learning potential, and have also provided working hypotheses and directions for many practitioners. These procedures can serve as a miniature model for intervention, and recommendations based on them can make more sense for educators, because they suggest practical guidelines and an integrative conceptualization of assessment and intervention processes. An important characteristic of interactive assessment is identification of specific obstacles that may be hindering cognitive performance, and specification of conditions under which intellectual performance can be facilitated (Feuerstein et al., 1979, 1987; Feuerstein, Hoffman, Jensen, & Rand, 1985, 1986; Feuerstein, Rand, & Rynders, 1988; Haywood, 1977, 1988).

The most articulated common characteristics of the various interactive assessment approaches are (a) the nature of examiner-examinee interaction in the assessment process, and (b) a belief in the plasticity and modifiability of the thinking processes of human beings. The most prominent figures in the development of interactive assessment approaches have been Vygotsky and Feuerstein. Vygotsky's approach is described by Guthke and Wingenfeld (Chapter 3, this volume). In the following section of this chapter Feuerstein's theoretical approach is described, especially in relation to the Learning Potential Assessment Device (LPAD). This is followed by a presentation of research using the LPAD with different groups, and the extension and application of interactive assessment to preschool children.

Feuerstein's Theory of Structural Cognitive Modifiability and Mediated Learning Experience

Feuerstein's approach to dynamic assessment has as its core the theory of structural cognitive modifiability (SCM) and mediated learning experience (MLE). The SCM theory (Arbitman-Smith, Haywood, & Bransford, 1984; Feuerstein et al., 1979, 1985, 1987, 1988; Feuerstein, Rand, Hoffman, & Miller, 1980; Feuerstein, Rand et al., 1986) is based on the assumption that human beings have the unique capacity to modify their cognitive functions and adapt to changing demands in life situations. This basic assumption shifts the responsibility for an individual's modifiability from the assessed or treated person to an examiner or mediator. Cognitive modifiability is considered possible irrespective of three conditions very often considered as barriers to change: etiology, age, and severity of condition. Feuerstein has described three main characteristics that define structural modifiability: permanence, pervasiveness, and centrality. Permanence refers to the endurance of the cognitive changes over time, that is, durability. Pervasiveness is related to a "diffusion" process in which changes in one part affect the whole. Centrality reflects the self-perpetuating, autonomous, and self-regulating nature of cognitive modifiability. The basic assumptions of the SCM theory are that (a) human beings are open systems amenable to cognitive changes that affect their functioning, and (b) cognitive modifiability is best explained by the MLE theory.

MLE refers to an interactional process in which adults, usually the parents, interpose themselves between children and the world and modify a set of stimuli by affecting their frequency, order, intensity, and context. Mediators arouse in children vigilance, curiosity, and sensitivity to the mediated stimuli, and create for and with the children temporal, spatial, and cause-effect relationships among stimuli. Feuerstein et al. (1979, 1980, 1987, 1988) suggested 11 characteristics of MLE; however, only the first three are considered as necessary and sufficient for any interaction to be classified as a mediated interaction: intentionality and reciprocity, meaning, and transcendence. Some authors consider only the first five or six criteria to be important dimensions of MLE (Haywood, 1987; Klein, 1988; Missiuna & Samuels, 1989; Tzuriel & Eran, 1990; Tzuriel & Ernst, 1990). In the following paragraphs the first six MLE criteria are described. For a more detailed description of all of the criteria that Feuerstein has suggested, see Feuerstein et al. (1987, 1988) and Tzuriel, Samuels, and Feuerstein (1988).

Intentionality and reciprocity. The first criterion refers to a mediator's intentional efforts to produce in a child a state of vigilance in order to help him/her to register some information. Intentionality can be observed at a very early age in dynamic mother-child interactions and is marked by many signs of reciprocity. The reciprocity aspect is conceptualized as essential for the development of basic feelings of competence and self-determination. Interactions imbued with reciprocal intentionality assist children to realize that their actions influence other people's behavior and foster their organismic belief that they can be agents of change.

Mediation of meaning. Mediation of meaning has long been recognized as a powerful determinant in effective learning processes (Ausubel, 1968; Postman & Weingartner, 1969). Mediation of meaning refers to interactions in which the presented stimuli pose affective, motivational, and value-oriented significance. The mediator does not convey a neutral attitude toward the stimuli but rather attaches importance and even enthusiasm. This is done both nonverbally and verbally. Nonverbal mediation of meaning can be expressed in voice intonation, body and face gestures, and repetition of activities and rituals. Verbal mediation can be expressed by relating a current event, activity, or learned context to past experiences or simply emphasizing its importance and value. It is assumed that a child who has experienced mediation of meaning will initiate attachment of meaning to newly acquired information rather than passively waiting for meaning to come.

Mediation of transcendence. Transcendence refers to both the character and the goal of MLE interactions. The objective of the MLE is to transcend the immediate needs and specific situation and reach out for goals that might have nothing to do with the original activities. Mediation of transcendence can be seen, for example, when a mediator uses daily activities such as planning a trip or playing a game to develop basic thinking and problem solving strategies such as planning or summative behavior. Although transcendence depends to a large degree on intentionality, the combination becomes a powerful means of widening the child's need system.

Mediation of feelings of competence. The mediator communicates to the child in various verbal and nonverbal ways that the child is capable of functioning independently and successfully. The mediator organizes opportunities for success and rewards the child not only for successful performance but also for attempts to master a problem. Another essential aspect of this criterion is communicating to the child in quite specific terms the nature of the child's correct or incorrect performance.

Regulation of behavior. In mediating for control of behavior, the mediator controls the system of the child's response prior to overt behavior in order to inhibit impulsive behavior or to accelerate the child's activity, depending on the task's characteristics and children's responses. Regulation of behavior can be done by modeling, by eliciting metacognitive strategies, analyzing the problem components, and arousing awareness of the nature of the task and appropriate response patterns.

Mediation of sharing. Sharing behavior both determines and is determined by the quality of the affective relationship between a child and his/her primary love objects. Sharing is the energetic component that permits transmission of information, and is considered to be "the spearhead of all the mediation which, by virtue of its affective, emotional quality ensures the effectiveness of the mediator in his or her mediational interactions with the child" (Feuerstein et al., 1985, p. 49).

An adequate MLE, often between a child and his/her parents, facilitates acquistion of cognitive functions, mental operations, learning sets, and need systems that permit the child later to benefit from learning experiences and be cognitively modified from learning opportunities. In other words, the child internalizes the learning mechanisms acquired in the process of mediation and uses them independently in the future. MLE is conceptualized as a proximal factor that helps to explain individual differences in cognitive performance. Distal factors such as poverty, emotional instability of parent or child, organic factors, and socioeconomic status are not thought to be causes of differences in learning ability, but are merely correlates of such individual differences. They must exert their effects through their influence on the proximal factors (MLE).

On the basis of SCM and MLE theory, Feuerstein and his colleagues have designed their dynamic approach and constructed a battery of tests called the Learning Potential Assessment Device (LPAD). Dynamic assessment goals according to the LPAD model are not restricted to peripheral, episodic, and fragmental components of the individual's functioning, such as test wiseness and familiarity with contents, but rather refer to modifiability of a structural nature that can be produced within a dynamic assessment procedure and not merely discovered or enhanced when they are within the "zone of proximal development" (Vygotsky, 1978). The structural changes are then interpreted as representing what the assessed individual can achieve if he/she would get in the future adequate mediation to help to stabilize and consolidate his/her learning.

Feuerstein et al. (1987) have drawn a distinction between functional cognitive modifiability and structural cognitive modifiability. Functional modification refers to intervention aimed at changing a person's functioning as it relates to interaction with a specific task. Models of intervention such as coaching (Budoff, 1969) or those used in assessment of "zone of proximal development" (Vygotsky, 1978) and graduated prompting (Campione & Brown, 1987) are referred to as functional, because a limited aspect of the person's functioning is targeted for change. The functional assessment is conceived as relatively limited in terms of the quantity and quality of changes that are the target of intervention. Missiuna and Samuels (1989) suggested that although the clues and aids given in functional assessment are contingent upon the child's performance, they are not individually modified for the child's unique needs; that is, the help given a child is more-or-less standardized. Because of these limitations some important questions are left unresolved, such as who is affected and in what dimension one is best affected by the intervention. Budoff's approach to learning potential assessment is criticized from this perspective because of its classifying those who benefit from teaching ("gainers") and those who do not show improvement ("nongainers"). It is only a short step from this classification approach to the search for some stable, fixed, and pervasive intellectual characteristic.

The concept of SCM, as opposed to functional cognitive modifiability, is aimed at producing and seeking changes of a structural nature. Structural changes are pervasive and determine cognitive functioning in a broad array of mental activities.

Feuerstein and his colleagues have suggested a list of deficient cognitive functions at the input, elaboration, and output phases of "the mental act" that serve as a guideline for observation and mediational efforts. Identification of deficient cognitive functions, the level of their modifiability, and the mediation required to change them are considered to be of critical importance for prescription of future learning. Examples of deficient cognitive functions at the input phase are blurred and sweeping perception, impaired systematic exploratory behavior, impaired verbal tools for processing of information, impaired need for precision and accuracy, impulsivity in gathering of information, and difficulty in simultaneous consideration of two or more sources of information. Deficient cognitive functions at the elaboration level include episodic grasp of reality, "narrowness" of the mental field, and impairments in spontaneous comparative behavior, need for pursuing logical evidence, hypothetical thinking, planning, and interiorization. At the output phase some deficient cognitive functions are egocentric modality of communication, trial-and-error responses, blocking behavior, deficient projection of virtual (implied or projected) relationships, impulsivity, and impaired precision and accuracy in communication. A review and detailed description of Feuerstein's list of deficient cognitive functions has been given by Feuerstein et al. (1979, 1980) and Feuerstein, Haywood, Rand, Hoffman, and Jensen (1986), and in a somewhat different interpretation by Haywood (1986).

Feuerstein's classification of deficient cognitive functions into input, elaboration, and output phases was validated recently by Jensen (1990) using a factor analysis of teachers' ratings of students who participated in a cognitive education program, Instrumental Enrichment (Feuerstein et al., 1980). Other studies related to the reliability of ratings of deficient cognitive functions as revealed by different tasks from the LPAD as well as their modifiability in different clinical groups have been reported by Samuels, Tzuriel, and Malloy-Miller (1989) and by Vaught and Haywood (1990), and are discussed in our section on LPAD research.

Dynamic assessment requires four major changes from static conventional testing: (a) change in the nature of the tasks, (b) change in the testing/interactional situation, (c) shift from product to process orientation, and (d) change in interpretation of results (Feuerstein, Rand, & Hoffman, 1979; Feuerstein, Haywood, Rand, Hoffman, & Jensen, 1986; Jensen & Feuerstein, 1987).

The tasks should address higher mental processes, be relatively accessible to change, and have an optimal level of complexity. Because the focus is on signs of modifiability, the tasks in the LPAD are not addressed to usual or familiar domains of content, such as academic tasks, and are specially constructed to require, permit, and enhance learning. The examiner observes specific cognitive functions and motivational factors that may relate to learning. The LPAD tasks are constructed to be sensitive to change by offering variations in task complexity and abstractness. Small changes in subjects' functioning can be amplified and interpreted as evidence of the possibility of future changes. The tasks are also constructed to motivate subjects to perform well and to enhance opportunities for successful interaction and experiences of competence.

The second change from standard testing is related to the test situation or more specifically to the examiner-subject interaction. The interaction is free of the constraints imposed in the standard situation with its neutrality and fixed roles. In the LPAD, examiners use the MLE criteria in their interactions. They behave flexibly so as to explore the meaning of successes or failures, provide feedback, and be ready to correct deficiencies, remove obstacles, and seek avenues for problem solving. Examiners are totally engaged in the activity, and intervene by giving feedback on performance, restraining impulsivity, focusing and preparing for difficult problems, requiring explanations and justifications, summarizing experiences, and encouraging reflective, insightful thinking. In using these mediational processes, examiners are alert to subjects' reactions and convey to them the feeling that the tasks are difficult but manageable, and that the subjects are capable of mastering the tasks. Feelings of competence, challenge, and interest are aroused by using various mediational procedures. The result of this active teaching process is often a change in the subjects' active exploration, task-intrinsic motivation, independence, pleasure, and insight.

The third change from standard testing is the shift from a product orientation to a process orientation. Examiners use dysfunctional responses as well as successful responses as working hypotheses both for targeting areas that need remediation and for required mediational processes. Failures are not necessarily attributed to lack of ability but rather to unfamiliarity with the task, inadequate development of operations required to solve the task, level of complexity or abstraction above the subject's present level, inefficiency of prerequisite components required for solving a problem (such as information), and nonintellective factors (such as motivation) that depress the subject's responses.

The fourth shift from standard testing and also from other dynamic approaches (Feuerstein et al., 1987) is in the interpretation of results. The examiner focuses on peaks of the individual's performance, which may appear as isolated or unpredicted performance among other low-level performance. Such unpredicted results are not seen as chance or overlearned behavior and therefore irrelevant to the assessment, but rather as indications of the person's potential development. The examiner's role is to generate hypotheses to explain the absence of other high-level results. Such hypotheses can be related to modality of input or output, level of task complexity, and degree of intervention needed to bring about success. Peak results are regarded as subjects for future study, with active attempts to produce insight into the conditions that brought about their appearance and to evaluate their generality and significance. The interpretation of results is also characterized by attempts to discover the sources of success or failure and relate them to a subject's intelligence and modifiability. Examiners use the list of deficient cognitive functions, which reflect the structure of a person's functioning, and the "cognitive map," which enables one to locate the function (for a detailed description of the cognitive map see Feuerstein et al., 1979; Feuerstein, Rand, et al., 1986). For example, subjects who fail on a task because of impulsivity at the input phase are very different from those who fail because they have difficulties in elaboration (operating upon information that is already encoded). Lack of familiarity with a task as a source of failure is very different from not having acquired a particular cognitive operation or from difficulty in using the required level of abstraction to solve the problem.

Modifiability can be interpreted along three dimensions: the domain in which the change has occurred, the quality of the achieved change, and the change in the amount and nature of the mediation required to produce the structural modification. Such a profile makes it possible to specify change in the following areas: (a) deficient cognitive functions, (b) specific content areas and operations, (c) nonintellective components (i.e., motivation, feelings of competence), and (d) degree of efficiency across the assessed functions.

Interactive-Dynamic Assessment Research

Interest in the clinical uses of interactive assessment has grown steadily over the last decade, but research on its characteristics, efficacy, and applications has not kept pace. Research using the LPAD or other interactive assessment approaches has been focused primarily on modifiability of different groups with learning difficulties such as culturally deprived and/or educable mentally retarded (EMR) persons (Feuerstein et al., 1979; Luther & Wyatt, 1989; see also Tzuriel & Feuerstein, Chapter 7 in this volume) learning-disabled children (Samuels, Tzuriel, & Malloy-Miller, 1989) learning-disabled adults (Barr & Samuels, 1988; see also Samuels, Lamb, & Oberholtzer, Chapter 11 in this volume) deaf children (Keane, 1983, 1987; Keane & Kretschmer, 1987), different minorities and ethnic groups such as Ethiopian Jewish immigrants and native Candians or Americans (Emerson, 1987; Gamlin, 1989; Kaniel & Tzuriel, 1990; Kaniel, Tzuriel, Feuerstein, Ben-Shachar, & Eitan, in press; Williams, 1990), intellectually handicapped children (Vye, Burns, Delclos, & Bransford, 1987), and penitentiary inmates (Waksman, Silverman, & Weber, 1983).

Special efforts have been made recently to extend interactive assessment to preschool children (Burns, 1983; Lidz & Thomas, 1987; Mearig, 1987; Missiuna & Samuels, 1989; Savron, 1989; Tzuriel, 1989a, 1989b; Tzuriel & Caspi, in press; Tzuriel & Eran, 1990; Tzuriel & Ernst, 1990; Tzuriel & Klein, 1985, 1987).

In the following sections research related to the LPAD model is discussed, followed by discussion of research on interactive assessment with preschool children. Research based on Vygotsky's concepts, such as the "graduated prompt" method (Campione & Brown, 1987) and the Lerntest approach (Guthke, 1982) is reported elsewhere (e.g., Guthke & Wingenfeld, Chapter 3 in this volume; Lidz, 1987a), as is work related to the approaches of Budoff (1967) and the testing-the-limits methods of Carlson and Wiedl (1978, 1979; see also Carlson & Wiedl, Chapter 6 in this volume). These additional sources should be consulted in order to get a complete view of work done on this topic.

LPAD Research

Feuerstein et al. (1979) compared educable mentally retarded (EMR) persons to a heterogeneous group of "culturally deprived," low-achieving adolescents who had been referred to a clinic for psychological assessment. The authors reported generally higher levels of performance by the culturally deprived group on all tests. The EMR group demonstrated significant improvement in performance on a retest given 2 months after the first administration.

Several case studies have shown the utility of the LPAD with special education students. Skuy, Archer, and Roth (1987) demonstrated that the LPAD was useful in identifying deficient cognitive functions and specifying effective mediational strategies in the development of an individualized educational program.

Kaniel and Tzuriel (Chapter 17 in this volume) reported that the LPAD was clinically useful with a borderline psychotic adolescent. The LPAD not only revealed cognitive potentials that otherwise were not found by standardized testing, but also functioned as a basis for a cognitive-psychotherapeutic approach (Haywood, 1989).

In a single case study, Katz (1984) used the LPAD with a 14-year-old deaf girl who scored 85 on the Wechsler Intelligence Scale for Children, Revised (WISC-R) Performance scale. The LPAD was found to be useful in delineating cognitive deficiencies and cognitive potentials as well as generating prescriptive recommendations for instructional planning.

Keane (1987) studied a group of severely and profoundly deaf children, comparing their performance on three experimental teaching conditions: mediation, elaborative feedback, and standard administration. Two static tests were used to compare conditions before and after the experimental conditions. The findings of this study indicated the superiority of the mediational style used regularly in LPAD testing over the other two conditions. The mediational style enhanced significantly the children's performance on the LPAD tests as well as the transfer of the learning to novel but comparable tasks used in the static posttest phase.

Samuels, Lamb, and Oberholtzer (Chapter 11 in this volume) used the LPAD with nonliterate adults who had learning difficulties. The mediation process within the LPAD administration revealed that their subjects had difficulties in organization, flexibility, and planning, as well as motivational and affective variables. These "nonintellective" factors were not apparent from standardized testing. Similar results were reported by Barr and Samuels (1988). The LPAD differentiated between adults who had primary emotional difficulties and those who had learning difficulties. Differential diagnosis is especially important in view of the emotional difficulties and social adjustment problems that occur in learning-disabled adults.

Haywood and Menal (in press) used LPAD to identify deficient and intact cognitive functions in a mildly mentally retarded and delinquent adolescent girl, did "cognitive-developmental psychotherapy" (Haywood, 1989) with her on the basis of the identified deficiencies and strengths, and then repeated LPAD as part of the evaluation of the therapy. The LPAD yielded information that was not available from standardized testing, and provided a useful foundation for treatment.

In most dynamic assessment studies, a test-teach-test model has been used, usually with group administration. Mediation has usually been provided for a single brief period regardless of whether changes have been observed or not. Although this group administration is methodologically and statistically more convenient, it does not permit examination of learning processes and mediational strategies as they are intended by the LPAD model. In addition, the test-teach-test model does not allow for mediation within the test phase. Such mediation while testing is an important source of information (e.g., how securely a subject has learned principles and strategies of problem solving, how investment will be required to extend the observed gains).

The LPAD has been used in a group dynamic assessment situation in several studies and has been shown to be effective (e.g., Tzuriel & Feuerstein, Chapter 7 in this volume). Although the group administration does not yield all the information needed for educational decisions and teaching processes, it has several advantages: (a) it enables one to examine a large number of persons simultaneously, and then to identify those who might require individual assessment; (b) it facilitates investigation of theoretical problems and hypotheses in controlled situations and in line with the experimental tradition, such as effects of mediational processes in groups, classroom composition, and educational policies; and (c) it facilitates establishment of the psychometric properties of the instruments. For a detailed discussion of group interactive assessment and empirical findings in different groups see Rand and Kaniel (1987) and Tzuriel and Feuerstein (Chapter 7 in this volume). In general, group administration has been found to be a useful screening procedure, especially for socially and economically disadvantaged children who have not often been confronted with cognitive tasks, and who might not have acquired the prerequisite cognitive functions to solve logic problems.

In a recent study, group interactive assessment was carried out with adolescent Ethiopian immigrants to Israel. Prior to their recent exodus from Ethiopia, most of them had lived in small villages, had very little exposure to technology, and had been relatively isolated from Western society. Several LPAD tests were given to a "mediation" group as part of a dynamic group assessment for 25 hours, and to a comparison group who performed on the LPAD tests without mediation (Kaniel et al., in press; Kaniel & Tzuriel, 1990). Both groups were tested on Raven's Standard Progressive Matrices (RSPM) before and after the LPAD administration. The results showed in general higher performance and higher transfer abilities for the mediation than for the comparison group. Furthermore, the Ethiopian 14- and 15-year-old immigrants performed after mediation at a level comparable to that of nonimmigrant 9- and 10-year-old Israeli children. Correlation of pre- to post-LPAD performance on the RSPM was significant for the comparison group but not for the mediation group. This last result was interpreted as an indication that mediation in the LPAD had changed the pattern of performance in the mediation group rather than just raising the performance level across all subjects. The 4- to 5-year gap in mental age seemed to reflect the educational deprivation of the immigrants. The gains from pre- to post-LPAD on the RSPM were as much as 22 points, as compared to 5 to 7 points for culturally deprived nonimmigrant adolescents. The Ethiopians' improvement after only 25 hours of mediation was equivalent to 3 years of mental age, a result that suggested significantly higher potential than was shown in their initial performance. Behavioral observation during testing showed that the subjects had high aspirations for success, task-intrinsic motivation, and seeking of challenges. For example, two weeks after administration of the Complex Figure, an LPAD test, the examiners found when they came back to continue testing that the subjects wanted to continue working on the figure and to practice drawing it. That kind of observations, not usual in standard testing procedures, is very important for understanding this interesting group and for recommending educational programs.

The utility of group testing was also reported by Luther and Wyatt (1989), who studied a group of vocational school English as a Second Language (ESL) students, using several of the LPAD tests. Their findings suggested that the LPAD was a better predictor of school success than was the WISC-R score. The LPAD was also useful in identifying students who would later function successfully in regular high school classes.

In a recent clinical study, Samuels, Tzuriel, and Malloy-Miller (1989) studied cognitive performance, deficient cognitive functions, amount and type of mediation required to improve performance, and certain nonintellective factors, in four groups of children. The four groups, ages 12 to 14 years, had previously been identified as (a) learning disabled without attention deficit (LD), (b) learning disabled with attention deficit disorder (LD/ADD), (c) educable mentally handicapped (EMH), and (d) normally achieving children. Results of the WISC-R failed to show differences between the LD and LD/ADD groups (mean WISC-R of 96.3 and 96.1, respectively) but did show significantly lower scores for the EMH group (mean WISC-R of 67.4).

The children were assessed by three trained examiners on eight tests from the LPAD. Mediation was given throughout the test phase, but only when necessary for correct performance. The mediation provided at the discretion of the examiner included teaching of content, language, rules and strategies necessary for the tasks, regulation of behavior (controlling impulsivity, overcoming blocking), arousing awareness and insights (metacognition), and providing feedback to crystallize learning and mediate feelings of competence.

All LPAD sessions were videotaped and careful records were kept of performance and mediation. After each teaching and testing session the examiners rated the subjects on three rating scales for type and severity of deficient cognitive functions (DCF), type and amount of mediation required, and nonintellective variables.

The overall agreement among examiners for the ratings of DCF and for ratings of mediation was 87.6% and 91.6%, respectively. These figures are much higher than those reported by Vaught (1989), who asked experts to observe dynamic assessment on a videotape and make inferences about the presence or absence of specific deficient cognitive functions as well as their severity, and the amount of mediation required to modify them. Vaught suggested that there is a need to develop a better classification of basic cognitive processes and deficiencies before broad clinical reliability can be achieved.

One of the serious problems posed by the teach-test model is that mediation during testing is given at the discretion of the examiner, who might have intervened more often than was actually necessary or have given less mediation than was needed. In other words, a child's performance might be a function of an examiner's style of mediation rather than the child's cognitive status.

Other problems derive from examiners' subjective perceptions and judgments of subjects' deficient cognitive functions, variations in examiners' own mediation, and the various nonintellective factors (e.g., need for mastery, resistance to mediation). This study by Samuels et al. (1989) is the first attempt that we know of to achieve reliability measures of the examiners' ratings as well as comparing actual performance scores to examiners' ratings of deficient cognitive functions, type and amount of mediation, and nonintellective factors.

In the study by Samuels et al., consistent patterns of performance were found across all groups. This lead the authors to suggest that examiner effects are probably not a major factor in the LPAD assessment. The performance scores indicated that the normally functioning children and the LD children made the highest scores on almost all tests, whereas the LD/ADD group consistently scored lower than did the LD and normally functioning groups. The EMH group demonstrated the poorest performance on all tests but also showed significant gains on every test with mediation. The findings on deficient cognitive functions showed a striking consistency across all categories. The normally functioning children showed the least deficiencies—sometimes none at all—in all categories.

The highest percentage of children rated as deficient was in the EMH group; in most categories (14 out of 19) more than 60% of the children were rated as deficient. The percentage of children in the LD/ADD group was consistently higher than those in the LD group. The group differences were primarily in degree rather than in kind. Another finding was a consistent drop in percentage of children rated as deficient, in all groups, from the training phase of the LPAD to the testing phase, with the exception of the language and communication categories, which remained high for all the clinical groups.

One of the most important observations from dynamic assessment is the type and amount of mediation required during testing. It is essential to investigate whether one of the groups required more restraint of impulsivity, metacognitive questioning, mediation of meaning, teaching of rules and strategies, teaching of language and concepts, or mediation of competence than did other groups. As expected, the EMH group required the greatest amount of mediation across all categories followed by the LD/ADD, the LD, and the normally functioning group. The LD group required less mediation than did either the LD/ADD or EMH group, except for mediation of competence. Mediation of competence was used extensively in both the training and test phases with children with learning disabilities. The most frequent mediational strategies required for the EMH group (and to a lesser degree to the LD/ADD and LD groups) were focusing, prompting, promoting metacognitive awareness, teaching rules and strategies, and mediation of competence.

Interactive Assessment of Young Children

Interactive assessment of young children is especially important in view of the early educational decisions that might determine their future learning. It is important to develop as early as possible procedures that will help to identify risk factors, and efficient mediational strategies to overcome learning difficulties (Lidz & Thomas, 1987; Mearig, 1987; Tzuriel, 1989a; Tzuriel & Klein, 1987). Several attempts have been made to design preschool measures and study their effectiveness with different groups of children (Bryant, Brown, & Campione, 1983; Burns, 1983; Lidz & Thomas, 1987; Mearig, 1987; Tzuriel, 1989a, 1989b, 1989c; Tzuriel & Caspi, in preparation; Tzuriel & Eran, 1990; Tzuriel & Ernst, 1990; Tzuriel & Klein, 1985, 1986, 1987).

In designing tests for young children one has to consider unique developmental factors that influence assessment. Young children are vulnerable to their environment, cannot effectively communicate their thoughts and experiences, and show inconsistency in performing tasks (Lidz, 1983). Young children are also influenced by stage-related aspects of biological development (e.g., attention span), misinterpretation of problems, distractibility, and a natural inclination for play.

Mearig (1987) has suggested several principles for development of preschool interactive assessment procedures, including clear directions, visual and auditory focusing, limiting the information to be dealt with simultaneously, familiarity with materials, specification of stimulus arrays, relating cognitive processes to curriculum concepts, preventing blocking of responses, and instigating feelings of competence. Tzuriel & Klein (1987) suggested that tasks should include manipulation of objects as a means of "bridging" from the concrete to the abstract. Mearig constructed a simplified version of some of the LPAD instruments for use with preschool and primary age slow-learning children. She also suggested a list of emerging cognitive functions to be observed in each instrument. So far, we know of no research on this version.

Lidz and Thomas (1987) suggested an extension of the Kaufman Assessment Battery for Children (K-ABC) by administering two subtests (Triangles and Matrices) before and after a session of teaching. These subtests were selected because they provided opportunities for mediation and because of their relative lack of demand for verbalization and vocabulary knowledge. Recording sheets were also developed to help in observation of cognitive functions and intervention successes and failures. Both subtests were administered to experimental and control preschool children from underprivileged backgrounds. The experimental group received mediation whereas the control group was exposed to the materials for the same length of time. Two transfer tasks from the K-ABC were given, and all children were rated by their teachers on the California Preschool Competency Scale. The children who got mediation between pretest and posttest phases showed higher gains on the Triangles and Matrices subtests than did children who did not get mediation. Correlations of the cognitive subtests with the social competency measure were higher for the mediated group than for the control group. This result was interpreted as an indication of a greater ability to predict adaptive behavior by dynamic than by static measures. No differences were found between groups on the transfer tasks.

Burns (1983) compared a mediational strategy derived from the LPAD approach to a "graduated prompt" strategy (Brown & Ferrara, 1985) in a sample of "high-risk" preschool children using the Stencil Design Test (Arthur, 1947). The mediation strategy was the most effective of the three approaches, especially on transfer tasks. The children performed better on both interactive tests than on static-normative tests.

Recently, three preschool dynamic measures have been developed by Tzuriel and Klein (1985, 1986, 1987) and Tzuriel (1989a, 1989b): (a) the Children's Analogical Thinking Modifiability (CATM), (b) the Frame Test of Cognitive Modifiability (FTCM), and (c) the Children's Inferential Thinking Modifiability (CITM). All three tests can be administered clinically where mediation can be provided for each item or in a research form where mediation is given only in the teaching phase; preteaching and postteaching phases are given with no intervention, although some regulation of behavior can be used. The CATM and the

FTCM contain two scoring methods, "all-or-none" and "partial credit." Each method provides different information and the gap between the two scores may provide indications of integrative capacities. In all three tests there is a preliminary baseline phase of familiarity with the instruments' physical dimensions and rules for solving problems. Different deficient cognitive functions can be identified as well as motivational-affective factors and mediational strategies that affect performance.

Materials for the CATM test are 18 blocks varying in color, shape, and size. Each of the preteaching, teaching, and postteaching phases contains 14 analogical problems arranged in increasing difficulty. The CATM has been used with different groups of "regular," disadvantaged, deaf, and special education kindergarten children with a variety of problems (Missiuna & Samuels, 1989; Tzuriel, 1989b, 1989c; Tzuriel & Klein, 1985, 1987; Tzuriel & Caspi, in press; Tzuriel & Ernst, 1990; Tzuriel, Menashe, & Shemesh, 1990). In general, the children have shown large gains from preteaching to postteaching phases, and higher performance in both phases than in Raven's Coloured Progressive Matrices (RCPM) given as a static-conventional test. In Tzuriel and Klein's (1985) original study, the highest gains were made by regular and disadvantaged groups, whereas the gains of the special education and mentally retarded (MR) (older children with kindergarten-equivalent mental age [MA]) groups were very small. The MR groups, however, showed improvement when a partial scoring method, in which credit was given for each dimension (color, shape, size) that was done correctly, was applied. Higher levels of functioning were also found on the CATM than on the RCPM especially when the analogical abstract items of the RCPM (items B8-B12) were compared to the analogical performance on the CATM. For example, the RCPM percentage score of the "regular" and disadvantaged children averaged 39 and 44%, respectively, as compared to 69 and 64% on the CATM postteaching test. This result was repeated in another study with hearing and deaf preschool children The percentage score of hearing and deaf children on the RCPM was 42 and 39%, respectively, as compared to 66 and 54% on the CATM ("all-or-none" method) postteaching test (Tzuriel & Caspi, in press). Percentage scores of the CATM using the "partial" scoring method were 86 and 81% for the hearing and deaf groups, respectively. These CATM findings indicate the existence of a higher level of learning potential than is indicated by static test scores.

Missiuna and Samuels (1989) tried to explain why the special education group showed no improvement in Tzuriel and Klein's (1985) study by randomly assigning preschool handicapped children to two treatment conditions. The first condition, "instruction," was similar to the original teaching phase in that children were getting the same nonprescribed teaching. The second condition, "mediation," was tailored to the unique difficulties of each child. The CATM preteaching test was given three times, the first two times with no teaching between the two administrations. The reason for that was to rule out modifiability as a function of test familiarity. The CATM postteaching test was given then, to both treatment groups, after the treatment condition. The findings supported the hypotheses: no changes were found between the first two standard administrations but significant improvement was found after the treatment phase only for the "mediation" group. The improvement of the mediation group was more impressive with the "partial credit" method of scoring than with the "all-or-none" method. Also, the mediation group required significantly more time to solve the postteaching problems than did the instruction group, a result that was explained by better control of impulsivity and awareness of different options for problem solving strategies. The "instruction" group showed minor improvements similar to those reported by Tzuriel and Klein (1985). Missiuna and Samuels's (1989) conclusion was that dynamic assessment should be tailored to the unique learning difficulties of subjects rather than applying a general standardized teaching method.

In a recent study (Tzuriel & Caspi, in press), preschool deaf children were compared on several dynamic and standard tests to hearing children who were pair-matched on variables of age, sex, and a developmental visual-motor measure. The deaf children performed lower in the CATM preteaching phase than did the hearing children, but showed greater improvement after the teaching phase; the two groups scored similarly in the postteaching phase. The CATM postteaching score was significantly predicted, in the deaf group, by family variables such as mother's occupation and the overall score on the Home Observation for Measurement of the Environment (HOME) inventory (Bradley, Caldwell, & Elardo, 1979), and by the CATM Preteaching score ($R^2 = .70$). In the hearing group only a static measure of analogies, a subscale from Snijders and Snijders-Oomen (1970), was found to be a significant predictor ($R^2 = .62$). Those results indicate that the contribution of family variables, which reflect level of cognitive stimulation and emotional support, was more meaningful in the deaf group than in the hearing group as environmental determinants that counter the mediational barriers. For deaf children, cognitive stimulation and emotional support at home appear to be more important in determining cognitive modifiability than for hearing groups. Similar psychometric qualities of both tests (analogies) take precedence over the family variables.

The importance of family variables was examined more closely in a study in which "mediated" interactions between mothers and their preschool children were compared to the children's cognitive modifiability (Tzuriel & Ernst, 1990). The main objective of this study was to examine a basic assumption of the SCM and MLE theory of Feuerstein et al. (1979, 1980, 1987, 1988). MLE is seen as a proximal etiological condition for differential modifiability. Distal etiological factors (e.g., genetic disorder, poverty, emotional problem) are seen as insufficient to explain cognitive development, although they are correlated with adequate or inadequate MLE. Mother-child interactions were videotaped for 30 minutes and analyzed later using Klein's (1988) MLE Observation scale. The sample consisted of 48 children and their mothers from low, medium, and high socioeconomic status (SES). All children were given the RCPM and the CATM and all mothers were given the Raven's Standard Progressive Matrices (RSPM). The CATM-postteaching score was taken as an indicator of cognitive modifiability. Distal factors were the SES level and the mothers' intelligence (RSPM), and proximal factors were MLE category scores. A model of distal and proximal factors was constructed to explain causal paths and analyzed by a structural equation model (SEM) using the LISREL 6 version (Joreskog & Sorbom, 1986). The CATM-postteaching score was significantly associated with the MLE category of Transcendence (i.e., going beyond the concrete, teaching of rules, strategies, and principles) and the CATM-preteaching score was associated with the MLE category of Meaning (i.e., labeling, mediation of importance and value of information). None of the children's cognitive scores was significantly associated with SES; however, SES level was significantly associated with four out of five MLE categories. Children's RCPM scores were not predicted by any of the distal or proximal factors. The results supported the SCM and MLE theory by showing in general that proximal factors (MLE) predict cognitive modifiability and cognitive performance more strongly than do distal factors.

The utility of the CATM was also demonstrated in two intervention studies of cognitive education (Samuels, Killip, MacKenzie, & Fagan, Chapter 10 in this volume; Tzuriel, 1989b; Tzuriel, Menashe, & Shemesh, 1990). In the first study by Samuels et al., an experimental group of preschool handicapped children received the Cognitive Curriculum for Young Children (CCYC; Haywood, Brooks, & Burns, 1986) for 1 year and were compared to a control group that received a good but noncognitive program. At the end of the program both groups were given the CATM as a dynamic test and the RCPM and Peabody Picture Vocabulary Test, Revised as a static test. The findings did not reveal any significant treatment effects. In a following assessment stage, 2 years later, an outcome unobtrusive measure of regular versus special education class attendance was taken. Of all measures taken at the end of the program 1 year earlier, only the CATM-postteaching score significantly predicted class attendance. Children attending regular classes had higher CATM-postteaching scores than did children who ended up attending special education classes. This result supported the notion that postmediation scores are better predictors of future learning than is initial performance on a static measure. Children who had participated in the CCYC, although functioning at lower levels at the beginning of the study, were less likely than were comparison children to be placed in special education classes.

In the second intervention study the CATM was given a few months after the start of the Thinking and Learning Ability Program (TLAP; Tzuriel, Menashe, & Shemesh, 1990) to experimental and control children. All children were in first grade and came from disadvantaged low-income families. No significant group differences were found on the CATM, a finding that was explained by lack of assimilation of teaching effects. Correlations of the CATM pre- to postteaching scores revealed a higher correlation in the experimental ($r = .83$, $p < .001$) than in the control ($r = .63$, $p < .001$) groups. These results were explained as indicating higher integrative capacity characterizing the experimental group more than the control group. Also higher correlations were found between the CATM and the CITM test given at the end of the intervention in the experimental than in the control group. The CITM/CATM correlations at the preteaching phase were .40 ($p < .001$) and .06 (ns) for the experimental and control groups, respectively. The correlations at the post-teaching phase were .76 ($p < .001$) and .17 (ns) for the experimental and control groups, respectively (using the "all-or-none" method of scoring; the results were essentially the same in the "partial credit" method). These findings were interpreted as indications of higher coherence of different cognitive processes in the experimental group than in the control group. This coherence increased from pre- to postteaching phases in both groups, although significant correlations were found only in the experimental group.

The FTCM, unlike the CATM, taps different domains of knowledge or understanding (e.g., numerical, spatial orientation) and requires different operations (e.g., numerical progression). The FTCM is composed of five square frames, 40 colored beads (red, yellow, blue, green), and three sets of problems for preteaching, teaching, and postteaching phases. The problems require identification of colors and numbers, location of beads in the frames, understanding the principle that governs the problem presented in the first three frames, and completing the pattern of beads in the fourth frame. The fifth frame is used for the teaching phase to demonstrate the principle according to which beads are arranged in the frames (Tzuriel & Klein, 1988). The validity and reliability of the FTCM has been demonstrated with children in preschool and first grade classrooms (Tzuriel & Klein, 1986).

The third interactive preschool measure developed by Tzuriel (1989a, 1989b, 1989c, 1990) is the Children's Inferential Thinking Modifiability Test (CITM). The CITM was designed to assess young children's modifiability in problems that require inferential-hypothetical thinking, use of cognitive strategies, inductive analytical reasoning, and understanding of "negation." Deficient cognitive functions can be identified, such as impaired systematic exploratory behavior, impaired spontaneous comparative behavior, and impaired simultaneous consideration of multiple sources of information. The CITM items are of three kinds. The first is a set of sentences or premises, each sentence containing information about the possible placement of objects (in pictures) inside houses. The houses are distinguished by their colored roofs; colors are in the same order across all sentences. The second is a set of big houses with same-colored roofs at the top of a page. The third is a set of 20 cards with pictures of objects.

The required task is to infer according to the information given in the sentences which objects should be placed in which houses. The information presented in each sentence is partial, and in order to solve the problem, one must compare the information across successive sentences and infer the correct location. Finally, the correct cards must be placed in the houses at the top.

In a study comparing socially disadvantaged to advantaged children, Tzuriel (1989a) reported (a) high improvement from preteaching to postteaching scores in both groups, (b) higher performance scores for advantaged than for disadvantaged children, and (c) higher scores for first grade than for kindergarten children. The disadvantaged children benefited more from the teaching than did the advantaged children, especially in the kindergarten subgroup. Teaching was found also to be more effective in improving performance on complex tasks than on simple tasks. Relative scores were higher on the CITM, the dynamic/interactive test, than on RCPM, the static test, especially for young children and for disadvantaged children. A higher correlation was found between preteaching and postteaching scores in the advantaged group ($r = .51$, $p < .001$) than in the disadvantaged group ($r = .07$, ns). The phenomenon of differential gains for advantaged and disadvantaged children found in different studies across samples and task domains might suggest that the initially low scores are due to nonintellective factors and that mediation helped those children in terms of learning habits, and peripheral cognitive dysfunctions (e.g., timidity, impulsivity, task-extrinsic motivation) that can be relatively easily modified. More detail on studies with these interactive assessment instruments for young children has been presented by Tzuriel (1989a, 1989b, 1989c, 1990; Tzuriel & Eran, 1990).

Tzuriel and Eran (1990) used the CITM to investigate the relation between mother-child MLE interactions and young children's cognitive modifiability (CM). Kindergarten and grade 1 to 3 children with their mothers were videotaped (each pair individually) for 20 minutes in a free-play situation. Their interactions were analyzed later using Klein's (1988) MLE Observation scale on five MLE categories. All children were given the RCPM and the CITM tests. A series of stepwise multiple regression analyses was carried out on the CATM preteaching, post-teaching, and gain scores. In each of these analyses, the RCPM (static) and MLE-total (sum of mediated interactions) scores were used as predictors. The power of the CITM score, relative to the MLE-total score, to predict the RCPM score gradually decreased from preteaching to postteaching score and from postteaching to gain score. The predictive power of the MLE-total score, on the other hand, gradually increased across the analyses. The results were explained by referring to the level of mediation reflected in each of the CITM scores. In the preteaching phase, only the RCPM was a significant predictor ($R = .40$, $F_{1,45} = 8.84$, $p < .004$), as both scores are derived from a conventional-static test. This result verifies what is commonly known in psychometric terms, that the common variance of two cognitive tests is higher than the common variance of a cognitive test with some observational measure (i.e., mother-child interactions). The CITM-postteaching score was significantly predicted by both the RCPM and the MLE-total scores ($R = .69$, $F_{1,44} = 19.80$, $p < .001$). The authors suggested that the children's postteaching performance had two components: (a) previously acquired skills, which were also shown in the preteaching score and which affected the common variance with the RCPM, and (b) what had been acquired in the mediation process within the testing situation. Both components, the previously acquired cognitive skills and the incremental part of learning during testing, were represented in the predictor variables. The results of the regression analysis carried out on the gain score revealed that only MLE-total was a significant predictor ($R = .43$, $F_{1,44} = 10.43$, $p < .002$). Thus, it seems that the more the criterion score was saturated with mediation effects, given within the testing situation, the more variance was contributed by MLE processes.

Applications and Future Research

In spite of an increasing awareness of the need for interactive assessment approaches, only a few clinical settings and graduate programs have adopted them in regular practice. The difficulties in integrating interactive approaches seem to be related to old conceptions about the structure and nature of human intelligence (Haywood et al., 1990; see also Haywood, Tzuriel, & Vaught, Chapter 2 in this volume), the subjective components involved in the assessment, lack of models of change (Jensen, 1990), practical concerns about the extensive investment required for both training of examiners and the assessment process, difficulties in finding appropriate criteria to be compared to assessment findings, and lack of solid empirical evidence to justify the extensive investment.

The necessity to change our conceptions of human capabilities from immutable to plastic and modifiable has been greatly emphasized by several contemporary theorists. Such a shift requires us to adopt a set of values and beliefs about human modifiability, and an active-modificational approach rather than a passive-recipient approach to apparent disability (Feuerstein, 1970, Feuerstein et al., 1988).

The quest for new concepts of intelligence and human functioning is intimately related to needs for new methods of assessment that are beyond the interactive approach, such as a transactional perspective on psychoeducational assessment (see Haywood, Tzuriel, & Vaught, Chapter 2 in this volume), holistic evaluation (Smith, 1989), views of multiple intelligence (Gardner, 1983; Sternberg & Wagner, 1987), and process assessment (Meyers, Pfeffer, & Erlbaum, 1985).

Some complaints raised frequently about interactive assessment concern the extensive time and effort required to train examiners, and the very interactive nature of the assessment process itself. Proponents of the interactive approach, however, comment that the long-range benefits to be derived from an optimistic, accurate, prescriptive assessment that is also expensive should be weighed against the relatively shorter, inexpensive, and less demanding standard approach that is very often pessimistic, inaccurate, and of limited direct relevance to school learning. Meyers (1987) referred to this problem by stating that "productivity" is defined very often as number of completed evaluations per time unit rather than a more meaningful criterion such as change in learning or teaching effectiveness.

The requirement to conceptualize human beings in terms of modifiability is more demanding intellectually and methodologically, but it also represents more accurately the alloplastic nature of the developing human being. The shift from a model of stability to a model of change (Jensen, 1990) seems to be an inevitable trend that will be blended with holistic and transactional assessment models. Feuerstein et al. (1987) and Jensen (1990) have suggested for example a profile for structural cognitive modifiability that relates to the domain in which changes have occurred, the quality of achieved change, and the change in the quality and quantity of mediation required for modifiability. Changes can be attributed to remediation of knowledge and habit aspects, to changes in the affective-motivational domain, and to "hard core" structural cognitive changes. Jensen (1990) has suggested for example a change model in terms of acquisition/retention of information, resistance/flexibility in confronting novel tasks, and transformability/generalizability in applying learned rules to new situations.

The subjective component of the assessment is integral to the mediational process and can be monitored by developing accurate rating scales based on specific indicators of deficiencies and strengths, and establishing appropriate categories of observation. The subjectivity problem is related to the fact that the examiner has a double role of mediator and observer. These two roles require special training techniques.

Meyers (1987) has mentioned some major dilemmas related to training in dynamic assessment. Among these are: freedom versus constraint given to trainees in experimenting with instruments and techniques, scientific versus practical orientation, labeling versus intervention, process versus product, observation versus teaching, and realistic versus idealistic approach. These dilemmas are not confined to training and relate to the assessment process itself.

The arguments concerning lack of solid evidence for the usefulness of interactive assessment have become weaker with the recent and rapid increase in research on this topic. A promising indication of rising awareness of and need for empirical validation of interactive assessment is the appearance of two new journals: the *International Journal of Dynamic Assessment and Instruction*, and the *International Journal of Cognitive Education and Mediated Learning*, both devoted to issues of interactive assessment, mediation, and cognitive intervention.

Parallel to efforts to apply interactive assessment methods in various settings, research should be focused on some unresolved questions that have both theoretical and applied aspects.

A critical problem in implementing research with interactive assessment is that of specifying a criterion of validity, especially when the assessment is not followed by the prescribed intervention aimed at remediation of learning difficulties and actualization of the examinee's potential. In the absence of appropriate follow-up mediation, the indications for cognitive modifiability shown during testing might never appear and thus might seem to refute the examiner's conclusions. Feuerstein et al. (1979) commented that extrinsic criteria for dynamic assessment are valid only when the prescribed remedial strategies have been used. Haywood (1988) suggested that the optimistic conclusions that arise often from dynamic/interactive assessment can do more harm than good if the conditions that have been found (by the assessment) to be necessary for improved performance are not actually carried out. It should be mentioned here that several studies have already shown the superiority of dynamic assessment findings over IQ in prediction of response to educational intervention (Camp, 1973; Carlson & Wiedl, 1979; Luther & Wyatt, 1989).

One of the persistent questions about interactive assessment is to what extent cognitive modifiability is generalized across knowledge or content domains. Cognitive modifiability was conceptualized by Feuerstein and his colleagues in general terms, although certain parameters related to modalities of performance (visual, spatial, numerical), content areas (numbers, words) and operations (analogy, seriation, syllogism) were taken into account in constructing dynamic tests. It is important to find out to what extent cognitive modifiability is "domain specific." Does it change developmentally? How do environmental and interactional factors affect its generalizability? What are the necessary and sufficient conditions for realization of the cognitive modifiability suggested by dynamic/interactive assessment? What are the effects of interactive assessment on parents' and teachers' attitudes toward children or even on their own values and teaching philosophies? The ultimate question about the utility of these approaches is whether full implementation of an interactive assessment approach changes the quality of education for assessed persons.

Acknowledgment. Parts of this paper were written while the first author was a visiting professor in the Department of Educational Psychology and Special Education at The University of British Columbia.

References

Arbitman-Smith, R., Haywood, H. C., & Bransford, J. D. (1984). Assessing cognitive change. In P. Brooks, R. Sperber, & C. McCauley (Eds.), *Learning and cognition in the mentally retarded* (pp. 433–471). Hillsdale, NJ: Erlbaum.

Arthur, G. (1947). *A point scale of performance tests.* New York: Psychological Corporation.

Astin, A. (1971). Open admissions and programs for the disadvantaged. *Journal of Higher Education*, *42*, 620–647.

Ausubel, D. P. (1968). *Educational psychology: A cognitive view.* New York: Delta Books.

Baily, D. B., & Harbin, G. L. (1980). Nondiscriminatory evaluation. *Exceptional Children*, *46*, 590–596.

Baker, F. (1971). Automation of test scoring, reporting and analysis. In R. Thorndike (Ed.), *Educational measurement* (pp. 202–236). Washington, DC: American Council on Education.

Barr, P., & Samuels, M. (1988). Dynamic assessment of cognitive and affective factors contributing to learning difficulties in adults. *Professional Psychology: Research and Practice*, *19*, 6–13.

Boorstein, D. (1974). *The Americans: The democratic experience.* New York: Vintage. Bradley, R. H. & Caldwell, B. M. (1979). Home Observation for Measurement of the Environment: A revision of the preschool scale. *American Journal of Mental Deficiency*, *84*, 235–244.

Bradley, R., Caldwell, B., & Elardo, R. (1979). Home environment and cognitive development in the first two years: A cross-lag panel analysis. *Developmental Psychology*, *15*, 246–250.

Bronfenbrenner, U. (1979). *The ecology of human development.* Cambridge, MA: Harvard University Press.

Brown, A. L., & Ferrara R. A. (1985). Diagnosing zones of proximal development. In J. Wertsch (Ed.), *Culture, communication and cognition: Vygotskian perspectives* (pp. 273–305). New York: Cambridge University Press.

Bryant, N. R., Brown, A. L., & Campione, J. C. (1983, April). *Preschool children's learning and transfer of matrices problems: Potential for improvement.* Paper presented at the Society for Research in Child Development, Detroit.

Budoff, M. (1967). Learning potential among institutionalized young adult retardates. *American Journal of Mental Deficiency*, *72*, 404–411.

Budoff, M. (1969). Learning potential: A supplementary procedure for assessing the ability to reason. *Seminars in Psychiatry*, *1*, 278–290.

Budoff, M. (1987). Measures of assessing learning potential. In C. S. Lidz (Ed.), *Dynamic assessment* (pp. 173–195). New York: Guilford.

Burns, M. S. (1983). *Comparison of graduated prompt and mediational dynamic assessment and static assessment with young children.* Unpublished doctoral dissertation, Vanderbilt University, Nashville, Tennessee.

Camp, B. W. (1973). Psychometric tests and learning in severely disabled readers. *Journal of Learning Disabilities*, *6*, 512–517.

Campione, J. C., & Brown, A. L. (1987). Linking dynamic assessment with school achievement. In C. S. Lidz (Ed.), *Dynamic assessment: An interactional approach to evaluating learning potential* (pp. 82–115). New York: Guilford.

Carlson, J. S., & Wiedl, K. H. (1978). Use of testing-the-limits procedure in the assessment of intellectual capabilities in children with learning difficulties. *American Journal of Mental Deficiency*, *82*, 559–564.

Carlson, J. S., & Wiedl, K. H. (1979). Toward a differential testing approach: Testing-the-limits employing the Raven Matrices. *Intelligence*, *3*, 323–344.

Coxhead, P., & Gupta, R. M. (1988). Construction of a test battery to measure learning potential. In R. M. Gupta & P. Coxhead (Eds.), *Cultural diversity and learning effiency* (pp. 118–140). London: Macmillan.

Cremin, L. (1964). *The transformation of the school*. New York: Vintage.

Eisenberg, L., & Connors, C. K. (1966). *The effect of Head Start on developmental process*. Paper presented at the 1966 Joseph P. Kennedy, Jr. Foundation Scientific Symposium on Mental Retardation, Boston.

Emerson, L. (1987, June). *Tradition, change and survival: Cognitive learning process, culture and education*. Paper presented at World Conference: Indigenous People's Education, Vancouver, British Columbia.

Feuerstein, R. (1970). A dynamic approach to the causation, prevention, and alleviation of retarded performance. In H. C. Haywood (Ed.), *Social-cultural aspects of mental retardation* (pp. 341–377). New York: Appleton-Century-Crofts.

Feuerstein, R., Haywood, H. C., Rand, Y., Hoffman, M. B., & Jensen, M. R. (1986). *Learning Potential Assessment Device Manual*. Jerusalem: Hadassah-WIZ0-Canada Research Institute.

Feuerstein, R., Hoffman, M. B., Jensen, M. R., & Rand, Y. (1985). Instrumental Enrichment: An interventional program for structural cognitive modifiability: Theory and practice. In J. W. Segal, S. F. Chipman, & R. Glaser (Eds.), *Thinking and learning skills* (Vol. 1, pp. 43–82). Hillsdale, NJ: Erlbaum.

Feuerstein, R., Rand, Y., & Hoffman, M. B. (1979). *The dynamic assessment of retarded performers: The Learning Potential Assessment Device: Theory, instruments and techniques*. Baltimore: University Park Press.

Feuerstein, R., Rand, Y., Hoffman, M. B., & Miller, R. (1980). *Instrumental Enrichment*. Baltimore: University Park Press.

Feuerstein, R., Rand, Y., Jensen, M. R., Kaniel, S., & Tzuriel, D. (1987). Prerequisites for assessment of learning potential: The LPAD model. In C. S. Lidz (Ed.), *Dynamic assessment* (pp. 35–51). New York: Guilford.

Feuerstein, R., Rand, Y., Jensen, M. R., Kaniel, S., Tzuriel, D., Ben-Shachar, N., & Mintzker, Y. (1986). Learning potential assessment. *Special Services in the Schools*, *2*, 85–106.

Feuerstein, R., Rand, Y., & Rynders, J. E. (1988). *Don't accept me as I am*. New York: Plenum Press.

Gamlin, P. (1989). Issues in dynamic assessment/instruction. *International Journal of Dynamic Assessment and Instruction*, *1*, 13–25.

Garber, H., & Heber, R. (1981). The efficacy of early intervention with family rehabilitation. In M. Begab, H. C. Haywood, & H. Garber (Eds.), *Psychological influences in retarded performance* (Vol. 2, pp. 71–87). Baltimore: University Park Press.

Gardner, H. (1983). *Frames of mind: The theory of multiple intelligences.* New York: Basic Books.
Gould, S. I. (1981). *The mismeasure of men.* New York: Norton.
Gray, S. W., & Klaus, R. A. (1965). An experimental preschool program for culturally deprived children. *Child Development, 36*, 887–898.
Gupta, R. M., & Coxhead, P. (1988). (Eds.) *Cultural diversity and learning efficiency.* London: Macmillan.
Guthke, J. (1982). The learning test concept—an alternative to the traditional static intelligence test. *German Journal of Psychology, 6*, 306–324.
Haney, W. (1981). Validity, vaudeville, and values: A short history of social concerns over standardized testing. *American Psychologist, 36*, 1021–1024.
Haussermann, E. (1958). *Developmental potential of preschool children.* New York: Grune & Stratton.
Haywood, H. C. (1977). Alternatives to normative assessment. In P. Mittler (Ed.), *Research to practice in mental retardation: Proceedings of the 4th Congress of the International Association for the Scientific Study of Mental Deficiency: Vol. 2, Education and training* (pp. 11–18). Baltimore: University Park Press.
Haywood, H. C. (1984, October). *Psychoeducational assessment of minority children: The issues.* Paper presented at meeting of the Association for Public Policy Analysis and Management, New Orleans.
Haywood, H. C. (1986). On the nature of cognitive functions. *The Thinking Teacher, 3*(1), 1–3.
Haywood, H. C. (1987). A mediational teaching style. *The Thinking Teacher, 4*(1), 1–6.
Haywood, H. C. (1988). Dynamic assessment: The Learning Potential Assessment Device. In R. Jones (Ed.), *Psychoeducational assessment of minority group children: A casebook* (pp. 39–63). Richmond, VA: Cobb & Henry.
Haywood, H. C. (1989, August). *Cognitive-developmental psychotherapy: An application of mediated learning.* Paper presented at the Second International Conference on Mediated Learning Experience (MLE), Knoxville, TN.
Haywood, H. C., Brooks, P., & Burns, S. (1986). Stimulating cognitive development at developmental level: A tested, non-remedial preschool curriculum for preschoolers and older retarded children. In M. Schwebel & C. A. Maher (Eds.), *Facilitating cognitive development; Principles, practices, and programs* (pp. 127–147). New York: Haworth Press.
Haywood, H. C., Brown, A. L., & Wingenfeld, S. (1990). Dynamic approaches to psychoeducational assessment. *School Psychology Review, 19*, 411–422.
Haywood, H. C., Filler, J. W., Shifman, M. A., & Chatelanat, G. (1975). Behavioral assessment in mental retardation. In P. McReynolds (Ed.), *Advances in pscyhological assessment* (Vol. 3, pp. 96–136). San Francisco: Jossey-Bass.
Haywood, H. C., & Menal, C. (in press). Psychothérapie cognitive-développementale: Etude d'un cas individuel [A case study of cognitive-developmental psychotherapy]. *International Journal of Cognitive Education and Mediated Learning.*
Haywood, H. C., & Switzky, H. N. (1974). Children's verbal abstracting: Effects of enriched input, age, and IQ. *American Journal of Mental Deficiency, 78*, 556–565.

Haywood, H. C., & Switzky, H. N. (1986). The malleability of intelligence: Cognitive processes as a function of poloygenic-experiential interaction. *School Psychology Review*, *15*, 245–255.

Jensen, M. R. (1990). Change models and some evidence for phases and their plasticity in cognitive structures. *International Journal of Cognitive Education and Mediated Learning*, *1*(1), 5–16.

Jensen, M. R., & Feuerstein, R. (1987). The learning potential assessment device: From philosophy to practice. In C. S. Lidz (Ed.), *Dynamic Assessment* (pp. 379–402). New York: Guilford.

Joreskog, K. G., & Sorbom, D. (1986). *LISREL VI: Analysis of linear structural relationships by the method of maximum likelihood*. Chicago: National Educational Resources.

Kamin, L. J. (1974). *The science and politics of IQ*. Potomac, MD: Erlbaum.

Kaniel, S., & Tzuriel, D. (1990). Dynamic assessment: learning and transfer abilities of Ethiopian immigrants to Israel. *The Thinking Teacher*, *5*(1), 6–9.

Kaniel, S., Tzuriel, D., Feuerstein, R., Ben-Shachar, N., & Eitan, T. (in press). Dynamic assessment, learning and transfer abilities of Jewish Ethiopian immigrants to Israel. In R. Feuerstein, P. S. Klein, & A. Tannenbaum (Eds.), *Mediated learning experience*. London: Freund.

Karier, C. (1976). Testing for order and control in the corporate liberal state. In N. Block & G. Dworkin (Eds.), *The IQ controversy* (pp. 339–373). New York: Pantheon.

Katz, M. (1984). Use of the LPAD for cognitive enrichment of a deaf child. *School Psychology Review*, *13*, 99–106.

Keane, K. J. (1983). *Application of mediated learning theory to a deaf population: A study in cognitive modifiability*. Unpublished doctoral dissertation, Columbia University, New York, NY.

Keane, K. J. (1987). Assessing deaf children. In C. S. Lidz (Ed.), *Dynamic Assessment* (pp. 360–378). New York: Guilford.

Keane, K. J., & Kretschmer, R. E. (1987). Effect of mediated learning intervention on cognitive task performance with a deaf population. *Journal of Educational Psychology*, *79*, 49–53.

Klein, P. S. (1988). Stability and change in interaction of Israeli mothers and infants. *Infant Behavior and Development*, *11*, 55–70.

Kohlberg, L., & Zigler, E. (1967). The impact of cognitive maturity on the development of sex-role attitudes in the years four to eight. *Genetic Psychology Monographs*, *75*, 89–165.

Lidz, C. S. (1983). Dynamic assessment and the preschool child. *Journal of Psychoeducational Assessment*, *1*, 59–72.

Lidz, C. S. (Ed.) (1987a). *Dynamic assessment*. New York: Guilford.

Lidz, C. S. (1987b). Historical perspectives. In C. S. Lidz (Ed.), *Dynamic assessment* (pp. 3–51). New York: Guilford.

Lidz, C. S., & Thomas, C. (1987). The Preschool Learning Assessment Device: Extension of a static approach. In C. S. Lidz (Ed.), *Dynamic Assessment* (pp. 288–326). New York: Guilford.

Luther, M., & Wyatt, F. (1989). A comparison of Feuerstein's method of LPAD assessment with conventional IQ testing on disadvantaged North York high school students. *International Journal of Dynamic Assessment and Instruction*, *1*(1), 49–64.

Mearig, J. S. (1987). Assessing the learning potential of kindergarten and primary-age children. In C. S. Lidz (Ed.), *Dynamic assessment* (pp. 237–269). New York: Guilford.

Mercer, J. R. (1975). Psychological assessment and the rights of children. In N. Hobbs (Ed.), *Issues in the classification of children* (Vol. 1, pp. 130–158). San Francisco: Jossey-Bass.

Messick, S. (1980). Test validity and the ethics of assessment. *American Psychologist*, *35*, 1012–1027.

Meyers, J. (1987). The training of dynamic assessment. In C. S. Lidz (Ed.), *Dynamic Assessment* (pp. 403–425). New York: Guilford.

Meyers, J., Pfeffer, J., & Erlbaum, V. (1985). Process assessment: A model for broadening assessment. *Journal of Special Education*, *19*, 73–89.

Minick, N. (1987). Implications of Vygotsky's theories for dynamic assessment. In C. S. Lidz (Ed.), *Dynamic assessment* (pp. 116–140). New York: Guilford.

Mischel, W. (1968). *Personality and assessment*. New York: Wiley.

Missiuna, C., & Samuels, M. (1988). Dynamic assessment: Review and critique. *Special Services in the Schools*, *5*(1–2), 1–22.

Missiuna, C., & Samuels, M. (1989). Dynamic assessment of preschool children with special needs: Comparison of mediation and instruction. *Remedial and Special Education*, *10*(2), 53–62.

Paour, J.-L. (1979). Apprentissage de notions de conservation et induction de la pensée opératoire concrète chez les débiles mentaux [Learning of conservation concepts and induction of concrete operatory thought in mentally retarded persons]. In R. Zazzo (Ed.), *Les débilités mentales* (pp. 421–465). Paris: Armand Colin.

Penrose, L. S. (1963). *The biology of mental defect*. London: Sidgwick & Jackson.

Phillips, D. (1984). The illusion of incompetence among academically competent children. *Child Development*, *55*, 2000–2016.

Postman, N., & Weingartner, C. (1969). *Teaching as a subversive activity*. New York: Delta Books.

Ramey, C. T., Collier, A. M., Sparling, J. J., Loda, R. A., Campbell, F. A., Ingram, D. L., & Finkelstein, N. W. (1976). The Carolina Abecedarian Project: A longitudinal and multidisciplinary approach to the prevention of developmental retardation. In T. Tjossem (Ed.), *Intervention strategies for high-risk infants and young children* (pp. 629–665). Baltimore: University Park Press.

Ramey, C. T., & MacPhee, D. (1981). A new paradigm in intellectual assessment. *Contemporary Psychology*, *26*(7), 507–509.

Rand, Y., & Kaniel, S. (1987). Group administration of the LPAD. In C. S. Lidz (Ed.), *Dynamic assessment* (pp. 196–214). New York: Guilford.

Reschly, D. J. (1980). Psychological testing in educational classification and placement. *American Psychologist*, *36*, 1094–1102.

Samuels, M., Tzuriel, D., & Malloy-Miller, T. (1989). Dynamic assessment of children with learning difficulties. In R. T. Brown & M. Chazan (Eds.), *Learning difficulties and emotional problems* (pp. 145–165). Calgary: Detselig Enterprises.

Savron, B. (1989). Modifying similarity thinking: Implications for the generalization of knowledge. *International Journal of Dynamic Assessment and Instruction*, *1*(1), 27–48.

Scarr, S. (1981). Dilemmas in assessment of disadvantaged children. In M. Begab, H. C. Haywood, & H. Garber (Eds.), *Psychological influences in retarded performance* (Vol. 2, pp. 3–16). Baltimore: University Park Press.

Seitz, V., Abelson, W. D., Levine, E., & Zigler, E. (1975). Effects of place of testing on the Peabody Picture Vocabulary Test scores of disadvantaged Head Start and non-Head Start children. *Child Development*, *46*, 481–486.

Sewell, T. E. (1987). Dynamic assessment as a nondiscriminatory procedure. In C. S. Lidz (Ed.), *Dynamic assessment* (pp. 426–443). New York: Guilford.

Skodak, M., & Skeels, H. M. (1945). A follow-up study of children in adoptive homes. *Journal of Genetic Psychology*, *66*, 21–58.

Skuy, M. S., Archer, M., & Roth, I. (1987). Use of the learning potential assessment device in assessment and remediation of learning problems. *South African Journal of Education*, *7*(1), 53–58.

Smith, L. (1989). Towards a more holistic view of learning and evaluation. *International Journal of Dynamic Assessment and Instruction*, *1*(1), 3–12.

Snijders, J. T., & Snijders-Oomen, N. (1970). *Non-verbal intelligence tests for deaf and hearing subjects*. Groningen, Netherlands: Walters-Noordhoff.

Sternberg, R., & Wagner, R. (Eds.) (1987). *Practical intelligences*. New York: Cambridge University Press.

Sutton, A. (1981). Cultural disadvantage and Vygotsky's stages of development. *Educational Studies*, *6*, 199–209.

Sutton, A. (1987). L. S. Vygotsky: The cultural-historical theory, national minorities and the zone of next development. In R. M. Gupta & P. Coxhead (Eds.), *Cultural diversity and learning efficiency* (pp. 89–117). London: Macmillan.

Tuddenham, R. (1962). The nature and measurement of intelligence. In L. J. Postman (Ed.), *Psychology in the making: histories of selected research problems* (pp. 469–525). New York: Knopf.

Tzuriel, D. (1989a). Inferential cognitive modifiability of young socially disadvantaged and advantaged children. *International Journal of Dynamic Assessment and Instruction*, *1*(1), 65–80.

Tzuriel, D. (1989b). Dynamic assessment of learning potential in cognitive education programs. *The Thinking Teacher*, *5*(1), 1–3.

Tzuriel, D. (1989c). Dynamic assessment of learning potential: Novel measures for young children. *The Thinking Teacher*, *5*(1), 9–10.

Tzuriel, D. (1990). *The Children's Inferential Thinking Modifiability Test (CITM): Instruction Manual*. Ramat-Gan, Israel: Bar Ilan University.

Tzuriel, D., & Caspi, N. (in press). Comparison of cognitive modifiability and cognitive performance of deaf and hearing preschool children. *Journal of Special Education*.

Tzuriel, D., & Eran, Z. (1990). Inferential cognitive modifiability as a function of mother-child mediated learning experience (MLE) interactions among kibbutz young children. *International Journal of Cognitive Education and Mediated Learning*, *1*, 103–117.

Tzuriel, D., & Ernst, H. (1990). Mediated learning experience and cognitive modifiability: Testing the effects of distal and proximal factors by structual equation model. *International Journal of Cognitive Education and Mediated Learning*, *1*(2), 119–135.

Tzuriel, D., & Klein, P. S. (1985). Analogical thinking modifiability in disadvantaged, regular, special education, and mentally retarded children. *Journal of Abnormal Child Psychology*, *13*, 539–552.

Tzuriel, D., & Klein, P. S. (1986, July). The dynamic method: A different approach to decision-making about cognitive modifiability of young children. Paper presented at the 28th World Congress of OMEP, Jerusalem, Israel.

Tzuriel, D., & Klein, P. S. (1987). Assessing the young child: Children's analogical thinking modifiability. In C. S. Lidz (Ed.), *Dynamic assessment* (pp. 268–282). New York: Guilford.

Tzuriel, D., & Klein, P. S. (1988). *The Frame Test of Cognitive Modifiability: Manual*. Ramat-Gan, Israel: Bar Ilan University.

Tzuriel, D., Menashe, B., & Shemesh, D. (1990, July). The Thinking and Learning Abilities Program (TLAP). Paper presented at the Second Congress of the International Association for Cognitive Education, Mons, Belgium.

Tzuriel, D., Samuels, M. T., & Feuerstein, R. (1988). Non-intellective factors in dynamic assessment. In R. M. Gupta & P. Coxhead (Eds.), *Cultural diversity and learning efficiency* (pp. 141–163). London: Macmillan.

Vaught, S. (1989). *Interjudge agreement in dynamic assessment: Two instruments from the Learning Potential Assessment Device*. Unpublished master's thesis, Vanderbilt University, Nashville, TN.

Vaught, S., & Haywood, H. C. (1990). Interjudge reliability in dynamic assessment. *The Thinking Teacher*, *5*(2), 2–6.

Vernon, P. E. (1979). *Intelligence: heredity and environment*. San Francisco: W. H. Freeman.

Vye, N. J., Burns, M. S., Delclos, V. R., & Bransford, J. D. (1987). *Dynamic assessment of intellectually handicapped children*. Unpublished manuscript. (Technical Report #4, Learning Technology Center). Nashville, TN: Vanderbilt University.

Vygotsky, L. S. (1929). The problem of the cultural development of the child. *Journal of Genetic Psychology*, *36*, 415–434.

Vygotsky, L. S. (1962). *Thought and language*. Cambridge, MA: MIT Press.

Vygotsky, L. S. (1978). *Mind in society: The development of higher psychological processes*. (M. Cole, V. John-Steiner, S. Scribner, & E. Souberman, Eds. and Trans.) Cambridge, MA: Harvard University Press.

Waksman, M., Silverman, H., & Weber, K. (1983). Assessing the learning potential of penitentiary inmates: An application of Feuerstein's Learning Potential Assessment Device. *Journal of Correctional Education*, *34*(2), 63–69.

Weaver, T. R. (1946). The incidence of maladjustment among mental defectives in military environments. *American Journal of Mental Deficiency*, *51*, 238–246.

White, B. L. (1975). *The first three years of life*. Englewood Cliffs, NJ: Prentice Hall.

White, S. (1981). *How could testing offer more help to schooling*? Unpublished manuscript.

Williams, L. (1990). Feuerstein's Instrumental Enrichment curriculum: A means to address issues in first nations education. *International Journal of Cognitive Education and Mediated Learning*, *1*, 73–78.

Windle, C. (1962). Prognosis of mental subnormals. *American Journal of Mental Deficiency*, *66*, (Monograph Supplement No. 5).

Zigler, E., Abelson, W. D., & Seitz, V. (1973). Motivational factors in the performance of economically disadvantaged children on the Peabody Picture Vocabulary Test. *Child Development*, *44*, 294–303.

Zigler, E., & Butterfield, E. C. (1968). Motivational aspects of changes in IQ test performance of culturally deprived nursery school children. *Child Development*, *39*, 1–14.

Zigler, E., & Seitz, V. (1982). Social policy and intelligence. In R. J. Sternberg (Ed.), *Handbook of intelligence*. New York: Cambridge University Press.

2
Psychoeducational Assessment from a Transactional Perspective

H. Carl Haywood, David Tzuriel, and Susan Vaught

Psychological assessment takes place within a logical context that is at least conceptual, and ideally theoretical, whether or not that conceptual context is explicit and well understood by practitioners. Psychological assessment that is done for educational purposes, that is, psychoeducational assessment, is undertaken in a special context: the effort to construct effective programs of education based upon individual characteristics and needs of students. On the assumption that the ability to profit from school experience varies as a function of individual differences in intelligence, school and educational psychologists and educators have traditionally spent the largest portion of their assessment time assessing ability. Unfortunately, such persons often are not operating on the basis of explicitly stated concepts of the nature and development of ability, or of what latent variables underlie individual differences in school achievement. Thus, practitioners may set out to assess individual differences in ability without actually understanding what they themselves believe to be the nature, modes of development, and various manifestations of the very ability that they seek to assess!

It is highly desirable, if not essential, that practitioners of the art of psychoeducational assessment, and certainly developers of the instruments of such assessment, hold, and be aware of, explicit, systematic concepts of the nature and development of intelligence, including ontogenesis, variety of manifestations, development of individual differences, susceptibility to modification, interaction with "nonintellective" variables, and correlation with important criterion variables. Further, it is especially desirable that theoretical understanding precede the development of assessment instruments, because such instruments should reflect consistent notions of the nature of what they are supposed to assess, that is, the latent variable. In accordance with this view, the goal of this chapter is to present one particular view, a transactional one, of the nature and development of human ability, and to suggest that such a view leads more logically to some psychoeducational assessment practices than to others. In doing so, we examine first some of the basic characteristics and problems of psychoeducational assessment, especially of individual differences in intelligence, then present our approach to the nature and acquisition of logical thought, and finally discuss particular assessment procedures that are conceptually consistent with that theoretical approach.

Nature and Problems of Psychoeducational Assessment

Psychologists agree generally that psychoeducational assessment has at least the following goals (Haywood, 1984; see also Utley, Haywood, & Masters, Chapter 19 in this volume):

1. to classify schoolchildren according to their aptitude for school learning;
2. to assist in grouping children by aptitude, the notion being that differential pedagogical techniques will be used for the different groups so formed;
3. to identify individual need for educational remediation in specific domains;
4. to construct prescriptive programs of education, either individually or for classified groups.

According to Haywood, Brown, and Wingenfeld (1990), these admirable goals, unfortunately for the children, have most often been collapsed into a primary emphasis on the first, classification. Classification itself has multiple goals, including group planning for the use of available resources in school systems and individualized educational programming. Classification in education is pursued for the same reasons as diagnosis in the health and mental health fields: the notion that effective treatments are known, are more-or-less automatically related to diagnoses, and will be implemented in cases of all persons who fit a particular diagnostic category. The corresponding pedagogical notion is that effective education can be achieved to the extent that instruction is "pitched" at just the right level for each child, i.e., if the level of difficulty is not too far above or below each child's learning aptitude. Three broad tracks have emerged from this approach: specialized instruction for exceptionally talented or "gifted" students, regular classes for the majority of students whose general learning aptitude is within two standard deviations of the population mean, and specialized instructional services for children who have low learning aptitude scores, as in the case of mentally retarded children, or quite special needs, such as children with impaired hearing or vision or with specific learning disabilities (Haywood, 1984). There are significant problems with the use of normative, standardized tests for these purposes, even when all of the purposes are pursued. The following discussion of these problems is borrowed heavily from Haywood (1984) and Haywood, Brown, and Wingenfeld (1990).

Whatever their predictive validity in a group or correlational sense (which might be differential with respect to ethnic group membership), standardized and normative tests have less success when applied to prediction in individual cases. This may be especially true when the scores of individual children in minority ethnic groups are compared with norms derived from samples of the majority population (Elliott, 1988; Gregory & Lee, 1986; see also Jensen, 1980, for a contrary view).

It is not merely a question of making certain that minority groups are proportionally represented in normative samples; indeed, the situation is inherently inappropriate even when the normative samples of the tests contain subjects from different ethnic groups in exact proportion to their numbers in the population. Haywood (1984) observed that

> It is scant comfort that the score of a black child is compared with that of the "average" child of comparable age in the normative sample, when that "average" child is a statistical abstraction made up of 80% white children, 11% black children, and some smaller percentages of children from other ethnic groups. One might observe that such a comparison is 11% correct in the case of a black child, and never more than 80% correct in the case of a white child. (p. 2)

The point is not one of differential effectiveness by ethnic group with respect to the tests' predictive (classificatory) validity when group comparisons are being made. The problem is not so much with the tests themselves (see discussion by Utley, Haywood, & Masters, Chapter 19 in this volume), because they do not appear to show predictable biases or differential predictability. The use of the tests in a normative way, that is, to compare the performance of individual children with that of the average performance of similar children in a normative sample, is the problem. Even though group data fail to reveal lower predictive validity for children who are like the smallest proportion of the normative sample, these "normative" comparisons are still inherently inappropriate because establishing children's rank order with respect to a normative sample is not very helpful either in estimating what those children can do or in constructing educational programs for them.

Assessment based primarily on normative tests and used primarily for classification may lead to misclassification that is not distributed equally over population subgroups (see, for example, Mercer, 1970, 1973, 1975). The direction of misclassification about which people are most concerned is placement in special education. Such misclassification is the joint product of test error, of overreliance on test data in the assessment process, and of the fact that variables other than intelligence itself may influence the learning and school performance of children; i.e., intelligence as a predictor of school performance is only one of several relevant predictors, albeit a major one. Even if the effects of individual differences in intelligence were distributed uniformly, the other predictors (e.g., individual differences in intrinsic motivation; Haywood & Switzky, 1986a) may exert differential influence depending upon the subcultural experiences of the children.

Another problem is that most standardized, normative tests, being used primarily for classification, are not prescriptive. Being derived from a "static" testing situation (one in which children are expected to answer questions and solve problems without help), scores on these tests contain little information about performance in a criterion situation, that is, one in which there actually is teaching. Knowing that a child lacks certain information or takes too long to solve a particular problem tells one little about how to teach the child to perform more adequately in that domain of functioning, or about why such deficiencies exist.

The notion that proper classification leads to proper treatment has not been broadly supported in the educational realm, especially with respect to the placement of children in special classes for educable mentally retarded children (Hobbs, 1974). Even when children have been "correctly" classified according to psychometric criteria, the promise of enhanced opportunities to learn is often not fulfilled (Dunn, 1968; Lilly, 1982). This statement simply calls attention to the critical difference between "need for special services" and "probability of deriving benefit from special services." In the case of most children who make low scores on standardized normative ability tests, the need for special services is apparent. The probability that they will benefit from special services depends upon the extent to which such services have been constructed on the basis of diagnostic and prescriptive information that is relevant to criterion (classroom learning) situations. In such situations, the problem may reside less in the predictor than in the criterion!

Another problem is that most standardized normative tests of ability do not reflect contemporary knowledge of cognitive and intellectual development and thus are based on outmoded models of the nature and development of ability factors (Haywood et al., 1990). The knowledge base has exploded in the last 20 years. Assuming an average lag of 20 years in the transition from theory/knowledge gains to their applications in practice, as Gallagher (1983) and Glaser (1976) have suggested, the earliest advances in this knowledge explosion are just now being reflected in the newest tests. Current concepts of the nature and development of ability (e.g., Gardner, 1983; Haywood & Switzky, in press; Horn, 1972; Sternberg, 1985) and of the relation between intellectual aptitude and other variables, must be taken into account in the construction of assessment procedures and instruments (Haywood & Switzky, 1986a).

Together with new knowledge has come a new set of assessment questions, demanding new approaches to finding the answers. Traditional normative tests are based principally on assessment of achievement (Anastasi, 1987; Reschly, 1981). These tests lead one to ask and answer such questions as how much a subject has learned, assuming equal opportunities to learn, and what kinds of things that person cannot do well.

Given contemporary knowledge of intellective and cognitive development, it is now possible to ask process questions: how persons go about defining, analyzing, and solving problems, what specific processes of thought appear to be working well, which ones are less adequately developed. More radically different, and even more important, questions concern how much investment an examiner has to make in order to stimulate a higher level of performance, and the nature of subjects' response to teaching of generalizable principles and strategies (e.g., Feuerstein, Rand, & Hoffman, 1979; Haywood, 1988; Haywood et al., 1990). By addressing these questions, examiners change the focus from children to precesses, environments, and strategies. One asks what processes must be taught and learned, what environmental conditions must exist, and how strategies must be changed, in order to produce an acceptable level of learning and performance. Such questions are in sharp contrast to the more traditional question of what persons who take tests *are*, and they require quite different assessment strategies.

Use of standardized normative tests may lead to self-fulfilling prophecies: children get low scores on predictive tests, these scores go to their teachers, and the children are taught at the level of the scores rather than being held to a higher potential level of learning. Because they are taught at a low level, they achieve at a comparably low level, thus completing the self-fulfilling prophecy (Brophy & Good, 1970; Cooper & Good, 1983). Even though there is controversy associated with the research on "Pygmalion" effects (e.g., Kellaghan, Madaus, & Airasian, 1982; Pelligrini, & Hicks, 1972; Raudenbush, 1984; Thorndike, 1968), the fundamental phenomena have been demonstrated repeatedly (e.g., Rosenthal, 1974; Rosenthal & Babad, 1985; Rosenthal, Baratz, & Hall, 1974; Rosenthal & Jacobson, 1968; Rosenthal & Rubin, 1971; Weinstein, Marshall, Sharp, & Botkin, 1987).

Failure-following-the-test may be paralleled by failure-within-the-test, leading to similar results over the short range. Many standardized normative tests of intelligence use a "ceiling item" procedure of administration, in which examiner and subject may leave a particular subtest only after a prescribed number of consecutive failures. The effect of this may be twofold: (a) successive item failures leave children with the notion that they are incapable of getting correct answers, so their enthusiasm for academic-like tasks decreases; and (b) motivation within the test is impaired, because each new subtest is begun with the taste of failure left over from the end of the preceding subtest. As a result, children may not approach assessment tasks enthusiastically or confidently.

Standardized normative ability tests do not do a poor job; they simply may not do the job that needs to be done. They do an excellent job of what they were designed to do, that is, to predict subsequent school achievement and to classify children according to those predictions. Those goals are no longer the most appropriate ones. We now have the ability to ask more sophisticated questions, such as: "What specific deficiencies or strengths in thinking processes are revealed by this performance?"; "Is there a simple explanation for any apparent deficiencies in ability, such as lack of essential information?" (i.e., a distinction between ignorance and inability); "What level of performance would be possible under optimal conditions, and what conditions must exist in order to produce that level of performance?" (Haywood et al., 1990). These are more challenging questions, questions of a transactional nature, and they require new goals as well as new techniques of assessment (Feuerstein et al., 1979; Haywood & Switzky, 1986b, 1986c). Some of these are discussed in later sections of the chapter.

A Transactional View of the Nature and Development of Ability and Thinking

The transactional perspective can be summarized as a list of assumptions about the nature of intelligence and its development, the nature of cognitive processes, comparison of these two constructs, the role of motivational and affective variables in the development of each, and the modifiability of intelligence and cognition. The following statements constitute the core of the transactional perspective. Following discussion of these, we take up the essential question of what gives this point of view its transactional character.

1. Intelligence is multifaceted.
2. Intelligence is multidetermined.
3. Individual differences in intelligence are understood well according to a polygenic model.
4. There are biologically determined trajectories of individual development to which each person seeks to adhere and to return.
5. Intelligence, understood as "native ability," is not sufficient to explain individual differences in effective thought, perception, learning, problem solving, and social interaction.
6. Whatever one's individual level of intelligence, certain more-or-less-formal modes of thinking, perceiving, learning, and problem solving must be acquired in order for subsequent effective thinking and learning, across a wide range of content and contexts, to occur.
7. The application of intelligence never occurs in any person at 100% of that person's capacity or potential.
8. The application of intelligence to thinking, perceiving, learning, problem solving, and social interaction can always be improved.
9. The development of modes of formal thought depends to some extent on conditions of motivation, especially "intrinsic" motivation, as well as on other affective and attitudinal states.

10. Intelligence is modifiable only modestly and with great investment, but cognitive processes are readily modifiable and their modification produces changes in performance.

Intelligence is Multifaceted

The multifaceted nature of intelligence refers to two phenomena. The first is the repeated finding of "structuralists" in psychometric research that there are several "clusters" of abilities, representing general, group, and specific factors (Horn, 1972; Kaufman, 1975; McCall, Hogarty, & Hurlburt, 1972; Meyers & Dingman, 1966; Meyers, Dingman, Orpet, Sitkei, & Watts, 1964; Stott & Ball, 1965). The second is the correlated clinical observation that persons seldom if ever present "flat" profiles of ability across different kinds of tasks—i.e., different kinds of ability seem to be required to comprehend and acquire proficiency in different kinds of performance (such as using words, understanding social relations, solving math problems, perceiving spatial relations, and making sense of seemingly ambiguous stimuli). If groups of persons are rank-ordered on one aspect of intellectual functioning, e.g., vocabulary, it is quite unlikely that they will retain the same ranks on a second aspect, e.g., block design or map reading or coding. This is not to deny the existence, at some level, of the "g" factor, or general intelligence. It is clear that to the extent that one has very high global intelligence one is more likely than are those with low global intelligence to be able to do all of these things well (see, e.g., Jensen, 1984, 1987). It is nevertheless useful to emphasize the intraindividual variability in intellectual *pattern* rather than some notion of intraindividual homogeneity. Gardner (1983) has focused attention most sharply on the differences, rather than the similarities, among the kinds of ability required to learn and perform different qualities of tasks such as doing mathematical operations, using words to create images, playing musical instruments, manipulating objects in space in an orderly manner, and understanding analogies. In a developmental sense, different types of ability appear to become increasingly differentiated with increasing age of children (e.g., Harwood & Naylor, 1971; Lienert & Croth, 1964; Nesselrode, Schaie, & Baltes, 1972). Guilford's structure of intellect model (Guilford, 1967; Guilford & Hoepfner, 1971) has relied most heavily upon, and in return given support to, a multidimensional view of the nature of intelligence.

Intelligence is Multidetermined

The multidetermined nature of intelligence is by now axiomatic, even to those who choose to emphasize one or another source. Switzky and Haywood (1984) have discussed four models of the development of intelligence: the genetic model, the environmental model, the genetic-environmental interaction model, and the transactional model. The two main effects (genetic and environmental) models were shown to rest on some valid observations but to be both conceptually and empirically inadequate to incorporate what is known about individual differences in intelligence. The interaction model incorporates more of the existing data, but is also inadequate. The most promising model was shown to be a transactional one, in which individual differences in intellectual development and expression are seen to be products of genetic endowment engaged in a series of "transactions" with environmental circumstances, and with a person-characteristic trajectory of development for each individual. Deviations from personal trajectories may be brought about by disease, injuries, and extreme deprivation of learning opportunities, but there are "self-righting tendencies" that make it possible, and not always difficult, to return individual development to its genetically determined trajectory (Waddington, 1957, 1962, 1966). According to this transactional model, then, any person's intellectual level at any moment is a product of that person's (genetically determined) personal developmental trajectory, presence of absence of extreme environmental events, and availability of learning opportunities and social-ecological supports (Sameroff & Chandler, 1975). More detailed discussions of this general point of view, with different emphases, have been presented by Haywood and Switzky (1986b), McCall (1981), Sameroff and Chandler (1975), Switzky and Haywood (1984), and Waddington (1957, 1962, 1966).

Polygenic Determination

The prevailing (but clearly not exclusive) view is that the development of intelligence is understood well according to a polygenic model. According to this concept (see, e.g., Gillespie & Turelli, 1989; McAskie & Clarke, 1976; Paul, 1980; Scarr, 1981; Scarr & Weinberg, 1983), individual differences in intelligence are the result of the action of several genes, none of which individually and solely determines the gross phenotypic variable of 'intelligence." In fact, each of several genes may be associated with the possibility of a different level of intelligence. Each person carries genes representing a limited portion of the complete range of intellectual possibilities. Thus, the different offspring of the same couple will have different intelligence levels sampled grossly from the same broad range. Because intelligence is not a single-gene trait (Bouchard & McGue, 1981), its different genetic determinants may be differentially affected by environmental change. In fact, Rice, Cloninger, and Reich (1980) presented a model of familial resemblance in ability that allows for polygenic inheritance, "cultural transmission," assortative mating, effects of common environments, and parental effects. This model is not only polygenic, it is quite consistent with a transactional view of the nature and development of individual differences in ability. Zigler and Hodapp (1986) have provided an easy-to-understand explanation and illustration of the polygenic model.

Intelligence is Not Sufficient

Haywood (1989) has distinguished sharply between intelligence and cognitive processes. He has maintained that the question of whether or not, or to what extent, intelligence is modifiable by experience is a less important question than its history of debate and research would suggest, precisely because intelligence alone is never sufficient to understand individual differences in criterion variables: effectiveness and efficiency of thinking, learning, problem solving, and gathering and applying knowledge. Intelligence is seen as largely genetically determined, difficult to modify substantially, and relating primarily to the relative ease with which persons acquire formal processes of thinking. This distinction is similar in some respects to that between "fluid" and "crystallized" intelligence (Cattell, 1980; Cattell & Horn, 1978; Hakstian & Cattell, 1978; Horn, 1980; Horn & Cattell, 1982), and even to notions of "practical" intelligence (Sternberg & Wagner, 1986; Wagner & Sternberg, 1985). The essence of the distinction is that, however many (or few) IQ points one has, it is still necessary to develop durable and generalizable modes of thinking (the "cognitive structures" that Piaget explored) in order to apply effectively the intelligence that one has. According to Haywood and Switzky (1986a), good environments do not create intelligence, but they have the potential to support the acquisition of essential cognitive processes. Further, "bad" environments do not destroy intelligence (unless they destroy a large number of brain cells), but they may function so as to block access to one's intelligence and render it "unavailable" for application to learning and problem-solving situations. The kinds of formal cognitive processes that must be acquired through experience include the cognitive "structures" that the Piagetians refer to (e.g., Piaget, 1970, 1985), as well as more sharply focused strategies for thinking in more specific situations.

Acquisition of Cognitive Processes

According to this distinction, both children who are high in genetic intelligence and those who are quite low must acquire certain cognitive processes in order to be effective in academic and social learning. Feuerstein and Rand (1974; Feuerstein, Rand, Hoffman, & Miller, 1980) have made a further distinction between the mechanisms by which children acquire such basic thinking modes: "direct exposure," and "mediated learning experience." It seems clear that children who are genetically predisposed to have a high level of intelligence will acquire relatively more of their essential cognitive processes through direct exposure, that is, through successive interactions with environmental events. Children who are genetically predisposed to have a low level of intelligence will require relatively more mediated learning (through the intervention of adults or other more cognitively competent persons), that is, will need more help, in order to acquire their basic cognitive processes. Haywood's (1989) distinction is summarized in Table 2.1.

According to this comparison, intelligence is largely genetically determined, whereas cognitive processes must be acquired. Intelligence is modestly modifiable, but cognitive processes are highly modifiable (having been acquired through learning in the first place). Components of intelligence include general, group, and specific factors—all related to "pure" ability variables, but components of cognitive processes may include both cognitive "structures" and motivational/attitudinal/affective variables. The principal role of parents in the development of intelligence is to contribute genes, nutrition, safety, and a supportive environment, whereas the role of parents in the acquisition of cognitive processes is to provide "mediated learning experiences" (see Arbitman-Smith, Haywood, & Bransford, 1984; Feuerstein et al., 1979; Haywood, 1987). According to this transactional perspective, intelligence is an outmoded and inadequate concept and should be replaced by more specific concepts such as focused cognitive processes.

Modifiability

In addition to strong evidence for very substantial genetic determination, there is also strong evidence for the possibility of modifications brought about by experience (see, e.g., Haywood, 1967; Haywood & Switzky, in press; Haywood & Tapp, 1966; Hunt, 1961, 1979; Kamin, 1974; Uzgiris,

TABLE 2.1. Comparison of intelligence and cognitive processes.

Dimension	Intelligence	Cognitive processes
Source	Largely genetic	Must be taught/learned
Modifiability	Modest, with great effort	High, with teaching
Character	Both global and specific; equals ability to learn	Generalized across content domains
Assessment	Achievement; products of past learning	Process assessment; learning in teaching situations; dynamic
Composition	Intellectual aptitudes (verbal, spatial, memory, quantitative, etc.)	Mix of "native" ability, work habits, attitudes, motives, strategies
Parents' role	Genes, nutrition, health, safety	Mediated learning; active, directed teaching

Note. From "Multidimensional Treatment of Mental Retardation" by H. C. Haywood, 1989, *Psychology in Mental Retardation and Developmental Disabilities* (Division 33, American Psychological Association), *15*(1), pp. 1–10. Copyright 1989 by American Psychological Association. Reprinted by permission.

1970). The question of what it is that is modified by experience remains open; i.e., is it intelligence ("native" ability) or is it cognitive processes (acquired modes of thinking) that one can change by educational programs, environmental deprivation, or environmental support? We know that well-conceived and studiously applied programs of early education can result in significant, if sometimes temporary, IQ increases, and that "graduates" of such programs do better than do their uninstructed counterparts in quite long-range criteria such as staying in school through high school, not being retained in grade, and avoiding special education placement (Royce, Lazar, & Darlington, 1983; Schweinhart & Weikart 1988). Because IQ gains do tend to disappear (usually not by going back down, but by having untreated children catch up), it seems reasonable to assume that what has been changed is not intelligence but the children's access to their intelligence and their ability to apply it. In other words, they have acquired a more effective set of fundamental cognitive processes than have "control" children, and they use those effective thinking modes in both academic and social learning. Thus, it should be possible to bring about durable improvement in children's learning and performance effectiveness without necessarily changing their "intelligence."

Everybody Needs Intellectual "Tuning"

The most common observation in clinical practice is that a given client is "functioning below potential." Reviewing psychological diagnostic reports in a psychiatric hospital, Haywood (unpublished) found that in over 70% of the cases the psychologists had concluded that the patients' intelligence had been underestimated by individually administered standardized intelligence tests! About 60 years age, Vygotsky (1929, 1962, 1978; see also Guthke & Wingenfeld, Chapter 3 in this volume) observed that persons are usually functioning below their intellectual potential and devised a method of estimating the potential intelligence as well as the relative degree of underfunctioning at a given time. He would typically give a test in the standard way (without help) and call the result "performance." He then would help the subjects to learn thinking and problem solving processes required for solving the kinds of problems represented in the test. Finally, he would give a "posttest" in order to determine to what extent the subjects had learned the principles and generalized them to the solution of further problems that required the same kinds of thought processes. Rey (e.g., 1934, 1962) used similar approaches to try to quantify and establish evidence for the discrepancy between performance and potential that clinicians were always suspecting. These early clinical efforts led to the Lerntest movement in Germany (Guthke & Wingenfeld, Chatper 3 in this volume), to the elaboration of Rey's work at Geneva, and to Feuerstein's elaboration of dynamic assessment in his Learning Potential Assessment Device. In the context of a transactional perspective on the nature and development of ability, the relevant implication is that intelligent and effective behavior requires native ability, but it also requires access to one's intelligence as well as systematic modes of generating, selecting, applying, and evaluating thinking, learning, and problem solving strategies. It is the relative availability and application of such strategies that constitute individual differences in the magnitude of the difference between performance and potential, and it is that area (Vygotsky's "zone of proximal development") that is eminently modifiable.

Cognition and Motivation

To paraphrase Julius Caesar, *Omnia conscientia divisi est in partes tres.* According to the philosophical forefathers of contemporary psychology (Boring, 1950), the three divisions of consciousness were said to be cognition, conation, and volition. Translating "cognition" into "intelligence," we have traditionally made a sharp separation between intellective and affective (conative) variables—while denying volition altogether, thanks to the combined influences of Sigmund Freud and John B. Watson! In making tests, psychologists have been careful to remove consideration of motives, attitudes, and feelings from assessment of intelligence. At the same time, we have certainly been aware that individual differences in performance effectiveness and efficiency are often observed to be the interactive products of both intellective and such "nonintellective" variables. Our position is that processes of thinking, learning, and problem solving develop in transactional relation with motivation, especially "task-intrinsic" motivation, attitudes about learning and thinking, self-concept variables, and habits of working, thinking, and learning (see Tzuriel, 1990). Haywood and Burke (1977) suggested a "motivational theory of cognition" in which there is a reciprocal relation between ability variables and intrinsic motivation. Contrasting children who are genetically predisposed to high ability with those of low genetic potential, they observed the following:

> The early attempts at exploration of relatively competent children meet with proportionately higher rates of success (pleasure) than the exploratory attempts of relatively incompetent children. In the first weeks after birth, normally developing children greet stimulus change with an orienting reflex, the relatively vigorous feedback from which is experienced as pleasurable mild arousal. Other children may be relatively unresponsive and may not exhibit the orienting reflex to the same levels of stimulation that were effective with normally developing children, or . . . may not experience sensory feedback from it. Thus, from the very outset, some children are experientially deprived relative to the experience of normally developing children [and] . . . may require more repetitions of stimulus events in order to form perceptual-cognitive schemata . . . These children then have increasing difficulty assimilating new information, since the initial store of cognitive

> structures is limited. To the extent that cognitive structures (schemata) are unavailable for the assimilation of new information, accommodation must occur, and radical accommodation . . . may lead to an unacceptably aversive level of arousal. Thus, novelty may come to be avoided systematically, and the initial disadvantage of relatively incompetent children is compounded many times by this succession of experiences. . . . One child may try unsuccessfully to explore and to gain mastery, and that failure is experienced as punishment. Another child tries to gain behavioral competence and meets with intermittent success, and that success is reinforcing. Increasingly, the second child gets the idea that there is some degree of satisfaction in taking in new information, in exploring the environment, in taking limited risks, in undertaking tasks, and in achieving some mastery. . . . Failing to find satisfaction in novelty and in task-related events, the child whose initial attempts at exploration and mastery have been frustrated may stop seeking satisfaction and withdraw into a pattern of seeking only to avoid disappointment by concentrating his attention upon nontask aspects of the environment . . . The child who has learned the rewards of engagement with novelty and with tasks becomes a predominantly intrinsically motivated child who is, relative to his general ability, efficient at learning and performance. The child who has failed to find satisfaction in novelty and in task orientation becomes an extrinsically motivated child and is, relative to his general ability, inefficient at learning and performance. (pp. 257–258)

According to this kind of analysis, the trait of intrinsic motivation develops in part as a consequence of the relation between environmental challenges and one's abilities to meet those challenges, but cognitive structures are acquired also in part as a function of changes in intrinsic motivation. There is strong evidence (e.g., Haywood & Switzky, 1986a) for at least an interactive relation, and perhaps for a transactional one, between these "intellective" and "nonintellective" variables—such consistent relations that it would seem inappropriate to continue to ignore the "conative" variables in the assessment of individual differences in "cognitive" variables. Tzuriel, Samuels, and Feuerstein (1987) have begun to specify the role of such variables in dynamic assessment. The relations among nonintellective factors and deficient cognitive functions, type and amount of mediation, and objective scores have been investigated recently on four clinical groups using a dynamic assessment approach (Samuels, Tzuriel, & Malloy-Miller, unpublished). A model of the relations among MLE processes, cognitive modifiability, and affective-motivational processes has been discussed by Tzuriel (1991). Basically, the affective-motivational factors are thought of as an essential substrate for the proposed relation between the components of MLE and cognitive modifiability. The transactional nature of the relationship is characterized by the reciprocal effects of all components (factors) and by the complex circular process. Whereas in interaction one factor (A) has an effect on a second factor (B), and vice versa, in transactional relations B, being changed or transformed by A, affects A in return in a different way than had the original B. For example, efficient mediation by parents can facilitate affective-motivational processes which, in turn, encourage the mediators to adjust both the quality and the quantity of their mediation to match the child's responses (e.g., reduce efforts for child's engagement).

What Makes This Approach Transactional?

There are several essentially "transactional" aspects of the general view of human ability presented here. The most important is the observation that *none* of the predisposing, precipitating, or consequent (criterion) variables is constant—a fact that makes the relations among them dynamic, constantly changing, and of a transactional character. Second, ability is seen as a series of *processes* that are constantly changing, that vary with respect to the nature of their own applications, and that respond to qualities from quite different domains of human functioning (that is, to cognitive processes, motivational traits and states, attitudes, habits, social histories). The following statements summarize the transactional nature of this view and its particular application to psychoeducational assessment.

1. If C is a joint product of A and B, then A and B *interact* in such a way that a different level and/or quality of C is produced by B for each of >1 qualities or levels of A, and/or vice versa. Such an interaction can be static in nature, i.e., time or sequence may not necessarily be critical to the interaction.
2. In order to be *transactional* rather than merely *interactive*, the relationship must be between/among variables that change over time, in such a way that the interactive relation of A and B to C changes in quality and/or level as changes occur in A, B, or C. Such changes may reflect development, or the effects of other variables.
3. The essence of a transactional view of the nature of ability is the notion of a *dynamic* (i.e., constantly changing) relationship between ability and environmental influences. This qualitatively unstable relationship is embodied in the notion of genetically determined "trajectories" of development, the "canalization" of certain important cognitive and affective components, and the differential effects of powerful environmental events upon development (Switzky & Haywood, 1984; Waddington, 1957, 1962, 1966), depending upon (a) the level of the established developmental trajectory, (b) the specific nature of the "powerful" events, and (c) the quality of the ("ordinary" or posttraumatic) environment (Sameroff & Chandler, 1975). All three sets of conditions exert their effects, but the effect of each is moderated, amplified, or rendered qualitatively different by the actions of the other two conditions. In psychoeducational assessment, the particularly relevant qualities of environments are circumstances that militate for or against the learning of specific generalizable modes

of perceiving, thinking, learning, and problem solving; i.e., specific cognitive functions that will be required both now and later to support the understanding and learning of a wide variety of both social and academic content.

4. Transactional interpretations of ability are addressed to *processes* rather than to states; therefore, *assessment* rather than *measurement* is the appropriate task.
5. A transactional approach to psychoeducational assessment implies a dynamic relationship among subject, assessor, materials, and tasks, such that each influences the others, including effects of subject variations on the behavior of examiners, and even subject and examiner influences on the meaning of tasks and materials. Added to the notion that what is to be assessed is processes rather than states or products, these dynamic relationships make assessment an extremely intricate enterprise. Such transactional enterprises can be understood as dynamic lattices in which the immediately prior value of each interacting variable affects the contemporary and next values of each of the other variables.
6. A transactional approach to assessment, then, is one that (a) is based upon a transactional view of the nature and development of human abilities and performance, (b) is able to reflect *processes*, e.g., thought processes, as well as changes in those processes under changing conditions of assessment; (c) incorporates deliberate change as an essential part of the assessment technique; (d) incorporates motivational and affective components of behavior.

Different Assessment Approaches that are Compatible with a Transactional Model

Dynamic Assessment

The philosophy, goals, methods, and interpretation of what has come to be called "dynamic" assessment follow quite naturally from a transactional perspective on the nature and development of ability. Dynamic (or "interactive" as we have called it in this book) assessment is characterized by: (a) an emphasis on the processes of perceiving, thinking, learning, and problem solving, as opposed to emphasis on the *products* or outcomes of these processes; (b) recognition of the constantly changing nature of the processes of logical thought; (c) belief in the modifiability of the fundamental processes of logical thought, and in the ability of persons to bring about such modification; (d) use of assessment methods in which some sort of teaching/helping is part of the testing, often in a test-teach-test sequence; (e) interpretation of the difference between unassisted performance and performance after teaching as indicative of modifiability or potential development; (f) teaching/learning of generalizable cognitive processes; (g) attempts to specify obstacles to effective learning and performance; (h) attempts to specify conditions that will permit or encourage more effective performance; (i) distinction between performance and potential, or between ignorance and inability (Haywood et al., 1990). This approach is called "dynamic" (or interactive) both because of its emphasis on processes that are constantly changing and because it involves deliberate attempts to modify those processes.

The essence of interactive/dynamic assessment is its reliance on the strategy of producing change in order to describe otherwise unobservable events. In the case of psychoeducational assessment, one tries to infer "learning potential" or potential performance by creating and applying conditions that support more nearly optimal performance. For example, a subject may be given a set of matrix problems such as Raven's Standard Progressive Matrices, as a "pretest," in a usual, standard, static mode. The score from that administration suggests the subject's usual independent performance. Training may then be given in the principles, concepts, and strategies of thinking and problem solving that may be required for successful performance on such tasks. Records are kept of the kinds and amount of teaching or "mediation" (Feuerstein et al., 1979) given and such variables as spontaneous corrections. Posttests are then given to determine the extent to which the subject has learned and can generalize those principles, concepts, and strategies to the solution of new problems of the same kind. Four important kinds of information are derived from these procedures: (a) initial level, or "performance," i.e., without help; (b) kind and amount of help/teaching/mediation needed to produce improved performance; (c) response to mediation, i.e., postteaching performance; (d) identification of the specific deficient cognitive processes that have impeded adequate performance. This last inference is based on the notion that if one applies a solution and performance is then improved, the nature of the original problem must have been related to the solution. The most important outcome is specification of the conditions that will support improved performance (Haywood, 1988).

These general principles of dynamic/interactive assessment have been incorporated in several assessment traditions and specific approaches. The most fully developed of these is the Learning Potential Assessment Device (Feuerstein et al., 1979; Feuerstein, Haywood, Rand, Hoffman, & Jensen, 1986; see also Tzuriel & Haywood, Chapter 1 in this volume). Strongly related bodies of work include Lidz's Preschool Learning Assessment Device (Lidz, 1990; Lidz & Thomas, 1987), and several instruments specifically focused on dynamic assessment of young children, such as Children's Analogical Thinking Modifiability (Tzuriel & Klein, 1985, 1987), the Frame Test of Cognitive Modifiability (Tzuriel & Klein, 1986), and the Children's Inferential Thinking Modifiability test (Tzuriel, 1989; Tzuriel & Eran, 1990), and procedures developed by Mearig (1987).

In addition to these procedures that are conceptually closely related to the theories and methods of Feuerstein, there is a substantially different tradition of interactive assessment in other parts of the world. For a description and history of the Lerntest approach, see Chapter 3 by Guthke and Wingenfeld, this volume. Other methods, developed and used primarily for research rather than for clinical use, include the "graduated prompt" procedure of Brown, Campione, and their colleagues (Brown & Ferrara, 1985), and the coaching methods of Budoff and associates (e.g., Budoff & Friedman, 1964; Budoff, Meskin, & Harrison, 1971). See also the chapters in this volume by Tzuriel and Haywood (Chapter 1), Carlson and Wiedl (Chapter 6), Samuels, MacKenzie, and Fagan (Chapter 10), and Samuels, Lamb, and Oberholtzer (Chapter 11) for more detailed discussions of different dynamic assessment methods and their use with different populations of subjects.

Dynamic assessment is not the only approach that is consistent with a transactional perspective on ability. In fact, there are several quite complementary assessment strategies that can fit comfortably under this conceptual umbrella. Following are brief discussions of just two of these: neuropsychological assessment and curriculum-based assessment.

Neuropsychological Assessment

The use of behavioral observations to make inferences about the integrity of the nervous system is called neuropsychological assessment (Deysach, 1986; Haywood, 1968; Reitan, 1962). Lewis and Sinnett (1987) observed that "These assessments allow the identification of patients whose cognitive deficits have been underestimated or overestimated by other diagnostic procedures and provide clinically relevant information about potential for and specific means to promote recovery" (p. 126). Haywood (1977) has observed that clinical neuropsychological assessment is different in important ways from standardized, normative assessment, and in many of those same ways is similar to dynamic assessment.

Neuropsychological assessment rests in part on the assumption that intelligence, although largely genetically determined, may not be accessible for a variety of reasons (especially because of injury or subfunctioning of some parts of the brain). Because of this assumption, neuropsychologists search for maximal performance rather than for typical performance; that is, they try to elicit each subject's best possible performance on a variety of tasks. Further, recognizing the multidimensionality and the complexity of ability, they use a substantial variety of diagnostic tasks rather than trying to base diagnostic inferences on "narrow-band" tests. Neuropsychologists recognize a discrepancy between performance and potential, so they search both for ways to define "potential" and for the conditions that will promote the realization of that potential. They are typically at least as interested in comparisons among different aspects of functioning within persons as in comparisons of their subjects' performance with some normative standard. In making such within-subject comparisons, neuropsychologists frequently compare functions that are centrally mediated on different sides of the brain, for example, language functions with visual-spatial-perceptual functions, as well as sensory and motor functions (mediated in the posterior and anterior portions, respectively, of the cerebral hemispheres). Observing the changing nature of brain functions, they also compare performances in the same domains over time.

Although one of the major traditions in neuropsychology, the Halstead-Reitan approach (Reitan, 1962), is based upon use of "objective" data gathered in standardized ways and evaluated by comparison to normative standards (Lewis & Sinnett, 1987), another major tradition rests on the work of A. R. Luria (see, e.g., Christensen, 1975), who made extensive use of qualitative information and "tailored" his tests and his procedures to the individual characteristics, abilities, and requirements of his subjects (Lewis & Sinnett, 1987). Thus, at least in one of its major traditions, clinical neuropsychology shares a part of a transactional perspective as well as this aspect of dynamic assessment. In both of these traditions, clinical neuropsychologists search for the cognitive processes that their subjects employ in solving the test items rather than merely for correct (or incorrect) responses.

Curriculum-Based Assessment

A somewhat newer approach in psychoeducational assessment is curriculum-based assessment (CBA; Deno, 1985; Fuchs & Fuchs, 1986; Fuchs, Fuchs, & Stecker, 1989), so named because the material that one assesses with CBA is the very content of a local school curriculum (Deno, 1987; Fuchs, 1987; Tucker, 1985). CBA is an outgrowth of dissatisfaction with the use of nationally standardized school achievement tests, which, although allowing for comparison of local students' performance with that of students in many other places, might not reflect what is actually taught in any particular classroom. Its primary objective is to "obtain a reliable and valid measure of student achievement" (Deno, 1987, p. 41), while providing data for frequent modification of goals and teaching methods. Deno (1987) defined CBA as "any approach that uses direct observation and recording of a student's performance in the local school curriculum as a basis for gathering information to make instructional decisions." It is in many ways a *formative* evaluation technology, in that its users take frequent samples of students' performance and use the data to make inferences about learning processes and to adjust teaching methods, rates, and contents.

Fuchs (1987) has outlined four steps in CBA. These are (a) identifying the long-range goal; (b) creating the pool of test items; (c) measuring pupil performance; and (d) evaluating the data base. The first step, identifying the long-range goal, requires teachers/evaluators to define in quite concrete terms the performance standard that they expect of each student. The second step requires them to identify the precise body of content that is to be learned, and to sample that content for test items. The third, measuring pupil performance, repeated as often as two or more times per week, requires systematic sampling from the "goal-level material" (Fuchs, 1987, p. 42) and charting the scores. Evaluating the data base is the heart of the method: rates of learning and projected (goal-established) rates are compared so that teachers may do what is necessary to conform the students' rates of progress to the slope of the goal-established curve. By examining the concordance or discrepancy of the empirical and projected progress curves and relating data points to corresponding teaching/learning strategies, evaluators can make some inferences about learning processes. Special sections of *Exceptional Children* (Tucker, 1985, guest editor) and *Teaching Exceptional Children* (Deno, 1987) have been devoted to these methods, and they contain especially instructive papers.

Although it clearly has not been derived from a specifically transactional concept of human ability, CBA is in many important ways consistent with such a view, and is also consistent with the conceptual basis of dynamic assessment. Characteristics of CBA that seem consistent with a transactional view include (a) view of learning ability as modifiable; (b) assumption that performance does not necessarily equal potential; (c) emphasis on identification and modification of processes of learning; (d) comparison of individuals' performance with other samples of their own performance rather than with norms; (e) use of assessment as a basis for educational prescription and change; and (f) use of direct intervention as part of the assessment procedure. Indeed, dynamic assessment and CBA could be quite complementary. Dynamic assessment is focused upon the search for and modification of quite fundamental and generalizable cognitive processes, that is, processes of thinking that cut across a wide variety of content domains. Many cognitive psychologists question the utility of the concept of broadly generalizable basic cognitive processes, preferring instead the notion of relatively domain-specific or domain-relevant cognitive strategies. With its emphasis on specific academic content, CBA could be a very useful addition.

There are other assessment approaches whose use would be entirely consistent with a transactional perspective. These include "diagnostic classrooms" and "ecological assessment." Because the rest of this volume is devoted to interactive methods of psychological and psychoeducational assessment, these methods are not discussed here. The primary point of these examples is that a transactional view of human ability can lead one to specific assessment strategies.

Summary

We have argued that psychoeducational assessment is done on the basis of either implicitly or explicitly held theories of the nature and development of human ability, that such theories should be made explicit, and that assessment methods and strategies should be clearly based on them. We have presented a brief discussion of a "transactional" perspective on the nature and development of human ability, and tried to show that such a view demands certain assessment strategies while not leading naturally to others.

The following were said to be characteristics of a transactional perspective on human ability: (a) it is multifaceted; (b) it is multidetermined; (c) intelligence is an inadequate concept; (d) cognitive processes are acquired, and therefore are modifiable; (e) there is always a difference between performance and potential; (f) ability has motivational, affective, and attitudinal components; and (g) the relation between ability and environmental influences on it is constantly changing.

"Dynamic" or "interactive" approaches to assessment have been shown to be consistent with such a transactional perspective, as have neuropsychological and curriculum-based assessment. Assessment that is based on a transactional perspective must (a) be addressed to processes; (b) use intervention as an assessment strategy; (c) make use of a dynamic relationship among subject, assessor, materials, and tasks; (d) incorporate motivational and affective aspects of behavior as part of ability; and (e) identify the necessary and suffidient conditions for modifiability of the cognitive processes that one is assessing.

References

Anastasi, A. (1987). *Psychological testing* (6th ed.). New York: Macmillan.

Arbitman-Smith, R., Haywood, H. C., & Bransford, J. D. (1984). Assessing cognitive change. In P. Brooks, R. Sperber, & C. M. McCauley (Eds.), *Learning and cognition in the mentally retarded* (pp. 433–471). Hillsdale, NJ: Erlbaum.

Boring, E. G. (1950). *A history of experimental psychology* (2nd ed.). New York: Appleton-Century-Crofts.

Bouchard, T. J., & McGue, M. (1981). Familial studies of intelligence: A review. *Science*, *212*, 1055–1059.

Brophy, J., & Good, T. L. (1970). Teachers' communications of differential expectations for children's classroom performance: Some behavioral data. *Journal of Educational Psychology*, *61*, 365–374.

Brown, A. L., & Ferrara, R. A. (1985). Diagnosing zones of proximal development. In J. Wertsch (Ed.), Culture, Communication, and cognition; Vygotskian perspectives. (pp. 273–305). New York: Cambridge University Press.

Cattell, R. B. (1980). The heritability of fluid, g-sub(f), and crystallized, g-sub(c), intelligence, estimated by a least squares use of the MAVA method. *British Journal of Educational Psychology*, *50*, 253–265.

Cattell, R. B., & Horn, J. L. (1978). A check on the theory of fluid and crystallized intelligence with description of new subtest designs. *Journal of Educational Measurement*, *15*(3), 139–164.

Christensen, A. L. (1975). *Luria's neuropsychological investigation*. New York: Spectrum.

Cooper, H. M., & Good, T. L. (1983). *Pygmalion grows up: Studies in the expectation communication process*. New York: Longman.

Deno, S. L. (1985). Curriculum-based measurement: The emerging alternative. *Exceptional Children*, *52*, 219–232.

Deno, S. L. (1987, Fall). Curriculum-based measurement. *Teaching Exceptional Children*, *18*, 41–42.

Deysach, R. E. (1986). The role of neuropsychological assessment in the comprehensive evaluation of preschool-age children. *School Psychology Review*, *15*(2), 233–244.

Dunn, L. M. (1968). Special education for the mildly retarded—Is much of it justifiable? *Exceptional Children*, *35*, 5–22.

Elliott, R. (1988). Tests, abilities, race, and conflict. *Intelligence*, *12*, 333–335.

Feuerstein, R., Haywood, H. C., Rand, Y., Hoffman, M. B., & Jensen, M. (1986). *Examiner manual for the Learning Potential Assessment Device*. Jerusalem: Hadassah-WIZO-Canada Research Institute. [Available from HWCRI, 6 Karmon Street, Jerusalem, Israel.]

Feuerstein, R., & Rand, Y. (1974). Mediated learning experiences: An outline of proximal etiology for differential development of cognitive functions. *International Understanding*, *9–10*, 7–37.

Feuerstein, R., Rand, Y., & Hoffman, M. B. (1979). *Dynamic assessment of retarded performers: The Learning Potential Assessment Device, theory, instruments, and techniques*. Baltimore: University Park Press.

Feuerstein, R., Rand, Y., Hoffman, M. B., & Miller, R. (1980). *Instrumental Enrichment: An intervention program for cognitive modifiability*. Baltimore: University Park Press.

Fuchs, L. S. (1987, Fall). Program development. *Teaching Exceptional Children*, *18*, 42–44.

Fuchs, L. S., & Fuchs, D. (1986). Curriculum-based assessment of progress toward long-term and short-term goals. *Journal of Special Education*, *20*(1), 69–81.

Fuchs, L. S., Fuchs, D., & Stecker, P. M. (1989). Effects of curriculum-based measurement on teachers' instructional planning. *Journal of Learning Disabilities*, *22*(1), 51–59.

Gallagher, J. J. (1983). The uses of social policy analysis with mental retardation. In K. T. Kernan, M. J. Begab, & R. B. Edgerton (Eds.), *Environments and behavior* (pp. 37–54). Baltimore: University Park Press.

Gardner, H. (1983). *Frames of mind: The theory of multiple intelligences*. New York: Basic Books.

Gillespie, J. H., & Turelli, M. (1989). Genotype-environment interactions and the maintenance of polygenic variation. *Genetics*, *121*, 129–138.

Glaser, E. (Ed.) (1976). *Putting knowledge to use*. Los Angeles: Human Interaction Research Institute.

Gregory, S., & Lee, S. (1986). Psychoeducational assessment of racial and ethnic minority groups: Professional implications. *Journal of Counseling and Development*, *64*, 635–637.

Guilford, J. P. (1967). *The nature of human intelligence*. New York: McGraw-Hill.

Guilford, J. P., & Hoepfner, R. (1971). *The analysis of intelligence*. New York: McGraw-Hill.

Hakstian, A. R., & Cattell, R. B. (1978). Higher-stratum ability structures on a basis of twenty primary abilities. *Journal of Educational Psychology*, *70*, 657–669.

Harwood, E., & Naylor, G. (1971). Changes in the constitution of the WAIS intelligence pattern with advancing age. *Australian Journal of Psychology*, *23*, 297–303.

Haywood, H. C. (1967). Experiential factors in intellectual development. In J. Zubin & G. A. Jervis (Eds.), *Psychopathology of mental development* (pp. 69–104). New York: Grune & Stratton.

Haywood, H. C. (1968). Introduction to clinical neuropsychology. In H. C. Haywood (Ed.), *Brain damage in school age children* (pp. 3–19). Washington, DC: Council for Exceptional Children.

Haywood, H. C. (1977). Alternatives to normative assessment. In P. Mittler (Ed.), *Research to practice in mental retardation: Proceedings of the 4th Congress of the International Association for the Scientific Study of Mental Deficiency. Vol. 2, Education and training* (pp. 11–18). Baltimore: University Park Press.

Haywood, H. C. (1984, October). *Psychoeducational assessment of minority children: The issues*. Paper presented at the Association for Public Policy Analysis and Management, New Orleans.

Haywood, H. C. (1987). A mediational teaching style. *The Thinking Teacher*, *4*(1), 1–6.

Haywood, H. C. (1988). Dynamic assessment: The Learning Potential Assessment Device. In R. L. Jones (Ed.), *Psychoeducational assessment of minority group children: A casebook* (pp. 39–63). Richmond, VA: Cobb & Henry.

Haywood, H. C. (1989). Multidimensional treatment of mental retardation. *Psychology in Mental Retardation and Developmental Disabilites* (Division 33, American Psychological Association), *15*(1), 1–10.

Haywood, H. C., Brown, A. L., & Wingenfeld, S. (1990). Dynamic approaches to psychoeducational assessment. *School Psychology Review*, *19*, 411–422.

Haywood, H. C., & Burke, W. P. (1977). Development of individual differences in intrinsic motivation. In I. C. Uzgiris & F. Weizmann (Eds.), *The structuring of experience* (pp. 235–263). New York: Plenum.

Haywood, H. C., & Switzky, H. N. (1986a). Intrinsic motivation and behavior effectiveness in retarded persons. In N. R. Ellis & N. W. Bray (Eds.), *International review of research in mental retardation* (Vol. 14, pp. 1–46). New York: Academic Press.

Haywood, H. C., & Switzky, H. N. (1986b). The malleability of intelligence: Cognitive processes as a function of polygenic-experiential interaction. *School Psychology Review*, *15*, 245–255.

Haywood, H. C., & Switzky, H. N. (1986c). Transactionalism and cognitive processes: Reply to Reynolds and Gresham. *School Psychology Review*, *15*, 264–267.

Haywood, H. C., & Switzky, H. N. (in press). Ability and modifiability: What, how, and how much? In J. S. Carlson (Ed.), *Cognition and educational practice*. Greenwich, CT: JAI Press.

Haywood, H. C., & Tapp, J. T. (1966). Experience and the development of adaptive behavior, In N. R. Ellis (Ed.), *International review of research in mental retardation* (Vol. 1, pp. 109–151). New York: Academic Press.

Hobbs, N. (1974). *The futures of children: Categories, labels and their consequences*. Report of the Project on Classification of Exceptional Children. Nashville: Vanderbilt University.

Horn, J. L. (1972). Structure of intellect: Primary abilities. In R. M. Dreger (Ed.), *Multivariate personality research*. Baton Rouge, LA: Claitor.

Horn, J. L. (1980). Concepts of intellect in relation to learning and adult development. *Intelligence*, *4*(4), 285–317.

Horn, J. L., & Cattell, R. B. (1982). Whimsy and misunderstanding of gf-gc theory: A comment on Guilford. *Psychological Bulletin*, *91*, 623–633.

Hunt, J. McV. (1961). *Intelligence and experience*. New York: Ronald.

Hunt, J. McV. (1979). Psychological development: Early experience. In M. R. Rosenzweig (Ed.), *Annual review of psychology* (Vol. 30, pp. 103–143). Palo Alto, CA: Annual Reviews, Inc.

Jensen, A. R. (1980). *Bias in mental testing*. New York: Free Press.

Jensen, A. R. (1984). Test validity: g versus the specificity doctrine. *Journal of Social and Biological Structures*, *7*(2), 93–118.

Jensen, A. R. (1987). Psychometric g as a focus of concerted research effort. *Intelligence*, *11*(3), 193–198.

Kamin, L. J. (1974). *The science and politics of IQ*. Potomac, MD: Erlbaum.

Kaufman, A. S. (1975). Factor structure of the McCarthy scales at five age levels between 212 and 812. *Educational and Psychological Measurement*, *35*, 640–656.

Kellaghan, T., Madaus, G. F., & Airasian, P. W. (1982). *The effects of standardized testing*. Boston: Kluwer-Nijoff.

Lewis, L., & Sinnett, E. R. (1987). An introduction to neuropsychological assessment. *Journal of Counseling and Development*, *66*, 126–130.

Lidz, C. S. (1990). *Preschool Learning Assessment Device (PLAD), Curriculum-Based Dynamic Assessment, and Mediated Learning Experience Rating Scale Manuals*. Philadelphia: Temple University. [Available from author.]

Lidz, C. S., & Thomas, C. (1987). The Preschool Learning Assessment Device: Extension of a static approach. In C. S. Lidz (Ed.), *Dynamic assessment: An interactional approach to evaluating learning potential* (pp. 288–326). New York: Guilford Press.

Lienert, G., & Croth, H. (1964). Studies of the factor structure of intelligence in children, adolescents, and adults. *Vita Humana*, *7*, 147–163.

Lilly, S. M. (1982). Toward a unitary concept of mental retardation. *Education and Treatment of Children*, *5*, 379–387.

McAskie, M., & Clarke, A. M. (1976). Parent-offspring resemblances in intelligence: Theories and evidence. *British Journal of Psychology*, *67*(2), 243–273.

McCall, R. B. (1981). Nature-nurture and the two realms of development: A proposed integration with respect to mental development. *Child Development*, *52*, 1–12.

McCall, R. B., Hogarty, P. S., & Hurlburt, N. (1972). Transitions in infant sensorimotor development and the prediction of childhood IQ. *American Psychologist*, *27*, 728–748.

Mearig, J. S. (1987). Assessing the learning potential of kindergarten and primary-age children. In C. S. Lidz (Ed.), *Dynamic assessment* (pp. 237–267). New York: Guilford.

Mercer, J. R. (1970). Sociological perspective on mild mental retardation. In H. C. Haywood (Ed.), *Social-cultural aspects of mental retardation* (pp. 378–391). New York: Appleton-Century-Crofts.

Mercer, J. R. (1973). *Labeling the mentally retarded*. Berkeley: University of California Press.

Mercer, J. R. (1975). Psychological assessment and the rights of children. In N. Hobbs (Ed.), *Issues in the classification of children* (Vol. 1, pp. 130–158). San Francisco: Jossey-Bass.

Meyers, C. E., & Dingman, H. F. (1966). Factor analytic and structure of intellect models in the study of mental retardation. *American Journal of Mental Deficiency*, *70*(4), 7–25 (Monograph Supplement).

Meyers, C. E., Dingman, H. F., Orpet, R., Sitkei, E., & Watts, C. (1964). Four ability-factor hypotheses at three levels in normal and retarded children. *Monographs of the Society for Research in Child Development*, *29*, (5, Serial No. 96).

Nesselrode, J., Schaie, W., & Baltes, P. (1972). Ontogenetic and generational components of structural and quantitative changes in adult behavior. *Journal of Gerontology*, *27*, 222–228.

Paul, S. M. (1980). Sibling resemblance in mental ability: A review. *Behavior Genetics*, *10*(3), 277–290.

Pelligrini, R., & Hicks, R. (1972). Prophecy effects and tutorial instruction for the disadvantaged child. *American Educational Research Journal*, *9*, 413–419.

Piaget, J. (1970). *Le structuralisme*. Paris: Presses Universitaires de France. (*Que sais-je?*, No. 1311).

Piaget, J. (1985). *The equilibration of cognitive structures: The central problem of intellectual development* (T. Brown & K. Julian Thampy, Trans.). Chicago: University of Chicago Press.

Raudenbush, S. W. (1984). Magnitude of teacher expectancy effects on pupil IQ as a function of the credibility of expectancy induction: A synthesis of findings from 18 experiments. *Journal of Educational Psychology*, *76*, 85–97.

Reitan, R. M. (1962). Psychological deficit. *Annual Review of Psychology*, *13*, 415–444.

Reschly, D. J. (1981). Psychological testing in educational classification and placement. *American Psychologist*, *36*, 1094–1102.

Rey, A. (1934). D'un procédé pour évaluer l'éducabilité (quelques applications en psychopathologie) [A procedure for assessing educability (applications to psychopathology)]. *Archives de Psychologie*, *24*, 297–337.

Rey, A. (1962). *Etudes des insuffisances psychologiques. II. La systématisation des observations* [The study of psychological deficits. II. Systematization of observation]. Neuchâtel: Delachaux et Niestlé.

Rice, J., Cloninger, C. R., & Reich, T. (1980). Analysis of behavioral traits in the presence of cultural transmission and assortative mating: Applications to IQ and SES. *Behavior Genetics*, *10*(1), 73–92.

Rosenthal, R. (1974). *On the social psychology of the self-fulfilling prophecy: Further evidence for Pygmalion effects and their mediating mechanisms* (Module 53). New York: MSS Modular Publications.

Rosenthal, R., & Babad, E. Y. (1985). Pygmalion in the gymnasium. *Educational Leadership*, *43*(1), 36–39.

Rosenthal, R., Baratz, S., & Hall, C. M. (1974). Teacher behavior, teacher expectations, and gains in pupils' rated creativity. *Journal of Genetic Psychology*, *124*, 115–121.

Rosenthal, R., & Jacobson, L. (1968). *Pygmalion in the classroom*. New York: Holt, Rinehart, & Winston.

Rosenthal, R., & Rubin, D. B. (1971). Pygmalion reaffirmed. In J. D. Elashoff & R. E. Snow (Eds.), *Pygmalion reconsidered* (pp. 289–334). Worthington, OH: Charles A. Jones.

Royce, J. M., Lazar, I., & Darlington, R. B. (1983). Minority families, early education, and later life chances. *American Journal of Orthopsychiatry*, *53*, 706–720.

Sameroff, A. J., & Chandler, M. J. (1975). Reproductive risk and the continuum of caretaking casualty. In F. D. Horowitz, M. Hetherington, S. Scarr-Salapatek, & G. Siegel (Eds.), *Review of child development research* (Vol. 4, pp. 187–244). Chicago: University of Chicago Press.

Scarr, S. (1981). *Race, social class, and individual differences in I.Q.* Hillsdale, NJ: Erlbaum.

Scarr, S., & Weinberg, R. A. (1983). The Minnesota adoption studies: Genetic differences and malleability. *Child Development*, *54*, 260–267.

Schweinhart, L. J., & Weikart, D. P. (1988). Early childhood education for at-risk four-year-olds? Yes. *American Psychologist*, *43*, 665–667.

Sternberg, R. J. (1985). *Beyond IQ: A triarchic theory of human intelligence*. New York: Cambridge University Press.

Sternberg, R. J., & Wagner, R. K. (Eds.), (1986). *Practical intelligence: Nature and origins of competence in the everyday world*. New York: Cambridge University Press.

Stott, L., & Ball, R. (1965). Infant and preschool mental tests: Review and evaluation. *Monographs of the Society for Research in Child Development*, *30*(3), Whole No. 101.

Switzky, H. N., & Haywood, H. C. (1984). A biosocial ecological perspective on mental retardation. In N. E. Endler & J. McV. Hunt (Eds.), *Personality and the behavioral disorders* (2nd ed., Vol. 2). New York: Wiley.

Thorndike, R. L. (1968). Review of *Pygmalion in the classroom. American Educational Research Journal*, *5*, 708–711.

Tucker, J. A. (1985). Curriculum-based assessment: An introduction. *Exceptional Children*, *52*, 199–204.

Tzuriel, D. (1989). Dynamic assessment of learning potential: Novel measures for young children. *The Thinking Teacher*, *5*(1), 9–10. [Available from author.]

Tzuriel, D. (1991). Cognitive modifiability, mediated learning experience and affective-motivational processes: A transactional approach. In R. Feuerstein, P. S. Klein, & A. Tannenbaum (Eds.), *Mediated learning experience*. London: Freund.

Tzuriel, D., & Eran, Z. (1990). Inferential cognitive modifiability of kibbutz young children as a function of mother-child mediated learning experience (MLE) interaction. *International Journal of Cognitive Education and Mediated Learning*, *1*(2), 103–117.

Tzuriel, D., & Klein, P. S. (1985). Analogical thinking modifiability in disadvantaged, regular, special education, and mentally retarded children. *Journal of Abnormal Child Psychology*, *13*, 539–552.

Tzuriel, D., & Klein, P. S. (1986). *The dynamic method: A different approach to decision-making about cognitive modifiability of young children.* Paper presented at the 28th World Congress of OMEP (Organisation Mondiale de l'Education Préscolaire [World Preschool Education Organization]), Jerusalem, July 13–17. [Available from authors.]

Tzuriel, D., & Klein, P. S. (1987). Assessing the young child: Children's Analogical Thinking Modifiability. In C. S. Lidz (Ed.), *Dynamic assessment: An interactional approach to evaluating learning potential* (pp. 268–282). New York: Guilford Press.

Tzuriel, D., Samuels, M. T., & Feuerstein, R. (1987). Non-intellective factors in dynamic assessment. In R. M. Gupta & P. Coxhead (Eds.), *Cultural diversity and learning efficiency*. London: Macmillan.

Uzgiris, I. C. (1970). Sociocultural factors in cognitive development. In H. C. Haywood (Ed.), *Social-cultural aspects of mental retardation* (pp. 7–58). New York: Appleton-Century-Crofts.

Vygotsky, L. S. (1929). The problem of the cultural development of the child. *Journal of Genetic Psychology*, *36*, 415–434.

Vygotsky, L. S. (1962). *Thought and language*, Cambridge, MA: MIT Press.

Vygotsky, L. S. (1978). *Mind in society: The development of higher psychological processes*. Cambridge, MA: Harvard University Press.

Waddington, C. H. (1957). *The strategy of the genes*. New York: Macmillan.

Waddington, C. H. (1962). *New patterns in genetics and development*. New York: Columbia University Press.

Waddington, C. H. (1966). *Principles of development and differentiation*. New York: Macmillan.

Wagner, R. K., & Sternberg, R. J. (1985). Practical intelligence in real-world pursuits: the role of tacit knowledge. *Journal of Personality and Social Psychology*, *49*, 436–458.

Weinstein, R. S., Marshall, H. H., Sharp, L., & Botkin, M. (1987). Pygmalion and the student: Age and classroom differences in children's awareness of teacher expectations. *Child Development*, *58*, 1079–1093.

Zigler, E., & Hodapp, R. M. (1986). *Understanding mental retardation*. New York: Cambridge University Press.

3 The Learning Test Concept: Origins, State of the Art, and Trends

JÜRGEN GUTHKE and SABINE WINGENFELD

Historical Roots and Theoretical Foundations

Since the advent of intelligence tests, there has been a heated controversy among psychologists, educators, and the public about their practical value and theoretical foundations. In a letter to Eduard Spranger, Wilhelm Wundt already criticized intelligence testing of pupils for being too practice-oriented. Further suggestions for improvement, even for more dynamic assessment of intelligence, have been made for decades. Even so, the practice of intelligence testing has not undergone any fundamental, revolutionary changes since Binet.

During the 1960s and 1970s, researchers in Europe, the United States, and Israel proposed, largely independently of each other, an alternative to the conventional static intelligence tests. We have used the term "learning test" to distinguish these alternatives from conventional intelligence tests. This diagnostic method differs from conventional intelligence tests in that examiners record not only how persons solve particular test items without help by the examiner, but also to what extent they are able to improve their test performance, if they are provided with feedback, prompts, or even complete training programs between a pretest and a posttest. The focus on the learning process during a test procedure that optimizes performance (Wiedl, 1984) and the recording of learning gains are expected to provide additional diagnostic information. This information should enable diagnosticians (a) to make more reliable and valid differential diagnoses than with traditional intelligence tests (e.g., to distinguish between educable mentally retarded[1] and more severely retarded children), (b) to make more accurate predictions about the future mental development of subjects, and (c) to derive suggestions for psychoeducational interventions from the assessment itself.

---

[1] The term *educable mentally retarded* is used in this chapter, and includes persons whose IQ may be higher than the cutoff score for mild mental retardation used by the American Association on Mental Retardation.

The learning test concept has been well received by the professional public (cf. Groffmann, 1983), especially in light of the lively and controversial debate on the limits and dangers of traditional intelligence testing that took place all over the world during the 1960s and 1970s. The learning test concept appears to be a paradigm of recent origin that is little elaborated, and operationalized in only a few procedures. Its underlying idea, however, reaches far back in the history of our discipline. This idea is to conduct a comprehensive and detailed assessment of intellectual functioning by determining not only people's present level of ability, but also, in a dynamic way, their potential for improvement with help.

The roots of this idea and of the learning test concept can be found in folk wisdom and in the writings of many philosophers of the past. We are well aware of the fact that conventional intelligence testing does not allow individuals to learn from the mistakes they made during testing for solving the next test item. Traditional tests do not provide the feedback that is usually given in everyday life, whereas learning tests proceed from this point.

Vygotsky and His Influence on the Development of Learning Tests

Lev Semenovich Vygotsky[2] (1896–1934) is regarded by many contemporary authors as the true creator of the learning test concept. He might have been able to go beyond just formulating that idea to translating it into procedures applicable in practice, had not an untimely death prevented him from doing so (cf. pedology decree, below). Vygotsky was well aware of the requirements to be met in practice and had gained practical experience himself, particularly by examining schizophrenic persons and handicapped children. (He is considered to be the founder of "defectology" in the Soviet Union.) Vygotsky (1964) believed that psychologists should do practical work just as physicians do.

It was not until after 1956 in the Soviet Union, and only after about 1964 on an international scale (when his book *Thought and Language* was first published in the German Democratic Republic) that Vygotsky was rediscovered as one of the most outstanding, versatile, and creative psychologists of our century. His insights in many fields of psychology (e.g., developmental psychology, psychology of language and thought, neuropsychology, pathopsychology, psychology of art) are regarded not only as the true starting point for the development of Soviet psychology and a Marxist-based psychology (Leontiev & Luria, 1964), but also as valuable

[2] In this chapter, the spelling of Russian names is consistent with their spelling in the U.S. literature (e.g., Vygotsky instead of Wygotski; Leontiev instead of Leontjev).

achievements in and as inspiration to "world psychology" (e.g., Wertsch, 1985a). The publication of Vygotsky's work and that of his best-known students, Luria and Leontiev, in many different languages, as well as the increasing worldwide recognition of Vygotsky's work, indicate that Vygotsky is acknowledged internationally as an important pioneer. Jean Piaget (1962), whose work has been criticized constructively by Vygotsky, regretted very much in 1962 that he had not been able to read Vygotsky's work earlier and had never met this ingenious scholar, who, in Piaget's view, had understood many things much better than he himself had been able to do during the 1920s.

The Cultural-Historical School and the Pedology Decree

Vygotsky is considered to be the founder of the cultural-historical school within Soviet psychology. Initially, his ideas were received enthusiastically by his Soviet colleagues, and he became the recognized and leading figure of Moscow's Psychological Institute. According to the current Soviet view, this school later became subject to biased and indiscriminate criticism. One of the criticisms raised against the cultural-historical school was that it was un-Marxist, because it neglected the role of class conflict, was not focused enough on Soviet society, and followed a sociological line of thinking. Furthermore, though only partly justified, the school was equated with the questionable theories and practices of the "pedologists."

In the 1920s and the early 1930s, pedology had established itself in the Soviet Union as a science of child development with the goal of studying child development from an interdisciplinary (i.e., pediatric, psychological, and educational) vantage point. The pedologists were a sort of school psychologist but without thorough education in psychology. In their practice, they adopted uncritically the Western (Binet type) intelligence tests for selection purposes in large-scale investigations. Because they also adopted the genetic interpretation of test results used in other countries, many children were wrongly labeled "unintelligent" and incapable of learning. These unjustified findings applied especially to children from illiterate families or Asian backgrounds. In those ethnic groups, very low educational levels had prevailed during the czarist era, and the young Soviet state was still struggling with the consequences thereof. Millions of children and adults are said to have undergone psychometric aptitude testing, and the large-scale use of intelligence tests led to protests by parents and educators (note the similar contemporary debate on the use of intelligence tests and the ensuing discrimination against minorities and certain lower socioeconomic groups in the United States, e.g., Cordes, 1986).

Both the policy on industrialization of the country (many rural residents had to be trained to be industrial workers) and Lenin's policy of providing equal access to educational resources for all ethnic groups would be endangered if a large proportion of the population were shown to have low intelligence and little capacity for learning. These factors contributed to the pedology decree of the Central Committee of the Communist party of the Soviet Union in 1936, in which pedology was strongly condemned. We now know that the results of intelligence tests were erroneously equated with a person's intellectual ability or learning potential. Moreover, the role of environmental factors in the development of intelligence was largely ignored. The pedology decree therefore cannot simply be denounced as an intervention by the Party and the State into science. Rather, it reflects the very unfavorable circumstances for objective scientific discussions (e.g., the personal cult around Stalin, cf. Petrovskij, 1964). The ban of pedology, the discontinuation of many psychological and pedological journals in which Vygotsky had played a leading role as contributor, and the polemics against Vygotsky and, after Vygotsky's death, Luria and Leontiev as leading representatives of the cultural-historical school, must be evaluated in light of these circumstances (see also Rissom, 1981).

Vygotsky's writings were not republished in the USSR until 1956. Since then, leading Soviet psychologists (particularly Leontiev & Luria, 1964) have been emphasizing the leading role Vygotsky played in the development of Soviet psychology.

The Experimental-Genetic Method

Internalization

Vygotsky was by no means an uncritical supporter of traditional intelligence tests, nor an advocate of a fatalistic endogenous or sociologistic position on child development. Contrary to criticisms, he and his students did not hold extreme positions on the nature-nurture issue. In fact, the most important insight of the cultural-historical school was that it understood the nature and the development of mental processes and qualities (including intelligence) as resulting from the internalization of the socially determined cultural heritage by the active subject (cf. also Leontiev, 1978), with biological factors providing the framework of the capacity for internalization. In his writings on the social origins of individual mental processes, Vygotsky explicitly referred to Karl Marx's famous sixth thesis on Feuerbach and defined the psychological nature of human beings as the "aggregate of internalized social relations" (Vygotsky, 1981, p. 164; Wertsch, 1985b). Similar to Mead (1934), Vygotsky perceived the danger of individualistic and reductionistic psychologizing in traditional psychology. He assumed a close relationship between internalization and the social origins of individual psychological processes. He regarded internalization as a process during which interpsychological forms of higher mental functions developed through adult-child interactions become intrapsychological as the child internalizes the socially formed external world (Galperin & Leontiev, 1972; Wertsch, 1985a).

Experimental-Genetic Method

Vygotsky called for going beyond the purely fact-finding approach of traditional psychology, in which a person's present status at a given point in time is ascertained and usually interpreted as determined by biological maturation or genetic endowment. Instead, psychology should investigate the *process* of internalization in a dynamic way. He demanded that the purely confirmatory experiments of general psychology and developmental psychology be complemented with the *experimental genetic method*. Later, this idea reappeared in Rubinstein's (1958) call for a more educational orientation of psychological experiments. This important Soviet psychologist was otherwise critical of Vygotsky's work. These ideas are a specification of the epistemological postulate, inherent in Marxist philosophy, that persons will gain the best knowledge of the phenomena and objects in the world by actively trying to change them.

Vygotsky's student Leontiev (1931) used the experimental-genetic method in his memory research. He described the method as follows:

> The task of genetic (developmental) studies in psychology consists not only of showing the development of specific forms of behavior, by merely stating that one form has been replaced by other, new forms of development, but also of studying the process of transition to new forms. . . . this task can be designed so as to be conducted under artificial, laboratory condition. (p. 181)

In the German literature this procedure is frequently labeled *Ausbildungsexperiment* (educational experiment). Thus, neither Vygotsky's writings nor those of his well-known students showed any signs of fundamental rejection of or disregard for experiments or tests conducted under laboratory conditions (cf. also Leontiev, 1968). Contrary to claims by contemporary critics of psychological experiments and tests, Vygotsky did not regard observation of human beings in natural learning and instructional situations alone as the royal road to assessment of intelligence. Despite his critical attitude toward conventional static intelligence tests, Vygotsky was well aware of the advantages of a standardized, experimental, and psychometric approach in psychodiagnostics (cf. Vygotsky, 1935, p. 5). At the same time, he believed that the experimental-genetic method, appropriately modified, should be applied to psychodiagnostics (Guthke, 1972, 1977). Vygotsky elaborated this notion by distinguishing two zones—"the zone of actual development" and the "zone of proximal (potential) development."

The Zones of Development

The zone of actual development is characterized by the developmental and test tasks that children are able to solve by themselves, without assistance by adults. Vygotsky, however, stressed the importance of examining not only mature but also developing functions, as illustrated in his frequently quoted example of the gardener who

. . . would be acting wrongly if he evaluated the state of his orchard only on the basis of the apple trees which have matured and carried fruit, instead of taking into consideration the maturing trees. Like the gardener, the psychologist must take into consideration not only the functions that have matured, but also those that are in the process of maturing. He must consider not only the actual level of development, but also the zone of proximal development (Vygotsky, 1964, p. 212).

Vygotsky's focus on predicting future growth continues to influence Soviet psychology and distinguishes American from Soviet research (Wertsch, 1985a). In a conversation with Urie Bronfenbrenner, Leontiev stated that "American researchers are constantly seeking to discover how the child came to be what he is; we in the USSR are striving to discover not how the child came to be what he is, but how he can become what he not yet is" (Bronfenbrenner, 1977, p. 528).

What were Vygotsky's ideas for assessing the zone of proximal development? Based on his developmental notions about the internalization of the world through child-adult interaction and the transformation of interpsychological functions into intrapsychological ones, Vygotsky suggested that the zone of proximal development is manifest in the child's interaction with adults or more capable peers. He illustrated this view with the example of two children who reach a mental age of 8 years in a conventional Binet-type test. Both children would obtain help in the form of examples, leading questions, or even demonstrations of the correct solution by the examiner. (We did not find more detailed description of the educational phase of testing in Vygotsky.) Whereas one child attained a mental age of 9 years after intervention, the other child obtained a mental age of 12 years.

Vygotsky defined the zone of proximal development as the discrepancy between actual level of development, determined by the number of independently solved tasks, and the level that the child reaches with the assistance of an adult. He predicted that

. . . in school, there will be more differences between these two children resulting from the discrepancy in their zones of proximal development than there will be similarities based on their present level of development. This discrepancy will manifest itself primarily in the dynamics of their intellectual development, and their progress and performance in school. The study shows that the zone of proximal development influences the dynamics of intellectual development and the level of achievement more directly than the present level of the development." (Vygotsky, 1964, p. 212).

Assessing the Zone of Proximal Development

To our knowledge, Vygotsky himself never subjected this hypothesis to empirical study, nor did he develop detailed instructions for the diagnostic procedure he proposed. Following the pedology decree, psychometric procedures in the assessment of mental abilities were completely abandoned in the Soviet Union. Instead, *dynamic diagnostic examinations*, which frequently lasted for several weeks, were conducted as an attempt to explore the zone of proximal development in quasi-instructional situations (see e.g., Menchinskaya, 1974). Soviet defectologists (e.g., Vlasova & Pevzner, 1971) who made explicit reference to Vygotsky, considered responsiveness to assistance in learing to be an essential criterion for distinguishing between educable retarded and more severly mentally retarded children. This procedure was introduced in the German Democratic Republic in 1952 to overcome traditional ("bourgeois") assessment methods for admission to special education. For 1 week, children are observed in natural school situations.

Limitations

The limits and problems of this method became apparent soon: it was uneconomical and subjective. Learning situations were not standardized and norms for evaluation of results were lacking (cf. the similar contemporary debate in the United States, in which Feuerstein's Learning Potential Assessment Device (Feuerstein, Rand, & Hoffman, 1979) was criticized as too subjective, e.g., Cordes, 1986). Since the mid-1960s, we therefore have consistently been trying to combine psychometric principles with the idea of assessing the zone of proximal development (see Guthke, 1972, 1977, for an overview of the methodology and empirical results).

Changing Attitudes Toward Assessment

In Eastern Europe, a new view of tests was generally adopted at that time. Advantages and disadvantages of tests were compared more objectively and new directions in assessment methodology were sought. Consequently, attempts were made in the Soviet Union and other socialist countries, especially Hungary, although largely independently (see e.g., Ivanova, 1973; Kalmykova, 1975; Klein, 1978). At about the same time, psychologists in the Western countries (see, e.g., Budoff, Meskin, & Harrison, 1971; Feuerstein, 1972; Flammer, 1974; Hurtig, 1962) started to suggest procedures similar to learning tests in order to overcome the limitations or the purely status-oriented conventional intelligence tests, especially for the differential diagnosis of children with learning problems. In some of these publications, explicit references were made to Vygotsky.

Other Theoretical Foundations of the Learning Test Concept

Theory of Activity

Besides Vygotsky's work, our own work on the learning test methodology was also influenced by the theory of activity of Soviet psychology

(Leontiev, 1978). This theory grew out of the elaboration and continuation as well as criticism of Vygotsky's work (see, e.g., Rubinstein, 1958). In the theory of activity, mental processes and characteristics are conceived of as products of human activity. Particular importance is attached to the concept of age- and situation-specific dominant activity (Leontiev, 1978). By requiring that diagnostic procedures include activities that predominate in a given age range and in the demands of everyday life, this concept is similar to the principle of ecological validity in Western psychology (Pawlik, 1977). The assessment of schoolchildren therefore should be focused on learning as their dominant activity and not merely on the results of their learning.

The same diagnostic implication applies to adult learning. Despite the increasing importance of assessing adults' ability for learning new skills in occupational training and continuing education programs, conventional vocational aptitude assessment continues to be based on purely fact-finding performance measures.

A detailed discussion of other theoretical frameworks supporting the learning test concept is beyond the scope of this chapter. We therefore provide only a brief overview of those frameworks that are based on a completely different theoretical context and other subdisciplines of psychology (see Guthke, 1972, 1977).

Psychology of Learning

From the viewpoint of the psychology of learning, Ferguson (1954) postulated that a person's mental abilities in a given area of learning can only be determined reliably after an overlearning phase, that is, by testing the limits (see also the testing the limits concept by Schmidt, 1971). As early as the 1930s, the German psychologist Kern (1930) had written a book on research on the effects of practice. In this book, he was very critical of psychometric aptitude tests and other achievement tests that were used at that time. Kern assumed that initial inhibitions (*Anfangshemmungen*) frequently distort the results of the first testing session and called for the assessment of the capacity for practice (*Übungsfähigkeit*) as an index of future success. For several weeks, tests were administered repeatedly. The results of the first testing session were correlated with those obtained in subsequent testing sessions. Kern found significant shifts in the rank order, primarily up to the fifth testing session, after which results remained relatively stable. He concluded that the one-time administration of a test procedure does not lead to a definite prognosis and may lead to false conclusions in many individual cases (p. 463).

Cognitive Psychology

The development of learning tests also was influenced by research on thinking and problem solving (e.g., Klix & Lander, 1967; Rubinstein,

1961). In this field of psychology, one examines how more complex problems are solved across several trials and how the subjects make use of feedback, additional information, and problem solving strategies provided by the experimenter or a computer (see also Dörner, 1984).

Educational Psychology

Research on psychological aspects of teaching and learning contribute to the theoretical foundations of learning tests (e.g., Flammer, 1975; Pawlik, 1982). A consistent finding, especially for complex learning processes, has been that the success of instructional programs cannot be predicted well by the conventional confirmatory and often domain-unspecific tests. This led to the call for collecting samples of subjects' learning of instructional materials during "miniature learning situations" and for using these samples as predictors of the future learning potential in these domains (cf. also Roth, 1957). Thorndike (1926) and representatives of earlier educational psychology in the United States had emphasized (as did Rubinstein, 1958) that human intelligence or ability manifested itself primarily in how fast people can learn new information and how far they can transfer the new information to new situations (see also recently Brown & Ferrara, 1985).

Personality Psychology

Finally, we should mention general theoretical premises in personality psychology (Pawlik, 1982). Heiss (1964), for instance, called for a dynamic process-based view of personality characteristics instead of the prevailing static view. He criticized traditional personality tests as dominated by static thinking. In one of his widely known Zubin axioms, Zubin (1950) postulated that one should determine both the present level of each trait based on a single sample and the variance by taking many test samples.

Concepts of Intelligence

In research on intelligence, it is becoming customary to distinguish three meanings of intelligence: intellectual endowment, intellectual status, and intellectual potential (see, e.g., Baltes & Willis, 1982; Guthke, 1980a). *Intellectual endowment* (similar in meaning to "intelligence reserve," Baltes & Willis, 1982) refers to the biological conditions necessary for the development of intelligence that are determined at birth by anatomical and physiological characteristics that are different for each person. So far, these conditions cannot be determined exactly at birth by either biological or psychological methods. At most, one can make assumptions about the nature of these conditions, by determining a person's *intellectual status* or performance with intelligence tests. The utility of such assessments is limited, however, because the samples of intelligent behavior obtained from these tests are determined by the test structure and the test situation and are not representative of the person's full range of intelligent behavior. In addition, the results of a single intelligence test do not permit drawing direct inferences about characteristics of a person's intellectual endowment nor about future learning potential, because the test result is always the result of a dialectic interaction between environmental and "internal" factors, from conception onward. In psychodiagnostic practice, intelligence test results should be considered in the context of the child's learning and developmental history, which must be determined as accurately as possible, but this is difficult to achieve. Valuable additional diagnostic information can be gained, however, from assessment of both a person's intellectual status and *intellectual potential* in a controlled learning situation.

Baltes' (1983) definition of the intellectual potential resembles closely an earlier one by Guthke (1972, 1980a). The intellectual potential or "competence" refers to the range of performance that can be activated under alternative conditions (e.g., those facilitating learning and thinking as in the learning test) and available as a sample of behavior.

The assessment of intellectual potential through learning tests will not permit fully reliable inferences about the nature of the intellectual endowment on the one hand and the future learning potential on the other hand, because subjects' intellectual status and their learning and performance in a specific testing situation result from previous learning processes. Conclusions about intellectual potential will, however, have a higher degree of probability. This is the most we can expect to accomplish, given the complexity of conditions influencing prognoses in psychology.

State of the Art, Problems, and Prospects

Types of Learning Tests

As stated above, learning tests assess information processing not only with respect to the problem situations and tasks with which the subjects are confronted, but also with respect to the processing of assistance offered in the form of simple feedback, prompts, or as long-term teaching programs that train test-taking strategies. We have distinguished several types of learning tests according to the length of the training phase and have developed procedures that are representative of each type (cf. Guthke, 1972, 1980b, 1982; see the reviews by Flammer & Schmidt, 1982; Kormann, 1982; Wiedl, 1984).

Long-Term Learning Test

The classical learning test is the long-term learning test (LTL) consisting of a pretest, a training (or pedagogical) phase, and a posttest. The learning test battery *Reasoning* (see Guthke, Jäger, & Schmidt, 1983) is an example of this type of learning test. The test is standardized for grades 6 through 10. It is designed to assess the core factor of intelligence, reasoning, in the three basic domains (i.e., verbal, numerical, figural) in which reasoning manifests itself (cf. Jäger, 1984). The test consists of the kinds of verbal analogies, and numerical and figural sequences that are commonly used in other intelligence tests (see Guthke, 1980a, for more detailed description). Following the pretest, the students are given "semiheuristic" programmed instruction manuals during the training phase. Training can be individualized or take place in groups. Students are taught metacognitive strategies for solving the test items. After practicing the strategies, the students are presented with the posttest, a parallel test. Testing and training sessions can extend across several days.

Scoring of Long-Term Learning Tests

The scoring of learning tests and the measurement of change in a methodologically satisfactory way is an issue that has not yet been fully resolved (cf. Guthke, 1980b; Petermann, 1978; Rost & Spada, 1978). The simple difference between pretest and posttest is not a useful learning tests result due to (a) the dependence of difference scores on the initial scores (cf. Wilder, 1931, in Guthke, 1977), (b) the regression phenomenon, and (c) the unreliability of the difference scores (in which the two error values of the basic scores combine). Various conversion formulas, such as residual gain (Klauer, 1975; also see Guthke, 1977), did not provide satisfactory results. We therefore decided to regard the result of the posttest as the true learning test result, because the learning gain is reflected in the posttest.

Subjects can be classified twice (even three times if the residual gain is determined as the difference score) on the basis of separate norm tables for pretest and posttest. The pretest norm values indicate the students' standing within their reference group (e.g., 6th grade) with respect to their intellectual status in the domain examined. The posttest norm value, on the other hand, characterizes the students' position relative to their potential for development (intellectual potential) after a controlled educational intervention.

Short-Term Learning Tests

In contrast to long-term learning tests, in short-term learning tests the training phase is built directly into the test procedure. Short-term learning tests (STL) require only one testing session during which systematic feedback and assistance are given. Two types of short-term learning tests can be distinguished: (a) tests providing merely systematic feedback, and (b) tests during which extensive assistance is given in addition to simple feedback.

The *Sequence of Sets Test* ("Mengenfolgentest"; Guthke, 1983) represents the first type of STL, i.e., only systematic feedback is provided. Designed to assess the learning skills prerequisite for mathematics, the test is administered to children before entering elementary school. Following the presentation of the first three members of a series of sets (symbolized by cards differing in number and depicting little bears), for example, 6–5–4, the children make guesses about how to continue the series, selecting choices from a set of response cards. The test consists of a total of nine items. After each trial the subject is given feedback as to whether the card selected is correct or wrong. Wrong cards are turned, whereas correct cards are put into the sequence. The Sequence of Sets Test is an intensive learning procedure not only because subjects have a chance to learn from and correct their mistakes as they work each item, but also because each successfully completed item helps them gain experience for solving further items.

The *Raven Short-Term Learning Test* (Frohriep, 1978), designed primarily for early identification of mentally retarded children, represents the second type of short-term learning test by including both simple feedback and extensive help. The kinds of help provided are largely influenced by Galperin's learning theory (Galperin & Leontiev, 1972). First the children are given the original Raven's Coloured Progressive Matrices (Raven, 1956). Children who fail are given the same item in a puzzle form as the first intervention. Many children of normal intelligence are able to arrive at the correct solution when the item is presented in a more concrete manner. Children who still arrive at incorrect solutions are allowed to continue trying on their own. The children's insight into their mistakes determines the further course of the training. Children showing themselves capable of learning from the mistakes made are allowed to go on trying (second and third kinds of help). Children showing no insight are offered a fourth intervention right away: they are shown a card with the correct solution drawn into the matrix. After the card is removed, the children are expected to fill the space correctly by themselves. If they fail again, they are given the fifth and last kind of help, with the experimenter placing the correct piece in the space. After the piece has been removed and placed among the other alternatives with the children's eyes closed, the children are asked to repeat the solution.

Testing the Limits as Learning Tests

In the widest sense of the word, simple test repetitions such as the testing-the-limits strategy (Schmidt, 1971) might also be regarded as learning tests. Studies in Hungary (cf. Tringer, 1980) and in the German Democratic Republic (cf. Roether, 1986; Wolfram, Neumann, & Wieczorek, 1986) have shown that mere repetition of concentration and memory tests can lead to considerable increases in the validity and differential diagnostic utility of these procedures. Brain-damaged patients and low-achieving neurotic patients with no brain damage were found to differ more markedly in the posttest than in the pretest. Posttest scores were more strongly related to relevant neurological symptoms. One such concentration learning test (cf. Winkler, 1988) for children and adults with norms for ages 6 to 90 is currently being prepared for publication by our research group.

Assessing Learning Processes with Static Tests

Finally, one might try to use conventional static intelligence tests (i.e., without repetition) for assessing learning processes. For example, the Raven's Coloured and Standard Progressive Matrices (Raven, 1956, 1958) also require learning processes, though to a lesser extent than the Raven Short-Term Learning Test described above (Frohriep, 1978). Fischer and Scheiblechner (Fischer, 1972, 1974) have attempted to identify learning parameters in conventional tests on the basis of probabilistic test theory. This procedure has proved problematic, however, and has not yet been used in practice.

Main Empirical Findings

As an extensive description of the numerous and varied empirical findings on the learning test methodology has been provided elsewhere (cf. Flammer & Schmidt, 1982; Groffmann, 1983; Guthke, 1977, 1980a, 1982; Kormann, 1982; Wiedl, 1984), we want to highlight just a few points. First, we were able to demonstrate increased performance on all intelligence tests after training. These results had repeatedly been found both in earlier studies (cf. Dembster, 1954; Klauer, 1975; Selz, 1935) and in more recent research (e.g., Baltes & Brim, 1984). Moreover, we were able to show that these training effects, as measured in the posttest or in learning-gain indices, cannot be predicted from the pretest scores with sufficiently high probability. That is, training effects provide additional diagnostic information. In some cases, major changes in the rank orders of subjects were observed between the first and the second testing. This observation is important, because, according to Meili (1965; cf. also Kern, 1930), diagnostically relevant changes in rank order after repeated administration of tests (with or without interpolated training) occur only in very unreliable tests but not in highly reliable ones.

Similar to other authors, our initial attempts at developing learning tests were based on well-established conventional, highly reliable static intelligence tests such as the Intelligence Structure Test (Amthauer, 1953, 1970) and Coloured Progressive Matrices (Raven, 1956), for which we developed a training phase. At first, we wanted to test, in the "traditional" manner, if the learning tests yielded higher validity indices than the corresponding static tests. Although we were aware of the questionable value of teacher ratings of intelligence and of grades as external criteria of intelligence or intellectual potential, we initially calculated correlations with those external criteria in order to make comparisons. We found again and again that the posttest correlations were usually (though often not significantly) higher than the pretest correlations.

In later studies, we focused more on theory-guided construct validation and longitudinal studies (see Guthke & Gitter, 1987; Guthke & Lehwald, 1984; Hamers & Ruijssenaars, 1984, 1987; Wiedl, 1984). We found that learning tests (a) generally have higher factor validity than the corresponding static tests (cf. the specification hypothesis by Fleishman & Hempel, 1954), (b) are less sensitive to environmental factors, (c) are more strongly related to the results of strictly controlled learning experiments, (d) discriminate less strongly than do traditional tests between children taught by different kinds of instructional methods, (e) are more highly correlated with tests of creativity, and (f) partially reduce the effects of nonintellectual components (e.g., irritability, neuroticism) on the test result (cf. Wiedl, 1984).

Longitudinal studies, covering a period of 7 years, of the Sequence of Sets Test and the Raven Short-Term Learning Test revealed that predictive validity coefficients for the entire group were not significantly higher than those of conventional static tests. In the group of children with below-average intelligence, however, learning tests were clearly superior to static tests in predictive validity. Learning tests seem to be particularly suited for differential assessment of children with learning disabilities, handicaps, and irregular learning histories (Feuerstein, 1972; Flammer & Schmidt, 1982; Guthke, 1985). Recently, attempts have been made, however, to introduce learning test procedures in the entrance examinations to special schools for gifted students (cf. Wieczerkowski & Wagner, 1985).

In describing the major research findings, we should not ignore the fact that the lack of applicable procedures that was criticized by Flammer and Schmidt as recently as 1982 has been overcome in part. Since then, five learning tests have been published in the German Democratic Republic: (a) Sequence of Sets Test (Guthke, 1983), (b) Preschool Learning Test (Roether, 1983), (c) the learning test battery Reasoning (Guthke, Jäger, & Schmidt, 1983), (d) Situation Learning Test for selecting special education students (Legler, 1983), and (e) Test of Speed and Recall Capacity of Adults (Roether, 1984). The tests are available for use in diagnostic practice. Learning tests have been published in other countries as well (e.g., Hegarty, 1979; see Lidz, 1987, and other chapters in this volume).

Problems and Trends

The validity of learning tests, especially as compared to conventional intelligence tests, continues to be an issue that needs to be resolved. Learning tests are unlikely to predict the intellectual development of children better than conventional intelligence tests if the children continue to live in unfavorable home and/or school environments after the assessment. Wiedl and Herrig (1978) found that the predictive validity of learning tests was clearly superior for individualized instruction only. One might argue that the main purpose of learning tests should not be to predict school achievement or to correlate their results with teacher ratings of intelligence. Rather, they are designed to uncover children's learning potential, learning strategies, and sources of errors, in order to design classroom instruction or to provide special support for students (see also Carlson & Wiedl [Chapter 6] and Tzuriel & Feuerstein [Chapter 7] in this volume).

In this context, three central questions have to be raised: (a) Most learning test items have been derived from conventional intelligence test items and assumptions of classical test theory, without detailed, theory-based task analysis. *Does current task construction satisfy the requirements for process-oriented tests that focus on enhancing thinking and learning ability*? (b) Similar to conventional intelligence tests, many learning tests have been constructed to examine general, largely content- and domain-unspecific thinking ability. *How can we derive specific suggestions for enhancing intellectual ability from test performance if learning tests are not domain and subject specific*? (c) Usually, the training phase is relatively similar for all subjects to assure standardization. *Is the training phase sufficiently individualized to uncover individual process characteristics of learning*? We will discuss these three question in more depth in the next paragraphs.

Test Construction and Task Analysis

In our view, the future of the intelligence assessment lies in combining test construction and task analysis according to basic research principles with the learning test concept (for an extensive discussion see Berg & Schaarschmidt, 1984; Brown & French, 1978; Guthke, 1986; Klix, 1983). This way, both the procedural weaknesses of "conventional" learning tests and the conceptual shortcomings of conventional static intelligence tests will be overcome. Over the past few years, we have tried to develop *diagnostic programs* as a new kind of learning test that satisfies these requirements (see Guthke & Wohlrab, 1982). Diagnostic programs must

(a) provide an exact description of the test's demand structure, (b) be structured hierarchically, and (c) provide continuous feedback during the test.

Exact Description

The objective demand structure of the whole test and the test items must be exactly describable, as is required for content validation (Klauer, 1978). For this purpose, we have developed a variety of tasks that satisfy this requirement. We have used tasks drawn from propositional logic, because task complexity can be well described in terms of the required logical operations and their combination (cf. Wohlrab's Propositional Logic Program, described in Guthke, 1986). We also used concept formation tasks whose demand structure has been satisfactorily established by basic research on concept formation (cf. Diagnostic Programs for Assessment of Mental Retardation, Guthke & Löffler, 1983; Michalski, 1988). A program for assessing the ability of foreign students to learn foreign languages (cf. Guthke, Harnisch, & Caruso, 1986) that requires subjects to learn an artificial language also lends itself to an exact description of the complexity of the various items used. In our most recent work (cf. Guthke, Räder, Caruso, & Schmidt, 1988), a modified version of Buffart and Leeuwenberg's (1983) structural information theory has been used to determine objectively the complexity of sequence of figures test items. This theory allows not only for description of the objective demand structure of conventional sequence of figures test items, but also—much more importantly—for a theory-guided construction of items and multiple choice distractors, and error analyses (including even prediction of the most frequently occurring errors).

Hierarchical Structure

Diagnostic programs are structured hierarchically. The essential point about their structure is not the subjective index of difficulty common in classical test theory, but the degree of complexity obtained from logical/psychological analysis. As a rule, the initial items serve for testing and, if needed, teaching of elementary operations, which occur in increasingly complex combinations in later items.

Continuous Feedback

Like a programmed instruction manual, diagnostic programs provide continuous feedback and assistance. As is the case with the mastery learning strategy (Bloom, 1968), the next item cannot be started until subjects have solved all the preceding ones by themselves, or have reached the correct solution either through a system of standardized interventions or, if necessary, through demonstration by the experimenter or the computer.

Thus, the distinction commonly made in the "conventional" learning test between a test phase and a training phase becomes meaningless. Each item has both a test and a training function. The number and kinds of assistance given and the way it is provided, and the total amount of time taken by the subject during the test become the crucial parameters for analysis. We are currently trying to combine the learning test concept with the tailored testing or adaptive testing principle (e.g., Weiss, 1985). Contrary to traditional adaptive testing, our focus is not on the statistical indices of difficulty for a reference sample, but on errors and error sources occurring in the individual case. Although we attempt to individualize both the testing and the training, subjects always have to pass prop items. Included for the standardization of the procedure, these items serve to check previous learning and are reached directly, when the subjects do not require prompts or easier items. Furthermore, the path to be followed and the help to be given when certain types of errors are made are clearly specified in the program. There are many avenues, however, to the goal, i.e., the last prop item. Because such a test procedure is rather difficult to administer and score, we use microcomputers to administer and score the diagnostic programs.

Domain-Specificity of Learning Tests

The question of whether learning tests are sufficiently domain-specific to enable prediction of and suggestions for the development of intellectual ability touches on the role of both general (heuristic) and specific competences. This issue has been the subject of an ongoing, lively, and controversial debate not only among diagnosticians but also in research on problem solving, in instructional psychology (e.g., Neber, 1987), and in general and development psychology (e.g., Lishout, 1987). The earlier views which overemphasized either general or domain-specific knowledge, strategies, or competencies, now are being replaced by a more synthetic position that emphasizes the interaction of both general and specific abilities in the solving of test items and problems in work and school settings. Leontiev (1968), an advocate of the activity-oriented approach to assessment, also stressed the importance of assessing general intellectual abilities besides knowledge of and abilities in special school subjects.

Gurewitsch (1981) suggested that domain-specific ability and proficiency tests measure the influence of controlled instruction, whereas tests of general ability (such as intelligence tests) reflect primarily the effect of less-controlled everyday experience. Furthermore, Schladebach (1983) found that even domain-unspecific tests (in this case analogies) predicted performance in a particular school subject (biology) as reliably as did test items constructed for that subject (ones that involved biological terms). As a rule, however, domain-specific procedures will predict learning success in a given area or subject better than domain-unspecific tests (cf. Winkler, 1978).

Need for Domain-Specific Learning Tests

In view of current calls for learning tests that permit specific suggestions on how teachers might support and enhance student ability (e.g., Wiedl, 1984), special consideration must be given to domain-specific learning tests. During the last few years, increasing efforts have been made to develop support- or structure-oriented assessment procedures (Kormann, 1979; Kornmann, 1983; Kornmann, Meister, & Schlee, 1983; Matthes, 1978, 1983; Müller, 1978; Probst, 1982; Rüdiger, 1978; Schnotz, 1979). These authors attempt to define the structure of the domain to be assessed (e.g., the concept of number, generic concept formation, or reading process) through didactic means, the given specialty area (e.g., mathematics), and psychology (primarily developmental psychology). The structural definition then guides test presentation and interpretation in terms of specific learning processes. Theory-guided error analysis (cf. Küffner, 1981) is gaining importance for this approach. It is likely that test items, error analyses, and the kinds of assistance provided will be derived from neuropsychological knowledge (cf. Ayres, 1979; Jantzen, 1983; Luria, 1970; Rösler, Ott, & Richter-Heinrich, 1980) in the future (for preliminary work, cf. Graichen, 1975). Proponents of theory-oriented and interactive assessment frequently reject psychometric approaches (e.g., Probst, 1982). This course of action is problematic because, without statistical standardization, tests users have no comparison standards.

Test Practice

Since 1952, admission to special education in the former German Democratic Republic has been determined during a week-long admission procedure. Initially, admission was decided based on qualitative and observational data. Due to lack of quantitative standards, this practice was considered unsatisfactory and replaced with special test lessons in German, mathematics, and geography (Buss, Scholz-Ehrsam, & Winter, 1982). These lessons represent domain-specific learning tests (cf. Buss & Scholz-Ehrsam, 1973; Situational Learning Test by Legler, 1983), that incorporate statistical reference norms. During the last few years, our own research team also has developed a number of domain-specific learning tests. Nonetheless, such an approach raises several *critical issues.*

Need for a Large Number of Domain-Specific Tests. Even for a single school subject, such as German or mathematics, a whole range of subject-specific tests ought to be devised because the competence for solving algebra problems can be vastly different from that for solving geometrical problems. Who is going to construct the great number of procedures that would be required; who will ultimately apply them? The teachers' primary concern is teaching, not diagnosing. Being unfamiliar with many school subjects, psychologists might not be sufficiently trained for scoring and interpretation of these tests. A possible solution might be the concurrent teaching and assessment of the subject's current state of learning on the basis of computer-assisted intelligent tutorial systems (Mandl & Fischer, 1985). The learning test principle is incorporated in these systems because a diagnosis is made as subjects learn, and because of the use of feedback, prompts, and individualized information. Such technological advances may not be very instrumental, however, in resolving the second problem.

Emotional Blocking. Many low-achieving children feel frustrated, and are emotionally blocked in their thinking, simply because they are exposed to material that so far has always been associated with experiences of failure. But if they are given test items apparently unrelated to classroom tasks, such as Raven-type items, they often are very motivated to achieve and are much less inhibited. Without being limited by the specific gaps in their knowledge and by emotional blocking, they are likely to approach the test unprejudiced and to reveal their intellectual potential which rarely shows in their classwork.

Prediction of External Criteria. External criteria of a more general nature such as overall success in school usually can be predicted better by more general intelligence or learning tests than by highly domain-specific procedures. We think that for all the reasons mentioned, importance should be attached in the future to the construction of both general intelligence tests (i.e., tests that are not specific to school subjects or areas of learning) and highly domain- and curriculum-specific procedures. The choice of one procedure over the other should be guided by the referral question, be it the prediction of a child's general success in school, or a professional diagnostic consultation with teachers. As a rule, however, a combination of both may be indicated.

Is Training Sufficiently Individualized?

As mentioned above, diagnostic programs provide a higher degree of individualization than the "conventional" learning tests. Still, many other questions concerning the individualization of the training phase can be raised: (a) Is not individual learning success a function of the match between personality traits and characteristics of the methods used? In view of the large variety of individual "learning styles," is it not better to relinquish "external control" of the learning process (except for providing feedback information) in learning tests altogether? (b) Consistent with the theory of activity (Leontiev, 1978), in learning tests, is it not important to describe, measure, and train not only task-specific executive actions or operations but also an individual's orientational activity as defined by Galperin (cf. Heijden, 1986)? In this context, the role of metacognition, awareness, and learning strategy (cf. Flavell, 1979) during the learning test process becomes relevant. (c) Are we taking motivational and emotional problems involved in learning and their effects on the result of the learning test sufficiently into account during the training phase of learning tests? Although some empirical and theoretical work on these questions has been done (cf. Guthke & Lehwald, 1984; Wiedl, 1984), most of them remain unanswered. It is interesting and important to note, for example, that quest for knowledge influences the posttest result more strongly (i.e., the learning test), whereas irritability, intolerance of frustration, and anxiety affect the pretest (i.e., the conventional intelligence test) more strongly.

Concerning the degree of individualization of learning tests, diagnosticians are caught between a rock and a hard place. If the training phase is highly individualized, the administration and scoring of the test become more subjective, and the standardization and psychometric analysis of the test process become less meaningful. When confronted with a choice between two equally important requirements for diagnostic procedures, individualization and standardization, diagnosticians appear to have two options: (a) try to balance the two requirements, or (b) make a decision based on the primary diagnostic objective.

Expansion of the Use of Learning Tests

During the past few years, research on the learning test concept has gone beyond issues of intelligence and school settings. Members of our research group (e.g., Enger, 1987; Winkler, 1978, 1988) and members of other, clinically oriented research teams in Germany, who explicity based their work on the learning test concept (cf. Löwe & Roether, 1978; Roether, 1986; Wolfram, Neumann, & Wieczorek, 1986), have used procedures similar to learning tests in studies of intelligence, memory, and speed in adults in order to make inferences about vocational aptitude (cf. the trainability concept by Robertson & Mindel, 1980) and the performance of psychosomatic patients (especially cardiac infarction patients, cf. Günther & Günther, 1980), and to differentiate between low-achieving neurotic and brain-damaged patients. Baltes and associates (e.g., Baltes & Brim, 1984) have used learning test procedures as tools for gerontological research on the plasticity, resources, and the development of intelligence among healthy older persons. In addition, the learning test concept has been used in characterological research. Zimmermann (1987) developed a procedure for assessing aspects of people's social learning ability with an experimental two-person matrix games. Göth and Guthke (1985) successfully used learning test procedures specific to psychotherapy to predict therapy outcomes in hospital patients undergoing group therapy. Ettrich and Guthke (1988) found that simple repetition of personality inventories provided better diagnostic information on clinical issues. Learning tests are also being used in psychological assessment of driving ability (e.g., in aptitude tests of electric engine drivers).

Concluding Remarks

The range of areas in which the learning test concept could be and has already been used, could still be expanded. Further discussion of the various uses of the learning test concept will, however, exceed the scope of this chapter. We have tried to go beyond the original conception of learning tests as an alternative type of intelligence and performance test, and to adopt a larger theoretical framework in which the learning test concept is a concrete alternative used for psychological diagnostics of intraindividual variability (cf. Guthke, 1981). Instead of being regarded solely as a measuring error (that lowers test reliability) or as a fluctuation in a trait, intraindividual variation in different test situations becomes a valuable source of additional diagnostic information (cf. Pawlik, 1976).

Dynamic assessment is a possible avenue to this source, and learning tests represent one type of dynamic approach that holds much promise for the future. In the United States, Brown and French (1978) believe that the assessment of intelligence and achievement in the next millennium will be determined by a combination of learning tests and task analysis derived from basic research in psychology. In his much acclaimed book *Beyond IQ*, Sternberg (1985) observed—particularly with reference to Feuerstein's Learning Potential Assessment Device (Feuerstein, Rand, & Hoffman, 1979)—that the learning test concept represents one of a few highly innovative new directions in the assessment of intelligence. In the Soviet Union, psychologists regarded the combination of the learning test concept with an activity- and theory-based diagnostic approach as a chief priority for future intelligence assessment at the fourth nationwide Congress of Soviet Psychologists in Moscow (Awerin, 1984; Talysina, 1983). There appears to be a growing consensus on the goals of future research that is cutting across national and school boundaries. We have, however, only taken the first steps toward this goal, and may make detours or follow different paths while pursuing it. Our future attempts at developing dynamic approaches to assessment will profit if we look back and evaluate what we have achieved in the past. This chapter was prepared with that goal in mind.

References

Amthauer, R. (1953, 1970). *Intelligenzstrukturtest* [Intelligence structure test]. Göttingen: Hogrefe.

Awerin, A. V. (1984). Probleme der Psychologie in der UdSSR: Überblick über den VI. Allunionskongress der Gesellschaft für Psychologie der UdSSR [Problems of psychology in the USSR: Overview of the VIth All-Union Congress of the Society for Psychology of the USSR]. *Psychologie Information*, *2*, 2–12.

Ayres, A. J. (1979). *Lernstörungen. Sensorisch-integrative Dysfunktionen* [Learning disorders: Sensory-integrative dysfunctions]. Berlin: Springer.

Baltes, P. B. (1983). Zur Psychologie der Intelligenz im Alter—Nur Abbau oder Entwicklung? [The psychology of intelligence in old age: Deterioration only or development?]. In Max-Planck-Gesellschaft (Ed.), *Jahrbuch 1983* (pp. 53–72). Göttingen: Generalverwaltung der Max-Planck-Gesellschaft.

Baltes, P. B., & Brim, O. G. (Eds.). (1984). *Life span development and behavior* (Vol. 6). New York: Academic Press.

Baltes, P. B., & Willis, S. L. (1982). Plasticity of intellectual functioning in old age: Penn State's Adult Development and Enrichment Project (ADEPT). In F. I. M. Craik & S. E. Trehnts (Eds.), *Aging and cognitive processes* (pp. 353–389). New York: Plenum.

Berg, M., & Schaarschmidt, U. (1984). Überlegungen zu neuen Wegen in der Intelligenzdiagnostik [Reflections on new ways for intelligence assessment]. *Wissenschaftliche Zeitschrift der Humboldt-Universität zu Berlin. Mathematisch-naturwissenschaftliche Reihe*, *6*, 565–573.

Bloom. B. S. (1968). Learning for mastery. In *Evaluation Communications* (Vol. 1 [2]). Los Angeles, CA: Center for the Study and Evalution of Instructional Programs.

Bronfenbrenner, U. (1977). Toward an experimental ecology of human development. *American Psychologist*, *32*, 513–551.

Brown, A. L., & Ferrara, R. (1985). Diagnosing zones of proximal development. In J. V. Wertsch (Ed.), *Culture, communication, and cognition: Vygotskian perspectives* (pp. 273–305). New York: Cambridge University Press.

Brown, A. L., & French, L. A. (1978). The zone of potential development: Implications for intelligence testing in the year 2000. *Intelligence*, *3*, 255–277.

Budoff, M., Meskin, J., & Harrison, R. H. (1971). Educational test of the learning potential hypothesis. *American Journal of Mental Deficiency*, *76*, 159–169.

Buffart, H., & Leeuwenberg, E. (1983). Structural information theory. In H. E. Geissler, H. Leeuwenberg, & V. Sarris (Eds.), *Modern issues in perception* (pp. 48–72). Berlin: Deutscher Verlag der Wissenschaften.

Buss, A., & Scholz-Ehrsam, E. (1973). Unterrichtslektionen im Hilfsschuleaufnahmeverfahren [Lessons used in the admissions procedure for special education]. *Sonderschule*, *18*.

Buss, A., Scholz-Ehrsam, E., & Winter, K. (Eds.). (1982). *Handreichung (2) für den Hilfsschulpädagogen zur Auswahl von Kindern ohne vorherigen Schulbesuch für die Hilfsschule (Diskussionsmaterial)* [Guidelines (2) for special educators for the selection of children without prior school attendance for special education (Materials for discussion)]. Berlin: Ministerium für Volksbildung.

Cordes, C. (1986). The debate over how to help minority students. *APA Monitor*, *17*, 4.

Dembster, J. J. B. (1954). Symposium on the effects of coaching and practice in intelligence tests. Southampton investigation and procedure. *British Journal of Educational Psychology*, *24*, 1–4.

Dörner, O. (1984). Denken, Problemlösen und Intelligenz [Thinking, problem solving, and intelligence]. *Psychologische Rundschau*, *35*, 1–9.

Enger, C. (1987). *Zum Einsatz von Lerntests bei der Differentialdiagnostik hirnorganisch und neurotisch bedingter Leistungsbeeinträchtigung im Erwachsenenalter* [The use of learning tests for the differential diagnosis of performance deficits in brain damaged and neurotic adults]. Unpublished research report, Section Psychology, Karl Marx University, Leipzig.

Ettrich, K. U., & Guthke, J. (1988). Therapieorientierte Psychodiagnostik und Psychodiagnostik intraindividueller Variabilität [Therapy oriented psychodiagnostics and psychodiagnostics of intraindividual variability]. In H. Schröder & J. Guthke (Eds.), *Fortschritte der klinischen Persönlichkeitspsychologie und klinischen Psychodiagnostik. Psychotherapie und Grenzgebiete* (Vol. 9, pp. 95–105). Leipzig: Barth.

Ferguson, G. A. (1954). On learning and human ability. *Canadian Journal of Psychology*, *8*, 95–113.

Feuerstein, R. (1972). Cognitive assessment of the socioculturally deprived child and adolescent. In L. J. Cronbach & P. J. Drenth (Eds.), *Mental tests and cultural adaptation* (pp. 265–275). The Hague, The Netherlands: Mouton.

Feuerstein, R., Rand, Y., & Hoffman, M. B. (1979). *The dynamic assessment of retarded performers*. Baltimore: University Park Press.

Fischer, G. H. (1972). A step toward a dynamic test theory. *Research Bulletin, Psychologisches Institut der Universität Wien*, *10*.

Fischer, G. H. (1974). *Einführung in die Theorie psychologischer Tests* [Introduction to psychological test theory]. Bern-Stuttgart: Huber.

Flammer, A. (1974). Längsschnittuntersuchung mit Lern- und Transfertests [A longitudinal study with learning tests and transfer tests]. *Schweizerische Zeitschrift für Psychologie*, *33*, 14–32.

Flammer, A. (1975). *Individuelle Unterschiede in Lernen* [Individual differences in learning]. Weinheim/Basel: Beltz.

Flammer, A., & Schmidt, H. (1982). Lerntests: Konzept, Realisierung, Bewährung [Learning tests: concept, realization, and utility]. *Schweizerische Zeitschrift für Psychologie und ihre Anwendung*, *41*, 114–138.

Flavell, J. (1979). Metacognition and cognitive developmental inquiry. *American Psychologist*, *34*(10), 906–911.

Fleishman, E. A., & Hempel, W. E. (1954). Changes in factor structure of a complex psychomotor test as a function of practice. *Psychometrica*, *19*(3), 239–251.

Frohriep, K. (1978). Einige Ergebnisse zur prognostischen Validität eines neu entwickelten Kurzzeitlerntests für die Differentialdiagnostik entwicklungsrückständiger Vorschulkinder im Vergleich mit konventionellen Verfahren und Lanzeitlerntests [Some results on the prognostic validity of a newly developed short-term learning test for differential diagnostics of developmentally delayed children as compared to conventional procedures and long-term learning tests]. In G. Clauss, J. Guthke, & G. Lehwald (Eds.), *Psychologie und Psychodiagnostik lernaktiven Verhaltens. Tagungsbericht* (pp. 67–72). Berlin: Gesellschaft für Psychologie der DDR.

Galperin, A. N., & Leontiev, A. N. (Eds.). (1972). *Probleme der Lerntheorie* [Problems of learning theory]. Berlin: Volk und Wissen.
Göth, N., & Guthke, J. (1985). Therapiebezogene Psychodiagnostik-neue methodische Ansätze [Therapy-oriented psychodiagnostics: New methodological approaches]. *Psychologie für die Praxis*, *1*, 66–71.
Graichen, J. (1975). Kann man legastenische und dyskalkulatorische Schulschwierigkeiten voraussagen? [Can school difficulties due to dyslexia and dyscalculia be predicted?]. *Praxis der Kinderpsychologie und Kinderpsychiatrie*, *24*, 52–57.
Groffmann, K. J. (1983). Die Entwicklung der Intelligenzmessung [The development of measurement of intelligence]. In K. J. Groffmann & L. Michel (Eds.), *Enzyklopädie der Psychologie, Vol. 2: Intelligenz- und Leistungsdiagnostik* (pp. 2–74). Göttingen: Hogrefe.
Günther, C., & Günther, R. (1980). *Gesundheit und intellektuelle Lernfähigkeit* [Health and intellectual learning potential]. Unpublished doctoral dissertation, Wilhelm-Pieck Universität, Rostock.
Gurewitsch, K. M. (Ed.). (1981). *Psychologische Diagnostik* [Psychological diagnostics]. Moscow: Pädagogika (Russian).
Guthke, J. (1972, 1977). *Zur Diagnostik der intellektuellen Lernfähigkeit* [Assessment of intellectual learning potential]. Berlin: Deutscher Verlag der Wissenschaften; Stuttgart: Klett.
Guthke, J. (1980a). Ist Intelligenz meßbar? [Can intelligence be measured?]. Berlin: Deutscher Verlag der Wissenschaften.
Guthke, J. (1980b). *Veränderungsmessung und Psychodiagnostik intraindividueller Variabilität (Review)* [Assessment of change and psychological diagnostics of intraindividual variability: A review]. Paper presented at the XXII International Congress of Psychology, Leipzig.
Guthke, J. (1981). Zur Psychodiagnostik intraindividueller Variabilität [Psychological assessment of intraindividual variability]. In M. Vorwerg (Ed.), *Zur psychologischen Persönlichkeitsforschung 4* (pp. 9–33). Berlin: Deutscher Verlag der Wissenschaften.
Guthke, J. (1982). The learning test concept—an alternative to the traditional static intelligence test. *The German Journal of Psychology*, *6*(4), 306–324.
Guthke, J. (1983). *Mengenfolgentest* [Sequence of Sets Test]. Berlin: Psychodiagnostisches Zentrum der Humboldt Universität zu Berlin.
Guthke, J. (1985). Ein neuer Ansatz für die rehabilitations psychologisch orientierte Psychodiagnostik: das Lerntestkonzept als Alternative zum herkömmlichen Intelligenztest [A new approach to psychological diagnostics for rehabilitation: The learning test concept as an alternative to traditional intelligence tests]. In K. H. Wiedl (Ed.), *Rehabilitationspsychologie* (pp. 177–194). Mainz: Kohlhhammer.
Guthke, J. (1986). Grundlagenpsychologische Intelligenzforschung und Lerntestkonzept [Basis research on intelligence and the learning test concept]. In U. Schaarschmidt, M. Berg, & K. D., Hänsgen (Eds.), *Diagnostik geistiger Leistungen. Proceedings of a conference* (pp. 53–67). Berlin: Psychodiagnostisches Zentrum der Humboldt-Universität zu Berlin.
Guthke, J., & Gitter, K (1987). Zur Vorhersagbarkeit der Schulleistungsentwicklung in der Unter- und Mittelstufe auf Grund von Status und Lerntest-

resultaten in der Vorschulzeit [Predictability of the development of school achievement in elementary and middle school levels based on preschool learning test results]. In: Rektor der Universität (Ed.), *Risikobewältigung in der lebenslangen psychischen Entwicklung* (pp. 71–74). *Proceedings of the Third Baltic Sea Symposium on Clinical Psychology*. Rostock: Wilhelm-Pieck Universität.

Guthke, J., Harnisch, A., & Caruso, M. (1986). The diagnostic program of syntactical rule and vocabulary acquisition: A contribution to the psychodiagnosis of foreign language learning ability. In F. Klix & H. Hagendorf (Eds.), *Human memory and cognitive capabilities* (pp. 903–911). North Holland: Elsevier Science Publishers.

Guthke, J., Jäger, C., & Schmidt, J. (1983). *Lerntestbatterie "Schlußfolgerndes Denken" (LTS)* [Learning test battery "Reasoning"]. Berlin: Psychodiagnostisches Zentrum der Humboldt-Universität zu Berlin.

Guthke, J., & Lehwald, G. (1984). On component analysis of the intellectual learning ability in learning tests. *Zeitschrift für Psychologie*, *192*, 3–17.

Guthke, J., & Löffler, M. (1983). A diagnostic program (learning test) for the differential assessment of school failure in 1st grade pupils. In H.-D. Rössler, J. P. Das, & I. Wald (Eds.), *Mental and language retardation* (pp. 41–50). Berlin: Deutscher Verlag der Wissenschaften.

Guthke, J., Räder E., Caruso, M., & Schmidt, K. D. (1988). Entwicklung eines kontentvaliden computergestützten adaptiven Lerntests mit Hilfe der strukturellen Informationstheorie [Development of a content valid, computer-supported, adaptive learning test based on structural information theory]. *Diagnostica*.

Guthke, J., & Wohlrab, U. (Eds.). (1982). *Neuere Ergebnisse der Lerntestforschung: Diagnostische Programme als Lerntestvariante* [Recent results of learning test research: Diagnostic programs as alternatives to learning tests]. Unpublished research report. Leipzig: Karl-Marx-Universität, Sektion Psychologie.

Hamers, J. H. M., & Ruijssenaars, A. J. (1984). Leergeschiktheid en Leertest [Learning ability and learning test]. Unpublished doctoral dissertation, Nijmegen.

Hamers, J. H. M., & Ruijssenaars, A. J. (1987). *Learning potential tests and the prediction of school achievement.* Paper presented at the International Conference on Learning Disabilities, Amsterdam.

Haywood, H. C., Meyers, C. E., & Switzky, H. N. (1982). Mental retardation. *Annual Review of Psychology*, *33*, 309–342.

Hegarty, S. (1979). *Manual for the test of children's learning ability*. Windsor: NFER Publishing Company.

Heijden, M. K. v. d. (1986). *Assessment of learning strategies from an activity. Psychological Point*. Paper presented at the First International Conference on Activity Theory. Berlin (West).

Heiss, R., (1964). Über den Begriff des Verhaltens und das Modell der Persönlichkeit [On the concept of behavior and the model of personality]. In K. Gottschaldt, P. Lersch, F. Sander, & H. Thomae (Eds.), *Handbuch der Psychologie* (Vol. 6, pp. 960–974). Göttingen: Hogrefe.

Hurtig, M. (1962). *Intellectual performance in relation to "former learning" and "real" and "pseudo-mentally" deficient children*. Proceedings of the London Conference on the Scientific Study of Mental Deficiency, Dagosham.

Ivanova, A. (1973). *Das Lernexperiment als Methode der Diagnostik der geistigen Entwicklung der Kinder* [The learning experiment as diagnostic method for the mental development of children]. Moscow: Pedagogika (Russian).

Jäger, A. O. (1984). Intelligenzstrukturforschung: Konkurrierende Modelle, neue Entwicklungen, Perspektiven [Intelligence structure research: Competitive models, new developments, perspectives]. *Psychologische Rundschau, 35*(1), 21–35.

Jantzen, W. (1983). Diagnostik im Interesse des Betroffenen oder Kontrolle von oben? [Diagnostics in the interest of the person or control from above?]. *Forum Kritische Psychologie, 1*, 10–35.

Kalmykova, S. J. (Ed.). (1975). *Probleme der Diagnostik der geistigen Entwicklung der Schüler* [Problems of diagnostics of the mental development of pupils]. Moscow: Pedagogika (Russian).

Kern, B. (1930). *Wirkungsformen der Übung* [Effects of training]. Münster: Helios.

Klauer, K. J. (1975). *Intelligenztraining im Kindesalter* [Training intelligence during childhood]. Weinheim: Beltz.

Klauer, K. J. (1978). Kontentvalidität [Content validity]. In K. J. Klauer (Ed.), *Handbuch der pädagogischen Diagnostik* (Vol. 1, pp. 225–255). Düsseldorf: Schwann.

Klein, S. (1978). *Intelligence and learning potential theory and practice.* Paper presented at the XIXth International Conference on Applied Psychology, Munich.

Klix, F. (1983). Begabtenforschung—ein neuer Weg in der kognitiven Intelligenzdiagnostik [Research on gifted persons: A new approach in cognitive diagnostics of intelligence]. *Zeitschrift für Psychologie, 191*, 360–387.

Klix, F., & Lander, H. J. (1967). Die Strukturanalyse von Denkprozessen als Mittel der Intelligenzdiagnostik [The structural analysis of thought processes as tool of intelligence diagnostics]. In F. Klix, W. Gutjahr, & J. Mehl (Eds.), *Intelligenzdiagnostik* (pp. 245–279). Berlin: Deutscher Verlag der Wissenschaften.

Kormann, A. (1979). Lerntests—Versuch einer kritischen Bestandsaufnahme [Learning tests: An attempt of critical evaluation]. In L. H. Eckensberger (Ed.), *Bericht über den 31. Kongreß der Deutschen Gesellschaft für Psychologie in Mannheim 1978* (Vol. 2, pp. 85–95). Göttingen: Hogrefe.

Kormann, A. (1982). Möglichkeiten von Lerntest für Diagnose und Optimierung von Lernprozessen [Applicability of learning tests for diagnostics and optimization of learning processes]. In K. H. Ingenkamp, R. Horn, & R. S. Jäger (Eds.), *Tests und Trends 1982. Jahrbuch der pädagogischen Diagnostik* (pp. 97–118). Weinheim/Basel: Beltz.

Kornmann, R. (1983). Variation von Testbedingungen als förderungsdiagnostischer Ansatz [Variation of testing conditions as an approach to development-enhancing diagnostics]. In H. P. Trolldenier & B. Meissner (Eds.), *Texte zur Schulpsychologie und Bildungsberatung*, (Vol. 4, pp. 254–261). Braunschweig: Pedersen.

Kornmann, R., Meister, H., & Schlee, J. (Eds.). (1983). *Förderungsdiagnostik. Konzept und Realisierungsmöglichkeiten* [Development-enhancing diagnostics: Concept and possibilities]. Heidelberg: Schindele.

Küffner, H. (1981). *Fehlorientierte Tests: Konzept und Bewährungskontrolle* [Misoriented tests: Concept and control of verification]. Weinheim: Beltz.

Legler, R. (1983). *Situations-Lerntest (SLT)* [Situation learning test (SLT)]. Berlin: Psychodiagnostisches Zentrum der Humboldt-Universität zu Berlin.

Leontiev, A. N. (1931). *Entwicklung des Gedächtnisses* [Development of memory]. Moscow: Krupskaya Academia of Communist Education Press (Russian).

Leontiev, A. N. (1968). *Einige aktuelle Aufgaben der Psychologie* [Some current tasks of psychology]. Sowjetwissenschaft. Gesellschaftswissenschaftliche Beiträge.

Leontiev, A. N. (1978). *Activity, consciousness, and persomality*. Englewood Cliffs, NJ: Prentice Hall.

Leontiev, A. N., & Luria, A. R. (1964). Die psychologischen Anschauungen L. S. Wygotskis. Einführung. [The psychological views of L. S. Vygotsky. Introduction]. In L. S. Vygotsky: *Denken und Sprechen* (pp. 1–33). Berlin: Akademie-Verlag.

Lidz, C. S. (Ed.). (1987). *Dynamic assessment: An interactional approach to evaluating learning potential*. New York: Guilford.

Lishout, C. F. M. (1987). Learning and instruction: A part of development. In E. Corte & P. Span (Eds.), *Learning and instruction: European research in international context* (pp. 53–67). Oxford: Pergamon Press.

Löwe, H., & Roether, D. (1978). *Lernpsychologische Untersuchungen im Erwachsenenalter mit dem modifizierten RAVEN-test als Kurzzeitlerntest* [Psychological studies on adult learning using the modified RAVEN test as short-term learning test]. In G. Clauss, J. Guthke, & G. Lehwald (Eds.), *Psychologie und Psychodiagnostik lernaktiven Verhaltens. Tagungsbericht* (pp. 143–150). Berlin: Gesellschaft für Psychologie der DDR.

Luria, A. R. (1970). *Die höheren kortikalen Funktionen und ihre Störung bei örtlicher Hirnschädigung*. Berlin: Deutscher Verlag der Wissenschaften. [English Edition: (1966). Higher cortical functions in man. New York: Basic Books].

Mandl, H., & Fischer, P. M. (Eds.). (1985). *Lernen im Dialog mit dem Computer* [Learning by dialogue with computers]. Munich: Urban & Schwarzenberg.

Matthes, G. (1978). Zur Diagnostik individueller Verlaufsqualitäten der Lerntätigkeit beim Problemlösen [Diagnosis of individual processing qualities of learning while problem solving]. In G. Clauss, J. Guthke, & G. Lehwald (Eds.), *Psychologie und Psychodiagnostik lernaktiven Verhaltens. Tagungsbericht* (pp. 118–123). Berlin: Gesellschaft für Psychologie der DDR.

Matthes, G. (1983). Anwendungszusammenhänge und -voraussetzungen korrekturorientierter Diagnostik [Relationships and prerequisites for application of correction-oriented diagnostics]. *Psychologie für die Praxis*, *1*, 42–54.

Mead, G. H. (1934). *Mind, self, and society from the standpoint of a social behaviorist*. Chicago: University of Chicago Press.

Meili, R. (1965). *Lehrbuch der psychologischen Diagnostik* [Textbook of psychological diagnostics]. Bern: Huber.

Menchinskaya, N. A. (Ed.). (1974). *Besonderheiten des Lernens zurückgebliebener Kinder* [Particularities of learning among retarded children]. Berlin: Volk und Wissen.

Michalski, S. (1988). *Das diagnostische Programm "Begriffsanaloges Klassifizieren" (dP "BAK")—ein Lerntest für leistungsversagende Schüler erster Klassen* [The diagnostic program "Classification from conceptual analogy":

A learning test for pupils failing in first grade]. Unpublished doctoral dissertation, Karl-Marx-Universität, Sektion Psychologie, Leipzig.
Müller, K. H. (1978). Überprüfung verschiedener Ansätze für pädagogisch-psychologische Schulleitsungsmeßverfahren im Bereich der Mathematik (POS 6. Klasse "Gebrochene Zahlen) [Study of different approaches to psychoeducational assessment in mathematics]. In G. Clauss, J. Guthke, & G. Lehwald (Eds.), *Psychologie und Psychodiagnostik lernaktiven Verhaltens. Tagungsbericht* (pp. 96–102). Berlin: Gesellschaft für Psychologie der DDR.
Neber, H. (1987). Problemlösen und Instruktion [Problem solving and instruction]. *Psychologie in Erziehung und Unterricht*, *34*(4), 241–246.
Pawlik, K. (Ed.). (1976). *Diagnose der Diagnostik* [Diagnosis of diagnostics]. Stuttgart: Klett.
Pawlik, K. (1977). Ökologische Validität [Ecological validity]. In G. Kaminski (Ed.), *Umweltspychologie: Perspektiven, Probleme, Praxis* (pp. 59–72). Stuttgart: Klett.
Pawlik, K. (Ed.). (1982). *Multivariate Persönlichkeitsforschung* [Multivariate personality research]. Bern, Stuttgart, Wien: Huber.
Petermann, F. (1978). *Veränderungsmessung* [Measurement of change]. Stuttart: Kohlhammer.
Petrovskij, A. V. (1964). Über die Anfänge der marxistischen Psychologie [The beginnings of marxist psychology]. In *Fragen der Theorie und Geschichte der Psychologie* (pp. 5–12). Moscow: Moscow Pedagogical Institute "Lenin" (Russian).
Piaget, J. (1962). Comments on Vygotsky's critical remarks concerning "The language and thought of the child" and "Judgment and reasoning in the child." Cambridge, MA: MIT Press.
Probst, H. (1982). *Zur Diagnostik und Didaktik der Oberbegriffsbildung* [Diagnostics and didactics of abstracting]. Oberbiel: Solms.
Raven, J.C. (1956). *Coloured Progressive Matrices*. London: H. K. Lewis.
Raven, J. C. (1958). *Standard Progressive Matrices*. London: H. K. Lewis.
Rissom, J. (1981). Der Begriff des Zeichens in den Arbeiten L. S. Vygotskys [The concept of symbols in L. S. Vygotsky's work]. Unpublished doctoral dissertation, Marburg.
Robertson, I. T., & Mindel, R. M. (1980). A study of trainability testing. *Journal of Occupational Psychology*, *53*, 131–138.
Roether, D. (1983). *Vorschul-Lerntest (VLT)* [Preschool learning test]. Berlin: Psychodiagnostisches Zentrum der Humboldt Universität zu Berlin.
Roether, D. (1984). *Der Test "Tempoleistung und Merkfähigkeit Erwachsener" (TME)* [Test of speed performance and memory of adults]. Berlin: Psychodiagnostisches Zentrum der Humboldt Universtität zu Berlin.
Roether, D. (1986). *Lernfähigkeit im Erwachsenenalter* [Learning Potential of Adults]. Leipzig: Hirzel.
Rösler, H. D., Ott, J., & Richter-Heinrich, E. (1980). *Neuropsychologische Probleme der klinischen Psychologie* [Neuropsychological problems in clinical psychology]. Berlin: Deutscher Verlag der Wissenschaften.
Rost, J., & Spada, H. (1978). *Learning tests: Psychometric and psychological considerations on a method to get diagnostic information from process data.* Paper presented at the XIXth International Congress of Applied Psychology, Munich.

Roth, H. (1957). *Pädagogische Psychologie des Lehrens und Lernens* [Pedagogical psychology of teaching and learning]. Hannover: Schrödel.

Rubinstein, S. L. (1958). *Grundlagen der allgemeinen Psychologie* [Foundations of general psychology]. Berlin: Volk und Wissen.

Rubinstein, S. L. (1961). *Das Denken und die Wege seiner Erforschung* [Ways to the study of thinking]. Berlin: Volk und Wissen.

Rüdiger, D. (1978). Prozeßdiagnose als neueres Konzept der Lernfähigkeitsdiagnose [Process diagnostics as a recent concept for learning potential assessment]. In H. Mandl & A. Krapp (Eds.), *Schuleignungsdiagnose—Neue Modelle, Annahmen und Befunde* (pp. 66–83). Göttingen: Hogrefe.

Schladebach, G. (1983). *Über den Zusammenhang fachunspezifischer und fachspezifischer Fähigkeiten im schlußfolgernden Denken* [The relationship of subject-specific and nonspecific abilities in reasoning]. Unpublished doctoral dissertation, Karl-Marx Universität, Sektion Psychologie, Leipzig.

Schmidt, L. R. (1971). Testing the limits in Leistungsverhalten: Möglichkeiten und Grenzen [Testing the limits of achievement behavior: possibilities and limits]. In E. Duhm, (Ed.), *Praxis der klinischen Psychologie* (Vol. 2, pp. 9–29). Göttingen, Hogrefe.

Schnotz, W. (1979). *Lerndiagnose als Handlungsanalyse* [Diagnosis of learning as analysis for action]. Weinheim: Beltz.

Selz, O. (1935). Versuche zur Hebung des Intelligenzniveaus [Attempts at increasing the level of intelligence]. *Zeitschrift für Psychologie*, *134*, 236–301.

Sternberg, R. J. (1985). *Beyond IQ*. Cambridge, London: Cambridge University Press.

Talysina, N. F. (1983). *Theoretische Probleme der Psychodiagnostik der intellektuellen Tätigkeit* [Theoretical problems of psychological diagnostics of intellectual activity]. Paper presented at the 6th All-Union-Congress of the Psychological Society of the USSR, Mocsow (Russian).

Thorndike, E. L. (1926). *Measurements of intelligence*. New York: Columbia University.

Tringer, L. (1980). Regulationsstörungen der Aufmerksamkeit bei Neurosen [Problems of regulating attention with neurosis]. In H. D. Rösler, J. Ott, & E. Richter-Heinrich (Eds.), *Neuropsychologische Probleme der klinischen Psychologie* (pp. 56–59). Berlin: Deutscher Verlag der Wissenschaften.

Vlasova, T. A., & Pevzner, M. S. (1971). *Kinder mit Abweichungen in der Entwicklung* [Children with temporary retardation in development]. Moscow: Pädagogika (Russian).

Vygotsky, L. S. (1935). *Grundlagen der Pädologie* [Foundations of pedology]. Leningrad.

Vygotsky, L. S. (1964). *Denken und Sprechen*. Berlin: Akademieverlag. [English edition: Thought and language, 1962. Cambridge, MA: MIT Press].

Vygotsky, L. S. (1981). The genesis of higher mental functions. In J. V. Wertsch (Ed.), *The concept of activity in Soviet psychology* (pp. 144–188). New York: M. E. Sharpe.

Weiss, D. I. (1985). Adaptive testing by computer. *Journal of Consulting and Clinical Psychology*, *53*(6), 774–790.

Wertsch, J. V. (1985a). *Vygotsky and the social formation of mind*. Cambridge, MA: Harvard University Press.

Wertsch, J. V. (Ed.). (1985b). *Culture, communication, and cognition: Vygotskian perspectives*. Cambridge: Cambridge University Press.

Wieczerkowski, W., & Wagner, H. (1985). Diagnostik von Hochbegabung [Diagnostics of giftedness]. In R. S. Jäger, R. Horn, & K. H. Ingenkamp (Eds.), *Tests und Trends 4* (pp. 109–132). Weinheim: Beltz.

Wiedl, K. H. (1984). Lerntests: nur Forschungsmittel und Forschungsgegenstand? [Learning tests: Means and subject of research only?]. *Zeitschrift für Entwicklungspsychologie und Pädagagische Psychologie*, *16*, 245–281.

Wiedl, K. H., & Herrig, D. (1978). Ökologische Validität und Schulerfolgsprognose im Lern- und Intelligenztest: Eine exemplarische Studie [Ecological validity and prognosis of success in school in learning and intelligence tests: An exemplary study]. *Diagnostika*, *24*(2), 175–186.

Winkler, E. (1978). Psychodiagnostiche Untersuchungen zu Leistungs- und anderen Persönlichkeitsvariablen als Prädiktoren des Studienerfolges im Chemie-Grundstudium [Psychodiagnostic studies of achievement and other personality variables as predictors of success in basic studies in chemistry]. In G. Clauss, J. Guthke, & G. Lehwald (Eds.), *Psychologie und Psychodiagnostik lernaktiven Verhaltens. Tagungsbericht* (pp. 78–83). Berlin: Gesellschaft für Psychologie der DDR.

Winkler, E. (1988). *Testmanual "Konzentrationslerntest"* [Manual for the concentration learning test]. Unpublished manuscript, Karl-Marx Universität, Sektion Psychologie, Leipzig.

Wolfram, H., Neumann, J., & Wieczorek, V. (1986). *Psychologische Leistungstests in der Neurologie und Psychiatrie* [Psychological achievement tests in neurology and psychiatry]. Leipzig: Thieme.

Zimmermann, W. (1987). *Prozessdiagnostic prosozial-kooperativer Lernfähigkeit* [Process diagnostics of prosocial-cooperative learning potential]. Psychologia Universalis (Vol. 49). Frankfurt/M.: Athenäum.

Zubin, J. (1950). Symposium on statistics for the clinician. *Journal of Clinical Psychology*, *6*, 1–6.

4
Reflections on Remediation and Transfer: A Vygotskian Perspective

J. P. Das and Robert N. F. Conway

Theoretical Roots of Remediation: A Review

Remedial training for learning handicaps and for intellectual deficits is currently a popular topic in the field of exceptionality. We can see that it has four theoretical roots. These are the research in memory, especially into the structure and control processes; early experience and intellectual development, the research that was pioneered by Hebb; learning styles and teaching strategies in the tradition of aptitude-treatment interaction; and finally, Vygotsky's views on learning, maturation, and the role of instruction. Let us consider each one separately.

The first root is in a model of memory, its structure, and control processes. Atkinson and Shiffrin (1968) proposed a box model of long- and short-term memory that has since become quite influential. It had a great influence on researchers in the field of mental retardation insofar as they saw a possibility of improvement in memory of the retarded through the control processes suggested in the Atkinson-Shiffrin model (Belmont & Butterfield, 1971). The control processes serve a number of functions such as the maintenance of information in short-term memory (STM) and transfer of information from short- to long-term memory as well. Later research has begun to cast some doubt on the necessity of all information to first enter STM before they can be transferred to long-term memory. The control processes, which include rehearsal and chunking, still survive as basic mechanisms for enhancing memory. These processes were fully utilized in techniques for teaching strategies for better learning and memory by a number of researchers since 1971 (Belmont & Butterfield, 1971). Among these techniques are simple instructions to use some strategies, presenting materials in a specific form that will require the use of a particular strategy, modeling techniques where the experimenter demonstrates this strategy, and fading and prompting, all of which have been described previously (see Ellis, 1979, pp. 619–657). How useful have these techniques become is questionable, however. As several reviews, including Resnick's (1981) have pointed out, instructing individuals or letting them model strategies such as rehearsal, has not led to a transfer of the learned skill. Therefore, the same group of researchers joined by new ones such as Glaser and Bassok (1989) and Brown and Campione (1981), are formulating programs for future research that will emphasize the development of general learning skills. As expected in the current spirit of the times, metacognition has crept into most of those new techniques. Current research, therefore, considers transfer as the primary aim for training in control processes, and there is a great deal of speculation concerning the teaching of strategies.

The second root that can be identified lies in the work of Hebb and his associates and students on sensory deprivation. Sensory deprivation has a deleterious effect on cognitive growth in animals and is the obverse of early stimulation, which is shown to influence and accelerate cognitive development. Haywood and Tapp (1966) summarized this work. They mentioned three different kinds of deprivation conditions that have been tried on animals. These are (a) extreme sensory deprivations, which involve giving no opportunity for sensory stimulation through vision, hearing, and so on, (b) social isolation, and (c) unimodal deprivation, by which the animal is made insensitive to a particular kind of sensory stimulation such as hearing or vision. They then go on to cite the early work of J. McV. Hunt, who showed that not only rats but humans may profit from early stimulation. Following this review, Das (1973) has elaborated on the implications of cultural deprivation and its effect on cognitive competence. Das has critically examined the efficacy of early education and its relationship to sensory deprivation experiments, in which it was concluded that the disadvantaged individuals that we are likely to study for cognitive competence almost never are subjected to the extent of social and sensory deprivation that characterize studies on animals. However, education, early or late, as shown by Feurestein (Feurestein, 1979; Feurestein & Hamburger, 1965) does improve cognitive abilities that might have been adversely affected by cultural deprivation. Compensatory education for the disadvantaged children derives its impetus from the research on early experience.

The push for early stimulation as well as compensatory education have influenced the treatment of learning-disabled children who are not culturally disadvantaged. Diagnosis of dyslexia at an early preschool age, and treatment for the defective function have been widely recommended; Bradley and Bryant's (1983) work provides a recent instance of this prevalent trend. They noticed that the would-be reading-disabled preschoolers were deficient in detecting rhyming, and devised a program that strengthened the children's perception of rhyming words and increased their reading performance. Feuerstein, as mentioned above, attempts to remediate deficits in intentional learning by an interactive instructional procedure.

The third root of remedial training may lie in aptitude-treatment interactions. Learning styles and teaching strategies have been quite popular for some time because of the common sense notion that the two should fit. Cronbach and Snow (1977) have written masterly reviews of aptitude-treatment interaction. Most of the research results offer mild support for the effectiveness of matching aptitudes to treatments. However, the desire on the part of the researchers to consider the modification of instructional strategies, according to the individual differences in the aptitudes of the learners can have only a beneficial effect on the learner who is undergoing remedial instruction. Perhaps it is quite acceptable to state that a learner's knowledge base and aptitude should be taken into account during instruction. Through formal instruction, children acquire scientific concepts and are able to refine their experiential concepts. On the other hand, it is only through experience that scientific concepts acquire a broader base in the cognitive domain of the individual, which facilitates their application in new situations. Thus, the tradition of Vygotsky has influenced mediated training and dynamic testing approaches of Feuerstein. At the same time it has begun to direct our attention to the preconditions for transfer of training.

The fourth influential root is the work of Vygotsky, specifically his contention that learning is a collaborative effort, and instruction need not always follow the level of intellectual maturity of children. In fact, the purpose of education is to accelerate the cognitive development of the child. The existing level of children's cognitive competence may not indicate their potential, hence a teach-test-teach-test paradigm is recommended. "What children can do with assistance of others might be in some sense even more indicative of their mental development than what they can do alone." (Vygotsky, 1978, p. 85).

Such quotations from Vygotsky, and his notion that children are like raw fruits in the field yet to mature fully, and thus *their potential for development must be considered by any measure of their ability*, has led to much talk and some research on the efficacy of "dynamic testing" and "instrumental enrichment" (see Lidz, 1987). Instruction may take place in formal or informal settings; the mediators could be peers or adults. But the central point is that learned skills have a social origin, and even more broadly stated, cognitive processes have a sociohistorical origin, especially as these depend on a system of signs, which is commonly called language.

Following Vygotsky's leadership in the Soviet Union, new research and thinking on education have evolved, although the literature is almost entirely in Russian. As gleaned from the infrequent English articles of Vygotsky's intellectual successors such as Leontiev, Luria, Elkonin, and Davydov, research has shown that a *psychologically based instruction could highly stimulate the mental development of the child*, permitting younger children to acquire new forms of thinking (Leontiev & Luria, 1972).

Vygotskian Concepts and Implications for Remediation

Internalization and Mediation

Let us start with Vygotsky's two major notions, internalization and sociocultural mediation, which determine as well as characterize mental activity. Internalization or, to borrow a Freudian terminology, interiorization can be found at many levels of children's activity; two of these are internalization of instruction and of language. Children learn through collaboration with others. Whenever children are given external instruction, either by another person or from reading books and manuals, they have to make the instructions their own. They have to know it and realize its meaning, and feel thoroughly familiar with it so that the instructions become a part of their own thinking. In doing so, children transform the external to internal codes, changing and modifying the original, and thus stamping it with their unique cognitive character. The process of internalization takes long to develop (Wertsch & Stone, 1985). Internal speech is an excellent example of the process of internalization. It has its own code, it is a language system unique to an individual, and it is not isomorphic to external speech. The quality of internal speech, or in common language, *ideas*, determines the competence in thinking. Likewise, disturbances in the individual's inner speech are shown in thought disorders. Loss of internal speech codes is manifested as loss of language or aphasia.

Signs and Their Role in Internalization and Mediation

The process of internalization of activity is assisted by language, both external and internal. Language itself is a sociocultural product. It is a system of signs, a mental tool. The meaning of signs is acquired, of course, through work and experience. Because a man does not work alone, that is, in a vacuum without any context or purpose and without using tools of labor and products of thought, all human activities have sociocultural roots (see Vygotsky, 1978, and Wertsch, 1985 for elaboration and critique). The point of interest for remedial instruction is the *quality* of internalization—not how *much* internalization has taken place following instruction, but what is its quality. The ingredient that contributes most to a high quality is reflection on the material of instruction. Without reflection, rote learning of instruction does not qualify as internalization, and does not facilitate transfer of learning.

We think internalization can be understood as a matrix of meanings that regulates the individual's activities. The pattern of interactions within this matrix changes qualitatively and characterizes stages of development. The factors that contribute to the matrix are ontological in nature, entailing sociocultural and genetic influences; the latter may impose some limiting conditions, as in the case of the mentally retarded. Vygotsky recognized the existence of limiting conditions while accepting children's potential to improve their performance with the help of mediators such as their peers and instructors.

A man's activity assimilates the experience of humankind—this statement by Leontiev (Wertsch & Stone, 1985) is the essence of the theoretical context of Vygotsky and the other developmental psychologists after him who have improved his theory. To quote Vygotsky (Minick, 1987),

> Any function in the child's cultural development appears on the scene twice or on two planes. It appears first on the social plane and only then on the psychological. It appears first between people as an intermental category and then within the child as an intramental category. This is equally true of voluntary attention, logical memory, concept formation, and the development of volition.

Mental functions have both a historical and a personal basis. They first appear in collaborative social interactions. Thus, *mediation* appears as a blending of two separate factors, which are integration (assimilation in Piaget's sense) and the history of the individual's experience; the individual is a member of a social-cultural group. Mediation can be activated from within the individual when formal and informal learning has been interiorized. Therefore, what is required for mediation to arise from within is a psychological tool. This is provided by internal speech, a system of signs or symbols that has evolved in the history of the culture. Signs, or the system of meanings they represent, mediate between stimuli and responses (Davydov & Radzikhovskii, 1985). Signs can be as simple as mnemonic devices for remembering a list of disconnected words or as complex as words and sentences that represent complex matrices of relationships.

The psychological tool of systems of meanings bears a strong resemblance to Pavlov's second signal system (Pavlov, 1942). A system of signals of primary signals is how Pavlov described the verbal system. Vygotsky's sign-meaning is much more developed and refined, but the idea is essentially the same.

The foregoing discussion on internalization and the theoretical aspects of mediation serves two purposes for this chapter: it provides a fresh look at the "verbal deficit" of learning-disabled children, and it leads to a consideration of zones of proximal development as a key concept in remedial training.

Zones of Proximal Development

Zones of proximal development (ZPD) has become a central concept for understanding what remediation achieves, and hence, is a familiar topic in the remediation literature today. Rogoff and Wertsch (1984) offer a good description of the concept and its use in American research. They even offer a sociopolitical analysis of the concept by Bruner. Unfortunately, the original writings of Vygotsky on ZPD are not extensive. The concept could not be developed too well because, as the Russian researcher (Davydov et al., 1985) say, its theoretical superstructure did not exist. Vygotsky did not have much time to develop the concept because of his illness and premature death, although in spite of this, his writings run into six volumes in Russian. Contemporary American researchers by and large have not read the writings of Vygotsky. Minick (1987), an American researcher, is translating them, and has written a detailed review of the concept and its use by American researchers.

ZPD literally translated should be zone of nearest development (Minick, 1987). It is described by Vygotsky (1978, pp. 85–86) as follows:

> It is the distance between the actual developmental level as determined by independent problem solving and the level of potential development as determined through problem solving under adult guidance or in collaboration with more capable peers.

The earliest American research on ZPD was published by Budoff and Friedman in 1964; it used a test-train-test paradigm in order to obtain a quantitative measure of improvement or progress through ZPD. A recent book edited by Lidz (1987) contains many coherent treatments of ZPD. In this book, Campione and Brown (1987) report the use of a quantitative measure—the number of prompts required for the learner to progress through the task. They do not claim to be measuring ZPD. Minick does not think that the essential characteristics of ZPD have survived the American attempt to quantify it; the concept does not lend itself to quantitative measurement. He is correct in pointing out that "in outlining the concept of ZPD, Vygotsky was proposing a new theoretical framework for analyzing the child's current state of development and for predicting the next or the proximal level of development that the child might be expected to attain" (Minick, 1987, pp. 118–119).

We would argue that the two important purposes for using ZPD are as follows:

1. To study cognitive development as a product that is the consequence of the individual learning in collaboration with others. The context of learning is provided by the symbiotic relation between personal characteristics and social milieu. One is reminded here that in this relationship, the "natural" predispositions of the individual are confounded with sociocultural influences. ZPD cannot be measured; it has no baseline because it is not a part of the learner's characteristic. The product which is observable is cognitive activity. Cognitive activities are filtered through the prism of development (Luria, 1963), and thus have to be analyzed into basic components that may differ

at different stages of development. We should remember that development is an integration of sociohistorical and genetic factors.
2. Diagnosis is the second purpose of considering ZPD as a helpful concept. Budoff's early research was based on Luria's in which children who may have the same low score on a cognitive task at an initial testing may demonstrate small or large improvements after a period of intensive interaction with a mediator. Thus, ZPD "determines the domain of transitions that are accessible to the child" (cited in Minick, 1987). Luria was faced with the task of establishing a diagnosis of mental retardation (MR) for a large number of children whose initial intelligence scores were low. Some of these children improve substantially following what Feuerstein would call mediated experience, some show significant gains, and some show little improvement. The truly retarded are of the last category; they have also abnormal cognitive processing in addition to their failure to gain from mediated experience.

Learning Disability, Mental Retardation, and Cognitive Intervention

The learning disabled (LD) are regarded as normal in Soviet psychology, but temporarily retarded. They do not benefit from normal instruction and may have specific disabilities in cognitive processing. But the assumption is that the specific disability can be circumvented with the help of appropriate collaborative effort. LD children can use speech and language and can benefit from verbal instruction. In contrast, the MR (a) cannot use knowledge obtained in the course of speech communication, (b) are unable to assimilate verbal instructions in a generalized form, and (c) have limited ability to use language as a means of independent thinking (Luria, 1963). The way to improve MR's cognitive behavior is *not* through verbal instructions and "metacognitive" procedures because both rely heavily on a complex semantic system (sign-meanings in Vygotsky's terms).

Verbal deficits associated with learning disability are not general as in the MRs. They are specific and open to change. They are found in lexical access to phonology and semantics as well as in the knowledge of linguistic rules. But the deficits are not restricted to processing verbal material; they appear in nonverbal tasks such as figure copying as well (Das, Bisanz, & Mancini, 1984). The deficit, when found frequently involves both verbal and nonverbal domains. It involves certain aspects of using *signs*.

We have explained the types of these difficulties by the coding processes in our information integration theory (Das, Kirby, & Jarman 1979), relating the use of successive processing to learning of decoding skills and predominantly simultaneous processing to comprehension. "Whereas *both* processes are necessary at a lower level of competence in reading, it is *simultaneous* processing that makes for better comprehension rather than successive processing at higher levels where adequate vocabulary and decoding skills are required" (Das, 1984b, p. 39).

The question is, Can these significant processing skills be taught (mediationally) and internalized sufficiently enough to be a part of the learning-disabled child's own repertoire? Briefly, for the LD child, the answer is yes; training in the use of successive and simultaneous processes, together with attention and planning, improves decoding and comprehension.

Below is a summary of intervention studies done by our group using methods to improve simultaneous-successive coding, planning, and attention in LD and educable mentally retarded (EMR) samples.

Training in Coding, Attention, and Planning (CAP)

LD studies

The two initial studies within the Das et al. (1979) model utilized only successive strategy training tasks (Kaufman, 1978; Krywaniuk, 1974). A later study (Brailsford, 1981) incorporated both simultaneous and successive processing. All studies were conducted with elementary school–aged pupils who were either low achievers or reading disabled.

Krywaniuk Study

The initial study (Krywaniuk, 1974; see also Das et al., 1979; Krywaniuk & Das, 1976), used 11 training tasks that emphasized successive more than simultaneous processing, and that were context-free in that they did not reflect competence in any specific academic subject areas. The subjects were from grades 3 and 4 in a school located on a Canadian Indian reserve. All were considered underachievers. The training was conducted individually over a period of 14 hours. The control group received a total of 3 hours of interaction with the experimenter; no training was given during this period. During training, the teacher encouraged the pupil to verbalize his thinking. The teacher encouraged the use of appropriate strategies and attempted to point out the ways in which the strategies were of use in the solution of the problem. Tasks included Sequence Story Boards, Parquetry Boards, Serial Recall, Matrix Serialization (Number Matrix), and five filmstrips designed to focus on visual training skills (see Krywaniuk & Das, 1976).

The Sequence Story Boards required the pupil to arrange 12 pictures in a sequence to tell a story. Verbalization was encouraged as the pupil examined the pictures and arranged them in sequence. Following the completion of the task, the pupil was required to tell the story in the order of the scenes he had determined. Parquetry Designs involved the use of geometric shapes to build patterns, initially on the template and later using the template as a reference only. The patterns became increasingly different. Serial Recall was a memory task to recall 12 shapes that had been hidden, after exposure to the pupil. As the task required no specific order of recall and encouraged the grouping of objects to increase the chance of recall, the task could be perhaps termed *Free Recall of Associative Pairing*. The Coding task required the correct sequential recall of a series of hand and knee claps, whereas the Matrix Serialization was the same as the Matrix Numbers task used in the present study. The five filmstrips were commercially produced and covered visual discrimination and spatial orientation, visual-motor coordination, visual memory, figure ground discrimination, and visualization. The filmstrips were used with the minimum training group as their total (3-hour) training, but only as part of the program for the experimental group.

The posttesting results indicated that the experimental group had significantly higher scores than the control group in Serial Learning and Visual Short-Term Memory, the two successive tests in the battery. Improvement was also found in the Schonell Word Recognition Test, a result that was "unexpected" (Krywaniuk, 1974, p. 102). The results of the study indicated both near transfer to other nontaught examples of successive processing and far transfer to reading. In comparison to other studies claiming transfer, the results obtained by Krywaniuk represent strong examples of transfer. Additionally they illustrate that a training program focusing upon a weak skill can permit the pupil to more efficiently use that skill (Krywaniuk, 1974).

Kaufman Study

Kaufman (1978; see also Das et al., 1979; Kaufman & Kaufman, 1978), also conducted a predominantly successive strategy training program. A total of 17 above average and 17 below average pupils were assigned to experimental and control groups. The below average group can be considered to be a learning-disabled group (Das et al., 1979). The training group received 10 hours of individual training, using a total of 11 tasks. The tasks included the five filmstrips used previously by Krywaniuk, and in addition, People Puzzle, Matrix Letters, Numbers and Pictures (based on Krywaniuk's Matrix Serialization), Serial and Free Recall of Pictures, and Follow the Arrow.

The People Puzzle required the child to sort out the jumbled horizontal pieces of the puzzle and construct faces from it. In Serial Recall of pictures, the children were trained to recall an increasingly long series of picture cards, whereas in Free Recall the cards can be remembered in any order. Follow the Arrow was a confirmation of successive training;

here the children learned to join pictures with arrows to show the correct sequence of events. The sequence had been shown to the child before on the master card that was to be studied by the child.

The results of the training showed that the experimental group had significantly higher scores on all successive marker tests and one simultaneous test, which was Memory for Designs. Near transfer could be considered to have been obtained in the case of the successive marker tests, and far transfer in the case of the Schonell Word Identification Test. The experimental group's posttest score was significantly higher in the mathematical composite of the Metropolitan Achievement Test, reflecting far transfer to mathematics as well.

Brailsford Study

Brailsford (1981; see also Brailsford, Snart, & Das, 1984), incorporated both simultaneous and successive processing strategies in her training program with reading-disabled children from upper elementary classes. Twelve pupils were assigned to each of the experimental and control groups. The experimental group took part in 15 hours of training, conducted individually. Twelve simultaneous processing tasks were utilized, including four that were subtests in the trial edition of the Kaufman Assessment Battery for Children (K-ABC). In addition, six successive processing strategy tasks were included, which were Matrix Letters and Number, Picture Story Sequencing, Serial Recall, and Associative Pairing based on previous studies. Tasks such as Tracking I and II were taken from earlier Soviet studies that are described below. The tasks were devised by Venger and Kholmovska (1978) of Moscow, who include them in a preschool psychodiagnostic battery.

The training program focused not only on simultaneous and successive processing but also on verbalization. Children were encouraged to verbalize during the tasks and also to explain their strategies following the completion of the task. As with both previous studies, all tasks were context-free and were primarily designed to reflect either simultaneous or successive processing, although the verbalizations of children showed that individual processing did not always reflect Brailsford's anticipated task focus.

The posttest results for simultaneous marker tests indicated higher experimental group results in Memory for Design but not for Figure Copying. In all successive marker tests the experimental group was significantly higher. Far transfer was obtained for instructional reading levels as measured by the Standard Reading Inventory (McCracken, 1966). Far transfer to the Gates-MacGinitie Prose Comprehension subtest was not obtained. Brailsford explains the failure to obtain far transfer as possibly being due to the multiple-choice format of the test which constricts access to the text and "does not place reliance on the active organizational strategies emphasized in the training tasks" (Brailsford, Snart, & Das, 1984). In contrast, the Standard Reading Inventory, because of its requirements to read, reconstruct, and answer questions requires the utilization of the coding and retrieval strategies taught in the training program.

Studies with the Mentally Retarded

Parmenter Study

Parmenter (1984) trained educable mentally retarded late adolescents on four successive processing tasks. The sessions, totaling 50 hours of training, were held over a period of 4 months. The tasks selected had previously been successfully utilized in either the Kaufman or Krywaniuk study.

Following the completion of training, the group was unable to demonstrate transfer to either successive or simultaneous processing marker tasks, or to academic tests of reading. The failure to demonstrate either near or far transfer was explained by Parmenter as a failure by the learners to utilize the strategies in attempting marker tests, in favor of existing inefficient or inappropriate strategies. A further reason advanced was that the learners may have failed to learn the strategy to a level of proficiency that permitted them to apply it to an alternate task.

Conway Study

Conway (1985) incorporated an equal balance of simultaneous and successive processing tasks in a training study for EMR children attending special classes in two elementary schools. The training took part in small groups of four children over a total of 18 hours. The training model differed from the previous LD studies in that, following the introduction of two simultaneous and two successive processing strategy tasks, the children were reintroduced to one simultaneous and one successive task in order to teach discrimination between the two processing strategies, and to demonstrate that one strategy was more appropriate than the other for a given task. This concept of discrimination was considered an important skill in attempting alternate novel tasks.

As in the Brailsford study, the emphasis was on the child's solution to the task, not on rehearsing an adult-instructed verbal sequence. The role of the group was to provide both a more natural learning environment and to provide feedback and models for the training program. Like Brailsford, Conway found that the verbalization of some children revealed that the less appropriate processing strategy was employed to solve a particular task. The group situation provided the opportunity for another group member to demonstrate the more appropriate strategy using a language and conceptual framework understood by the group members.

The results of the study failed to demonstrate transfer either to other simultaneous or successive tasks or to academic tasks of reading and mathematics. The failure to demonstrate transfer was considered by Conway to be due to the inability of the children to perceive the need to apply the learned strategies to novel tasks.

The Success of LD Studies

The three LD studies conducted within our model of training have clearly demonstrated both near transfer to tests of simultaneous and successive processing, and *very far transfer* to reading and mathematics. Unlike many studies of transfer, the near transfer tasks are clearly different from the training tasks. Far transfer tasks require the application of strategies, learned in context-free tasks, to context-specific tasks of reading and mathematics, a far more substantial degree of transfer than has been demonstrated in other cognitive training programs. In addition, the studies have demonstrated the viability of teaching context-free processing strategies to low achievers and reading disabled.

The encouraging LD results have led us to begin working to extend the training program and to formalize it. Coding, attention, and planning are the three processes focused upon in the training program. In addition, specific process training for school-related skills such as spelling, decoding, and comprehension are being developed. A preliminary report on improving spelling is described in the next section.

From Global to Content-Specific Process Training: Bridging the Gap

General Objectives

The specific training program has as its primary aim the acquisition of processing strategies both within tasks in which content provides no difficulty and in which the processing strategies can be taught without the added difficulty of teaching the contextual information, and in the application of processing strategies within current academic tasks. Consequently, the program removes from the child the need to transfer learned strategies from a global training program to academic tasks. In some cases it may be appropriate to teach strategies directly within academic tasks rather than requiring a separate global strategy training program initially.

The program should ideally be taught in small-group situations. In line with Vygotsky's ZPD concept that social learning situations play an important role in skill acquisition, processing strategies are most appropriately taught in a shared learning environment. Group learning has advantages over individual learning, particularly in that it permits greater peer interaction in the learning process. The use of natural language by children within the group situation allows clarification of task, and natural language verbalization permits group members to become instructors of each other. The group situation allows the teacher to be seen less in an instructing role and as a dispenser of reinforcement, and more as a facilitator and mediator.

The training program does not contain a sequence of specific teacher-directed training steps as would be found in some of the verbal self-instruction or metacognitive literature. The aim is that each learner learns in collaboration with the teacher and other group members. Rigid instructional steps are avoided because they do not permit the learners to transfer instructions or strategies into their own language. The role of the teacher and other group members is to assist in the individual's mediation of the coding and planning strategies.

General Teaching Principles

The following general principles apply to CAP training.

1. The training program is not prescriptive and the teacher should use only those parts he requires. For example, if the learner is shown to be weak in successive coding, the teacher, in consultation with the school psychologist, will select more successive coding training tasks, while still using some simultaneous tasks to permit discrimination between the two coding strategies.
2. The program has been developed to meet the needs of those learners who require the development of coding and planning strategies free of the constraints or "fears" of academic content.
3. The training model is based upon the following sequence:
   (a) learning the strategy through structured teacher assistance;
   (b) practicing coding and planning by testing the strategy in both example and nonexample through both training tasks and other materials available;
   (c) bridging the strategy and planning to academic tasks through specific examples from both known and unknown academic content.
4. Materials and tasks specified in the training program serve only as starting points for teachers who are expected to make use of alternate resources available in classrooms and resource rooms. These additional materials provide valuable opportunities to demonstrate the wider application of the strategy and discriminate between appropriate and inappropriate use of the strategy.

5. Progress should be closely monitored at all times to ensure that each learner has acquired that skill and that a ceiling effect has not been reached.
6. There is no prescribed amount of time that should be allocated to the training of coding, attention and planning strategies in nonacademic tasks. At all times the relationship of coding strategies to academic tasks should be demonstrated so that the need to use nonacademic tasks can be ended as soon as possible. The program is designed to develop the ability to use appropriate strategies within academic tasks and the teacher must always see this as the primary aim of the program.

Specific Teaching Principles

CAP training is an interactional program in which the teacher's active participation is required. The teacher's role includes:

1. Introducing the task and explaining the task demands;
2. Guiding the individual learner within the group in attempting the solution of the task. The individual and group need to be challenged to see the relationships between the coding strategy used in each task and those of previous tasks, other nonacademic tasks, and specific academic tasks.
3. Providing opportunities for learner evaluation of the success of their strategy use and for initiating group discussion on the value of the appropriate strategy;
4. Identifying blockages in the learner's coding and planning and promoting discussion on alternate methods;
5. Providing sufficient alternate materials to allow practice of selection and application of the appropriate strategy;
6. Continued linking of coding and planning to known and unknown academic and everyday activities;
7. Maintenance of coding and planning strategies within academic programs.

Improvement of Spelling: A Study on Specific Process Training

Learning spelling requires attention to the letter sequences in the word which is to be spelled. Hence, successive processing is especially involved in spelling. A deficiency in successive processing is therefore observed in poor spellers. Given such a deficiency, the training program should promote successive processing. Planning, along with successive processing needs to be the object of training so that the process can be approximately organized and applied in learning the spelling for new words. The following study by Spencer (Spencer, Snart, & Das, 1989) attempted to test improvement in spelling by including both global and specific training. The global processes, successive coding and planning were chosen for remediation by selecting five CAP training tasks. The bridging tasks were five spelling tasks, which were modeled after the CAP tasks in keeping with the spirit of successive processing and planning. Twenty children between 8 and 12 years (mean 10.8 years) and very poor in spelling, served as subjects. Their spelling level was at some two-and-a-half grades below the level expected of their age. Ten of these children were placed in the group that received remedial training; the other ten continued to standard instructions in reading and spelling in the resource room.

As examples of the global and specific tasks, consider the following: Bead Threading ("watch it") requires the child to thread a bead pattern by recalling the order in which different beads were dropped by the teacher. The beads were large or small (size) and yellow, red, blue, or green (color). The teacher drops the beads in predetermined serial orders. The child copies the order using his/her frame, then checks if the order was correct by lifting the cover off the teacher's frame. Interactions between the child and the teacher occur frequently. These focus on the processing demands of the task, identification of blocks in processing, and providing an opportunity for verbalizing the processing strategies (but not forcing the child to verbalize).

The spelling task that models the above is described here in detailed steps to show how the "bridging" tasks are structured and given.
Spelling training: "Watch it."

1. The teacher will present a card with letters arranged on it and say "This word is friend," and then turn the card over immediately saying "Use the letters in front of you to make this word" (student places letter cards in a card holder). The teacher records the response and asks the student to mix up the letters.
2. The teacher presents a window chart to the student. Each window has a strip of paper with a letter on it. The teacher says "Watch carefully." The teacher then pulls the strips through the windows one at a time, saying the letter name. The letter is exposed for no longer than 5 seconds. The student is then asked to arrange the letters in front of him in the card holder as he remembers seeing them. The teacher records the response. The student checks his response by exposing the letters in the windows. Each letter is left exposed to allow the student to check. The student corrects errors as they are discovered.
3. The teacher takes the chart from the child. Holding up the chart for the child to see that the letters are still exposed, the teacher then says the name of each letter and then pulls the letter out of sight. The teacher says the whole word after the last letter has been named and pulled out of sight. The student is then asked to place the letter cards

in the holder in the correct order. The teacher records the response. The student is then given the window chart to check his response. The student checks his response by exposing the letters in the windows. Each letter is left exposed to allow the student to check. The student corrects errors as they are discovered.
4. Repeat step 3.
5. Repeat step 1.

The Problem of Transfer: Does the Vygotskian Perspective Help?

Developmental Considerations

Transfer is an integral part of not only learning, but development. When learning and development are considered to be inextricably blended together, transfer may become the essential ingredient for children's cognitive growth. "Development consists in part of going from the context-dependent state where resources are welded to the original learning situation to a *relatively* context-independent state where the learner extends the ways in which initially highly constrained knowledge and procedures are used" (Brown, Bransford, Ferrara, & Campione, 1983, p. 142).

Transfer need not be mediated by verbal instruction, nor does it need to be conceptualized by external speech, or even represented by inner speech. For if it were, animals could not be shown to transfer learning. Thus the question is not whether mentally handicapped children or learning-disabled children can transfer what they learn, but what kind of learning are we targeting for transfer?

Brown and Campione (1986) as well as Campione and Brown (1987, 1989) have discussed the conditions of successful transfers. They seem to emphasize principles as a target of transfer; these are based on inductive inferencing arising out of children's experience with the tasks rather than on the explicit teaching of principles. The children come up with the principle or the essential similarities between separate instantiations of the principle; even 3- and 5-year-old children can do this. Brown and Campione (1986) recommend, following Vygotsky, that learning takes place in collaboration with peers and experts. A scaffold, an adjustable and temporary support, is to be provided to children for promoting their conceptual understanding of a set of similar problems; then transfer of learning becomes possible.

If both learning and transfer are required in a complex system of *sign meanings*, mentally retarded children cannot be successful in either of them. Luria's (1963) observation in regard to their weakness in the verbal system is basically correct: Mentally retarded children cannot use the information obtained through speech for generalization or transfer, and they have only a limited capacity for using language for thinking. Perhaps that is why in our research on process training (Conway, 1985), we observed that the retarded children failed to benefit from remediation.

Spontaneous transfer does not appear even for individuals who are adept at using the verbal system (mathematical symbols and inner speech included). Brown et al. (1983) note its absence in problem solving situations such as in doing the Tower of Hanoi task. They recommend prompts and hints. The assumption is that individuals must be helped to see how a general principle may apply to a specific situation. Strategy-teaching is not enough unless we also teach where to use what strategy. This task becomes formidable if IQ is in the retarded range. Such children need to be prompted frequently. This itself decreases the chances for transfer. The greater the number of prompts during training, the lesser the transfer.

We are suggesting that in process training, the behavior targeted for transfer is to be guided by principles or rules that have been learned. How that learning should take place, whether deductively by explicit step-by-step instruction or through inductive inferencing, is to be discussed later. But let us distinguish between *three bases of transfer* following the ideas of E. L. Thorndike (Hilgard & Bower, 1975).

Basis of Transfer

Transfer of learning to a new situation may occur when the original and the new situations are (a) similar in content, (b) similar in procedure, or (c) share the same principle of learning. The greater the number of identical elements in the old and the new situation, the stronger is the transfer. That has been shown in strategy training studies on mentally retarded subjects by Belmont and Butterflied (1977) and many others (see Borkowski & Cavanaugh, 1979). Its application is limited because the transfer based on the number of identical elements is too narrow; hence the pessimism surrounding the generalizability of strategy training with the mentally retarded has become widespread (Das, 1985).

The second type of transfer can occur if the procedure of learning is similar, even if the content is different. For instance, serial recall shows the typical bowing curve in spite of differences in content of learning; training that concentrates on the rehearsal of the middle items (which are involved in the bow) may elevate the subject's recall score. Other tasks with procedural similarities but that are far different in content, are shown in common test-taking skills. Because of such similarities, subjects may improve in their test scores as they are exposed to more than one test, even if the tests are heterogeneous in content (i.e., memory and abstract reasoning). Feuerstein utilizes transfer of this type to a great extent in his instrumental enrichment procedures.

The third kind of transfer, of principle, is the aim of all "cognitive strategy" training because it should result in far transfer. General strategy training aims at far transfer; the tacit assumption here is that we can teach an overarching set of principles that helps the wary learner while traveling in a new land.

An Alternative to Strategy Training

As an alternative to general strategy training (cf. Borkowski & Cavanaugh, 1979; Glidden, 1979), it is proposed that *transfer of principle can be facilitated only when the subject has acquired the principle through his or her own experience.* Often the experiences have to be guided by an externally initiated structure. The procedure is identical to learning of new concepts, as Vygotsky (1962) has discussed. For instance, the child may start learning the concept of an airplane through a prototype, first getting to know it and gradually being exposed to varying shapes, sizes, and functional characteristics of airplanes. Alternatively, the child can be introduced to various airplanes, thus gradually acquiring knowledge about airplanes. Both procedures of concept learning lead to the acquisition of a comprehensive concept, passing through stages of imperfect and pseudoconcepts, as Vygotsky (1962) has discussed. But the learning is collaborative, and requires internal representation which involves transitions from intermental to intramental representations. Such learning facilitates inductive rather than deductive inferencing.

Cognitive strategy training does not follow the inductive route. Brown (under preparation) has conducted a series of exquisite studies on transfer of learning that, we think, facilitate inductive inferencing leading to the discovery of a rule or principle. She shows that abstract principles can be transferred to new instances when the skill is acquired in a flexible rather than a fixed context. A flexible use of strings, for example as a tool for measuring things, as material for sewing, for pulling people out of the water, etc., promotes transfer to a broader range of situations. In a fixed learning situation where children learn one general rule thoroughly, such creative uses of the tool are blocked; they develop a set, it becomes rigid, and results in negative transfer. It appears to be rooted in control process, and to a certain extent in fitting direct instruction to the aptitude of the learner. These are the first and third roots identified in the beginning of this chapter.

Strategy training (see the special issue of *Educational Psychologist*, 1986, for a sampler) comes in many forms, but essentially it is based on the *principle of deduction*. Some strategy is given to be applied in a set procedure. The learner has to identify the instance where the strategy is applicable, then follow the deductive procedure: All men are mortal; is Jack an instance of a man?; if so, he is mortal. The learner has not worked his or her way through experiences that lead to the eduction of the principle that "all men are mortal." The learner did not use the principles of induction. It seems reasonable to consider structuring the remedial training program in such a manner that *inductive inference* will occur spontaneously. The global process training experience in our remedial program perhaps allows this. The principle need not be verbalized in our training, and even cannot be verbalized accurately. But the learner has a sense of where it should apply. Training for cognitive processing has a better chance of leading to transfer in the mentally retarded when the inductive procedure through the structured experience provided by the remedial tasks is followed. Even then the retarded may not show far transfer. An "inductive leap" is required to educe a common principle, to go from particular instances to a general rule. The extent to which the retarded children can do this is determined by a complex set of conditions. The major one seems to be the quality of sign meanings or the inner speech. Even when they are put through the structured remedial program for the enhancement of cognitive processing, they cannot conceptually represent and analyze the experience. Citing Brown's paper again, young children (3 to 5 years) cannot understand complex explanations of the principle, although they have been able to derive it from their experience with a given set of problems. The limitation may be found in the elusive "quality of sign meanings." As Leontiev and Luria (1972) describe it,

> . . . at each stage, the developing word meaning requires a different *mental operation*. Thus, with a small child a basic role is played by immediate impressions (partly emotional); with a schoolchild this structure undergoes a deep change, and finally with an adult the mental operations required to process word meanings involves an extremely complex process of deep psychological changes. (p. 314)

The retarded children, like the young children of 5, had an immature sign-meaning system.

Does the "inductive" training program relate to the Vygotskian perspective? We think it does, and to the Piagetian notion that we learn by operating on reality. It is through *labor* that we learn, including the learning of symbolic tools such as language. And it is in collaboration with others that our cognitive development occurs. When a strategy or principle is articulated subsequent to experiences from which it is educed, it will have a better chance for application in "far" situations.

References

Atkinson, R. C., & Shiffrin, R. M. (1986). Human memory: A proposed system and its control processes. In K. W. Spence & J. T. Spence (Eds.), *The psychology of learning and motivation: Advances in theory and research* (Vol. 2). New York: Academic Press.

Belmont, J. M., & Butterfield, E. C. (1971). What the development of short-term memory is. *Human Development*, *14*, 236–248.

Belmont, J. M., & Butterfield, E. C. (1977). The instructional approach to developmental cognitive research. In R. Kail & J. Hagen (Eds.), *Perspectives on the development of memory and cognition*. Hillsdale, NJ: Erlbaum.

Borkowski, J. G., & Cavanaugh, J. C. (1979). Maintenance and generalization of skills and strategies by the retarded. In N. R. Ellis (Ed.), *Handbook of mental deficiency, psychological theory and research* (2nd ed., pp. 569–617). Hillsdale, NJ: Erlbaum.

Bradley, L., & Bryant, P. E. (1983). Categorising sounds and learning to read: A causal connexion. *Nature*, *301*, 419–421.

Brailsford, A. (1981). *The relationship between cognitive strategy training and performance on tasks of reading comprehension within a learning disabled group of children*. Unpublished master's thesis, University of Alberta, Edmonton.

Brailsford, A., Snart, F., & Das, J. P. (1984). Strategy training and reading comprehension. *Journal of Learning Disabilities*, *17*, 287–290.

Brown, A. L. (1989). Analogical learning and transfer: What develops? In S. Vosinadou & A. Ortony (Eds.), *Similarity and Analogical Reasoning* (pp. 369–412). New York: Cambridge University Press.

Brown, A. L., Bransford, J. D., Ferrara, R. A., & Campione, J. C. (1983). Learning, remembering, and understanding. In J. H. Flavell & E. M. Markman (Eds.), *Carmichael's manual of child psychology* (Vol. 3). New York: Wiley.

Brown, A. L., & Campione, J. C. (1981). Inducing flexible thinking: The problem of access. In M. P. Friedman, J. P. Das, & N. O'Connor (Eds.), *Intelligence and learning*. New York: Plenum.

Brown, A. L., & Campione, J. C. (1986). Psychological theory and the study of learning disabilities. *American Psychologist*, *14*, 1059–1068.

Budoff, M., & Friedman, M. (1964). "Learning potential" as an assessment approach to the adolescent mentally retarded. *Journal of Consulting Psychology*, *28*, 434–439.

Campione, J., & Brown, A. (1987). Linking dynamic assessment with school achievement. In C. Lidz (Ed.), *Dynamic Assessment* (pp. 82–115). New York: Guilford Press.

Conway, R. N. F. (1985). *The information processing model and the mildly developmentally delayed child: Assessment and training*. Unpublished doctoral dissertation, Macquarie University, Newcastle, Australia.

Cronbach, L. J., & Snow, R. E. (1977). *Aptitudes and instructional methods: A handbook for research on interactions*. New York: Irvington.

Das, J. P. (1973). Cultural deprivation and cognitive competence. In N. R. Ellis (Ed.), *International review of research in mental retardation* (Vol. 6, pp. 2–53). New York: Academic Press.

Das, J. P. (1984a). Intelligence and information integration. In J. Kirby (Ed.), *Cognitive strategies and educational performance* (pp. 13–31). New York: Academic Press.

Das, J. P. (1984b). Simultaneous and successive processing in children with learning disability. *Topics in Language Disorders*, *4*, 34–47.

Das, J. P. (1985). Remedial training for the amelioration of cognitive deficits in children. In A. Ashman & R. Laura (Eds.), *The education and training of the mentally retarded* (pp. 214–244). London: Croom Helm.

Das, J. P., Bisanz, G. L., & Mancini, G. (1984). Performance of good and poor readers on cognitive tasks: Changes with development and reading competence. *Journal of Learning Disabilities*, *17*, 549–555.

Das, J. P., Kirby, J. R., & Jarman, R. F. (1979). *Simultaneous and successive cognitive processes*. New York: Academic Press.

Davydov, V. C., & Radzikhovskii, L. A. (1985). Vygotsky's theory and the activity-oriented approach in psychology. In J. V. Wertsch (Ed.), *Culture, communication, and cognition*. New York: Cambridge University Press.

Ellis, N. R. (1979). *Handbook of mental deficiency, psychological theory and research* (2nd ed.). Hillsdale, NJ: Erlbaum.

Feuerstein, R. (1979). *The dynamic assessment of retarded performers*. Baltimore: University Park Press.

Feuerstein, R., & Hamburger, M. (1965). *A proposal to study the process of redevelopment in several groups of deprived early adolescents in both residential and non-residential settings*. Unpublished report, the Youth-Aliyah Department of the Jewish Agency, Jerusalem.

Glaser, R., & Bassok, M. (1989). Learning theory and the study of instruction. *Annual Review of Psychology*, *40*, 631–666.

Glidden, L. M. (1979). Training of learning and memory in retarded persons: Strategies, techniques, and teaching tools. In N. R. Ellis (Ed.), *Handbook of mental deficiency, psychological theory and research* (2nd ed., pp. 619–657). Hillsdale, NJ: Erlbaum.

Haywood, H. C., & Tapp, J. T. (1966). Experience and the development of adaptive behavior. In N. R. Ellis (Ed.), *International review of research in mental retardation* (Vol. 1, pp. 109–151). New York: Academic Press.

Hilgard, E. R., & Bower, G. H. (1975). *Theories of learning* (4th ed.). Englewood Cliffs, NJ: Prentice-Hall.

Jensen, A. R. (1969). How much can we boost I. Q. and scholastic achievement? *Harvard Education Review*, *39*, 1–123.

Kaufman, D. (1978). *The relationship of academic performance to strategy training and remedial techniques: An information processing approach*. Unpublished doctoral dissertation, University of Alberta, Edmonton.

Kaufman, D., & Kaufman, P. (1978). Strategy training and remedial techniques. *Journal of Learning Disabilities*, *16*, 72–78.

Krywaniuk, L. W. (1974). *Patterns of cognitive abilities of high and low achieving school children*. Unpublished doctoral dissertation, University of Alberta, Edmonton.

Krywaniuk, L., & Das, J. P. (1976). Cognitive strategies in native children: Analysis and information. *Alberta Journal of Educational Research*, *22*, 271–280.

Leontiev, A., & Luria, A. (1972). Some notes concerning Dr. Fodor's "Reflections on L. S. Vygotsky's Thought and Language". *Cognition*, *1*, 311–316.

Lidz, C. S. (1987). *Foundations of dynamic assessment*. New York: Guilford.

Luria, A. R. (1963). *The mentally retarded child*. New York: Macmillan.

McCracken, R. A. (1966). *Standard reading inventory manual*. Kalmath Falls, OR: Kalmath Printing Co.

Minick, N. (1987). The zone of proximal development. In C. S. Lidz (Ed.), *Foundations of dynamic assessment*. New York: Guilford.

Parmenter, T. R. (1984). Ph.D. Thesis. Macquarie University, Sydney, Australia.

Pavlov, I. P. (1942). *Lectures on conditioned reflex* (Vol. 2) (W. H. Gantt, Trans.). New York: International Publishers.

Resnick, L. B. (1981). Instructional psychology. *Annual Review of Psychology*, *32*, 659–704.

Rogoff, B., & Wertsch, J. V. (Eds.) (1984). *Children's learning in the "zone of proximal development."* San Francisco: Jossey-Bass.

Spencer, F., Snart, F., & Das, J. P. (1989). A process-based approach to the remediation of spelling in students with reading disabilities. *The Alberta Journal of Educational Research*, *35*(4), 269–282.

Venger, L. A., & Kholmovska, V. V. (1978). *Diagnostika umstennago razvitiya doshkolnivok*. Moscow: Pedgogika.

Vygotsky, L. S. (1962). *Thought and language*. Cambridge, MA: MIT Press.

Vygotsky, L. S. (1978). *Mind in society: The development of higher psychological processes*. Cambridge, MA: Harvard University Press.

Wertsch, J. V. (Ed.) (1985). *Culture, communication and cognition*. Cambridge, MA: Harvard University Press.

Wertsch, J. V., & Stone, C. A. (1985). The concept of internalization in Vygotsky's account of the genesis of higher mental functions. In J. V. Wertsch (Ed.), *Culture, communication, and cognition*. New York: Cambridge University Press.

Part 2
Research on Interactive Assessment and Related Issues

Chapters 5 through 10—the largest single section of the book—are focused on research. The research section could be even larger, given that some chapters have been placed arbitrarily in the next section, Applications, because they illustrate the diversity of applications of interactive assessment, even though they are also research reports.

These reports reflect two broad research strategies: research on the clinical instruments of interactive assessment, and the use of these clinical instruments as research tools in a more basic sense. In fact, both strategies have somtimes been used in the same work.

The chapters in this section are a diverse group, representing at least four broad theoretical orientations: neo-Piagetian, mediated learning, neuropsychological, and learning tests. Chapter 5, by Paour, is a good example of the use of a clinical technology as a research tool to get information about basic developmental processes. He and his collaborators have blurred the distinction between assessment and treatment in their "operatory learning" procedure—a distinction that is less sharp in interactive assessment than in more traditional psychometric approaches. In a series of studies, they have both located a developmental fixation and demonstrated durable and generalizable modifications in cognitive processes.

Three of the chapters are related, with varying degress of fidelity, to the "mediated learning" concept associated with Feuerstein: Chapter 7, by Tzuriel and Feuerstein; Chapter 9, by Klein; and Chapter 10, by Samuels, Killip, MacKenzie, and Fagan. Even within that group there is considerable diversity. In a very practical study, Tzuriel and Feuerstein show an important use of interactive assessment on a broad scale, contrast three levels of teaching intensity, and show differential effects on different socioeconomic groups. Klein's chapter addresses one of the most fundamental aspects of the mediated learning concept: the role of early parent-child interactions in cognitive development. In the process of examining that basic question, she has developed an observation protocol that can be used by others in different settings. Samuels, Killip,

MacKenzie, and Fagan report on the use of mediated learning technology (for dynamic assessment of young children) in program evaluation. Specifically, they have related these assessment procedures to an educational program, the Cognitive Curriculum for Young Children, that has been derived from a similar set of theory.

In Chapter 6, Carlson and Wiedl report on a research collaboration that spans a number of studies. They distinguish between native ability and cognitive competence, and try in their testing procedures to reveal cognitive competence by varying testing conditions such as verbalization (during and after problem solution) and feedback (also during and after the solution). Their work is at the intersection of clinical and experimental modes and represents a set of replicable procedures that can fit into different conceptual schemes.

The research of Das and Naglieri is rooted in yet another conceptual scheme, the neuropsychology of A. R. Luria that has been extended and elaborated by Das. In Chapter 8, they build upon previous work in which they have identified three principal components of information processing. In general, their experimental approach to interactive assessment is to associate cognitive inefficiency with one or more of these three components. They are less concerned than are the others with assessment of modifiability, but their procedures are clearly open to the teaching-within-the-test strategy, especially if the teaching is done after an initial no-teaching phase.

In general, these chapters seem to us to suggest the richness of research possibilities, both for research on the utility of interactive assessment and for the use of these clinical instruments as research tools.

5
Induction of Logic Structures in the Mentally Retarded: An Assessment and Intervention Instrument

Jean-Louis Paour

The notions of "training the intellect," and consequently of programs of cognitive education, depend to a large degree on the ability of psychologists and educators to assess or diagnose specific problems in cognitive development, to specify the conditions under which development, especially in those "deficient" processes, can be accelerated, and to provide the tools for both assessment and intervention.

We have been conducting research since 1968 on the induction of logic structures in mentally retarded persons (Castellan & Paour, 1968; Paour, 1975, 1978, 1979, 1980, 1981a, 1981b, 1982, 1985, 1986, 1988 Paour, Galas, Malacria-Rocco, & Soavi, 1985; Robeants, 1987; Soavi, 1986). In this chapter we try to demonstrate that the theory and method of this approach to assessing and stimulating cognitive development and functioning constitute important bases for the understanding and educational treatment of mental retardation. Taken sequentially, these studies on induction of logic structures have helped us to do several things:

1. to specify the structural and functional determinants of prolonged abnormal fixations at the preoperatory level that retard and impede the intellectual development of retarded persons;
2. to induce cognitive gains that seem to reflect functionally integrated structural change in mildly and moderately retarded persons;
3. to present evidence that such persons are characterized by a relative but quite real developmental plasticity;
4. to specify the conditions under which this induction constitutes an effective instrument for helping retarded persons to accede to the level of concrete operatory thought when they have not done so spontaneously.

We cannot present all of our studies in detail. Instead, we present the theoretical foundations of this type of assessment/intervention and discuss the nature and the significance of the cognitive gains so induced. Readers will find a more detailed discussion of our intervention methods in the case study section of this book (Paour & Soavi, Chapter 18).

Theoretical Basis of Induction of Logic Structures

Our current conception of the induction of logic structures rests on two principal bases. The first, *structural*, is borrowed from the description of the "logic of the preoperatory child" (Orsini, 1965; Orsini-Bouichou, 1975, 1982). The second, *functional*, comes from the increasingly detailed view of the cognitive difficulties of retarded persons that we have observed in our own induction studies.

Structural Aspects

Operatory Learning

The theory and practice of induction of logic structures is part of the more generic concept of *operatory learning*. Operatory learning is defined, first of all, by its goals. One asks whether or not it is possible, and if so under what conditions, to bring about deliberately those "operatory" behavior patterns that Piaget regarded as evidence of the construction of intelligence. In accordance with a Piagetian constructivist position, the term refers to a concept of learning that rests on the subjects' active treatment of situations that induce cognitive conflicts.

This stream of research arose from an epistemological problem regarding the nature of logico-mathematical knowledge. Piaget saw in this reliance on learning a means of demonstrating that the numerical, relational, physical, or spatial "invariants" (more-or-less universal understandings of stable phenomena in these realms) cannot be the results of empirical learning (observation, association, reinforcement), but are the products of a structural developmental progression that is itself the result of the coordination of actions. Studies conducted at the International Center for Genetic Epistemology have seemed to demonstrate that it is possible only with great difficulty to accelerate the appearance of concrete operatory behavior patterns in children who are developmentally at the preoperatory level (Greco, 1959; Morf, Smedslund, Vinh Bang, & Wohlwill, 1959).

These first studies contributed to the establishment of the paradigm of operatory learning and to the development of primary methods known as equilibration or reequilibration by induction of a cognitive conflict. They bear as well upon the thorny problem of how to interpret the gains that follow learning. For this type of intervention, the goal is the development of relatively general *processes* of information processing rather than the learning of specific responses; therefore, it is essential to use stringent criteria to assess the structural authenticity of any induced changes. Thus, the difficult problem of the generalization of acquired functions, that is today central to any attempt at cognitive education (Arbitman-Smith, Haywood, & Bransford, 1984; Baumeister, 1984; Borkowski &

Cavanaugh, 1979; Spitz, 1986), has always been at the heart of the problem of operatory learning.

After the initial Genevan studies, the epistemological debate was very quickly abandoned in favor of attempts to analyze the mechanisms by which preoperatory behavior patterns were transformed into operatory ones (Inhelder, 1966; Inhelder & Sinclair, 1969; Inhelder, Sinclair, & Bovet, 1974). A virtual swarm of research followed, with some investigators challenging the relevance of Piagetian analysis and others trying to support it by refining its descriptions. These studies were concerned essentially with the operatory behavior patterns of conservation of numerical and physical invariants and with quantification of class inclusion.

Attempts to synthesize and integrate this line of research have been only partially successful and sometimes contradictory. This is due in part to the large number of studies, the diversity of their methods and goals, the divergence of results (due to a great diversity in evaluation criteria), as well as the many controversies that they have stimulated (Brainerd, 1977; Flavell, 1970; Laurendeau & Pinard, 1966; Lefebvre & Pinard, 1976; Orsini-Bouichou, 1975; Paour, 1979; Pascual-Leone, 1976; Pinard, 1981; Strauss, 1972).

With the exception of a relatively recent interest in the social dynamics of cognitive equilibration (Doise, Mugny, & Perret-Clermont, 1975; Fraysse, 1987; Gilly & Roux, 1984), this research seems today to have died out. There are three reasons for this: (a) in the absence of sufficiently coherent data, operatory learning has not become "the royal road" that had been wished for the detailed study of developmental mechanisms (Inhelder, Sinclair, & Bovet, 1974); (b) interest in operatory behavior patterns has diminished considerably in favor of approaches that stress functional and procedural description rather than underlying cognitive structures; and especially (c) the inability to resolve the critical problem of the sequelae of learning (Bideaud, 1985; Laurendeau-Bendavid, 1985; Vinh Bang, 1985).

Paour (1979) has reported a large group of studies on operatory learning conducted with mentally retarded or low socioeconomic status (SES) subjects, and it is these studies that are referred to in the remainder of this chapter. The relative concordance of their results, compared with those from studies conducted with normally developing children, is no indication that they are free of methodological difficulties and problems of interpretation.

Operatory learning might not have attained the goals set for it; nevertheless, one can extract four points that are important for cognitive education:

1. It is demonstrably possible to hasten the development of operatory behavior patterns to a much greater extent than Piaget thought possible.

2. Learning conducted within a constructivist paradigm attests to the relevance of methods focused on an active approach to tasks that induce cognitive conflicts.
3. The pretraining level of development turns out to be the clearest determinant of the efficacy of teaching.
4. Researchers have neglected Piaget's (1974) requirement of evaluating the effects of learning with respect to its integration into the subject's cognitive and behavioral repertoire, i.e., its functional aspect.

From Learning to Induction of Logic Structures

Induction Versus Learning of Logic Structures

Our choice of the term *induction* is deliberate, signifying the type of "operatory learning" intervention that we have used here and presented elsewhere (Desprels-Fraysse, Fraysse, Orsini-Bouichou, & Paour, 1979; Orsini-Bouichou, & Malacria-Rocco, 1978). Our basic method is to accelerate the development of operatory thought in order to understand its determinants better. The *goal* of our induction methods is to foster our subjects' accession to concrete logic. The *method* is to try to bring about a confluence of structural and functional conditions that underlie the subjects' own acquisition of operatory behavior sequences, rather than to teach them directly. Therefore, induction underscores, on the one hand, the mediational character of the intervention, and, on the other hand, the fact that one seeks by it to stimulate a general developmental process rather than a specific cognitive conflict.

A Description of Preoperatory Abilities: General Rule Systems

This original conceptualization of operatory learning rests on Orsini-Bouichou's (Orsini, 1965; Orsini-Bouichou, 1975, 1982; Orsini-Bouichou & Paour, 1986) description of the cognitive abilities of preoperatory children between 4 and 7 years of age.

Piaget himself recognized (Piaget, 1970; Piaget, Grize, Szeminska, & Vinh Bang, 1968) that preoperational thought had been essentially described as the absence or negative state of concrete operatory thought. It is this tendency in genetic epistemology to define a positive state in essentially negative terms that, in our opinion, accounts for the difficulty in describing the competencies of preoperatory children. Indeed, we know that the specific observational situations and questions that Piaget used do not permit one to retrace the stages of the construction of a concept beyond the beginning of the children's ability to assimilate those situations.

Proceeding from the hypothesis that the spontaneous behavior patterns of children reflect their development, Orsini-Bouichou (Orsini, 1965; Orsini-Bouichou, 1975, 1978, 1982) performed a methodological reversal. In place of the responses of children to questions posed by experimenters, she substituted a focus on the questions that the children themselves posed spontaneously. Using this approach, she constructed different experimental tasks in which the subjects freely organized quite simple materials,[1] without preconceived direction. With each task, in children as young as 3 to 4 years of age, she has observed some regularities in their organization of objects that qualify as true rules in that they are replicable, relatively transposable, and verbalizable as such. The comparison of rules observed in different experimental tasks has permitted the abstracting of general rule systems (called operators), each corresponding to a level of invariant. The establishment of the hierarchical evolution of these systems has made it possible to delineate the cognitive development of preoperatory children between 3 and 7 years of age.

Level I. This system of elementary rules supports the repeated application of a given pattern of action to a given end previously identified by the child: the child acts repeatedly upon a particular object selected to reflect a "making the same" relation. He/she performs a series of spontaneous activities (alignment of objects, repetition of a similar graphic or auditory production) out of which the child selects a relationship for its own sake, while ignoring the other ones. At this level, the child identifies objects in terms of their relationships with (other) identical objects.

Level II. The emergence of this stage reveals the establishment of a "pairing relationship," within which the child contrasts or combines one relation with another. Its primordial importance has been stressed elsewhere by Wallon (1942) and Piaget (Piaget et al., 1968). Given that the level I operator can be related to the emergence of a relationship of absolute identity between objects, the level II operator is characterized by the creation of paired elements of relative similarity and difference. This development reveals the interplay of opposite relations, alternation by opposites, and initial attempts at grouping and seriation. This relation, created on the basis of a minimal difference between the elements of a pair, does not lead immediately to the abstraction of a general and generalizable relationship. The child will depart only slowly and progressively from the organizing principle of "pairing." Based on their experimental induction of a system of level III rules (see discussion below) in level II normally developing children, Desprels-Fraysse and Fraysse (1977,

---

[1] It is not possible to describe these situations fully here; nevertheless, one can get the general idea from the description of the training situation presented below.

1978) have been able to describe several steps in children's progressive liberation from the initially facilitating but limiting "pairing" context. Desprels-Fraysse (1980, 1985, 1986) has supported their relevance with cross-observations gathered outside of the induction paradigm. Based on their description (Desprels-Fraysse & Fraysse, 1977), we focus here on the two extreme steps (level IIa and level IIb):

> In level IIa, children begin to generate pairing relations on the basis of observed differences, and are able to abstract, from the observation of a number of objects, a rule of dependency that still relies on the specific characteristics of the objects from which it was derived and thus does not yet correspond to a general rule based on a totally abstract criterion (and therefore does not hold for all the objects) (p. 143).

In level IIb,

> children impose a dependency relation on an increasingly large number and diversity of objects. They are able to extract the relevant relations from the totality of the objects' characteristics. The dependency rule always refers to objects, although the children can clarify the intervening values (p. 144).

Level III. This level is shown by the application of a relation of correspondence (similarity or difference) capable of generating a series of pairings: "It is a question of maintaining a configural invariant, under conditions of more and more complex modifications" (Orsini-Bouichou, 1975). These abstract relations, however, remain dependent on configuration of objects. This (level III) operator would be at the same developmental level as the intermediate period observed in the classical operatory tests of conservation, seriation, and classification.

Level IV. This level appears with concrete operatory behavior and reflects the ability to coordinate several rules of correspondence. At this level, children operate by creating relations within a system of relations. The invariants at this level are therefore independent of the configuration of objects.

The regularities on which these proposed general systems of rules are based have been demonstrated by induction studies as well as by both cross-sectional and longitudinal observations (Cunha de Carvalho, Hurtig, & Orsini-Bouichou, 1984; Desprels-Fraysse, 1980, 1985, 1986; Florès & Orsini-Bouichou, 1979; Noizet, 1965; Orsini-Bouichou, 1975, 1982; Orsini-Bouichou, Malacria-Rocco, & Rohrer, 1985). Two recent studies confirm the relevance of this model for describing the cognitive development of mentally retarded children (Soavi, 1986), and of Haitian children living in extremely deprived environments (Robeants, 1987).

Because these rule systems reflect a very general competence applicable to extremely diverse contexts and objects, Orsini-Bouichou suggests that their emergence is related to an organizing function. The appearance of each of them exerts a determining influence by means of reorganizing cognitive behavior sequences that bring about accession to higher levels of reasoning.

This conceptualization has led to a whole series of experiments on precocious induction of the next higher rule system (Cunha de Carvalho, 1983; Desprels-Fraysse & Fraysse, 1977; Florès & Orsini-Bouichou, 1979; Fraysse & Desprels-Fraysse, 1978; Orsini-Bouichou, 1975, 1978, 1985; Robeants, 1987). Conducted on normal children of 5 to 6 years of age, these experiments have demonstrated the relevance of the structural approach, and have supported the hypothesis of the organizing quality of the induction of these general rule systems. These studies have shown that the induced appearance of a new rule system leads in fact to some relatively general cognitive gains across various conceptual domains (number, classification, seriation, physical quantity, spatial relations). Although at the time of their emergence these general rule systems can help to define children's competence levels, once they have been established they lose this diagnostic quality, becoming nothing more than very general cognitive tools, and therefore can no longer be considered developmental stages in the Piagetian sense.

Fixations at the Preoperatory Level in the Mentally Retarded

This very description helps us also to understand better the retardation in the development of operatory thought in the mentally retarded. The eleven induction studies that we have done with mentally retarded persons[2] show that on Piagetian tests the control subjects gained little or nothing between pretest and final posttest. The number of posttests and the long interest intervals in some of our studies allowed us to use the term *immobility* in describing our subjects, as shown, for example, in study number 7. In 27 months, the level of logical reasoning in 9 of 11 control subjects, assessed by a large group of operatory tests, did not increase at all; still, this group of tests revealed some modest cognitive gain relative to the developmental period within which we were testing (Paour, 1981a). This immobility was all the more striking because these subjects had attained at pretest a level of reasoning that we considered to be relatively close to concrete operativity, and that their chronological ages (8 to 10 years) would lead one to believe that they were still in a period of relative intellectual growth.

These experiences led us to interpret this immobility as *the consequence of an abnormally long fixation at the level of a rule system that the subjects could not surpass spontaneously* (within the temporal limits of our observations). We use the term *fixation* to indicate that it is more a

---

[2] The list and principal characteristics can be found in Tables 5.1 through 5.5.

question of a true arresting of development than of a slowing such as one may observe in the curve of mental age gains. In fact, even if the subjects should be still capable of acquiring isolated information, their fixation would be revealed by their persistence in a stereotyped mode of general functioning.

Our attempts at induction, not only those that succeeded but especially those that failed, taught us that these fixations result from the interaction of structural and functional determinants.

At the structural level, there are some developmental stages that require profound reorganization of the preexisting rule system, and those stages would have formed the basis of the fixations. Thus, we have observed (Paour, 1980) that two major structural obstacles impede our mentally retarded subjects' accession to concrete operativity. The first relates to the abstraction of relatively generalized relations between elements of a series of pairings (passage from level IIa to level IIb). The second relates to the construction of invariants depending on a system of qualitative compensations[3] (passage from level III to level IV). These obstacles have been confirmed, respectively, by longitudinal (Soavi, 1986) and cross-sectional (Robeants, 1987) observation. In this chapter we analyze the first obstacle, because it is undoubtedly responsible for the most severe fixations and it led us to develop the intervention presented below. Moreover, it is that one that is used in the case study (Paour & Soavi, Chapter 18 in this volume) that complements this chapter.

This kind of structural obstacle can be described as a chronic difficulty in spontaneously establishing or inferring a relation between objects, facts, or situations in the absence of any context (time, causality, function, or custom) that would explicitly point to a relational dependency. Thus, it is a question of chronic difficulty in establishing or inferring concrete arbitrary relations. This kind of "putting into relationship" indicates cognitive operations so fundamental that one can easily understand that their development and use would be a necessary condition for progress in intellectual development. The psychology of intelligence has in fact taught us that the abstraction of arbitrary relations and the analogical reasoning that it makes possible constitute fundamental tools of human thought. Moreover, we know that mentally retarded persons have difficulty abstracting this type of relation, as work with Raven's Progressive Matrices (Raven, 1948) with this population has demonstrated.

---

[3] Piaget wrote about qualitative compensations in the context of conservation of physical quantities such as liquids: the child would induce the conservation by compensating with the dimensions "higher but less wide"; such a compensation remains qualitative because it is not quantified. When this type of reasoning is sufficiently common (in the child's repertoire) at the time of accession to concrete operativity, one can speak of a system of qualitative compensation in the manner of a mode of reasoning.

Our observations made in the course of our induction studies (Paour, 1980; Soavi, 1986) have permitted us to distinguish several levels of structural difficulty that testify to these fixations.

The first (and prerequisite) developmental level is characterized by the ability to abstract differences between objects that are sufficiently stable to form the basis of a logical relation. One may note that the degree of complexity of the relation is not at issue here; rather, one asks whether or not the subject can establish relations on the basis of differences *that he himself has identified*.

The second level is a central one. It corresponds to the understanding of the concept of pairing, that is, to the *ability to abstract a relation in the propitious and fundamental context of the pairing* (level IIa). It is a question of creating or seeking out an abstract connection that transcends that of the action that actually brings together the elements; e.g., a connection based on spatial or temporal proximity in which the bringing together (pairing) can be accomplished. The problems that retarded persons experience in this kind of cognitive activity have led us to think that *the concept of pairing, understood as a system and the locus of dependencies, constitutes in fact the matrix for the representation (abstraction) of many contextual or arbitrary relations*.

The third level is the *extension of this abstraction to a group of pairings (levels IIb and III)*. It represents a relation that is capable of producing and regulating groupings, and of anticipating, deducing, and expressing this relation in the form of a clearly presented verbal rule.

The fourth level is related to *various degrees of complexity in the coordination of relations among themselves*, first through sequencing and then by qualitative compensatory changes (level IV).

It is not possible to understand the phenomenon of fixations solely on the basis of these different levels of *structural* complexity. We must also consider its *functional* components.

Functional Aspects: The Hypothesis of Chronic Deficient Functioning

The ability to organize and to understand the world through searching out and/or creating arbitrary relations among its elements is a cognitive attitude that is clearly related to curiosity, motivational orientation, a need system, in fact to what Nuttin (1980) has called "functional dynamism." To be able to overcome structural obstacles requires a level of functioning that is sufficiently effective to insure: (a) *the mastery of the antecedent system* that in turn, by virtue of its autonomy and of its automaticity, will become a true cognitive tool; (b) *its intense and diversified application* to sufficiently different, disturbing, and difficult contexts as to insure the emergence of the cognitive conflicts that define the limits of this system and bring about its transformation; (c) *the process of abstracting a new structure of understanding* on the basis of emergent responses born out of attempts to resolve conflictful situations.

The fact that a child has available a cognitive tool (for example, the concept of pairing) is not sufficient to insure that he will be able to use that tool in a variety of situations. We have learned this with our retarded subjects who do not *spontaneously* apply a given cognitive principle but who are nevertheless able to use it when they are explicitly asked to do so. Indeed, many of our trained subjects have learned very quickly (Soavi, 1986), suggesting to us that they had the necessary cognitive structure but needed help only in learning to apply that structure.

The effectiveness of our interventions (Paour, 1980; Paour et al., 1985), as well as the increasingly detailed observation of the functional characteristics of different populations of children,[4] has led us to propose the hypothesis that prolonged abnormal fixations at the preoperatory level reflect a chronic condition of deficient cognitive functioning (Paour, 1988).

On the cognitive level, retarded persons are therefore characterized primarily by a chronic discrepancy between their level of development of cognitive competencies and the resources available for applying them spontaneously. Whatever their level of intellectual development, they have great difficulty in mobilizing their cognitive tools effectively. The very chronicity of their deficient cognitive functioning, whatever its determinants might be, contributes in important ways to the maintenance, and, especially in mildly retarded persons, to the very essence, of the delays and fixations in intellectual development.

In this general sense, this hypothesis is not original; on the contrary, it is consistent with some widespread contemporary conceptions (Brown & Campione, 1986; Feuerstein, Rand, & Hoffman, 1979; Haywood, 1987; Paris & Haywood, 1973; Sternberg & Spear, 1985). It raises anew some old controversies (Zigler, 1969), and is reminiscent of issues in the competence-performance distinction and the concept of pseudo-retardation.

This point of view may be able to reconcile two diametrically opposed theses in which mental retardation has been characterized either as a simple slowing of development (developmentally similar to younger non-retarded children; developmental model) or as the expression of a specific

[4](a) Rapidly developing children (Planche, 1984a); (b) children who have been exposed to either flexible or rigid parental educational practices (Cunha de Carvalho, 1983); (c) socioeconomically disadvantaged children (Palacio–Quintin, 1987; Robeants, 1987); and (d) mentally retarded children in the course of induction of logic structures (Soavi, 1986), in experiments on LOGO programming (Paour, Cabrera, & Roman, 1985), and on treatment of an exploratory task not completed by the experimenter (Paour, 1988).

qualitative difference (deficit model). At the psychological level, mental retardation seems to us to be characterized simultaneously by a simple slowed development, i.e., in the development of cognitive structures, and by a difference in the manner in which the cognitive structures are ultimately applied.

Without wishing to emphasize an exclusively functional interpretation of mental retardation, we must recognize, within the Piagetian constructivest framework, the importance of cognitive functioning in integrating and serving as a mediator of other kinds and levels of determinants. This view of cognitive functioning as mediator implies that the cognitive structures develop independently of their initial determinants. This is why, together with Ellis and Cavalier (1982), Baumeister (1984), Sternberg and Spear (1985), and Kahn (1985), but contrary to the position of Zigler (1969, 1972), we do not believe that the experimental support of the hypotheses of similar sequence and similar structure between retarded and nonretarded persons (Weisz, Yeates, & Zigler, 1982; Weisz & Zigler, 1979) enables one to reject the deficit hypothesis. We do not, however, wish to rush to the interpretation of observed differences between retarded and nonretarded persons as the direct and immediate result of neurologic deficits. In this matter, cognitive functioning, through its mediating role, assures relative independence of etiologic conditions and intellectual efficiency (Feuerstein, Rand, & Hoffman, 1979; Haywood & Wachs, 1981; D'Erario & Pollicina, 1988), and compels us to take into account the role of noncognitive determinants. Even if Zigler would not totally support a motivational theory of mental retardation, he would agree that certain aspects of cognitive *functioning* have a very direct and permanent effect on the construction of cognitive *tools*. Only by employing a well-controlled intervention, focused on the modification of functioning rather than on the simplification of the tasks, can we begin to understand the differences in learning and performance efficiency[5] so frequently observed between retarded and nonretarded persons who are matched on mental age.

Our observations of functional difficulties suggest that these difficulties lie at the level of information input and the normative control of information processing (Paour, 1988). These observations are consistent with data from the experimental literature (Ellis, 1970; Spitz & Borys, 1984; Zeaman & House, 1979) and also with the observations of Feuerstein et al. (1979). These observations have contributed to the development of the intervention principles and techniques that we present in the next sections.

---

[5] It is clear that it is not a question of holding themselves to performances *per se* but to procedures and strategies that have been put into operation.

General Principles and Method of Induction of Logic Structures

We describe in this section the principles and method of induction of logic structures that we have used in our studies. In doing so we rely on the technique (D'Erario & Pollicina, 1988; Paour, 1975, 1980, 1985; Robeants, 1987; Soavi, 1986) that we call "training in abstraction and coordination of transformation rules."

Choosing Critical Objectives: Beginning with Fixations

As our studies on operatory learning have shown, any developmental treatment must take into account the initial level of the subjects. In our situations that means helping retarded persons to overcome their somewhat stereotyped use of rule systems that describe their fixations at the preoperatory level. The goal of our intervention is therefore to bring about effective use of cognitive systems that are already in place in order to stimulate the development of systems at the next higher level.

Inducing an Autonomous Knowledge Structure

In this intervention we try to induce the construction of the pairing concept as a prerequisite to the abstraction of arbitrary, contextual relations. We do not set out to solve our subjects' problems directly by helping or teaching them to solve such problems as Raven's matrices. Others have shown (Budoff, 1967; Feuerstein et al., 1979; Hurting, 1969) that it is quite possible to make rapid improvement in the performance of mildly retarded persons on this type of problem, and that such improvement bears witness to their cognitive potential. However, we are not so much seeking immediate success as a profound transformation in the subjects that will enable them ultimately to solve such problems by themselves, without need of specific help and in varied contexts. In other words, it is a question not only of stimulating their developmental potential, but also of helping them to apply that potential effectively.

The Intervention Situation

Our strategy is to present a situation in which the active treatment brings about a degree of understanding of *relations of dependency*, independent of any causal, functional, or spatial context. Toward this end, we have conceived a situation of transformation of an object into another object that meets three precise criteria: (a) to evoke a systematic comparison of the objects before and after the transformation, (b) to bring about the interpretation of the transformations as dependencies whose regularities can be observed and whose rules can be abstracted, and (c) to bring about the coordination of these rules by sequencing and then by way of compensatory changes.

The apparatus consists of a box that we call the "transformation box" (50 cm × 30 cm × 20 cm; see Figure 5.1) and several groups of varied objects that serve as transformation materials.

The transformation box has four compartments distributed as follows:

Subject side. (a) An opening on the top (entrance) for putting in the objects, and (b) an opening at the bottom (exit) for taking out the objects that the experimenter has substituted for those the subjects put in at the top. The bottom opening has a hinged door whose purpose is to keep the subjects' attention focused on the returned objects, at least at the beginning of the intervention.

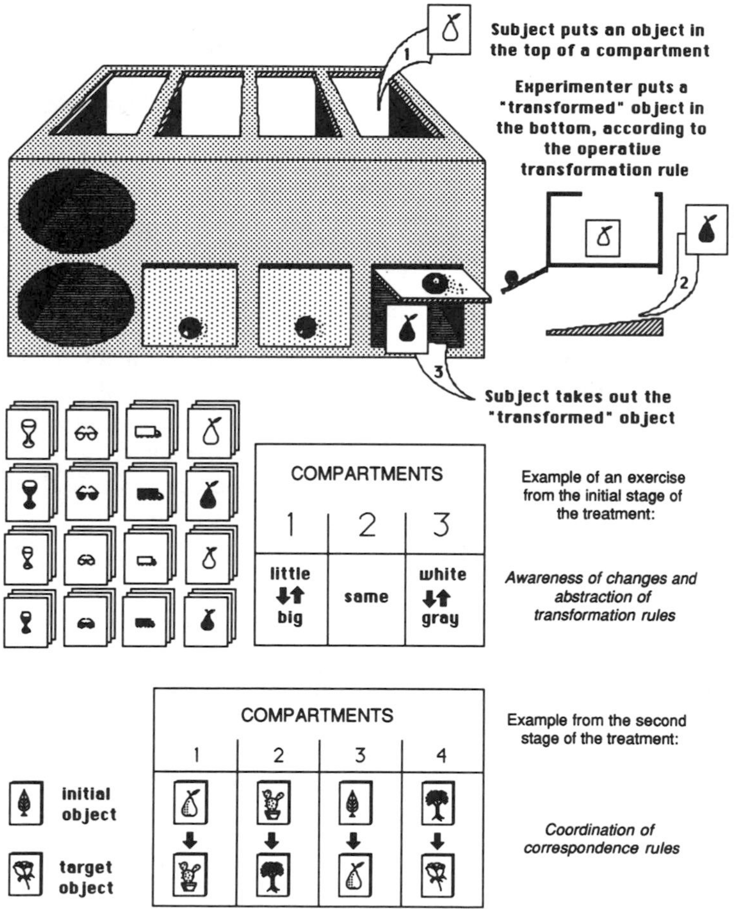

FIGURE 5.1. The transformation box.

Experimenter side. Two distinct levels: the objects that the subjects put in stay in the top level; the bottom level is for substituting the objects that the subjects then retrieve.

During practice, subjects only see their side of the box and therefore, do not witness the substitution of the objects that they have put in the box. Depending on the task, the compartments not in use are blocked by a piece of cardboard.

Subjects and experimenters have identical sets of objects. Depending on the task, each set may consist of: (a) small familiar objects (nails, pins, chalk); (b) little toys (beads, cars, figures); (c) cardboard forms (persons, animals); and (d) paper geometric figures.

For each compartment, throughout each game, there is a correspondence rule that relates the objects put in the box by the subjects to those given back by the experimenter. The difficulty of each exercise is a function of (a) the number of compartments in use, (b) the nature of the correspondence rules, (c) the kinds of objects, (d) the properties that are to be transformed, and eventually (e) the type of coordination required.

Practice Paradigm

During practice, this standard paradigm is employed, with adaptations appropriate to the objectives of the various phases of the intervention. Each exercise can include up to six phases, depending on each subject's success and on the level of difficulty of the problems.

Material Description and Organization

The objects are laid out in an unsystematic array, and the subjects are asked to describe them. When their descriptions lack precision or accuracy, the experimenter helps them by presenting pairs of objects chosen for their capacity to bring about the abstraction of the relevant properties of the objects. However, the experimenter never verbalizes the relevant characteristics.

Spontaneous Activity

Subjects organize their activity freely by placing the objects of their choice into the compartments of their choice, with the experimenter intervening only when necessary to keep the action going.

First Verbalization

Subjects are asked some general questions, such as "Tell me, what does the box do?" or "Explain to me what happens in each compartment." Without actually giving the answers, the experimenter gives feedback appropriate to the degree of relevance and generalization of each response, for example, "It's not quite that way, you have to think about it some more."

Guided Activity

Choice of objects and of compartments is always under the control of the subjects, but the experimenter tries to improve their functioning by using a series of prompts. These include pointing out that there are other compartments that can be explored, suggesting looking at an object before putting it into a compartment, asking for a description of an object, asking why a particular object has been selected, asking what object the subject thinks is going to be returned, suggesting use of rules that have been abstracted earlier in the exercise. The assistance provided is limited to the functional aspects of the task and never addresses its cognitive aspects.

Second Verbalization

One proceeds as in the first verbalization: "What does the box do?" "Explain to me what happens in each compartment."

Anticipation

Subjects must anticipate the outcome of a series of transformations of different kinds (direct, reverse, using new objects, using new and incongruous objects). Transformations are not actually made during this phase and correct answers are not provided. The purpose is to check the generality and solidity of the subjects' understanding of the principles they have learned up to that point.

Coordinations

As soon as the subjects are capable of abstracting sufficiently generalizable transformation rules, the experimenter presents exercises that require the coordination, either by succession or by compensation, of previously abstracted rules. *Coordination by succession* refers to exercises in which the subjects have to coordinate previously abstracted transformation rules where the task is to accomplish the necessary transformations, but in no particular sequence. Example: In one exercise there are three possible transformation rules (large ↔ small; red ↔ blue; thick ↔ thin), and the subjects must transform a red, large, and thick object into one that is red, small, and thin. It is sufficient to use only the large ↔ small and thick ↔ thin compartments. Sequence is irrelevant, and there is no type of qualitative compensation that one has to make just to carry out the two correct transformations. *Coordination by compensation* requires taking account of the order in which the transformations that the subjects have already abstracted are put into play. Example: The problem is to deepen the color (redder, for example) and increase the thickness; make the object larger; make the object less thick. The subjects must transform one object by deepening its color, by increasing its size, but not by changing its thickness. In this case, the order of the transformations is important because it is necessary to *compensate* the thickening that is necessarily linked to deepening the color.

Training Procedure

The training comprises five stages. Each stage consists of exercises of increasing difficulty. The number of exercises of the same degree of difficulty depends on the progress of the subjects. The sequence is shown in Figure 5.2.

1. The first step in this sequence is *to bring about the representation of changes* in terms of the relationship of dependency that ties the object that was put into the top of the box to the transformed object that comes out at the bottom, by (a) familiarizing the subjects with the task; (b) calling for systematic comparison of the object before and after transformation; and (c) bringing about the abstraction of the connection (between the objects) in the form of a change, a transformation, or an exchange, of which one can notice the regularities and abstract the rules.
2. The second step is to complete the abstract dependencies in terms of changes by the *abstraction of constant properties that remain in spite of the transformations* (for example, to understand that in Figure 5.2 the nature of the object does not change).
3. The third step is to bring about the abstraction of *subtle and relative dependent relations that lie on a continuum of transformation (more or less)*.
4. The fourth step is to obtain a given object *by successive transformations of an initial object*.
5. The fifth step is to obtain a given object *by compensation of transformation rules*: when the transformation rules in effect at a given moment work against the ability to obtain a designated object immediately, it is necessary to counterbalance their (the active rules') respective effects by being willing to distance oneself temporarily from the target object with respect to certain dimensions. (See previous explanation of *coordination by succession* and *coordination by compensation*.)

It is reasonable to ask how our intervention strategies actually follow principles derived from our conceptualization of the structural and functional aspects of fixation. Here are those principles:

1. Begin with fixations and set up training stages based on our knowledge of the genesis of rule systems that one seeks to induce.
2. Never give answers; change the initial task in case of persistent difficulty; leave to the materials the role of confirming the subjects' actions; assess continuously the degree of understanding and generalization of what has been learned.

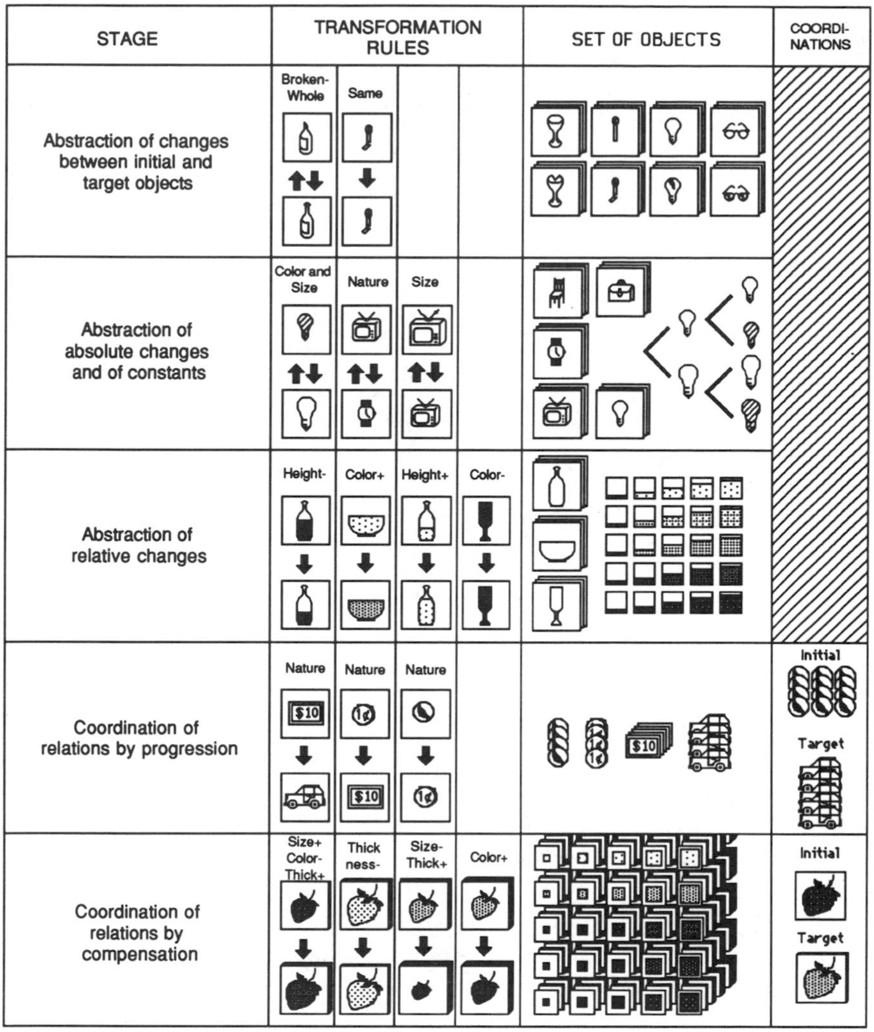

FIGURE 5.2. Sample exercise, showing each step in the intervention.

3. Support and guide the subjects' functioning by (a) individualizing the intervention, (b) clarifying the situation without at any time minimizing the planning and control aspects of the action, and (c) guiding the subjects' performance.

Studies

We have conducted 12 separate studies since 1967. The designs of these are presented in Tables 5.1 to 5.5. We emphasize here those methodological characteristics that may help readers to understand both the

TABLE 5.1. Studies: List and groups.

Study No.	Authors	Year[a]	Groups[b]	Sex M	Sex F	No. of Immigrants[c]	Institutions[d]	Status[e]
1	Castellan & Paour (1968)	67–68	NT = 20	20				
			NC = 20	20				
			RT = 35	35		6	CCA	12
2	Chevalier & Grimaldi (1972)	71–72	RT = 8	8		1	CCA	4
			RC = 8	8		1	CCA	4
3	Julien, Magagli, & Tosti (1972)	71–72	RT = 8	7	1		CCA	
			RC = 7	6	1		CCA	
4	Paour (1980)	74–76	RT = 20	9	11	4	SPC	
			RC = 22	11	11	3	SPC	
5	Chevalier & Grimaldi (Paour, 1980)	74–76	RT1 = 6	6			CCA	3
			RT2 = 6	6			WCA	3
			RC1 = 6	6			CCA	3
			RC2 = 6	6			WCA	3
6	Castellan, Grégoire, & Poli (1976)	75–77	NT = 10	8	2	1	CCA	
			RT = 10	8	2	3	CCA	6
7	Paour (1980)	76–79	NT = 6	3	3			
			NC = 6	3	3			
			RT = 11	8	3	0	CCA	5
			RC = 11	10	1	1	CCA	4
8	Paour (1982)	80–82	RT = 11	6	5	4	SSC	
			RC = 11	6	5	5	SSC	
9	Galas, Sidérakis, & Soavi (1981)	80–83	RT1 = 10	5	5	5	NIS	
			RT2 = 10	7	3	5	NIS	
			RC = 10	5	5	6	NIS	
10	Foul & Malika (1982)	81–82	RT = 8	4	4		CCA	
			RC = 8	4	4		CCA	
11	Soavi (1986)	82–84	RT = 11	7	4	4	NIS	
			RC = 11	6	5	3	NIS	
12	Colognola, D'Erario, Gigli, Grubar, Ferri, Pollicina, Paour, & Soavi (D'Erario & Pollicina, 1988)	86–88	RT1 = 5	5			CCA	5
			RT2 = 5	5			CCA	5
			RC1 = 5	5			CCA	5
			RC2 = 5	5			CCA	5

[a] Years of the study.
[b] N: nonretarded subjects; R: retarded subjects; T: trained; C: control.
[c] Subjects from North African immigrant families.
[d] CCA: private center for children or adolescents; SPC: special class in primary regular school system;
NIS: special nonintegrated school of the regular school system; SSC: special class in secondary regular school system; WCA: private work center for adults.
[e] Number living in the institution during the week.

meaning and the strength of our results. We are fully aware that it is not easy to gather irrefutable evidence on the subject of developmental plasticity and cognitive modifiability (Arbitman-Smith et al., 1984; Baumeister, 1984; Blackman & Lin, 1984; Bradley, 1983; Burden, 1987; Savell, Twohig, & Rachford, 1986; Spitz, 1986).

Aims

Although we do rely on common problems and methods, our research has also been characterized by systematic variations across studies that reveal their progression. These stages are (a) investigating first the developmental plasticity of mentally retarded persons who are fixated at preoperatory levels (studies 1, 2, and 3); (b) taking into account both chronological age and severity of retardation with children at the same initial level of preoperativity (studies 4, 5, 8, and 9); (c) comparison with nonretarded children of the same initial preoperativity level who are given the same training (6 and 7); (d) in-depth analysis of the induced gains at the level of functional characteristics (8, 11, and 12); (e) adaptation of the training procedures to a lower level of initial performance than in the early studies (10 and 11); (f) studying some organically retarded persons, and searching for neurophysiological concomitants of the induced gains (12); (g) steady improvement of the intervention through individualization (of the methods and sequences) and increasingly precise specification of the functional difficulties of our retarded subjects (8, 9, 11, and 12). These studies are listed in Table 5.1.

Subjects

By now we have worked with a total of 274 retarded subjects, of whom 164 were in the different experimental groups (and thus received training) and 110 were control subjects. Across all the studies, three-fourths were boys. The subjects' ages at pretest were between 6 and 20 years. Table 5.2 shows the medians and ranges of chronological age, mental age, and IQ of the subjects by study.

All of our subjects were in either public or private special education classes. The selection criterion that we added to that of special class placement was that they perform at a preoperatory level on a group of Piagetian tests. The general agreement that we observed, first among the Piagetian tests themselves, and then between the group of Piagetian tests and traditional psychometric criteria, led us to think that our subjects were characterized by relatively generalized and homogeneous developmental retardation.

In terms of IQ (see Table 5.2), scores on the New Metric Test of Intelligence (*Nouvelle Echelle Métrique de l'Intelligence*; Zazzo, Gilly, & Verba-Rad, 1966)[6] placed the majority of our subjects in the mildly retarded range. The others were for the most part scattered across the moderately retarded range, with a few posting IQs above 68. Our chief criterion was preintervention level with respect to general rule systems. Our training method required a minimal level of reasoning that, up to

---

[6] Revision of the Binet-Simon scales.

TABLE 5.2. Chronological age, mental age, and IQ (median and extreme values).

Study No.	Chronological age[a]			Mental age[b]			IQ[c]		
	Low	Med	High	Low	Med	High	Low	Med	High
1	6-3	6-6	6-9						
	6-3	6-6	6-9						
	8-0	12-0	16-0	*6-3*	*7-6*	*8-6*	*50*	*61*	*73*
2	10-7	11-6	12-9	7-0	7-7	8-0	57	65	72
	10-0	11-5	12-9	6-3	7-0	8-0	49	63	70
3	6-0	7-3	8-9	2-10	3-3	4-9	40	47	56
	6-0	7-3	8-9	2-9	3-6	4-6	38	45	58
4	8-0	9-4	10-8	5-3	6-6	7-6	55	67	76
	9-6	7-10	10-8	5-3	6-6	7-6	55	67	76
5	10-0	11-6	13-6	6-0	6-9	7-6	48	54	61
	15-4	19-0	20-0	6-3	7-2	7-6	42	43	52
	10-0	11-6	13-6	6-3	6-6	7-9	49	58	66
	15-6	19-2	20-0	6-0	6-9	8-0	40	45	53
6	5-1	5-5	5-9	5-0	5-5	5-10	95	99	107
	8-6	9-8	11-4	5-2	5-7	6-0	48	55	65
7	5-6	5-9	5-11	5-2	5-7	6-3	92	98	112
	5-4	5-8	5-10	5-0	5-7	6-6	87	99	116
	8-0	9-2	10-1	5-2	5-10	6-3	53	63	72
	8-3	9-3	10-8	5-0	5-10	6-6	47	60	73
8	14-2	14-8	15-1	6-6	7-6	8-6	51	65	73
	13-8	14-6	15-0	6-9	7-6	9-0	55	63	75
9	10-1	12-5	14-11	5-10	7-0	8-3	40	55	72
	10-0	12-6	14-9	6-3	6-11	8-9	45	55	68
	9-8	12-10	14-10	5-7	7-0	8-3	46	58	66
10	8-6	10-0	13-2	4-6	6-6	7-0	45	58	66
	9-0	10-2	13-0	4-8	6-6	6-9	42	55	67
11	8-5	10-4	13-10	4-7	6-6	7-6	47	60	67
	9-0	11-5	13-0	5-5	6-6	7-3	46	60	67
12	10-4	12-0	13-2	4-9	6-2	6-7	40	50	64
	8-0	13-0	14-0	4-9	6-2	6-7	39	51	60
	8-6	12-9	13-7	5-4	6-6	6-9	40	48	73
	9-10	10-9	14-9	5-0	6-0	6-9	45	50	60

[a] In years and months.
[b] NEMI (see the text); MA, in italics, derived from WISC (total score).
[c] NEMI; in italics, WISC Full Scale IQ.

now, has prevented us from working with subjects below the range of moderate mental retardation.

Except for study 12, in which 14 of the 20 subjects were diagnosed as having demonstrable organic pathology, we had no valid etiologic information. We can only say that virtually all of them lacked visible evidence of central nervous system pathology.

More than three-quarters of the subjects came from deprived socio-economic conditions but for the most part lived with their families. The percentage from North African immigrant families (who constitute a large part of the special education population in the south of France, comparable to "minority ethnic" status in the United States) varied across studies from 10 to 50.

Methodological Observations

With the exception of study 4, the samples in each study were rather small; however, their results appeared to be valid for the following reasons:

1. The number of studies, and especially their sequencing, permits us to specify some *replicable* conditions, that yield *reproducible* effects, of inducing logic structures in mentally retarded persons. We emphasize here that the relevance of an intervention is never as obvious as when it allows one to overcome a previously well-recognized cognitive obstacle. Thus, our final studies (9, 11, and 12) extend the training to subjects at an initial developmental level that in our previous studies (2, 6, and 10) would have been too low for the subjects to benefit from the intervention.
2. These studies (except study 9) avoid the major methodological problem of operatory learning and of attempts to enhance cognitive functioning and development. In fact, the induced gains correspond *by the nature of the tasks* to a far transfer inasmuch as: (a) the pretest and posttest instruments differed from the training situations with respect to materials, tasks, and types of questioning (for example, we do not use classic conservation questions such as "Is there more, the same, or less of ——— than of ———?"); (b) during training, we never teach the answers (except for group RT-1 of study 9).
3. The Piagetian operatory tests are indices of cognitive development that are known for their diagnostic validity and their reliability. In an intervention context, we have wanted to improve these measurement characteristics (reliability and validity) in the following ways: (a) each test has been designed to include several situations or questions (up to nine in the test of conservation of mass); (b) each test includes transformation of high-intensity stimuli; (c) any answer at the operatory level is followed routinely by a counterargument; (d) the level is inferred qualitatively from the totality of the answers (for example, to be assessed as conserving, the subjects must give only conservation answers and also refute all the counterarguments in a relevant fashion).
4. The literature on operatory learning suggests that the Piagetian tests are probably less sensitive to the effects of experimenters' expectations and attitudes than are intelligence tests. Moreover, the perseveration of relatively long-term fixations observed in our control groups, as well as in those of Lister (1969, 1970, 1972) and of Field (1974, 1977, 1979), suggests that practice effects are quite weak in these groups in spite of sometimes large numbers of posttests.

5. Because of the longitudinal follow-up after a number (often large) of training sessions (from 3 to 24, depending on the study) undertaken over long time periods (from $1\frac{1}{2}$ months to 17 months), we have been able to give detailed descriptions of the progress of individual subjects. Characteristics of these studies, content of pre- and posttests, nature of the control groups, and control for experimenter effects are listed in Tables 5.3, 5.4, and 5.5. As one can see from the case study (Paour & Soavi, Chapter 18 in this volume), we can relate the posttest results to the various indicators of development, efficiency, and functioning gathered during the intervention.
6. Several deferred posttests, separated by periods from 1 month to 1 and even 2 years after the end of the intervention (studies 7, 9), permitted us to assess the extended durability of the induced gains, and thus to confer on them some "ecological validity" (Baumeister, 1984).
7. Our results are otherwise largely corroborated by studies in which operatory learning of a more traditional nature has been used (Paour, 1979).

It is worth noting that study 12, still in progress, has been carried out by investigators (D'Erario & Pollicina, 1988) who are independent of our own research team, so one can perhaps have even more confidence in the conclusions.

Effectiveness and Limitations of the Method of Induction of Logic Structures

By comparison with control group subjects, most of whom remained fixated at their initial preoperatory levels, the trained subjects showed a relative but quite clear developmental plasticity. The training induced in them the construction of elementary logic structures that they had not constructed spontaneously. A large group of indices (explored in the following sections) point to the conclusion that these induced gains were of a truly structural nature.

Progression of the Training

Analysis of individual subjects reveals two strikingly different patterns of progression that point to an "all or nothing" effect.

The first pattern characterizes subjects who progressed little or not at all throughout the intervention. Their responses stayed at the same level from the first to the last session, and the Piagetian posttests confirmed this lack of gain. Neither the repetition of the exercises (from 3 to 24 times according to the study) nor the guiding of their functioning was sufficient to improve their solving and their understanding of the tasks.

TABLE 5.3. Characteristics of the intervention.

Study No.	Number of Subjects	Sessions Duration[a]	Sessions Staggering[b]	Sessions' content[c] 1	2	3	4	5	6
1	3	1.5	1.5				3		
	3	1.5	1.5				3		
2	20	10	4	7	7	3	3		
3	20	10	4	8	6	6			
4	20	10	5		7	10	3		
5	6	3	2.5				3	3	
	6	3	2.5				3	3	
6	6	3	2.5				6		
	6	3	2.5						
7	6	3	4				3	3	
	6	3	4				3	3	
8	6	3	4				6		
9	6	3	2.5						6
	6	3	2.5						6
10	6	3	2.5					6	
11	24	12	17		12	12			
12	24	12	6		12	6			
	24	12	6		12	6			

[a] Total duration of sessions in hours.
[b] Staggering from the first to the last session in months.
[c] 1: Equalization exercises by one to one correspondence and comprehension exercises of "more, same, and less" (Paour, 1980).
2: Abstraction of transformation rules (described in text).
3: Coordination of transformation rules (described in text).
4: Quantitative covariation exercises (Orsini-Bouichou, 1975, 1978).
5: Qualitative covariation exercises (Orsini-Bouichou, 1975, 1978).
6: Learning conservation of volume: group E1 (sessions adapted from Field, 1974); group E2 (Lefebvre & Pinard, 1972).

Moreover, our adherence to the principle of not giving the correct answers but instead allowing them to express their own constructions helps to explain the stereotypy of their behavior sequences. These subjects showed fixations comparable to those observed in the control groups. When the majority of the subjects failed to progress, as in studies 3 and 10, they confirmed the structural composition of their fixations by revealing that the training had not been adapted to the subjects' own developmental levels. This suggested that we should alter the intervention, as we did in studies 11 and 12 with our training on abstraction and on coordination of transformation rules.

The second pattern relates to *those subjects who did improve*. There were, to be sure, individual differences in magnitude of gains among those subjects who did progress; nevertheless, there was a sharp contrast between those who made gains, usually quite significant ones, and those who did not make gains. Like Anne, the subject of the case study in Chapter 18 (Paour & Soavi, this volume), the subjects who did make

TABLE 5.4. Pre- and Posttests content.[a]

Tests	Studies 1	2	3	4	5	6	7	8	9	10	11	12
Piagetian tests												
1. Number conservation												
Eggs & egg-cup							3					
Tokens			01	012		012	3		01234	01		01
Beads		01	01	012	012		0123	012	01234		01234	01
2. Physical quantities conservation												
Liquid						012						
Clay	01	01		012	012	012	0123	012	01234	01	01234	
Length	01						3					
Area									3		34	
Dissociation of weight/volume							3	02			34	
3. Class												
Classification		01	01	012			012					
Class inclusion		01		012	012		023	02				
4. Spatial relations												
Rotation of beads				012			0123					
Doll in landscape				012			0123					
Other tests												
NEMI		01		02	012	0	023	02	0	0	03	01
WISC	0		0	02								
Raven's Standard Matrices											0123	01
Passive sentences task				012								
Tower of Hanoi								02			0234	01

[a] Numbers in the table refer to pretest (0) and posttests (1 to 4) (see Table 5.5).

TABLE 5.5. Posttests, nature of control group, and experimenter effect.

Study No.	Number	Posttests[a] 1	2	3	4	Relations with control subjects[b]	Experimenter effect controlled[c]
1	2	2.5	3			No	No
	2	2.5	3			No	No
	1	3					
2	1	4.75					
	1	4.75				Yes	No
3	1	4.75					
	1	4.75				Yes	No
4	2	3.5	12				
	2	3.5	12			Yes	Total
5	2	3.5	12				
	2	3.5	12				
	2	3.5	12			Yes	No
	2	3.5	12			Yes	No
6	2	3.5	12				No
	2	3.5	12				No
7	3	7	15	27			
	3	7	15	27		Yes	Total
	3	7	15	27			
	3	7	15	27		Yes	Total
8	2	3.5	12				
	2	3.5	12			Yes	Partial
9	4	3	12	24	*36*		
	4	3	12	24	*36*		
	4	3	12	24	*36*	Yes	No
10	1	3.5					
	1	3.5				Yes	No
11	4	7	12	19	24		
	4	7	12	19	24	Yes	No
12	1	7	?				
	1	7	?				
	1	7	?			Yes	No
	1	7	?			Yes	No

[a] Interval in months from the beginning of the pretest; italics: indicates part of the initial group; ?: experiment still going on.
[b] Yes: the control subjects received the same number of individual sessions and time with an experimenter as the trained subjects.
[c] No: people who give the posttest tasks know to what group the subjects belong, partial: people giving the task are just informed about the general purpose of the research but not about the composition of the groups; total: people give the task without any relevant information.

gains often leapt past several targeted ontogenetic stages, and the posttests indicated that their cognitive gains were relatively generalized.

This bimodal effect is characteristic of the operatory learning situations for which we know the effectiveness of the intervention to be influenced by the subjects' initial level of development. A posteriori analysis of the results in terms of those at preoperatory levels, presented earlier, leads us to the same conclusion.

Thus, the data from studies 4, 5, 6, 7, 8, and 10, in which the initial level of preoperativity was evaluated *in terms of general rule systems* and in which the intervention comprised three and six sessions of exercises of quantitative covariations (Orsini-Bouichou, 1975; Orsini-Bouichou & Malacria-Rocco, 1978) permit us to reach the following conclusions:

1. None of the subjects ($N = 21$) whose initial level was less than level II made significant progress, whatever the number of training sessions.
2. Attainment of level IIb is apparently a sufficient condition for the effectiveness of this training. All of the subjects ($N = 19$) whose pretest level was at least IIb attained level IV (demonstrated by success on the test of conservation of mass) following the intervention.
3. Attainment of level IIa constitutes a necessary, but not sufficient, condition for the induction. Only 50% of these subjects ($N = 30$) attained level IV within the time limits of the longitudinal follow-up.

This last condition is itself relative to the characteristics of the intervention. In fact, the result of study 11 show that it is possible to improve the training designed for subjects at level IIa. The 10 subjects at this level made significant progess as a function of the training, previously described, on the transformation box. Further, some more conventional Piagetian learning (study 9) was shown to be quite effective at this level of preoperativity.

Effects of Training

Stable and Generalized Induction of Operatory Behavior Sequences

Induction of Authentic Operatory Behavior Patterns

The authenticity of the cognitive gains brought about by operatory learning has often been questioned. Pascual-Leone (1976) has interpreted, for example, the results of Lefebvre and Pinard (1972) as the product of a reduction in the degree of difficulty of the conservation tests. He claimed that by automatizing attention to the relevant dimensions of the tasks, the instruction would permit the solving of the conservation tasks with minimal mental effort. According to this point of view, the operatory behavior patterns that follow operatory learning would not have the same meaning as would behavior patterns that had been acquired spontaneously. The methodological precautions described previously in this chapter, as well as the difference between the training and the criterion tests used to measure the training effects, argue solidly against this interpretation.

Our interventions are the basis of a qualitative behavior gain that is subsequently reflected in the Piagetian tests. After the intervention, the subjects in fact exhibit concrete operatory behavior sequences, whereas at pretest they had shown typical preoperatory behavior. Table 5.6 shows these results on the conservation tests.

Three types of observations from our data support the conclusion that the subjects achieved a true understanding of the concepts in question. The first is the stability of the operatory behavior sequences in all the configurations of the same tests, and thus in the face of some extreme modifications. The second is their relevant refutations of the counter-arguments. The third is the diversity of the operatory arguments that the subjects used to support their responses to the conservation questions and to the counterartuments.

The magnitude of change, as well as the rapidity of progress attained, varied across subjects; however, looking only at the conservation tests, studies 2, 4, 5, 7, 8, and 11 offered us two important global results[7]:

1. The 65 trained subjects succeeded at the last posttest on three times as many of the conservation tests as did the 69 control subjects.
2. At the last posttest, 72% of the trained subjects, but only 17% of the control subjects, attained the operatory level on the conservation of mass test.

These gains seem important to us because acquisition of any *invariant*, whether qualitative, relational, numerical, or physical, represents a particularly decisive developmental step. Such a step is, first of all, a necessary step for the construction of the given ideational domain, and, once separated from the specific context in which it had been abstracted, it then becomes a general cognitive tool. The gains are important as well because they constitute evidence that it is possible to remove the structural and functional obstacles that are the basis of fixations at the preoperatory level of development.

Relatively Generalized Induction of Operatory Behavior

Considered individually, isolated gains do not necessarily lead to the conclusion that one has achieved truly structural changes. The appearance of an invariant can no longer be interpreted as an indicator of a generalized accession to a higher mode of reasoning. We present in the

[7] We do not include here the subjects from studies 2 and 8, nor from the RT-2 group of study 5, who did not receive an intervention adapted to their level (less than II or IIa), as well as subjects from study 12 from whom we do not yet have posttest data immediately following the end of their training.

TABLE 5.6. Results of conservation tasks[a].

Study			Pretest					Posttest 1					Posttest 2								Posttest 3								Posttest 4				
No.	Group	*n*	CH	BE	LI	CL	LE	CH	BE	LQ	CL	LE	CH	BE	LQ	CL	LE	SF	V1	V2	EG	CH	BE	CL	LE	SF	V1	V2	BE	CL	SF	V1	V2
1	NT	20				0	0				5	4																					
	NC	20				0	0				3	3																					
	RT	35				0	0				11	26																					
2	RT	8		0		0			6		6																						
	RC	8		0		0			1		1																						
3	RT	8	0	0				4	2																								
	RC	9	0	0				0	0																								
4	RT	20	4	3		0		14	12		5		19	16		16																	
	RC	22	7	9		0		10	10		1		13	11		6																	
5	RT1	6		0		0			6		6			6		6																	
	RC1	6		0		0			0		0			0		0																	
	RT2	6		0		0			0		0			0		0																	
	RC2	6		0		0			0		0			0		0																	
6	NT	10	2		0	0		2		0	0		4		3	1																	
	RT	10	1		0	0		2		0	0		5		3	2																	
7	NT	6		0		0			1		0			3		3					5	4	4	4	4		3	1					
	NC	6		0		0			0		0			4		4					6	5	5	5	5		4	0					
	RT	11		0		0			2		0			6		3					9	7	6	5	3		1	0					
	RC	11		0		0			1		0			1		0					3	3	1	1	0		0	0					

8	RT	11		4	0		7		5		10		7	7	6	1	5										
	RC	11		5	0		5		3		5		4	2	2	2	1										
9	RT1	10	1	0	0	7	9		6	9	8		7					9	8	7	4						
	RT2	10	2	0	0	6	6		2	7	7		4					7	7	4	0						
	RC	10	3	0	0	4	1		1	4	1		1					4	3	2	0						
10	RT	8	0		0	0			0																		
	RC	8	0		0	0			0																		
11	RT	11		0	0		3	3			0	3							8	4	4	1	8	7	5	0	3
	RC	11		0	0		0	0			0	0							0	0	0	0	0	0	0	0	0
12	RT1	5	0	0		2	1																				
	RT2	5	1	0		3	3																				
	RC1	5	0	0		0	0																				
	RC2	5	0	0		0	0																				

[a] Number of subjects passing each test (note we did not take into account intermediate answers that did not reach a complete operatory level; see our general criteria in the text).

CH: Number conservation of rows of nine tokens (Piaget & Szeminska, 1941).

BE: Number conservation of beads poured in jars (Piaget & Szeminska, 1941).

LI: Conservation of liquid poured in jars (Piaget & Szeminska, 1941).

CL: Conservation of mass (Piaget & Inhelder, 1941).

LE: Conservation of sectioned lengths (Piaget, Inhelder, & Szeminska, 1948).

SF: Conservation of area "fields and cows" (Piaget, Inhelder, & Szeminska, 1948).

V: Dissociation of weight from volume (Piaget & Szeminska, 1941); 1 refers to consistent answering based on weight and 2 refers to correct answering based on the height and the diameter of the cylinders.

EG: Conservation of the number of rows made of eggs and egg cups (Piaget & Szeminska, 1941).

succeeding paragraphs the observations that lead us to think that our intervention leads to a relatively generalized induction process.

Let us consider first study 9 (Paour, 1981b). In fact, two types of conventional operatory learning, the one taken from Field (1977) and the other from Lefebvre and Pinard (1972), reveal a classical generalization phenomenon. Following training on the conservation of liquids poured from one vessel to another, they have observed significant gains in other, different conservation tests (of number, mass, and area). These data accord well with those in the literature (Paour, 1979), especially those of Lister (1969, 1970, 1972) and of Field (1974, 1977, 1979). Although this type of intervention is not immune to some of the problems previously discussed, we can present some supplemental arguments in favor of the authenticity of the observed gains: (a) We have introduced at posttest some situations in which one does not have to answer with a conservation response. (b) All of the conserving subjects of group RT-1 gave at least one conservation argument that was different from the one used in the course of the learning. (c) The gains are still apparent 24 months after the end of the training. (d) An ultimate posttest[8] convinced us that the subjects who reached the "conserving" status following training could not be differentiated from "naturally" conserving subjects on tasks that were quite different from those of the training (transformation box, programming "turtle graphics" in LOGO).

In the other studies, any operatory gain corresponds to a generalization. Although we observed some individual differences in the total number of gains, we have shown (Table 5.7) that the subjects made general gains in several tests.

These gains reflect the construction of concepts from different domains: numerical and quantitative invariants (liquid, mass, length, area, weight, volume), classes and relations (studies 2, 4, and 7), and representation of spatial relations (studies 4 and 7). Table 5.8, in which we have presented the results obtained on the test used to assess class inclusion, shows the generality of the gains.

We conclude that our interventions can produce a relatively generalized development of reasoning corresponding to the appearance of concrete operatory behavior patterns observed across several quite central ideational domains.

The Induced Gains are Durable

Durability has always been considered to be one of the most solid criteria of structural cognitive change (Piaget, 1974; Vinh Bang, 1985). The

[8] We have had the opportunity to reexamine some of the subjects 12 months after their last posttest, in the context of their participation in a study on LOGO programming.

TABLE 5.7. Generalization of the induction effects in conservation problems.[a]

Hierarchical scale of conservation problems[c]	Experiment 7[b] Control ($n = 11$)	Experiment 7[b] Trained ($n = 11$)	Experiment 11[b] Control ($n = 11$)	Experiment 11[b] Trained ($n = 9$)
Number (rows of nine tokens)	2	3	2	1
Number (beads poured in jars)	—	1	—	1
Mass (balls of clay)	1	2	—	2
Area (fields and cows)	—	—	—	2
Dissociation of weight from volume (level 1)	—	2	—	—
Dissociation of weight from volume (level 2)	—	1	—	3

[a] Number of subjects at each level of the hierarchical conservation scale on last posttest.
[b] Taken into account because of the number of conservation tests.
[c] Inferred from the observed results in these two experiments.

solidity of the cognitive gains that we induce constitutes our third argument. In fact, cases of regression from one posttest to the next are rare; they have been observed in tests of conservation and classification of geometric forms with those subjects who have not completely reached the operatory (intermediate) level, i.e., subjects whose results are somewhat mixed across different tests. Once the children have reached the operatory level (consistently across different tests), we have never yet recorded any case of regression on tests of conservation of continuous quantity (mass,

TABLE 5.8. Results on class inclusion problem.

Study No.	Group	n	Pretest Incl.[a]	Pretest Gene.[b]	Posttest 1 Incl.	Posttest 1 Gene.	Posttest 2 Incl.	Posttest 2 Gene.	Posttest 3 Incl.	Posttest 3 Gene.
2	RT	8	1	?	8	?				
	RC	8	1	?	1	?				
4	RT	20	0		5	0	9	2		
	RC	22	0		1	0	1	0		
5	RT1	6	0		4	2	6	5		
	RC1	6	0		0	0	0	0		
	RT2	6	0		0	0	0	0		
	RC2	6	0		0	0	0	0		
7	NT	6	0		0	0	1	0	3	3
	NC	6	0		0	0	1	0	3	2
	RT	11	0		0	0	0		2	1
	RC	11	0		0	0	0		0	
8	RT	11	1	0			7	6		
	RC	11	1	0			3	2		

[a] Correct answers to question and counterargument with subclasses organized by objects.
[b] Correct answers to generalizations of the question (no material visible): "In the world are there more tulips or more flowers?"; "During springtime are there not more tulips?"; "Can we do something to get more tulips than flowers?"

length, area, weight-volume dissociation) and on the test of the quantitative aspects of class inclusion.[9] Finally, some of our studies support this relatively long-term stability (17, 20, and 21 months after the first posttest).

The Effects Are Maintained Beyond the Training Period

Not only are regressions virtually nonexistent, but our interventions have been found also to produce after-the-fact changes, that is, changes that evolve or are shown beyond the training period itself. In studies 4 and 7 especially, we observed a substantial progression between the first and subsequent posttest(s) in the absence of any further intervention. It has been suggested that after-the-fact changes are indications of true structural gains (Inhelder et al., 1974; Piaget, 1974; Vinh Bang, 1985). Piaget (1974) has characterized the effective mastery of an operation not only by its permanence but also by its ability to induce further changes without impeding the course of spontaneous development. The after-the-fact changes that we have observed support the induction theory and indicate that the intervention is the basis of a phenomenon of redevelopment or of relative remediation.

Effect of Chronological Age and of Etiology

When initial developmental level was held constant, our interventions were not less effective with older (12 to 16 years) than with younger (8 to 12) children. Indeed, we observed the opposite tendency: on the average, the gains for the older children were more numerous, more generalized, and faster. This observation led us to suggest the hypothesis that our intervention should have age-differential effects (Paour, 1980). With the younger children, it sets in motion a progressive structural development that is quite similar to what we have observed with nonretarded children. With older children, the same intervention seemed to trigger a restorative or unblocking type of process, as if the obstacles that had, up to that time, held back the development process had been suddenly removed.[10] This analysis requires cross-validation, because the training (both quality and number of sessions) was not exactly the same from one study to another. Whatever the validity of this analysis, these results clearly suggest that older children retain some developmental potential despite prolonged experience at the preoperatory level. The ideal of potential takes on added meaning because in the control group (without specific inter-

[9] As defined by the requirements listed previously.

[10] The RT-2 group from study 6 did not seem to us to contradict this interpretation, because they did not get an intervention adapted to their developmental level.

vention and for a given period of observation) the older subjects were the least likely to accede spontaneously to the operatory level (Paour, 1980).

With regard to etiology, on the basis of the first posttest data of study 12, currently in progress, it appears that with initial developmental level held constant it is possible to bring about some operatory gains in subjects whose retardation is clearly of organic origin.

We conclude that developmental plasticity, defined here as the ability to accede, with help, to the concrete operatory level of development, seems in essence to depend upon the initial level of preoperativity and on the type of intervention.

Functional Integration of Operatory Gains

Test of Production of Passive Sentences

In study 4, we have demonstrated very clear gains in the psycholinguistic task of understanding and producing sentences expressed in the passive voice (Sinclair 1968; Sinclair & Ferreiro, 1970) following induction (Paour, 1975, 1981a). This finding supports Sinclair's hypothesis: The ability to construct passive statements as a response to the test's constraints is related to firm accession to the level of concrete operations. We see this finding especially as evidence of the functional integration of cognitive gains.

Mental-Age Gains

Mental age and IQ were not our major dependent variables. They were used in the beginning to select subjects, and later in the posttests mostly as tools for the evaluation of the degree of integration and generalization of cognitive gains. Several studies (2, 4, 5, 7, 11, and 12) show that induced operatory gains can be accompanied by a large gain in mental age (Table 5.9). The median mental-age gain obtained on the New Metric Test of Intelligence ranged from 11 to 20 months in the trained groups, but from −1 to 8 months in the control groups. This general intellectual

TABLE 5.9. Median mental age gains (NEMI).

Study No.	Group: Trained	Group: Control	Number of months between pre- and last posttest
2	+11	+2	5
4	+18	+6	12
5	+13	−1	5
7	+20	+8	27
11	+18	+2	19
12	+14	+4	6

gain was supported by study 4, in which we also used the Performance scale of the Wechsler Intelligence Scale for Children, as well as by studies 11 and 12 in which we used Raven's Standard Progressive Matrices.

The mental-age gains of the subjects correspond to a rather modest average IQ gain of 6 points—well within the 10-point gain often found in compensatory education studies (Spitz, 1986). Even so, we interpret this modest gain as evidence of functional integration, for the following reasons. First, in most of the studies, the gains cannot be attributed to more favorable assessment circumstances, because the control subjects also had a prolonged individual interaction with an experimenter. Second, the average gain is of the same magnitude as that found in some control subjects who also progressed spontaneously on the Piagetian tests. Third, even though there is no apparent statistical connection between the magnitude of the IQ gains and that of the operatory gains, these gains do covary with operatory gains. Fourth, the intervention itself is not highly similar to the items on intelligence tests; further, the intervention is relatively modest compared to massive programs of compensatory education. For these reasons it seems reasonable to conclude that the IQ gains on the New Metric Test of Intelligence can be attributed to changes in the subjects' levels of logical development and to improvement in their cognitive functioning.

Raven's Standard Progressive Matrices

This test is interesting in several respects: as a test of general intelligence, and thus as a supplemental index of generalization, as well as a test of the generalization of the ability to form abstractions and to coordinate abstract relationships. We know also that this test is particularly difficult for mentally retarded persons, especially beginning with the B series where items requiring analogical reasoning first appear. It should be noted that our intervention does not include training in solving matrix problems; on the contrary, the transformation box is quite different from the Progressive Matrices items with respect to situation, materials, and dimensions of relationship. Table 5.10 shows the frequency distributions and mean scores on Raven's Standard Progressive Matrices (RSPM) for trained and control groups at pretest and at three posttests in study 11.

Studies 11 and 12 revealed a significantly greater gain for subjects in the trained groups than for those in the control groups. The groups were also clearly differentiated by the distribution of scores (see Table 5.10), which suggested that the trained subjects had clearly attained a developmental stage at which they could solve most of the items of series B as well as a number of items in the succeeding series at score levels well in excess of chance (mean = 9.2). Further, in study 11 the scores of the trained subjects increased between the last two posttests. An analysis of variance showed a significant trend from first to last posttest (F = 12.3,

TABLE 5.10. Raven's Standard Progressive Matrices Test (sets A and B), study 11: mean and distribution of the total score.

	Score																						
Group	2	3	4	5	6	7	8	9	10	11	12	13	14	15	16	17	18	19	20	21	22	23	Mean
Control																							
Pretest	—	1	—	—	2	1	1	1	3	2	—	—	—	—	—	—	—	—	—	—	—	—	8.27
Posttest 2	—	—	—	1	—	1	2	1	—	3	2	1	—	—	—	—	—	—	—	—	—	—	9.72
Posttest 3	—	—	—	1	—	1	1	1	1	3	—	2	1	—	—	—	—	—	—	—	—	—	10.18
Posttest 4	—	—	—	1	—	1	2	—	1	3	1	2	—	—	—	—	—	—	—	—	—	—	9.90
Trained																							
Pretest	1	—	1	—	1	—	2	2	2	1	1	—	—	—	—	—	—	—	—	—	—	—	8.09
Posttest 2	—	—	—	—	—	1	—	—	—	1	1	1	1	2	2	1	—	1	—	—	—	—	14.09
Posttest 3	—	—	—	—	—	—	—	—	—	1	—	1	1	—	—	1	2	1	1	—	1	—	16.88
Posttest 4	—	—	—	—	—	—	—	—	—	—	—	1	—	—	—	1	—	—	3	3	—	1	19.55

TABLE 5.11. Tower of Hanoi (3- disks and 2-transfers problem), study 8: mean and distribution of the total score.

Group	Score 0	1	2	3	4	5	6	7	8	9	10	Mean
Control												
Pretest	6	—	2	—	1	1	—	1	—	—	—	1.81
Posttest[a]	3	1	1	1	2	2	—	1	—	—	—	2.81
Trained												
Pretest	5	—	1	1	—	3	—	1	—	—	—	2.45
Posttest[a]	1	—	—	—	—	—	2	1	1	3	3	7.63

[a] Second posttest (12 months after pretest); the problem was not given at the first posttest.

$p < .002$; $F = 23.9$, $p < .00001$; and $F = 61.3$, $p < .00001$, respectively). This posttreatment increase supports the concept of the induction of logic structures as a generalized developmental process. Therefore, the RSPM results strengthen the interpretation that the training led to cognitive gains that were subsequently manifest in situations quite different from those of the training.

The Tower of Hanoi Problem

We chose this problem for two principal reasons. First, it is representative of a class of problems whose resolution requires planning and effective control of action. Moreover, Spitz and his collaborators (Borys, Spitz, & Dorans, 1982; Byrnes & Spitz, 1977; Spitz & Borys, 1984; Spitz, Webster, & Borys, 1982) have shown that retarded children perform on this problem at a significantly lower level than do nonretarded children of the same mental age. Specifically, they found that very few of their retarded subjects were able to solve the three-disks test with the minimum number of moves. By using this task we were able to extend our investigation of the degree of generalization beyond the construction of concepts to their ultimate application.

We used the method and scoring criteria that had been delineated by Byrnes and Spitz (1977). In particular, we did not allow for spontaneous corrections: any incorrect placement stopped the trial in which it occurred and was scored as a failure. This test was used in studies 8, 11, and 12[11], and the results are shown in Tables 5.11 and 5.12.

The performance of the control groups confirmed the findings of Spitz and collaborators, and showed us that repeated exposure to the problem (problems presented three times in study 11) did not significantly improve performance on the three-disks problem.

[11] We do not present those of study 12 in which the three-disks test has not yet been given.

Table 5.12. Tower of Hanoi (3-disks and 2-transfers problem), study 11: mean and distribution of the total score.

	Score											
Group	0	1	2	3	4	5	6	7	8	9	10	Mean
Control												
Posttest 2[a]	8	—	—	—	1	—	—	1	1	—	—	1.72
Posttest 3	10	—	—	—	—	—	—	—	1	—	—	0.72
Posttest 4	8	—	—	—	—	—	—	1	1	—	—	1.36
Trained												
Posttest 2[a]	3	—	—	1	—	2	—	2	1	1	1	4.90
Posttest 3	3	1	—	—	—	—	1	1	—	3	2	5.54
Posttest 4	1	—	—	—	—	1	—	—	2	1	4	7.77

[a] The 3-disks problem was not presented at pretest because of a general failure on the 2-disks problem.

By constrast, the trained groups showed very clear gains, as evidenced by:

1. A significant *mean difference* in the scores of the trained and control groups.
2. A very clear *difference in the score distributions* of the trained and control groups.
3. *Durable gains* from one posttest to another.
4. A tendency toward *improvement in scores from posttest to posttest.*
5. The *error-free performance* of several subjects on the 3- and even 4-disk problems.

These quantitative gains were accompanied by functional changes seen in: (a) the initial information input (spontaneously describing the materials and the task[12]), and (b) control in performing the task (following rules, pausing for reflection, inhibiting impulses to place a disk on a wrong post, spontaneously verbalizing intermediate goals).

The cognitive effectiveness shown by the trained subjects on the Tower of Hanoi problem confirms and corroborates our observation of steadily increasing cognitive effectiveness throughout the training sessions, especially during the intervention phases of coordination of relations.

Neurophysiological Concomitants

There is additional information from study 12 that promises to be important. The cognitive gains induced by the training were accompanied

[12] One can see here a generalization of the training method that systematically requires the subjects to describe the material before beginning to transform the objects.

by significant improvement of the REM sleep rate (Bergonzi et al., 1987), and that measure has already been shown (Grubar, 1983, 1986) to be correlated with individual differences in intelligence. This improvement was even stronger in the subjects who, in addition to the psychoeducational intervention, had also been given the drug butoctamide hydrogen succinate, but was significantly less in those who had not been given the chemical treatment. If these results are verified in subsequent posttests, we shall have additional evidence of the functional integration of the cognitive gains.

Limitations on the Induction of Logic Structures

The induction of logic structures encounters two major limitations that, given the present state of research in this field, seem more clearly related to the quality of the intervention than to the characteristics of our mentally retarded subjects.

As indicated previously, the first limitation relates to the initial level of development, because a minimal level of development is necessary for our training to be effective.

The second has to do with the effects of intervention itself. Even though the distal posttests have shown, on the one hand, that gains following intervention were quite durable, and on the other hand, that there were significant after-the-fact gains, the trained subjects did not progress further (within the time limits of the studies) to the next higher (preformal) developmental level. They became fixated at a new threshold that they did not seem able to surmount spontaneously. This observation ought not lead one to minimize the importance of the induced gains. By means of the intervention, we have been able to facilitate accession to a higher thinking mode, and this very accession actually changes, as we show in later paragraphs, a wide range of intellectual behavior patterns. Having said that, we must point out also that training procedures designed to induce the construction of elementary logical structures are not sufficient to bring about changes in functional characteristics to the extent of producing even more radical changes in the dynamics of the developmental process itself. The nature of this limitation seems to support, albeit negatively in this instance, the structural aspects of the induced cognitive gains.

Both limitations have led us to pursue the adaptation of the intervention for application to higher developmental levels. We work from the hypothesis that the guiding principles for the design of our method of induction of logical structures are equally relevant for the extension of this method to levels of development beyond those levels taken into account up to this point. On a more fundamental level, this adaptation consists in pursuing our study of developmental plasticity with mentally retarded persons.

Summary and Conclusions

Within the limits of this chapter, we have shown that the learning of logic structures can have a dual interest. At the theoretical level, it contributes to the understanding of mental retardation. On a clinical level, it constitutes an effective tool for both assessment and treatment.

Primarily because it rests on a developmental approach (Piagetian theory and general rule systems), the learning of logic structures permits one to construct training programs that are focused on precise developmental goals (induction of rule systems) and that are organized according to clearly specifiable general principles. Thus, one can study relatively clearly and reliably the conditions under which this approach can be effective, as well as the progressive attainment of its effects in the course of the intervention. From this point of view, this type of intervention seems clearly superior to more global educational interventions that, although intended to produce similar effects, represent such complex treatments that it is difficult to discern the reasons for their effectiveness. Thus, for example, even though one would not question the importance of individual interaction with the subjects, learning of logic structures allows us to relate the cognitive gains observed throughout the course of training to the summative gains revealed on the posttests (see Paour & Soavi, Chapter 18 in this volume).

Data from studies on the learning of logic structures help to clarify the processes of intellectual development in mentally retarded persons.

On a structural level, it appears to be true that the construction of different cognitive systems in the course of development presents different levels of difficulty. In fact, it is those developmental stages that require profound reorganization of previously established systems that are the basis of fixations. The mapping of critical developmental stages, although useful in educational intervention, is not adequate to explain the phenomena of fixation. One must still explain why retarded persons have particular difficulty in achieving these transformations. Inhelder (1943) had interpreted their temporary and definitive fixations as the result of a deficient constructive process. But later studies, focused on structural aspects, were not successful in specifying the precise nature of this deficit. For the most part they could only give rise to precise and static reports of systems organized into structures. Freeing the Piagetian approach to mental retardation from this impass would require a dynamic approach that rests on the functional application of logical operations and the study of the conditions under which they are modified. To advance the understanding of the phenomena of fixation, one must ask whether, to what extent, with what effects, and under what conditions both of subjects and of settings, it is possible to bring about, through teaching, accession to the next developmental stage when such accession has come about either too slowly or not at all.

By showing convincingly the possibility of inducing highly stable and generalizable cognitive gains, both conceptual and applied, the data from learning of logic structures attest that (a) the characteristics of the cognitive functioning of retarded persons (chronic deficient functioning) are fundamental to fixations, and (b) mentally retarded children and adolescents retain a relative but quite real developmental plasticity.

These two conclusions support and extend those of a number of other authors (Brown & Campione, 1986; Feuerstein, Rand, Hoffman, & Miller, 1980; Haywood, 1987) who have used other types of cognitive treatments. We maintain that our methodological requirements lead to especially solid evidence that it is possible to induce authentic structural cognitive gains in retarded persons. This possibility seems to meet quite well Spitz's (1986) requirement concerning evidence of cognitive change. Further, the induction of fundamental rule systems shows that such induced cognitive gains can be extremely generalized and firm. Thus, the learning of logic structures brings data decisively to bear upon two vital and presently controversial points in the debate over the educability of cognitive processes.

One must also point out that the developmental plasticity revealed by learning of logic structures is relative: (a) it remains to be demonstrated in persons who are initially at lower preoperatory levels, and (b) it is specific to our population (persons who have not been able to reach the concrete operatory level spontaneously). Finally, it remains "potential" to the extent that control group subjects continue to show its necessity (within the time limits of our interventions).

It is still important to ask whether our subjects are more intelligent or simply more knowledgeable. This is a difficult question whose answer requires that we continue to explore further the frontiers of developmental plasticity.

Accession to the concrete operatory stage, and the progressive mastery of its operations, constitute decisive developmental steps, for they determine quite directly the possibilities of scholastic and sociovocational adaptation. Although this step is normally transitory, it is the first of the conditions that are necessary for the construction of the most powerful tools of thinking. It will determine the conditions of acquisition, and, depending on the domain, the acquisition itself, of fundamental scholastic knowledge. Therefore, at the individual clinical level, it would seem to be important to be able, on the one hand, to assess the potential for accession to concrete operativity and, on the other hand, to have available an instrumentality by which to facilitate this accession. The induction method presented in this chapter meets these two requirements. The early training sessions make it possible to locate a subject's developmental level and functional modalities in relation to the cognitive requirement of the exercises and their progression; they can help us to specify particularly whether the subject has, or has not, reached a developmental level sufficient to derive benefit from teaching. Based on a developmental progression, the sequential arrangement of the induction exercises provides an intervention guide that is both extremely precise and also capable of adaptation to specific conceptual and functional problems. Finally, the concept of induction equips the intervenor with solid principles of intervention.

Thus, even though the method of learning of logic structures is still very much linked to quite basic concerns, it is likely that it can become an important part of cognitive education programs.

Acknowledgment. I am grateful to Francine Orsini-Bouichou for her wise suggestions on a previous version of this chapter, and I am deeply indebted to Carl Haywood, whose translation improved the original French manuscript.

References

Arbitman-Smith, R., Haywood, H. C., & Bransford, J. D. (1984). Assessing cognitive change. In P. Brooks, R. sperber, & C. McCauley (Eds.), *Learning and cognition in the mentally retarded* (pp. 433–471). Baltimore: University Park Press.

Baumeister, A. A. (1984). Some methodological and conceptual issues in the study of cognitive processes with retarded people. In P. Brooks, R. Sperber, & C. McCauley (Eds.), *Learning and cognition in the mentally retarded* (pp. 1–38). Baltimore: University Park Press.

Bergonzi, P., Colognola, R. M., D'Erario, C., Grubar, J.-C., Paour, J.-L., & Pollicina, C. (1987). *Effects of external stimuli on nocturnal sleep of mentally retarded subjects: Intensive learning sessions and oculomotor frequencies.* Paper presented at the 5th International Congress of Sleep Research, Copenhagen.

Bideaud, J. (1985). Le développement de connaissances logiques: l'apport des expériences d'apprentissage [The development of logical knowledge: the contribution of studies on learning]. *Archives de Psychologie*, *53*, 477–484.

Blackman, L. S., & Lin, A. (1984). Generalization training in the educable mentally retarded: Intelligence and its educability revisited. In P. Brooks, R. Sperber, & C. McCauley (Eds.), *Learning and cognition in the mentally retarded* (pp. 237–263). Baltimore: University Park Press.

Borkowski, J., & Cavanaugh, J. C. (1979). Maintenance and generalization of skills and strategies by the retarded. In N. R. Ellis (Ed.), *Handbook of mental deficiency: Psychological theory and research* (2nd ed., pp. 569–617). Hillsdale, NJ: Erlbaum.

Borys, S. V., Spitz, H. H., & Dorans, B. A. (1982). Tower of Hanoi performance of retarded yound adults and nonretarded children as a function of solution length and goal state. *Journal of Experimental Child Psychology*, *33*, 87–110.

Bradley, T. B. (1983). Remediation of cognitive deficits: A critical appraisal of the Feuerstein model. *Journal of Mental Deficiency Research*, *27*, 79–92.

Brainerd, C. (1977). Cognitive development and concept learning: An interpretative review. *Psychological Bulletin*, *84*, 919–939.

Brown, A., & Campione, J. C. (1986). Psychological theory and the study of learning disabilities. *American Psychologist*, *14*, 1059–1068.

Budoff, M. A. (1967). Learning potential among institutionalized young adult retardates. *American Journal of Mental Deficiency*, *72*, 404–411.

Burden, R. (1987). Instrumental Enrichment programme: Important issues in research and evaluation. *European Journal of Psychology of Education*, *2*(1), 3–16.

Byrnes, M. M., & Spitz, H. H. (1977). Performance of retarded adolescents and nonretarded children on the Tower of Hanoi problem. *American Journal of Mental Deficiency*. *81*, 561–569.

Castellan, E., Grégoire, A.-M., & Poli, J. (1976). *Comportements d'enfants déficients moyens et d'enfants normaux de 5-6 ans d'âge mental observés au cours d'éppreuves de conservation et en situation d'apprentissage de covariations quantitatives*. Unpublished master's thesis, University of Provence.

Castellan, M.-T., & Paour, J.-L. (1968). *Note de recherche à propos d'une analyse du passage de comportements préopératoires au comportements opératoires concrets* [Research note: An analysis of the progression from preoperatory to concrete operatory behavior]. Unpublished master's thesis, University of Provence, Aix-en-Provence, France.

Chevalier, B., & Grimaldi, D. (1972). *Essai d'apprentisage opératoire chez des enfants retardés moyens*. Unpublished master's thesis, University of Provence.

Cunha de Carvalho, L. (1983). *Structuration de l'environnement familial et développement cognitif: Etude différentielle et longitudinale* [Family environmental structure and cognitive development: Differential and longitudinal study]. Unpublished doctoral dissertation, University of Provence, Aix-en-Provence, France.

Cunha de Carvalho, L., Hurtig, M., & Orsini-Bouichou, F. (1984). Facteurs culturels, environnement familial, et apprentissage cognitif [Cultural factors, family environment, and cognitive learning]. *Psychologie Française*, *51*, 57–60.

D'Erario, C., & Pollicina, C. (1988). La promozione del "penserio operatorio-concreto" in soggetti con ritardo mentale medio e lieve: verifica del metodo di apprendimento induttivo "Scatolo di trasformazione" [Induction of concrete operatory thought in mildly and moderately mentally retarded children: Verification of the "transformation box" method of learning induction]. *Quaderni Oasi*, *13*, 9–38.

Desprels-Fraysse, A. (1980). Le schéma de covariation: moyen d'analyse du fonctionnement opératoire [The covariation schema: A method of analyzing operatory functioning]. *L'Année Psychologique*, *80*, 169–191.

Desprels-Fraysse, A. (1985). The sequence of development of certain classification skills. *Genetic Psychology Monographs*, *1*, 67–82.

Desprels-Fraysse, A. (1986). Domaine logique, domaine spatial, étude de quelques relations chez des enfants de quatre à huit ans [Study of some relations in the logical and spatial domains in 4- to 8-year-old children]. *Archives de Psychologie*, *53*, 439–446.

Desprels-Fraysse, A., & Fraysse, J. C. (1977). *Induction des structures logiques élémentaires chez des enfants d'âge préscolaire et analyse fonctionnelle des comportements observés* [Induction of elementary logic structures in preschool children and functional analysis of observed behavior]. Unpublished doctoral dissertation, University of Provence, Aix-en-Provence, France.

Desprels-Fraysse, A., & Fraysse, J.-C. (1978). Analyse fonctionnelle des comportements préopératoires [Functional analysis of preoperatory behavior]. *Cahiers de Psychologie*, *21*, 163–183.

Desprels-Fraysse, A., Fraysse, J.-C., Orsini-Bouichou, F., & Paour, J.-L. (1979). Genèse et déterminants de la pensée opératoire [Origins and determinants of operatory thought]. *Bulletin de Psychologie*, 340, 523–531.

Doise, W., Mugny, G., & Perret-Clermont, A. N. (1975). Social interaction and the development of cognitive operations. *European Journal of Social Psychology*, *5*, 367–383.

Ellis, N. (1970). Memory processes in retardates and normals. In N. R. Ellis (Ed.), *International Review of Research in Mental Retardation* (Vol. 4, pp. 1–32). New York: Academic Press.

Ellis, N., & Cavalier, A. R. (1982). Research perspectives in mental retardation. In E. Zigler & D. B. Balla (Eds.), *Mental retardation: The developmental-difference controversy* (pp. 121–152). Hillsdale, NJ: Erlbaum.

Feuerstein, R., Rand, Y., & Hoffman, M. B. (1979). *The dynamic assessment of retarded performers: The learning potential assessment device. Theory, instruments and techniques*. Baltimore: University Park Press.

Feuerstein, R., Rand, Y., Hoffman, M. B., & Miller, R. (1980). *Instrumental Enrichment*. Baltimore: University Park Press.

Field, D. (1974). Long term effects of conservation training with educationally subnormal children. *Journal of Special Education*, *7–8*, 449–461.

Field, D. (1977). The importance of verbal content in the training of Piagetian conservation skills. *Child Development*, *48*, 1583–1592.

Field, D. (1979). A comparision of the conservation acquisition of mentally retarded and nonretarded children. In Friedman, M. P., Das, J. P., & O'Connor, N. (Eds.), *Intelligence and learning* (pp. 491–496). New York: Plenum Press.

Flavell, J. H. (1970). Concept development. In P. H. Mussen (Ed.), *Carmichael's manual of child psychology* (pp. 983–1059). New York: Wiley.

Florès, C., & Orsini-Bouichou, F. (1979). *Induction et formation de la pensée logique chez l'enfant* [Induction and formation of logical thought in children]. Unpublished report, University of Provence, Aix-en-Provence, France.

Foul, G., & Malika, E. (1982). *Une experience d'apprentissage de covariations quantitatives chez des enfants retardés mentaux*. Unpublished master's thesis, University of Provence.

Fraysse, J.-C., (1987). Etude génétique de la prise en compte du partenaire dans la construction des opérations [Developmental study of awareness of the partner in the construction of operations]. *Bulletin de Psychologie, 382*, 915–922.

Fraysse, J.-C., & Desprels-Fraysse, A. (1978). Induction des structures logiques chez les enfants d'âge préscolaire [Induction of logic structures in preschool children]. *Cahiers de Psychologie*, *21*, 163–182.

Galas, D., Sidérakis, E., & Soavi, G. (1981). *Effet de deux types d'apprentissage opératoire sur la genèse des notions de conservation chez des enfants débiles mentaux*. Unpublished master's thesis, University of Provence.

Gilly, M., & Roux, J.-P. (1984). Efficacité comparée du travail en individuel et du travail en interaction socio-cognitive dans l'appropriation et la mise en oeuvre de règles de résolution chez des enfants de 11–12 ans [Differential effectiveness of individual and social-cognitive interactive work in the assimilation and application of problem-solving rules in 11- to 12-year-old children]. *Cahiers de Psychologie Cognitive*, *4*(2), 171–188.

Greco, P., & Piaget, J. (1959). *Apprentissage et connaissance* [Learning and understanding]. Vol. 7 of *Etudes d'épistémologie génétique*. Paris: Presses Universitaires de France.

Grubar, J.-C. (1983). Sleep and mental deficiency. *Review of E. E. G. Neurophysiology*, *13*, 107–114.

Grubar, J.-C. (1986). Approche psychophysiologique du potentiel intellectuel [A psychophysiological approach to intellectual potential]. *Enfance*, *1*, 85–90.

Haywood, H. C. (1987). The mental age deficit: Explanation and treatment. *Uppsala Journal of Medical Sciences*, Supplement 44, 191–203.

Haywood, H. C., & Wachs, T. D. (1981). Intelligence, cognition and individual differences. In M. J. Begab, H. C. Haywood, & H. Garber (Eds)., *Psychosocial influences in retarded performance. Vol. 1*: *Issues and theories in development* (pp. 95–126). Baltimore: University Park Press.

Hurtig, M. (1969). Une expérience d'apprentissage chez le débile [A learning study with mentally retarded persons]. In R. Zazzo (Ed.). *Les débilités mentales* (pp. 317–333). Paris: Armand Colin.

Inhelder, B. (1966). Développement, régulation et apprentissage [Development, regulation, and learning]. In F. Bresson & M. de Montmollin (Eds.), *Psychologie et épistémologie génétiques, thèmes piagétiens: Hommage á Jean Piaget* (pp. 119–188). Paris: Dunod.

Inhelder, B., & Sinclair, H. (1969). Learning cognitive structures. In P. Mussen, J. Langer, & M. Covington (Eds.), *Trends and issues in developmental psychology* (pp. 2–22). New York: Holt, Rinehart, & Winston.

Inhelder, B., Sinclair, H., & Bovet, M. (1974). *Apprentissage et structures de la connaissance* [Learning and the structuring of understanding]. Paris: Presses Universitaires de France.

Julien, C., Maglagli, D., & Tosti, M. (1972). *Essai d'apprentissage opératoire chez des enfants débiles mentaux moyens*. Unpublished master's thesis, University of Provence.

Kahn, J. V. (1985). Evidence of the similar-structure hypothesis controlling for organicity. *American Journal of Mental Deficiency*, *89*, 372–378.

Laurendeau, M., & Pinard, A. (1966). Réflexions sur l'apprentissage des structures logiques [Reflections on the learning of logic structures]. In F. Bresson & M. de Montmollin (Eds.), *Psychologie et épistémologie génétiques, thèmes piagétiens: Hommage à Jean Piaget* (pp. 191–210). Paris: Dunod.

Laurendeau-Bendavid, M. (1985). L'apprentissage des structures cognitives: Perspectives d'avenir après 25 années de recherche [The learning of cognitives structures: Perspectives on the future after 25 years of research]. *Archives de Psychologie*, *53*, 477–484.

Lefebvre, M., & Pinard, A. (1972). Apprentissage de la conservation des quantités par une méthode de conflit cognitif [Learning of conservation of quantity by a cognitive conflict method]. *Canadian Journal of Behavioural Science*, *4*, 1–12.

Lefebvre, M., & Pinard, A. (1976). Les expériences de Genève sur l'apprentissage: Un dossier peu convaincant (même pour un piagétien).

[Genevan studies on learning: an unconvincing collection, even for a Piagetian]. *Psychologie Canadienne*, *17*, 103–109.
Lister, C. (1969). The development of a concept of weight conservation in ESN children. *British Journal of Educational Psychology*, *39*, 245–252.
Lister, C. (1970). The development of a concept of volume conservation in ESN children. *British Journal of Educational Psychology*, *40*, 55–64.
Lister, C. (1972). The development of ESN children's understanding of conservation in a range of attribute situation. *British Journal of Educational Psychology*, *42*, 14–22.
Morf, A., Smedslund, J., Vinh Bang, & Wohlwill, J. (1959). *L'apprentissage des structures logiques* [The learning of logic structures]. Vol. 9 of *Etudes d'épistémologie génétique*. Paris: Presses Universitaires de France.
Noizet, G. (1965). Verbalisation et performance [Verbalization and performance]. *Cahiers de Psychologie*, *8*, 173–180.
Nuttin, J. (1980). *Théorie de la motivation humaine* [A theory of human motivation]. Paris: Presses Universitaires de France.
Orsini, F. (1965). Régularités et système de relations chez l'enfant [Regularities and system of relations in the child]. *Cahiers de Psychologie*, *8*, 143–155.
Orsini-Bouichou, F. (1975). *Régularités dans les organisations spontanées chez l'enfant et genèse des comportements cognitifs* [Regularities in children's spontaneous organizations and the origins of cognitive behavior]. Unpublished doctoral dissertation, Université René Descartes, Paris.
Orsini-Bouichou, F. (1978). Régularités et comportements de libres combinaisons, étude génétique [A developmental study of regularities and behavior in a free combinations task]. *Cahiers de Psychologie*, *21*, 123–138.
Orsini-Bouichou, F. (1982). *L'intelligence de l'enfant, ontogenèse des invariants* [The intelligence of the child and the ontogenesis of invariants]. Paris: Editions du Centre National de la Recherche Scientifique.
Orsini-Bouichou, F., & Malacria-Rocco, J. (1978). Des régularités à l'induction opératoire [Some regularities in induction of operatory thought]. *Cahiers de Psychologie*, *21*, 163–182.
Orsini-Bouichou, F., Malacria-Rocco, J., & Rohrer, B. (1985). Statut et autonomie de l'apprentissage, méthodes d'étude du fonctionnement et du développement cognitif [Status and autonomy of learning, methods for studying cognitive functioning and development]. *Archives de Psychologie*, *53*, 513–522.
Orsini-Bouichou, F., & Paour, J.-L. (1986). Cognitive change and behaviour. In P. van Geert (Ed.), *Theory building in developmental psychology* (pp. 259–292). Amsterdam: North-Holland.
Palacio–Quintin, E. (1987). *Apprendre les mathématiques, un jeu d'enfant*. Québec: Presses Universitaires du Québec.
Paour, J.-L. (1975). Effet d'un entraînement cognitif sur la compréhension et la production d'énoncés passifs chez des enfants déficients mentaux [Effect of cognitive training on the understanding and production of passive sentences in mentally retarded children]. *Etudes de Linguistique Appliquée*, *20*, 88–110.
Paour, J.-L. (1978). Une expérience d'induction des structures logiques chez des enfants déficients mentaux [A study of induction of logic structures in mentally retarded children]. *Cahiers de Psychologie*, *21*, 79–98.
Paour, J.-L. (1979). Apprentissage de notions de conservation et induction de la pensée opératoire concrète chez les débiles mentaux [Learning of conservation concepts and induction of concrete operatory thought in mentally retarded

persons]. In R. Zazzo (Ed.), *Les débilités mentales* (pp. 421–465). Paris: Armand Colin.

Paour, J.-L. (1980). *Construction et fonctionnement des structures opératoires concrètes chez l'enfant débile mental: Apport des expériences d'apprentissage et d'induction opératoire* [Development and application of concrete operatory structures in mentally retarded persons: Contribution from studies of learning and operatory induction]. Unpublished doctoral dissertation, University of Provence, Aix-en-Provence, France.

Paour, J.-L. (1981a). L'apprentissage des structures logiques comme instrument d'investigation du fonctionnement cognitif des arriérés mentaux: Illustration à partir d'une comparaison à long terme d'enfants normaux et arriérés soumis ou non à un entraînement opératoire [Learning of logic structures as a tool for studying the cognitive functioning of the mentally retarded: Description based on a long-term comparison of normal and retarded children who were or were not given operatory training]. *Neuropsychiatrie de l'Enfance et de l'Adolescence, 29*(1–2), 31–38.

Paour, J.-L. (1981b). Apprentissage des structures logiques et développement du langage chez les arriérés mentaux [Learning of logic structures and language development in the mentally retarded]. In J. A. Rondal, J.-L. Lambert, & H. H. Chipman (Eds.), *Psycholinguistique et handicap mental* (pp. 24–53). Brussels: Mardaga.

Paour, J.-L. (1982). El aprendizaje operatorio como instrumento de investigación y de intervención en retraso mental [Operatory learning as an investigative and intervention tool in mental retardation]. *Memoria del Primer Congresso Nacional sobre Deficiencia Mental* (pp. 45–65). Mexico City: Secretario de Educación Pública.

Paour, J.-L. (1985). De l'induction des structures logiques à la modification du fonctionnement [From the induction of logic structures to the modification of functioning]. *Revue Suisse de Psychologie, 44*(3), 135–147.

Paour, J.-L. (1986). Efficacité et limites de nouvelles technologies d'éducation de l'intelligence [Efficacy and limitations of new techniques for training the intellect]. *Schweizerische Heilpädagogische Rundschau, 9*, 207–215.

Paour, J.-L. (1988). Retard mental et aides cognitives [Mental retardation and cognitive aides]. In J.-P. Caverni, C. Bastien, P. Mendelsohn, & G. Tiberghien (Eds.), *Psychologie cognitive : modèles et méthodes*, (pp. 191–216) Grenoble: Presses Universitaires de Grenoble.

Paour, J.-L., Cabrera, F., & Roman, M. (1985). Educabilité de l'intelligence dans un environnement informatique à programmer: Intentions et conditions d'une recherche [Educability of intelligence in a computer programming environment: Objectives and conditions of investigation]. *Enfance, 2–3*, 147–158.

Paour, J.-L., Galas, D., Malacria-Rocco, J., & Soavi, G. (1985). L'apprentissage opératoire chez les retardés mentaux [Operatory learning in the mentally retarded]. *Archives de Psychologie, 53*, 477–484.

Paris, S. C., & Haywood, H. C. (1973). Mental retardation as a learning disorder. *Pediatric Clinics of North America, 20,* 641–651.

Pascual-Leone, J. (1976). On learning and development, Piagetian style. I. A reply to Lefebvre-Pinard. *Psychologie Canadienne, 17*, 270–288.

Piaget, J. (1970). Piaget's theory. In P. Mussen (Ed.), *Carmichael's manual of child psychology* (3rd ed., Vol. 1, pp. 103–128). New York: Wiley.

Piaget, J. (1974). Introduction. In Inhelder, B., Sinclair, H., & Bovet, M. *Apprentissage et structures de la connaissance*. Paris: Presses Universitaires de France.

Piaget, J., Grize, J. B., Szeminska, A., & Vinh Bang (1968). Epistémologie et psychologie de la fonction [Epistemology and psychology of functioning]. *Etudes d'épistémologie génétique*, Vol. 24. Paris: Presses Universitaires de France.

Piaget, J., & Inhelder, B. (1941). *Le développement des quantités physiques chez l'enfant*. Neuchâtel: Delachaux et Niestlé.

Piaget, J., Inhelder, B., & Szeminska, A. (1948). *La géométrie spontanée de l'enfant*. Paris: Presses Universitaires de France.

Piaget, J., & Szeminska, A. (1941). *La genèse du nombre chez l'enfant*. Neuchâtel: Delachaux et Niestlé.

Pinard, A. (1981). *Conservation of conservation*. New York: Academic Press.

Planche, P. (1984). *Fonctionnement et développement cognitif de l'enfant précoce: Etudes comparatives d'enfants précoces, moyens et retardés d'âge mental équivalent* [Functioning and cognitive development of the precocious child: Comparative studies of precocious, average, and retarded children of the same mental age]. Unpublished doctoral dissertation, University of Provence, Aix-en-Provence, France.

Raven, J. C. (1948). The comparative assessment of intellectual ability. *British Journal of Psychology*, *39*, 12–19.

Robeants, M.-J. (1987). *Etude du développement et du fonctionnement cognitif d'enfants Haïtiens* [A study of the cognitive development and functioning of Haitian children]. Unpublished doctoral dissertation, University of Provence, Aix-en-Provence, France.

Savell, J. M., Twohig, P. T., & Rachford, D. L. (1986). Empirical status of Feuerstein's "Instrumental Enrichment" (FIE) technique as a method of teaching thinking skills. *Review of Educational Research*, *56*(4), 381–409.

Sinclair, H. (1968). L'acquisition des structures syntaxiques [The acquisition of syntactic structures]. *Psychologie Française*, *13*, 167–174.

Sinclair, H., & Ferreiro, E. (1970). Etude génétique de la compréhension, production et répétition des phrases au mode passif [A developmental study of the understanding, production, and repetition of passive-voice sentences]. *Archives de Psychologie*, *15*, 1–42.

Soavi, G. (1986). *Une analyse du fonctionnement cognitif chez l'enfant retardé mental à propos de la genèse observée et provoquée de la relation de couple* [An analysis of cognitive functioning in the mentally retarded child with respect to the observed and induced origin of the pairing relation]. Unpublished doctoral dissertation, University of Provence, Aix-en-Provence, France.

Spitz, H. H. (1986). *The raising of intelligence: A selected history of attempts to raise retarded intelligence*. Hillsdale, NJ: Erlbaum.

Spitz, H. H., & Borys, S. V. (1984). Depth of search: How far can the retarded search through an internally represented problem space? In P. Brooks, R. Sperber, & C. McCauley (Eds.), *Learning and cognition in the mentally retarded* (pp. 333–358). Baltimore: University Park Press.

Spitz, H. H., Webster, N. A., & Borys, S. V. (1982). Further studies of the Tower of Hanoi problem solving performance of retarded young adults and nonretarded children. *Developmental Psychology*, *18*, 922–930.

Sternberg, R. J., & Spear, L. C. (1985). A triarchic theory of mental retardation. In N. Ellis & N. Bray (Eds.), *International review of research in mental retardation* (Vol. 13, pp. 301–326). New York: Academic Press.

Strauss, S. (1972). Inducing cognitive development and learning: A review of short-term training experiments. I. The organismic developmental approach. *Cognition, 1*, 329–357.

Vinh Bang (1985). La mesure de l'apprentissage en psychologie génétique [Assessment of learning in developmental psychology]. *Archives de Psychologie, 53*, 477–484.

Wallon, H. (1942) *L'évolution psychologique de l'enfant* [The psychological development of the child]. Paris: Armand Colin.

Weisz, J. R., Yeates, K. O., & Zigler, E. (1982). Piagetian evidence and the developmental-difference controversy. In E. Zigler & D. Balla (Eds.), *Mental retardation: The developmental-difference controversy* (pp. 213–276). Hillsdale, NJ: Erlbaum.

Weisz, J. R., & Zigler, E. (1979). Cognitive development in retarded and non-retarded persons: Piagetian test of the similar-sequence hypothesis. *Psychological Bulletin, 86*(4), 831–851.

Zazzo, R., Gilly, M., & Verba-Rad, M. (1966). *Nouvelle Echelle Métrique de l'Intelligence* [New Metric Test of Intelligence]. Paris: Armand Colin.

Zeaman, D., & House, B. J. (1979). A review of attention and retardates' discrimination learning. In N. R. Ellis (Ed.) *International Review of Research in Mental Retardation* (Vol. 4, pp. 63–120). New York: Academic Press.

Zigler, E. (1969). Developmental versus difference theories of mental retardation and the problem of motivation. *American Journal of Mental Deficiency, 73*, 536–556.

Zigler, E. (1972). Rigidity in the retarded: A reexamination. In E. Trapp & P. Himelstein (Eds.), *Readings in the exceptional child: Research and theory* (2nd ed., pp. 141–162). New York: Appleton-Century-Crofts.

6
The Dynamic Assessment of Intelligence

Jerry S. Carlson and Karl Heinz Wiedl

Even though the study of mental abilities is one of the most widely researched areas in psychology, a number of often related definitional and methodological issues remain unresolved. There are several reasons for this, including the complicated nature of the construct *intelligence*, measurement issues, and problems concerning how individual and group differences in measured intelligence are to be explained and interpreted.

Several decades ago, Boring offered the following definition of intelligence: "Intelligence is what the test measures" (Boring, 1923, p. 35). Were this definition acceptable, there would be little difficulty in interpreting test scores. Test results would accurately reflect an individual's mental ability, providing both the theory, although narrowly conceived in terms of a very restricted notion of operationalism, and the measurement of the construct. Although the definition used by Boring is still considered to be useful by some, most present research on intelligence is theory driven, with theory and measurement being mutually instructive, not simply interchangeable.

The interrelationship between theory and measurement is of particular significance where modifications in approaches to assessment are used. First, there must be some general, theoretical notion of what cognitive capacity is, and second, empirically verifiable evidence must be presented that the measurement approaches used allow better estimates of the cognitive capacity of the individuals or groups tested than would traditional psychometric approaches. In this chapter, we will address the issue of how the accuracy of the assessment of mental abilities can be increased through the use of selected dynamic testing procedures.

Our general model is consistent with the differentiations made by Hebb (1949) and elaborated on by Vernon (1962). Hebb considered Intelligence A to be theoretical, describing the general potential that an individual has to profit from environmental stimulation. It is largely neurobiological in nature, with genetic factors accounting for much of the variability. Intelligence B, on the other hand, was conceived by Hebb to be the actual intelligence that an individual uses in his daily behavior. It is seen as the product of complex genotype-environment interactions that cannot be reduced to either purely environmental or hereditary factors. It is assessed formally through what Vernon called Intelligence C, the actual performance on a test of intelligence. To the extent that Intelligence C is accurately measured, the theoretically more interesting Intelligence B can be estimated; even, perhaps, general estimates of Intelligence A can be made, although we are not sanguine on this point. (See Eysenck, 1982, for a representation of the view that good estimates of Intelligence A can be made from certain measures of Intelligence B, as well as from measures of evoked potential.)

For a test to be useful, of course, it must be valid. Cronbach (1971) has described two general types of validity. One type of validity, validity in the narrow sense, concerns the predictive qualities of a test. The other type of validity, validity in the larger sense, "examines the soundness of all the interpretations of a test" (p. 443). Accurate assessment of Intelligence C, and appropriate inference of Intelligence B or even Intelligence A, requires that the test be subjected to analysis of the criteria implicit in Cronbach's more broadly conceived notion of validity. Even though a test may meet the usual psychometric standards of reliability and have adequate predictive validity, it may fall short of providing an accurate estimate of Intelligence B—and from the perspective of construct validity, the test may be biased.

The debate concerning bias in mental measurement ranges from the classical test fairness concept of equal prediction described by Cleary (1968), Cleary, Humphreys, Kendrick, and Wesman (1975), and Eichorn and Bass (1971), to criteria involving group membership and cultural variables (Darlington, 1971), to the incorporation of sociological data in arriving at estimates of ability level (Mercer & Lewis, 1975). In our view, examination of construct validity is of particular importance when assessing potential bias and accuracy of inference concerning Intelligence B. As Cole (1980) has described it, this approach

> is to derive from the intended construct expectations or hypotheses of how a measure of that construct should behave (e.g., to what other variables it should and should not be related, what situations should or should not alter scores on it, or what interrelationships the items or subscores of the measures should have) and then to check whether the scores behave similarly and in expected ways in various groups of interest. (p. 1071)

Flaugher (1978) has suggested that test bias can result from many factors and that "tailored testing" may help reduce bias related to the atmosphere in which the test is administered. The notion of tailored testing can be extended to the use of a learning-oriented approach to assessment, where analysis can be made of gains individuals make under given conditions of test administration, and potential interactions of motivational, personality, and cognitive style factors may be studied (Resnick, 1979).

The usefulness of a test can also be seen from another perspective. Even when no attempt is made to assess Intelligence B or A, the assessment of intraindividual variation of performance—at the level of Intelligence C—may be helpful in itself. By making individual difference factors that affect performance evident, valuable information concerning potential interventions will be gained. This is especially significant for the special education and rehabilitation fields.

Traditional testing approaches do not incorporate modifications aimed at increasing levels of performance into their procedure; nor do they tend to take into account intraindividual variability on a number of dimensions that may affect test performance (Brown & French, 1979; Feuerstein, Rand, & Hoffman, 1979; Feuerstein, Rand, Hoffman, & Miller, 1980; Guthke, 1982). Accordingly, the results, though reliable, may not adequately reflect an individual's cognitive competence (Overton & Newman, 1982), and inferences concerning Intelligence B may be systematically biased. In addition, indications for intervention remain sparse.

Dynamic assessment addresses these problems. In the following sections of this chapter, we will describe some of the work on dynamic testing that has been done in our laboratories. Special consideration will be given to aspects of construct validity, as described by Cronbach and Cole, and to issues related to the study of individual differences.

First, we will describe a set of studies aimed at finding out which of a variety of within-test modifications in testing procedure yield scores that seem to reflect more accurately Intelligence B, or an individual's cognitive competence, than those obtained by traditional psychometric approaches. This will include studies that have used samples of children drawn from a variety of populations. Second, a series of studies will be summarized that provide closer analysis of the internal and external conditions that mediate performance change. Third, research concerning the efficacy of the approach for children from different ethnic groups will be discussed. Fourth, a theoretical model designed to conceptualize the phenomenon of performance change will be presented. Fifth, a summary of our most recent work will be given.

Approaches to Dynamic Assessment

In most of our work on dynamic assessment, we employed a testing paradigm that incorporates modifications of testing procedure into the test situation. While recognizing the value of approaches that involve training and transfer, exemplified by the work of Brown and Campione (Brown & Campione, 1986; Campione & Brown, 1984; Ferrara, Brown, & Campione, 1986), and Feuerstein and his colleagues (Feuerstein et al., 1979; Feuerstein et al., 1980), we have, nonetheless, concentrated our efforts on studying how modifications in test performance can be brought about by variation within the testing procedure itself. Our approach is practical and directly applicable for use by psychological practitioners. It avoids problems related to the measurement of change and it allows for direct analysis of how and to what extent sources of individual differences on putatively noncognitive variables affect test performance.

Testing Conditions Leading to Increased Performance

General Population

Although a number of investigations have been carried out that have assessed the effects of a variety of testing approaches on test performance, to our knowledge no systematic comparison of these approaches had been made prior to the 1979 Carlson and Wiedl (1979) study. (A partial exception to this is a study by Radford, 1966.) Our approach was to isolate the various modes of test administration and compare them with each other and with standard testing procedures. In the initial set of studies, we used Raven is Coloured Progressive Matrices (RCPM; Raven, 1976) as our testing instrument. The reason for choosing this instrument was that it is appropriate for the age groups we were interested in and, most importantly, it is a culture-fair test that is a reliable indicator of general intelligence or "g" (Jensen, 1980). In the 1976 study, our basic interest was to find out which of a variety of testing procedures yielded scores that seemed to be better estimates of Intelligence B, or an individual's cognitive competence, than those obtained by traditional testing approaches.

The testing procedures used are described below. It is important to note that all testing was done individually and that the *initial* answer the child gave was the answer scored. This implies that when verbalization is involved, it may affect performance on the item under consideration; when feedback without verbalization is involved, the effect can only be on items subsequent to the one under consideration. The testing procedures are as follows:

C_1. Standard procedure.

C_2. Verbalization during and after solution: requires the child to describe the main stimulus pattern prior to searching for the correct answer and then, after a particular alternative is chosen, to explain why he/she made that choice.

C_3. Verbalization after solution: involves the child describing the reasons for his/her choice after the choice is made.

C_4. Simple feedback: where the child is informed after the choice has been made whether or not it was correct.

C_5. Elaborated feedback: involves, in addition to simple feedback, an elaboration by the test administrator of the reasons why the chosen answer was correct or incorrect; the principles involved in the task are pointed out.

C_6. Elaborated feedback plus verbalization during and after solution: is a combination of conditions C_2 and C_5; it involves verbalization (description of the pattern to be completed), and after a choice has been made, the child's explanation for the reasons for solution chosen and elaborated feedback by the testor, informing the child of the correctness of the response and explaining the principles involved in the task.

An example of the Raven's Coloured Progressive Matrices is given in Figure 6.1. Factor analysis of this test (Carlson & Jensen, 1980) has

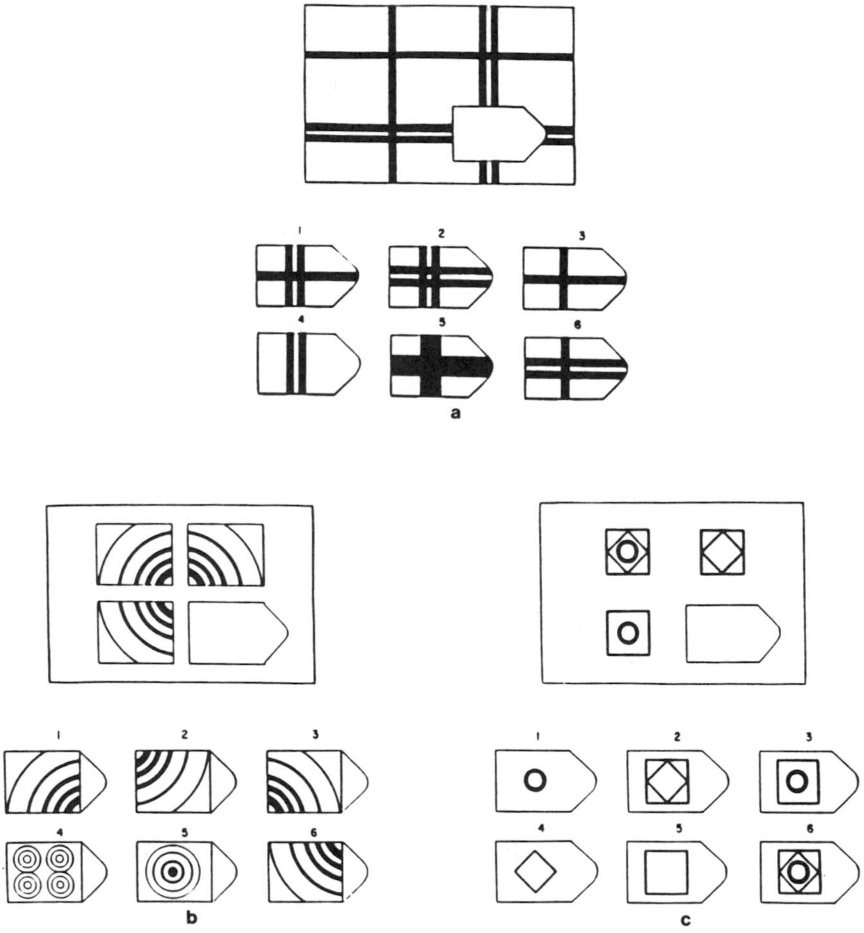

FIGURE 6.1. An example of Raven's Coloured Progressive Matrices: (a) simple pattern completion; (b) closure; (c) analogical reasoning

shown that it has three factors: simple pattern completion, pattern completion through closure, and analogical reasoning.

In the first study (Carlson & Wiedl, 1976), 434 second- and fourth-grade children were randomly assigned to one of the six testing conditions. All subjects were tested individually. Half were given the regular booklet form of the RCPM; half were given the puzzle version of the test. The puzzle version allows the subject to use overt trial-and-error procedures as he/she searches for the solution. The results of the investigation showed that conditions C_5 and C_6 were beneficial for the second graders, whereas conditions C_2 and C_6 led to higher performance for the fourth graders.

Although for the salient testing conditions higher levels of performance were found for the total RCPM score, the gains were the result of marked improvement on the relatively difficult reasoning by analogy items. Since the abstract reasoning by analogy items constitute the most heavily "g"-loaded part of the test, this finding is of particular interest as it substantiates the significance of the effective testing conditions. The lack of effect of C_2 for the second graders is most likely related to the fact that younger children tend not to profit from the guidance function that overt verbalization offers (Jensen, 1966). The puzzle version of the test was not effective in improving performance for the fourth graders, but it did lead to higher scores for the second-grade children. Not surprisingly, the improvement was traced to higher performance on the pattern completion and closure items. When the task involves relatively easy perceptual processes, younger children seem to profit from the use of overt trial and error; older children, on the other hand, do not profit from this as they apparently can use covert processes more effectively than can the younger children.

On the basis of the results of the above investigation, three types of studies were conducted. In one type of study (described in detail in the section immediately below), the goal was to ascertain the generality of the findings with populations of children with special characteristics such as mild retardation, specific learning disability, and deafness. In a second type of study (described in the second part of this chapter), the goal was to examine the question of *why* the salient testing conditions yield levels of performance that appear to be better estimates of Intelligence B than those obtained under traditional approaches. In a third type of study (described in the third part of this chapter), the goal was to examine the issue of potential compensations that dynamic assessment could bring about in performance of children from different ethnic groups.

Children with Special Characteristics

In a study of the applicability of the above-described testing approaches for children with mild mental retardation, we (Carlson & Wiedl, 1978) administered the RCPM to 108 special-placement children. The mean age of the sample was 10.5 years; the mean Wechsler Intelligence Scale for Children (WISC) IQ was 70.8. The subjects were randomly assigned to one of the six testing conditions described above. The results of the investigation were similar to those of the first study, with testing conditions C_2, C_5, and C_6 yielding higher levels of performance than the other conditions. Once again, the salient testing conditions were effective in improving performance on the reasoning by analogy items only. The results of this study were replicated in a subsequent investigation involving 134 mildly retarded subjects (Wiedl & Carlson, 1981). The only difference in results was that the verbalization condition, C_2, did not result in higher performance than obtained under the standard testing condition. Accordingly, doubt was cast on the efficacy of verbalization for mildly retarded children, although there is most likely a "threshold" mental ability level above which mildly retarded children can profit from verbalization procedures.

In a study focusing on nonretarded, learning disabled children, one of us (Carlson, 1983a) administered the RCPM Section C of the Raven's Standard Progressive Matrices (RSPM; Raven, 1962) and the Cattell Culture Fair Test (CCFT; Cattell & Cattell, 1960) to 229 fourth- and fifth-grade children; 75 of these children had been classified by their school district as having specific learning disability, and the remaining 154 had been given no special classification. The testing procedures employed were the standard C_1, verbalization C_2, and elaborated feedback C_5 conditions. The results pertinent to the main effects of the testing conditions showed that for both the learning-disabled and non–learning-disabled groups, and for both Raven tests and the Cattell test, verbalization (C_2) was the most effective testing condition. Elaborated feedback (C_5) was also effective, resulting in performance higher than that obtained under the standard condition (C_1). For the RSPM, performance on the reasoning by analogy items was most affected by the salient testing conditions. Differences between the learning-disabled and non–learning-disabled groups tended to be negligible regardless of the test used or testing condition employed.

In a study involving 6- to 12-year-old deaf children, Carlson and Dillon (1978) found that testing conditions beneficial in enhancing performance on the RCPM involved elaborated feedback plus "verbalization" (American sign language). Similar results were reported in an extension of this work by Dillon (1979).

In summary, although slight differentiations must be made according to the age and special characteristics of the children, testing procedures that involve either problem verbalization or elaborated feedback seem to provide the most effective approaches for improving test performance. These approaches appear to yield estimates of intellectual ability that are better indicators of cognitive competence than those obtained under standard, traditional testing procedures.

Factors That Explain Increased Test Performance

In our first studies (Carlson & Wiedl, 1976; Carlson & Wiedl, 1978), evidence was obtained that indicated that performance effects were related to specific individual-difference variables, particularly cognitive impulsivity/reflectivity, anxiety, and neuroticism. Subsequent studies were carried out to investigate these relationships further. The results of these studies are summarized below.

Test Anxiety, the Test Situation, and Visual Search Behavior

Two studies (Bethge, Carlson, & Wiedl, 1982; Wiedl, Bethge, & Bethge, 1982) were conducted to investigate the relationship between procedural characteristics, orientation variables (see A Theoretical Model, below) and the performance-optimizing conditions: problem verbalization and elaborated feedback. Both studies employed third-grade samples. The RCPM was used to measure cognitive ability. Orientation variables were conceptualized as subjects' evaluations of the test situation and test anxiety. Procedural characteristics included exactness and planfulness (see Das & Varnhagen, 1986). The hypothesis guiding the investigations was that the effects of the optimizing testing conditions could be at least partially explained through changes in orientation as well as in procedural characteristics. In other words, changes brought about in the "noncognitive" variables were hypothesized to contribute to improved cognitive performance.

The orientation variables were operationalized by two scales: one measured the helpfulness of the testing procedures as perceived by the subject; the other was a traditional measure of state test anxiety, patterned after the work of Mandler and Sarason (1952). The procedural characteristics, exactness and planfulness, were operationalized through subjects' visual search behavior as they solved the items on the RCPM.

Although verbalization as well as elaborated feedback led to higher levels of performance than those elicited under the standard testing condition, the findings related to the orientation and procedural characteristic variables are of primary importance. The optimizing testing conditions led to reduced test anxiety, more positive evaluation of the testing situation, and more planful and exact visual scanning behavior. These results suggest the efficacy of performance-improving testing conditions may lie, at least partially, in their effects on variables that in themselves are "noncognitive" but that affect performance on cognitive tasks.

The visual scanning behavior under verbalization and elaborated feedback testing conditions is depicted in Figure 6.2. Examination of

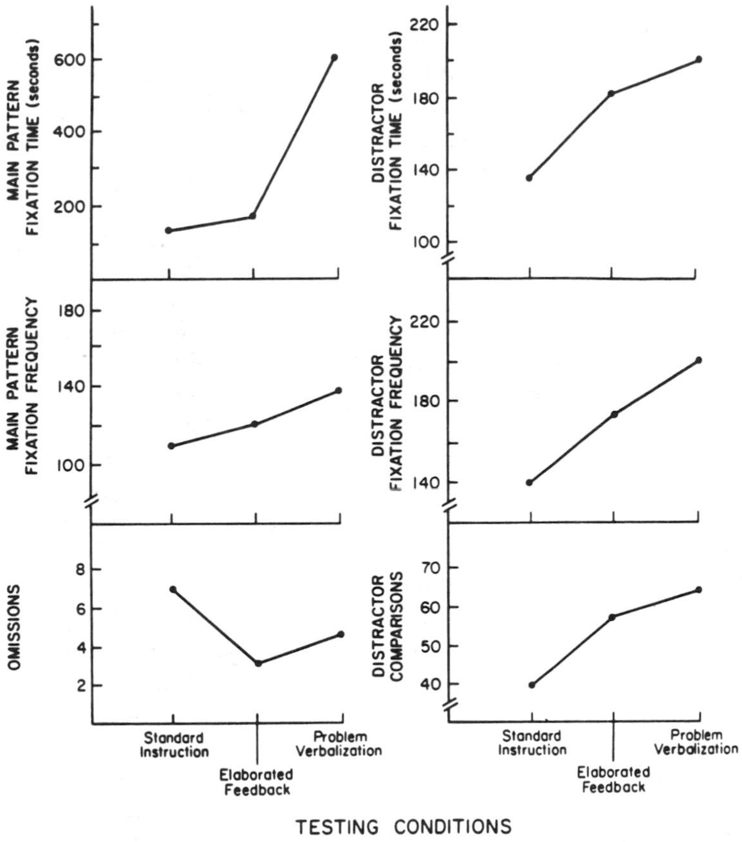

FIGURE 6.2. The visual scanning behavior under verbalization and elaborated feedback testing conditions. Results of eye movement measures are summed across all RCPM items for the three testing conditions.

Figure 6.2 will show marked changes in visual search behavior related to the verbalization condition: the subjects spent more time on both the main stimulus pattern of the RCPM and on the test's answer alternatives than they did under the standard or elaborated feedback condition. Similarly, the number of comparisons the subjects made between the main pattern and the answer alternatives increased significantly in the verbalization condition. These results are consistent with those obtained by Wagner and Cimiotti (1975), who showed that the subjects' overt verbalization while solving the tasks of the Matching Familiar Figures Test (MFFT) results in much more systematic search and comparison strategies than is evident for subjects who are given the MFFT in the traditional manner.

Impulsivity and Reflectivity

Impulsivity-reflectivity constitutes another, though not independent, dimension of what we term *procedural characteristics*. We hypothesized that the testing conditions that had been found to improve performance on the Raven matrices would be particularly effective for children who tended to be impulsive. If this were the case, another source of variability in performance on cognitive tasks would be partially explained by variability in an essentially "noncognitive" variable.

To investigate the hypothesis, one of us, Wiedl (1980), administered the MFFT to 150 second-grade children. Based on a median-split on the error scores on the test, the subjects were divided into two groups defined as impulsive or reflective. The subjects from both groups were individually administered the RCPM under one of four testing conditions: standard (C_1), verbalization (C_2), elaborated feedback (C_5), and verbalization and elaborated feedback (C_6). The results showed that the impulsive group scored significantly lower on the RCPM than did the reflective group when the test was administered under the standard condition. Under C_2 and C_5, however, the performance of the impulsive group improved significantly, matching that of the reflective group. The testing condition involving elaborated feedback (C_6) resulted in improved performance for both the impulsive and reflective groups. It did not result in compensatory effects for the impulsives, however.

Confirmation of the above results was obtained in a replication study (Wiedl & Bethge, 1981) that involved third-grade children who were classified as impulsive or reflective based on the latency score of the MFFT. Once again, whereas significant differences in performance between the two groups were observed under the standard testing procedure, compensations for the impulsive children were obtained under C_2 and C_5.

The general conclusion drawn from these two investigations was that impulsive behavior can be modified effectively through verbalization and feedback and that more accurate estimates of intellectual performance of impulsive children can be obtained through salient dynamic testing techniques than through traditional testing approaches.

With this in mind, the main question we asked was, Why do such compensations take place? To address this question, an investigation was designed to analyze how visual search behavior of the impulsive children may be affected by the salient testing conditions. The study involved administering the RCPM to 72 third-grade children who had been classified as impulsive or reflective by a median split on the latency measure of the MFFT (Wiedl & Bethge, 1983). In addition to the standard approach, the two dynamic testing conditions found to be effective in the previously described study were employed (C_2 and C_5). Using the measures of fixation time on the main stimulus of the RCPM and fixation

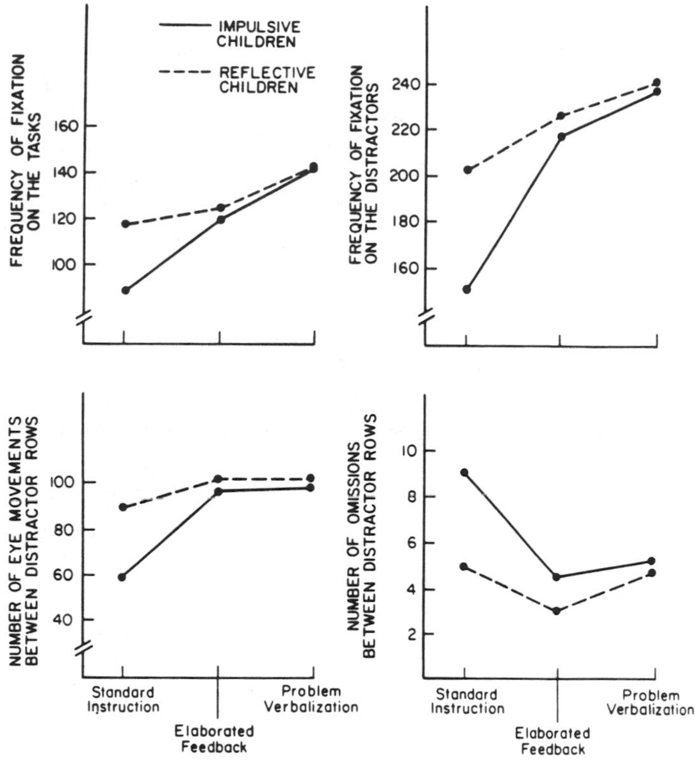

FIGURE 6.3. Results of measures of fixation time on the main stimulus of the RCPM and fixation time on the test's answer alternatives. —, effects of testing conditions on the visual search strategies of impulsive children; ----, of reflective children.

time on the test's answer alternatives, the results showed that the dynamic testing procedures had two effects: (a) they raised the impulsive children's general level of inspection time, and (b) they increased the differential amount of time that the impulsive children spent on items with higher levels of difficulty. Taken together, these results, which are summarized in Figure 6.3, suggest that the positive effects of the effective dynamic testing conditions are at least partially brought about by changes in relevant procedural characteristics as inferred through patterns of visual search behavior.

Compensations in Performance Across Ethnic Groups

There has been a good deal of research, discussion, and debate surrounding similarities and differences in mental abilities of members of different American ethnic groups (see, e.g., Eysenck & Kamin, 1981;

Jensen, 1985; Scarr, 1981). The issues most hotly debated concern test bias and the explanations used to account for the discrepancy between white and black performance on tests of mental abilities. It is not within the scope of this chapter to deal with the many methodological, theoretical, and sociological issues involved in assessment of black-white performance on IQ tests. Rather, we will discuss briefly how the dynamic assessment approach we use may be useful in addressing issues related to ethnic group differences in measured intelligence

In the previous section it was pointed out that "nontarget," i.e., putatively noncognitive, procedural and orientation variables play a role in performance on tests such as the Raven matrices. For example, performance-reducing effects of lack of motivation, anxiety, and impulsivity can be compensated for by salient dynamic testing approaches, especially overt verbalization. It seems clear that these particular "nontarget" variables, plus variables yet to be considered, play an important role in explaining individual differences in measured intelligence within a single ethnic group. In parallel fashion, it is fruitful to establish the extent to which these variables may contribute to observed group differences in performance on "g"-loaded tests of intelligence. Accordingly, application of dynamic testing procedures to black populations may help provide some insight into, and perhaps some revision of, the generalized finding that black Americans, on the average, score about one standard deviation lower than white Americans on standard IQ tests (Jensen, 1985).

To study the potential compensatory effects of the dynamic assessment approach for children from different American ethnic groups, Dillon and Carlson (1978) administered the RCPM as well as various Piagetian tests (matrices and order of appearance) to 189 white, black, and Hispanic children between the ages of 5 and 10 years. Three testing conditions were employed: standard (C_1), verbalization during and after solution (C_2), and verbalization during and after solution plus elaborated feedback (C_6). The sample was divided into three age groups (5 to 6 years of age, 7 to 8 years of age, and 9 to 10 years of age) and randomly assigned to testing conditions. Because the results were essentially the same for both the Raven and Piagetian tests, they are summarized in Table 6.1 for the Piaget matrices test only.

Inspection of Table 6.1 will show that significant differences in performance noted between the ethnic groups under standard conditions (C_1) were reduced under conditions C_2 and C_6. As had been found previously, although the verbalization condition was not effective for younger children, it was effective for children over 8 years of age. Elaborated feedback, on the other hand, was effective in improving scores regardless of age group. These results were encouraging as they offered some indication that compensations in test performance can be obtained for children of different ethnic groups. We did not conclude

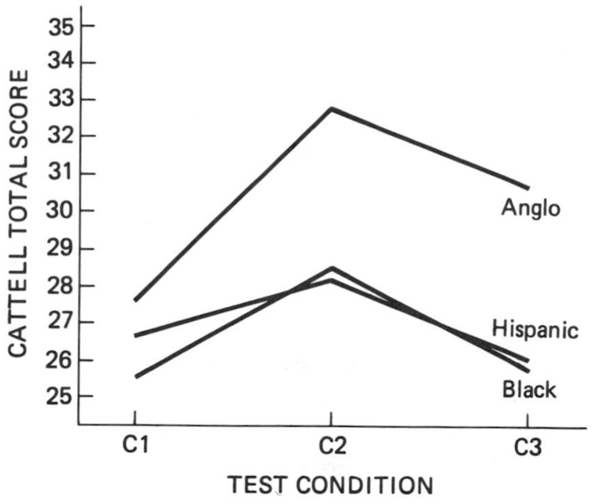

FIGURE 6.4. Results of administering the Cattell Culture Fair Test to 147 white, black, and Hispanic fourth- and fifth-grade children.

from this study that dynamic testing would eliminate group differences in tested intelligence; rather, we viewed the results heuristically, suggesting that certain compensations in performance can be manifested through dynamic assessment, which may affect various ethnic groups differentially and help compensate for what might be systematic underestimation of the mental ability of certain individuals from low-scoring groups.

In a follow-up to the above study, the Cattell Culture Fair Test (Cattell & Cattell, 1960) and the Raven matrices were administered to 147 fourth- and fifth-grade children (Carlson, 1983b). The sample consisted of 67 white children, 37 black children, and 43 Hispanic children. The subjects

TABLE 6.1. Means and standard deviations of Anglo, Mexican-American, and black children for the Piaget matrices administered under three conditions.

	Age: 5–6			Age: 7–8			Age: 9–10		
	C_1	C_2	C_6	C_1	C_2	C_6	C_1	C_2	C_6
Anglo									
Mean	1.29---	.71——	2.43	3.43---	2.43——	4.29	4.14——	6.00---	6.29
SD	.95	1.11	2.23	2.37	1.51	95	2.80	1.73	1.60
Mex-Am									
Mean	.57---	1.71——	2.43	2.14---	2.71——	4.00	4.29——	5.71---	6.14
SD	.98	1.70	2.23	.90	1.50	1.41	2.29	1.38	1.07
Black									
Mean	.57---	.86——	2.00	1.43---	2.71——	4.14	2.71——	5.72---	6.00
SD	.79	.85	1.83	1.40	1.60	90	1.38	1.25	1.00

--- difference not significant.
—— difference significant.

were randomly assigned to three testing conditions: standard (C_1), verbalization (C_2), and elaborated feedback (C_5). The results of the investigation showed that, for both that Raven and Cattell, the verbalization condition was particularly effective in improving scores. The Cattell results, summarized in Figure 6.4, show that although the dynamic testing procedures did lead to improvements in performance for the Hispanic and black subjects over their performance in standard conditions, improvements of equal magnitudes were also made by the white subjects tested. Accordingly, a differential compensatory effect was not found for the black children tested.

Although the results of the two studies confirm that verbalization can lead to higher performance of minority children on commonly used measures of general intelligence, the issue of whether compensatory effects can be obtained by the salient testing conditions remains open. What would seem to be critical to investigate is the distribution of the performance-affecting orientation and procedural variables in the ethnic groups of interest. Assuming that the distributions of these variables across ethnic group are not equal, studies should be undertaken to determine the relative amount of between-group variability attributable to these factors and how dynamic assessment could be used to yield estimates of intellectual ability that are as free of the performance-reducing effects of "nontarget" variables as possible.

A Theoretical Model

The investigations summarized in the previous sections were based on the assumption that the best estimates of Intelligence B can be made by the use of testing procedures that enhance performance and reduce the effects of noncognitive factors on cognitive tasks. To the extent that dynamic assessment approaches are effective, individual differences in test performance should be related principally to differences in cognitive competence and not to differences in factors that affect test performance in a variety of unspecified ways. If the effects of performance-affecting noncognitive variables can be taken into account through the use of effective dynamic testing procedures, the validity of the test should be increased and greater confidence in observed individual and group differences gained. Although terms such as "learning potential" (Budoff, 1970), "learning ability" (Guthke, 1982), and "plasticity" (Baltes & Baltes, 1982) have been used in the dynamic assessment literature, they leave open the central question of explaining why some individuals improve under certain test conditions whereas others do not. Accordingly, a theoretical model is required to explain and predict how modifications in testing procedures can yield results that are accurate estimates of the cognitive ability putatively assessed. The model should meet three criteria: (a) it should be able to specify how solution strategies vary with regard to various test items; (b) it should be complex enough so that test performance can be understood in terms of the contribution of both cognitive and noncognitive factors; and (c) it should be able to suggest a variety of interventions that can be used to optimize cognitive functioning.

We (Carlson & Wiedl, 1980) formulated a theoretical model that meets the above criteria by considering the theoretical work of Rubenstein (1958) and the expansion of this work by Lompscher (1975). In the model, a summary of which is depicted in Table 6.2, we do not conceive of test performance as a necessarily veridical indicator of a latent ability; rather, we conceptualize performance as a result of a dynamic interaction between the individual, the test materials, and the test situation. Variations in how the test is given affect this interaction and provide insight into individual-difference factors that affect test performance.

In the model, three levels of analysis can be made. These involve personal factors, task requirements, and diagnostic or intervention approaches.

Personal factors involve (a) cognitive components that reflect an individual's basic mental ability, (b) procedural characteristics that an individual employs in the task of problem solving, and (c) orientation variables that reflect how an individual approaches the test situation. The latter includes such variables as confidence, motivation, and anxiety.

Task requirements reflect the demands of the test itself. They can range from physical activity requiring overt processes to purely mental

TABLE 6.2. A conceptual schema for the analysis of test performance and change.

I. Personal factors
  - Cognitive component
    - Basic mutual abilities
    - Procedural characteristics (e.g. planning and strategic behavior)
    - Orientation variables (e.g., task-specific orientation, test anxiety)

II. Task requirements
  - Levels
    - Material for practical activity
    - Material for indirect perception
    - Material for linguistic-conceptual knowledge

III. Diagnostic approaches
  - Modification
    - Implicit/explicit
    - Predetermined/self-determined
  - Compensation
    - Prosthetic
    - Catalytic
  - Inhibition
    - Complicating factors

activity involving covert processes as well as specific linguistic and/or conceptual knowledge.

Diagnostic approaches involve three factors: (a) modification in relatively long-term changes in specific individual characteristics such as use of strategic rules or metacognitive processes; (b) compensation of situation-specific, i.e., short-term strategies (prosthetic compensation refers to the elimination or reduction of those characteristics that tend to hinder performance; catalytic compensation refers to the activation of latent personal characteristics that aid performance); (c) inhibition of cognitive performance through situational factors.

The model implies that a number of factors related to the individual, the test, and the conditions of test administration interact in complex and usually unmeasured ways. Our research has shown that specific modes of test administration can affect procedural and orientation variables in such a way that the individual's strategic approach to the tasks presented is modified, resulting in performance levels that offer what appear to be better estimates of ability than would be obtained using traditional psychometric approaches. A good deal of research is necessary before the several variables suggested by the model are operationalized and evaluated in terms of their theoretical and practical significance; nonetheless, the model can serve as a heuristically important guide in the quest to gain veridical estimates of group and individual differences in mental ability.

Summary of Most-Recent Work

Our present work concerning diagnostic approaches to intelligence assessment focuses on issues related to construct validity, a more differentiated perspective on methodological issues, and a better conception of the processes of change in test performance.

The empirical work is oriented by intrinsic and extrinsic validation strategies. The first strategy incorporates investigations designed to ascertain the fundamental mental components involved in processing the information presented by tasks such as those found in the Raven, Cattell, or Wechsler scales. Using chronometric and mathematical modeling approaches to establish the basal information-processing components involved in solving tasks from the Raven matrices, for example, Schoettke, Gediga, and Wiedl (1987) have shown that individual differences in performance are related to basic mental components and to the specific characteristics of the test items.

A second strategy involves further development of the assessment methodology and general model described in the previous sections of this chapter. Because test performance is conceptualized to be the result of the dynamic interaction between the individual, the test materials, and the test situation, with these interactions having differential effects on various subcategories of the problem-solving process, "diagnostic programs" (see Guthke, 1982) were and are being developed and tested. These programs take into account the various aspects of the general model, the requirements of the task, and the characteristics of the individuals being tested. At present we are working on such a program for the Wechsler Intelligence Scale for Children, although a program for the Raven matrices has already been developed (see Wiedl & Carlson, 1986) and applications of the program are now being made to geriatric and psychiatric patients.

Another focus of the dynamic assessment research being done in our laboratory now involves the use of latent class analysis to assess which individual difference characteristics are related to changes in test performance. This will allow for finer classification of the categories described by Budoff (1970) ("high scorer," "changer," and "nonchanger") as well as provide a more satisfactory theoretical explanation concerning the reasons for observed change or lack of change in individual test performance as a result of dynamic testing approaches.

Summary

In this chapter a number of studies were described which have, we believe, demonstrated the usefulness of dynamic assessment for measuring intellectual ability. The dynamic assessment approach we have used is practical and can be used for a variety of populations. It does not require specific training of the individual being tested or pre- and posttest designs. Furthermore, it avoids methodological problems related to the measurement of change. Although intelligence assessment continues to be plagued by a plethora of theoretical, methodological, social, political, and practical problems, the dynamic assessment approach described in this chapter provides an alternative to the traditional methods of assessment.

References

Baltes, P., & Baltes, M. (1982). Plasticity and enhancement of intellectual functioning in old age. In F. Craig & S. Trehub (Eds.), *Aging and cognitive processes* (pp. 353–389). New York: Plenum.

Bethge, H.-J., Carlson, J. S., & Wiedl, K. H. (1982). The effects of dynamic assessment procedures on Raven matrices performance, visual search behavior, test anxiety, and test orientation. *Intelligence*, *6*, 89–97.

Boring, E. G. (1923). Intelligence as the test measures it. *The New Republic*, *35*, 35–37.

Brown, A. L., & Campione, J. C. (1986). Academic intelligence and learning potential. In R. J. Sternberg & D. K. Dettermann (Eds.), *What is intelligence? Contemporary viewpoints on its nature and definition*. New York: Ablex.

Brown, A. L., & French, L. (1979). The zone of potential development: Implications for intelligence testing in the year 2000. *Intelligence*, *3*, 255–273.

Budoff, M. (1970). Learning potential: Assessing ability to reason in the educable mentally retarded. *Acta Paedopsychiatrica*, *37*, 293–309.

Campione, J. C., & Brown, A. L. (1984). Learning ability and transfer propensity as sources of individual differences in intelligence. In P. H. Brooks, R. D. Sperber, & C. McCauley (Eds.), *Learning and cognition in the mentally retarded* (pp. 265–294). Baltimore: University Park Press.

Carlson, J. S. (1983a). *Dynamic assessment in relation to learning characteristics and teaching strategies for children with specific learning disability*. Final report: U.S. Department of Education, Grant #6008100426, CFDA, 84,023E.

Carlson, J. S. (1983b). *Applications of dynamic assessment cognitive and perceptual functioning of three ethnic groups*. Final report: National Institute of Education, Grant #NIE-G-0081.

Carlson, J. S., & Dillon, R. F. (1978). The effects of testing-the-limits procedures on Raven matrices performance of deaf children. *Volta Review*, *4*, 216–224.

Carlson, J. S., & Dillon, R. F. (1979). The effects of testing conditions on Piaget matrices and order of appearance problems: A study of competence versus performance. *Journal of Educational Measurement*, *16*, 19–26.

Carlson, J. S., & Jensen, C. M. (1980). The factorial structure of the Raven Coloured Progressive Matrices: A reanalysis. *Journal of Educational and Psychological Measurement*, *40*, 1111–1116.

Carlson, J. S., & Wiedl, K. H. (1976). Modes of presentation of the Raven Coloured Progressive Matrices test: Toward a differential testing approach. *Trier Psychologische Berichte*, *3*, 1–78.

Carlson, J. S., & Wiedl, K. H. (1978). The use of testing-the-limits procedures in the assessment of intellectual capabilities in children with learning difficulties. *American Journal of Mental Deficiency*, *82*, 559–564.

Carlson, J. S., & Wiedl, K. H. (1979). Towards a differential testing approach: Testing-the-limits employing the Raven matrices. *Intelligence*, *3*, 323–344.

Carlson, J. S., & Wiedl, K. H. (1980). Applications of a dynamic testing approach: Empirical results and theoretical formulations. *Zeitschrift für Differentielle und Diagnostische Psychologie*, *4*, 303–318.

Cattell, R. B., & Cattell, A. K. S. (1960). *Culture Fair Scale 2*. Champaign, IL: Institute of Personality and Ability Testing, Inc.

Cleary, T. A. (1968). Test bias: Prediction of grades of Negro and white students in integrated colleges. *Journal of Educational Measurement*, *5*, 115–124.

Cleary, T. A., Humphreys, L. G., Kendrick, S. A., & Wesman, A. (1975). Educational uses of tests with disadvantaged students. *American Psychologist*, *30*, 15–41.

Cole, N. S. (1980). Bias in testing. *American Psychologist*, *36*, 1067–1077.

Cronbach, L. J. (1971). Test validation. In R. L. Thorndike (Ed.), *Educational measurement* (2nd ed.). Washington, DC: American Council on Education.

Darlington, R. B. (1971). Another look at "culture fairness." *Journal of Educational Measurement*, *8*, 71–82.

Das, J. P., & Varnhagen, C. K. (1986). Neuropsychological functioning and cognitive processing. *Child Neuropsychology*, *1*, 117–140.

Dillon, R. F. (1979). *The effects of elaborative testing conditions on the assessment of cognitive abilities in deaf children*. Unpublished doctoral dissertation, University of California, Riverside.

Dillon, R. F., & Carlson, J. S. (1978). Testing for competence in three ethnic groups. *Educational and Psychological Measurement*, *38*, 436–443.

Eichorn, H., & Bass, A. (1971). Methodological considerations relevant to discrimination in employment testing. *Psychological Bulletin*, *75*, 261–269.

Eysenck, H. J. (1982). *A model for intelligence*. New York: Springer.

Eysenck, H. J., & Kamin, L. (1981). *The intelligence controversy*. New York: Wiley.

Ferrara, R. A., Brown, A. L., & Campione, J. C. (1986). Children's learning and transfer of inductive reasoning rules: Studies of proximal development. *Child Development*, *57*, 1087–1099.

Feuerstein, R., Rand, Y., & Hoffman, M. (1979). *The dynamic assessment of retarded performers: The learning potential assessment device, theory, instruments, and techniques*. Baltimore: University Park Press.

Feuerstein, R., Rand, Y., Hoffman, M., & Miller, R. (1980). *Intrumental Enrichment*. Baltimore: University Park Press.

Flaugher, R. L. (1978). The many definitions of test bias. *American Psychologist*, *33*, 671–679.

Guthke, J. (1982). The learning-test concept: An alternative to the traditional static intelligence test. *German Journal of Psychology*, *6*, 306–324.

Hebb, D. O. (1949). *The organization of behavior*. New York: Wiley.

Jensen, A. R. (1966). Verbal mediation and educational potential. *Psychology in the Schools*, *3*, 99–109.

Jensen, A. R. (1980). *Bias in mental testing*. New York: Free Press.

Jensen, A. R. (1985). The nature of the black-white difference on various psychometric tests: Spearman's hypothesis. *Behavioral and Brain Sciences*, *8*, 193–219.

Lompscher, J. (1975). *Theoretische und experimentelle Untersuchungen zur Entwicklung geistiger Fähigkeiten*. Berlin: Volk und Wissen.

Mandler, G., & Sarason, S. (1952). A study of anxiety and learning. *Journal of Abnormal and Social Psychology*, *47*, 166–173.

Mercer, J. R., & Lewis, J. P. (1975). *System of multicultural pluralistic assessment: Technical manual*. Unpublished manuscript, University of California, Riverside.

Overton, W. F., & Newman, J. L. (1982). Cognitive development: A competence-activation/utilization approach. In T. Field, A. Houston, H. Quay, L. Troll, & G. Finley (Eds.), *Review of human development*. New York: Wiley.

Radford, J. (1966). Verbalization effects in a nonverbal intelligence test. *British Journal of Educational Psychology*, *36*, 33–38.

Raven, J. C. (1962). *The Advanced Progressive Matrices* (3rd ed.). London: Lewis.

Raven, J. C. (1976). *The Coloured Progressive Matrices*. London: Lewis.

Resnick, L. (1979). The future of IQ testing in education. *Intelligence*, *3*, 241–253.

Rubenstein, S. L. (1958). *Grundlagen der allgemeinen Psychologie*. Berlin: Deutscher Verlag der Wissenschaften.

Scarr, S. (1981). Testing *for* children: Assessment and many determinants of intellectual competence. *American Psychologist*, *36*, 1159–1166.

Vernon, P. E. (1962). *The structure of human abilities* (2nd ed.). London: Methuen.

Wagner, I., & Cimiotti, E. (1975). Impulsive und reflexive Kinder prüfen Hypothesen: Strategien beim Problemlösen, aufgezeigt an Blickbewegungen. *Zeitschrift für Entwicklungspsychologie und Pädagogische Psychologie*, *7*, 1–15.

Wiedl, K. H. (1980). Kompensatorische Interventionen im Rahmen intelligenzdiagnostischer Untersuchungen bei kognitive impulsiven Kindern. *Zeitschrift für Klinische Psychologie*, *9*, 219–231.

Wiedl, K. H., & Bethge, H.-J. (1981). Zur Auswirkung regulationsfördernder Situationsveränderungen auf Intelligenzleistung und Blickverhalten kognitiv impulsiver Kinder. *Zeitschrift für Entwicklungspsychologie und Pädagogische Psychologie*, *2*, 127–141.

Wiedl, K. H., & Bethge, H.-J. (1983). Die Anpassung der aufgabenbezongenen Betrachtungszeit an variierende Aufgabenschwierigkeiten: Diskriptive und veränderungsbezogene Analysen bei kognitive impulsiven und reflexiven Kindern. *Zeitschrift für Differentielle und Diagnostische Psychologie*, *4*, 67–77.

Wiedl, K. H., Bethge, H.-J., & Bethge, H. (1982). Die Anpassung der aufgabenbezongenen Betrachtungszeit an variierende Aufgabenschierigkeiten: Diskriptive und veränderungsbezogene Analysen bei kognitive impulsiven und reflexiven Kindern. *Zeitschrift für Differentielle und diagnostische Psychologie*, *4*, 67–77.

Wiedl, K. H., & Carlson, J. S. (1981). Dynamisches Testen bei lernbehinderten Sonderschülern mit dem Farbigen Matrizentest von Raven. *Heilpädagogische Forschung*, *9*, 19–37.

Wiedl, K. H., & Carlson, J. S. (1986). The dynamic testing approach: Theoretical conceptions and practical applications. In G. d'Ydewalle (Ed.), *Cognition, information processing, and motivation*. Amsterdam: North Holland.

7
Dynamic Group Assessment for Prescriptive Teaching: Differential Effects of Treatments

David Tzuriel and Reuven Feuerstein

The concept of cognitive modifiability, its nature, antecedents, and applications for assessment and intervention, has been recently the focus of interest for many psychologists and educators. The interest in cognitive modifiability has been broadened mainly because of the comprehensive work of Feuerstein and his colleagues on assessment of learning potential and the development of the Learning Potential Assessment Device (LPAD) and the Instrumental Enrichment program for modification of the intellectual level of functioning (Feuerstein, Rand, Hoffman, 1979; Feuerstein, Rand, Hoffman & Miller, 1980; Feuerstein, Haywood, Rand, Hoffman, & Jensen, 1986). An important characteristic of the LPAD, which is the most extensive dynamic approach known in the literature, is the fact that both the assessment method and the systematic interventional program are intrinsically linked to the same theoretical framework.

Previous attempts to assess the true capacity of retarded performers by conventional psychometric methods have been found to be inadequate. Psychometric test results of retarded performers only confirm what is already known—that their manifest level of functioning is low. The conventional tests bring about a vicious circle (process) in which inferences of low functioning are made by demonstration of poor performance, thus confirming the impression of stability of functioning and consequently preventing any serious attempts to change the course of development. In contrast, the assessment of cognitive modifiability is based on the induction of changes in examinees' thinking processes within the testing situation and assessing their modified performance in tasks that become gradually more complex and/or more abstract. The criterion for success in school learning and achievements of retarded performers is their level of cognitive modifiability rather than their level of actual performance. Their achievements in school depend of course on the amount and nature of investment given after the assessment procedure.

The assessment of cognitive modifiability requires an investment in attacking the cognitive impairments, deficient learning habits, and motivational patterns that are responsible for the poor performance. This assessment has special significance for disadvantaged and special needs children, who are jeopardized by conventional psychometric methods. The unique characteristics of the dynamic assessment of learning potential are discussed elsewhere (Feuerstein, et al., 1979). Most discussions refer to the individual assessment situation, which involves a complex interactional process. In the current study the focus is on group assessment of cognitive modifiability. Although group testing is much less effective in causing change and yields less information than does individual assessment, its merit is that it can provide preliminary indications about children's learning potential and specific difficulties that necessitate later in-depth individual assessment, and it is more economical. Other advantages are its utility in the description of groups or where entire classes present similar problems. In these cases the use of the dynamic approach might be very helpful in searching for educational, didactic, or organizational answers.

Dynamic group testing differs from conventional static testing by activating learning processes prior to test performance. It also differs by mediation during the testing itself whenever the tester considers that some basic prerequisites are still not available to the examinees. Feuerstein, et al. (1986) emphasized that there are three conditions necessary for group dynamic approach: (a) the results obtained in a group assessment are considered valid only if they demonstrate that the examinees are able to use the training provided in the test situation; (b) the test structure should permit dynamic measurement of individual modifiability; and (c) the teaching phase before testing should be presented in a manner that will ensure the maximum possible efficiency.

Besides the actual importance of dynamic group assessment as indicative of learning potential and of specific cognitive deficiencies, it also has theoretical importance for understanding the nature and conditions under which children's cognitive functioning is modified, as well as prescriptive implications for actual teaching in school.

It should be emphasized that dynamic group assessment does not replace individual testing, nor is it used as the sole measure for decision making for either placement or teaching strategies. Rather, dynamic assessment is used as a screening device to detect those students who will later need in-depth individual assessment. The LPAD group assessment is composed of eight tests (see Feuerstein et al., 1986, for specifications). In most cases a battery of three or four tests is used depending on the testing goals and examinee characteristics. In the current study two tests were investigated: Set Variations I and Set Variations II (see descriptions in Measures, below).

The objectives of the current study were: (a) to investigate cognitive modifiability under three experimental conditions—low teaching (LT), high teaching (HT), and no-teaching (control, NT); (b) to study the differential effectiveness of teaching levels for three different groups who differed in initial performance level; and (c) to study effectiveness of teaching conditions for disadvantaged as compared to regular schoolchildren.

Our main expectations were that the HT condition would be more effective in modifying cognitive performance of initially low-performing subjects than of students with initial medium or high performance level. We also expected children from schools labeled as disadvantaged to benefit more from teaching than would regular schoolchildren, especially in the HT condition.

Method

Subjects

The sample consisted of Israeli pupils (689 boys and 705 girls) from the fourth to ninth grades. Subjects came from 30 classes in 14 schools labeled by the Ministry of Education as serving disadvantaged or "culturally deprived" children (N = 595), and 23 classes in 8 regular schools (N = 799). Children in nonintegrative schools in Israel usually come from a homogeneous socioeconomic status level. The average number of years of education of fathers of disadvantaged and regular children was 9.49 and 12.48, respectively. The parallel average years of education for mothers was 9.43 and 12.53, respectively. Most of the fathers (40%) and mothers (17%) of regular schoolchildren had technical or professional occupations (e.g., teachers, academics, artists, qualified technicians) as compared to fathers (11%) and mothers (9%) of disadvantaged schoolchildren. Only 5% of the fathers and 24% of the mothers of the regular schoolchildren were manual laborers, held jobs in the service occupations, or worked in unskilled positions as compared to 40% of fathers and 47% of mothers of disadvantaged children.

Measures

Raven's Standard Progressive Matrices (RSPM; Raven, 1947) is a test of reasoning ability based on figural stimuli. The test measures the ability to form comparisons, to reason by analogy, and to organize spatial perceptions into systematically related wholes. The RSPM consists of 60 items grouped into five sets of 12 items each. In each item the examinees are asked to complete the matrix by selecting the correct answer from six to eight alternatives. For some problems the solution requires a Gestalt approach in which the internal structure of the stimulus is discovered perceptually. For other problems the solution is discovered by an analytic approach using logical operations. In addition to the total score, two more scores were derived: from the RSPM a score on items B8 to B12 (5 items), and a score composed of items B8 to B12 and C7, C8, C12, D12, and E12 (10 items). These scores were used because of their similarity to the Set Variations test. The objective was to assess the degree of modifiability on these derived scores, which were closely similar to the teaching conditions.

Set Variations I consists of 35 items divided into five parts; each part contains one example and six other problems based on the same principles for solution as in the example. Within each set the items' difficulty increases progressively. The tasks are similar to items B8 to B12 of the RSPM (see example in Figure 7.1).

The problems must be solved by applying analogical operations. Examinees must supply the missing part in the problem out of eight distractors by deducing the relationship between the two objects in the upper row or between objects in the left column and applying it to the lower row or to the right column, respectively. Set Variations II consists of 63 items divided into five parts; each part contains one example and 10 to 15 problems based on the same principles for solution as in the example. The tasks are similar to items C7, C8, C12, D12, and E12 of the RSPM (see example in Figure 7.1). In general, problems in Set Variations II are more difficult, complex, and abstract than are problems in Set Variations I. The strategies of finding the solution, number of distractors, and many required cognitive functions for solution are similar in both Set Variations. Split-half reliabilities of LPAD Set Variations I and II were .82 and .98 in a high teaching (HT) condition, respectively. (See Procedure, below, for explanation of conditions.) In a low teaching (LT) condition the parallel reliabilities were .90 and .93, respectively. The correlations between the RSPM and Set Variations in HT and LT conditions were .18 (ns) and .78 ($p < .001$), respectively. The parallel correlations for Set Variations II were .49 ($p < .05$) and .85 ($p < .001$), respectively. It should be noted that the correlations between the Set Variations and RSPM scores were much higher in the LT than in the HT condition.

Procedure

Classes in each grade were randomly assigned to one of three experimental conditions: LT, HT, and NT. A basic before-after design was used with identical (RSPM) tests given before and 2 weeks after the intervention. The reason for retesting the subjects 2 weeks after the intervention was to determine whether cognitive changes, manifested in actual performance, would be more-or-less stable and not affected by experimental artifacts immediately after the intervention or by spontaneous temporal changes.

The RSPM was administered to all subjects before the intervention as a static measure. In the second phase the LT and HT condition were

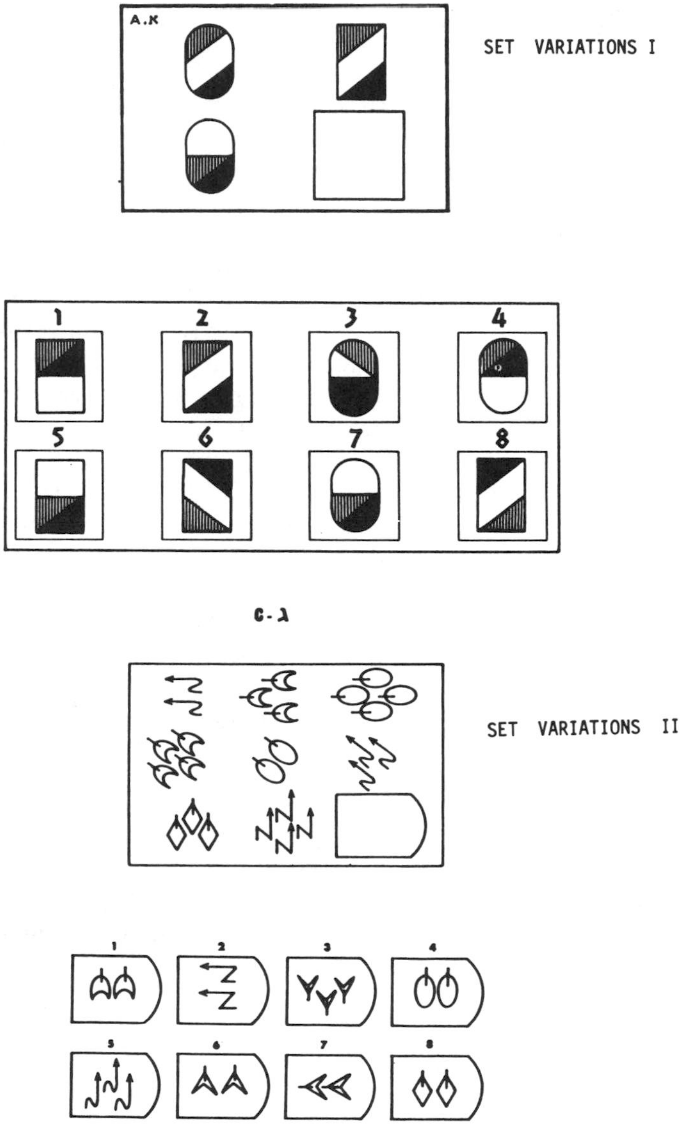

FIGURE 7.1. Example of matrix problems.

applied; no treatment was given to the NT group. The difference between the LT and the HT conditions was in the degree of teaching. Whereas in the HT condition subjects received a set of five exemplar problems and were taught intensively how to solve these problems, subjects in the LT condition were taught only one exemplar problem. A placard of each problem was displayed in front of the class.

The teaching of each sample task involved probing questions and eliciting responses as well as direct teaching of principles. The tester-teacher repeated and summarized the responses if necessary to ensure that they had been heard and understood by all subjects. In explaining how to solve the problems (see exemplar problems in Figure 7.1) the tester used principles of change or transformation, showing that any change that occurs in the first row (or column) will also occur in the second row (or column). All five exemplar tasks were explained to the children one after the other prior to the independent work on the Set Variations. Special care was taken to demonstrate the process of elimination of wrong distractors, focusing on relevant cues, considering several sources of information given in a problem (e.g., form, color, direction, number), and learning the meaning of basic verbal tools such as "row" and "column" that are necessary to find the correct answers. Emphasis was also given for systematic, organized, and nonimpulsive search of the correct answers.

Although subjects worked independently in the Set Variations, they could ask questions. The only assistance that the tester could offer was to point to the pairs of items in the task from left to right or from top to bottom, and to focus the subjects' attention on the process of systematic search. While pointing, the tester might say only "What happens here must also happen here." There was no time limit for work on the Set Variations. Time of teaching and practice lasted about 1 hour for the LT condition and about 3 hours for the HT condition.

The intervention procedures were generally similar across all grade levels (4 to 9), except for the use of Set Variations I in grades 4 to 6 and Set Variations II in grades 7 to 9. This division was crucial because subjects' level of cognitive development had to correspond to the nature of intervention. Although both Set Variations require abstract analogical thinking and deductive reasoning and both are aimed at modifying deficient cognitive functions, Set Variations II contains problems with higher levels of complexity and abstraction and requires in some parts more difficult operations (e.g., projection of virtual relations) than the Set Variations I.

In the last phase of the study, 2 weeks after the intervention, all groups including the NT group were given the RSPM.

Results

Subjects in each grade were divided into three performance level groups (low, medium, high) according to their initial score on the total RSPM pre-intervention performance. The cutoff scores for dividing subjects into three levels were differential by grade. This division was made to investigate the effectiveness of the different teaching conditions for subjects who initially functioned on different levels. In some analyses the initial performance level was the actual score on items B8 to B12 (grades 4 to 6) or on B8 to B12 and C7, C8, C12, D12, and E12 (grades 7 to 9). These two groups of items will be referred to as B8-B12 and B8-E12. The reason for carrying out an additional set of analyses using the B8-B12 or the B8-E12 scores was to investigate in detail the subjects' performance on RSPM items upon which the Set Variations I (B8-B12) or Set Variations II (B8-E12) are based. These analyses allowed us to evaluate near-transfer effects of the intervention procedures.

Separate analyses were carried out on Set Variations (I and II) and on gain scores on the RSPM (total, B8-B12, and B8-E12). One of the problems we faced in evaluating the effectiveness of teaching conditions on subjects who initially performed on a low, medium, or high level was the problem of ceiling effect. The initially low-performing group might show relatively high achievements or high gains following intervention just because they had enough room to increase their performance. On the other hand, initially high-performing subjects might show relatively smaller gains because they were close to the "ceiling" and did not have much "room" to make progress. To overcome this problem we used in most analyses the initial score on the RSPM as a covariate. We tried to control the ceiling effect in two ways: first, by classifying subjects into low, medium, or high performance levels, and second, by using the initial performance level as a covariate.

In some analyses we could not use the initial score as a covariate because the values of the independent variable of initial performance were composed of exactly the same covariate score. For example in analyses in which we used the initial performance level on B8-B12 the value range was 0 to 5. In this case we could not use the same variable as a covariate. Only in analyses in which subjects were grossly classified into high, medium, and low groups based on interval scores could we use the more detailed score as a covariate.

In the following section descriptive data on Set Variations I and II, the RSPM's pre- and postteaching scores, and gain scores on RSPM are presented. In Tables 7.1 and 7.2 the initial performance level is based on the RSPM total score, whereas in Tables 7.3 and 7.4 the B8-B12 and B8-E12 scores were taken as initial performance level. Statistical analyses of the reported data are then presented using Teaching Condition, Initial Performance Level, and Type of School as independent variables and performance on Set Variations or RSPM gain scores as dependent variables. The difference score was computed by substracting the initial B8-B12 percentage score from the Set Variations percentage score. It should be noted that Set Variations I items are based exactly on the B8-B12 items, hence the appropriateness of computing this subtraction. Also, all subjects who scored 0 on B8-B12 received a 0% score. In the same way, all subjects who scored 1, 2, 3, 4, and 5 received a percentage score of 20%, 40%, 60%, 80%, and 100%, respectively. In the NT condition no

TABLE 7.1. Percent of correct answers on RSPM pre- and postteaching and on Variations I by Teaching Condition and Initial Performance Level (Grades 4–6).

Initial RSPM level	*n*	RSPM-1	Set Variations I	RSPM-2	Gain
			High Teaching		
Low	96	40.31	51.32	53.51	13.20
Medium	74	63.47	73.33	69.05	5.58
High	86	74.11	79.07	74.55	.44
Total	256	58.36	67.01	65.07	6.71
			Low Teaching		
Low	49	46.55	52.45	53.67	7.12
Medium	62	64.11	60.43	67.69	3.58
High	73	76.44	79.68	77.15	.71
Total	184	64.33	65.94	67.71	3.38
			No Teaching		
Low	67	45.12	—	50.97	5.85
Medium	69	64.03	—	66.47	2.44
High	69	74.00	—	74.18	.18
Total	205	61.39	—	64.00	2.61

scores are reported for Set Variations I since by definition in NT condition this test was not administered.

Descriptive Data

Cognitive modifiability was operationalized in two ways: (a) the RSPM gain score from pre- to postintervention tests and (b) the Set Variations scores. With regard to the Set Variations scores, the RSPM initial score cannot always be used as a baseline criterion for modifiability because the Variations items are different from the RSPM items. Furthermore, some parts to the Variations, especially Variations II, contain more difficult items than does the RSPM. The criterion for assessment of cognitive modifiability in the case of the Set Variations is comparison to the prototype items upon which the variations are based. Thus, Variation I are compared to RSPM B8-B12 scores and Variations II are compared to RSPM B8-E12 scores.

In Table 7.1 (grades 4 to 6) and Table 7.2 (grades 7 to 9) we present the results on RSPM pre- and postteaching scores, the gain score, and the Variations score. To compare the Variations score to the RSPM, all scores were converted to percentages. The results in Table 7.1 refer only to grades 4 to 6 where the examinees received Variations I, and the results in Table 7.2 refer only to grades 7 to 9 where the examinees received Variations II. Unlike the initial B8-B12 score the prescores (1 to 5) here were not automatically converted into 0% to 100%. Each

TABLE 7.2. Percent of correct answers on RSPM Pre- and Postteaching and on Variations II by Teaching Condition and Initial Performance Level (Grades 7–9).

Initial RSPM level	*n*	RSPM-1	Set Variations II	RSPM-2	Gain
			High Teaching		
Low	113	48.57	40.71	62.03	13.46
Medium	114	69.71	58.55	75.64	5.93
High	107	78.96	75.49	80.86	1.90
Total	334	65.52	57.94	72.71	7.19
			Low Teaching		
Low	49	51.46	33.74	59.56	8.10
Medium	61	71.56	56.42	75.79	4.23
High	57	80.17	69.12	81.73	1.56
Total	167	68.60	54.10	73.05	4.45
			No Teaching		
Low	26	50.38	—	55.77	5.39
Medium	30	72.61	—	74.78	2.17
High	55	79.61	—	78.76	−.85
Total	111	70.87	—	72.30	1.43

category of the B8-E12 contained two to three points, thus allowing more variance of scores within each category.

The results in Table 7.1 and Table 7.2 are very similar in indicating that both teaching level and initial performance level affected performance on the Set Variations and on the RSPM. Highest gains in the HT condition were found especially for the initially low-performing students. The gains decreased with the decrease in the teaching level. The difference between teaching conditions was higher in the initially low-performing group than in the medium- or high-performing group in which the differences were minute. Comparison of the Set Variations I score to RSPM scores (Table 7.1) revealed that in the HT condition the Set Variations I scores were higher than RSPM-1 score in all performance level groups, whereas in the LT condition it was true only for the low-performance group. The parallel comparison in grades 7 to 9 (see Table 7.2) reveals that RSPM-1 scores were higher than were Set Variations II scores. However, the gap between RSPM-1 and Variations II scores was much smaller in the HT group than in the LT group.

In Table 7.3 the postteaching scores for each initial performance level on B8-B12 score (0–5) is compared to both Set Variations I and postteaching score on B8-B12. Again, all scores were converted to percentages.

As can be seen from Table 7.3, the lower the initial performance level the higher the gain score as well as the Set Variations I score in all teaching conditions, and especially in the HT condition. For the highest performing subjects there was even a statistical regression phenomenon: the postteaching scores were actually lower than the preteaching scores.

Table 7.3. Percent of correct answers on RSPM B8-B12 scores, on LPAD Set Variations I, and gain scores by initial B8-B12 scores and Teaching Condition.

Initial B8-B12 level	n	Set Variations I	B8-B12 post	Difference
			High Teaching	
0 (0%)	63	48.7	54.6	54.6
1 (20%)	17	58.6	80.0	60.0
2 (40%)	24	61.1	80.0	40.0
3 (60%)	38	71.7	86.8	26.8
4 (80%)	49	76.1	88.2	8.2
5 (100%)	64	79.6	91.6	−8.4
Total	255	66.9	79.2	12.4
			Low Teaching	
0 (0%)	32	47.4	50.0	50.0
1 (20%)	7	48.1	65.7	45.8
2 (40%)	4	55.0	74.2	34.1
3 (60%)	18	57.0	84.4	24.4
4 (80%)	45	71.8	84.9	4.8
5 (100%)	68	77.3	90.0	−10.0
Total	174	65.9	79.1	6.5
			No Teaching	
0 (0%)	35	—	46.9	46.9
1 (20%)	9	—	53.3	33.3
2 (40%)	18	—	58.9	18.9
3 (60%)	34	—	75.9	15.9
4 (80%)	51	—	86.1	6.1
5 (100%)	57	—	88.4	−11.6
Total	204	—	74.8	6.1

[a] Difference (in %) between B8-B12 (post) and Set Variations I.

High gains were found also for the NT condition especially for the initially low-performing subjects. The Set Variations I scores were higher than the initial B8-B12 scores but lower than the postteaching B8-B12 scores.

In Table 7.4 the pre- and postteaching scores on B8-E12 items (10) are presented together with the gain scores and the Set Variations II scores. All results refer to grades 7 to 9 where the examinees received Set Variations II. The initial performance level is based on five interval scores (0–1, 2–3, 4–5, 6–7, and 8–10) in order to maximize the number of subjects in each cell.

The results in Table 7.4 indicate that the gain scores and Set Variations II scores were generally higher for initially low-performing subjects than for initially high-performing subjects. Higher performances were achieved in the HT condition than in the LT condition and higher in the LT condition than in the NT condition. Similar to results in Table 7.3, higher gains were achieved in the NT condition for initially low-performing subjects than for other performance groups.

TABLE 7.4. Percent of correct answers on RSPM B8-E12 pre- and postteaching scores and on Set Variations II scores by initial B8-B12 scores and Teaching Condition.

Initial B8-E12 score	*n*	Pre	Set Variations II	B8-E12 post	Difference[a]
			High Teaching		
1	44	3.9	35.3	42.7	38.9
2	34	23.8	42.8	55.3	31.5
3	76	46.1	54.6	66.8	20.6
4	147	64.5	65.2	76.3	11.8
5	33	81.8	78.8	87.4	5.6
Total	334	50.0	57.9	68.7	18.7
			Low Teaching		
1	12	7.5	18.97	35.0	27.5
2	12	26.7	32.47	35.8	9.2
3	33	47.0	50.89	64.5	17.6
4	91	64.6	58.49	71.1	6.5
5	19	84.7	74.50	86.8	2.1
Total	167	56.6	54.10	66.5	9.9
			No Teaching		
1	12	5.0	—	29.2	24.2
2	3	26.7	—	36.7	10.0
3	22	46.8	—	54.1	7.3
4	49	66.1	—	69.6	3.5
5	25	85.6	—	75.6	−10.0
Total	111	59.0	—	62.6	3.6

[a] Difference (in %) between B8-E12 (post) and Set Variations II.

Analyses of Covariance of Set Variations I and II

The Set Variations I and II were analyzed separately for grades 4 to 6 and 7 to 9, respectively. In both analyses the independent variables were Teaching Condition, Initial Performance Level, and Type of School. The covariate was initial RSPM total score. The results of both analyses are presented in Table 7.5.

The results for Set Variations II indicate that subjects in the HT condition achieved higher scores than did subjects in the LT condition and that regular schoolchildren scored higher than did disadvantaged children. All main effects were modified by the interaction of Initial Performance Level with Teaching Condition and of Teaching Condition with Type of School. These interactions are presented in Figures 7.2 and 7.3.

As seen from Figure 7.2 the medium-performing group had the greatest benefit from the HT condition, whereas all other performance groups showed no significant changes.

The interaction shown in Figure 7.3 indicates that the difference between regular schoolchildren and disadvantaged schoolchildren was higher in the HT condition than in the LT condition.

TABLE 7.5. Analyses of covariance of Set Variations I and Set Variations II by RSPM Initial Performance Level, Teaching Condition, and Type of School.

	Set Variations I			Set Variations II		
Source of variation	df	MS	F	df	MS	F
Initial Performance Level (A)	2	18.75	.74	2	563.79	8.20***
Teaching Condition (B)	1	389.47	15.40***	1	3264.89	47.47***
Type of School (C)	1	438.70	17.34***	1	2045.53	29.74***
A × B	2	121.87	4.82**	2	30.08	.64
A × C	2	30.56	1.21	2	40.13	.58
B × C	1	252.34	9.98**	1	743.17	10.81***
A × B × C	2	28.74	1.14	2	25.33	.37
Covariate (RSPM-Initial)	1	2601.96	102.87***	1	6500.33	94.51***
Error	560	25.59		488	68.78	

$^{**}p < .01$. $^{***}p < .001$.

Results on Set Variations II given to grades 7 to 9 show that all main effects were significant. Thus, subjects in the high-performance level achieved the highest scores, followed by the medium group who achieved intermediate scores, and the low-performance group who achieved low

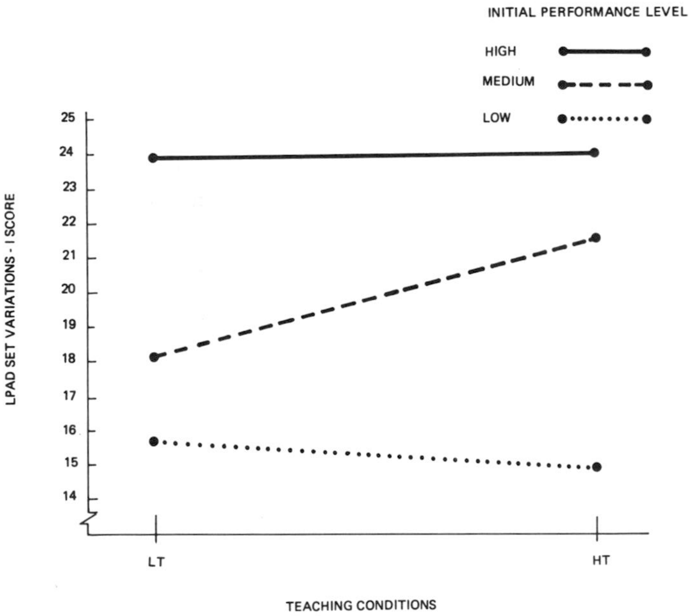

FIGURE 7.2. Performance on the LPAD Set Variations I of groups whose preteaching scores were high, medium, or low, under conditions of either low-intensity teaching or high-intensity teaching.

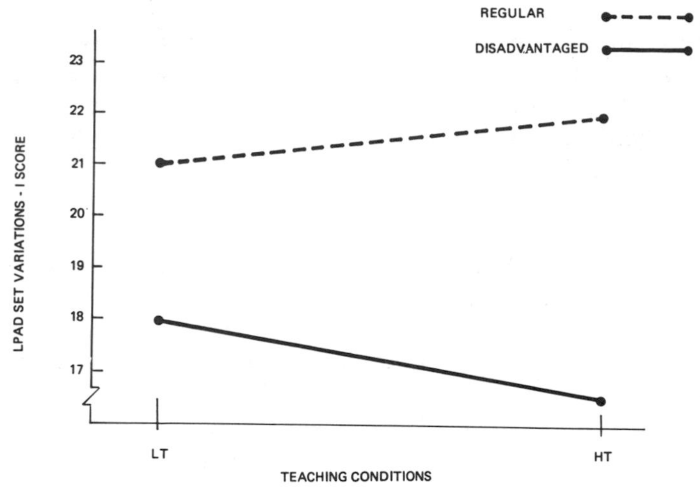

FIGURE 7.3. Differential performance on the LPAD Set Variations I of "regular" and "disadvantaged" groups under low or high teaching conditions.

scores (see Table 7.2 for actual scores). The interaction of Teaching Condition with Type of School (see Figure 7.4) indicates that the difference between regular and disadvantaged schoolchildren was much lower in the HT condition than in the LT condition. Comparison of this

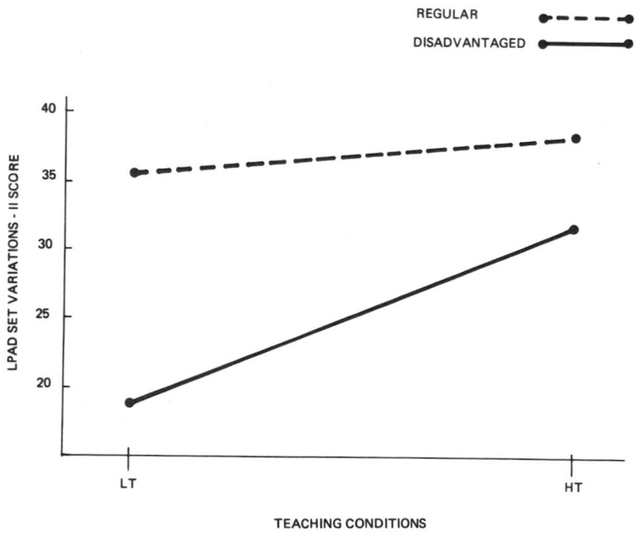

FIGURE 7.4. Performance on LPAD Set Variations II of "regular" and "disadvantaged" groups under low or high teaching conditions, showing the interaction between teaching condition and social group.

interaction to the same interaction found for Set Variations I (see Figure 7.3) reveals opposite findings. These differences are discussed later.

A second set of analyses was carried out on the Set Variations scores using the B8-B12 and B8-E12 variables as finer scales of initial performance level than the RSPM total score. Another reason for these analyses was, as mentioned before, to tap the near-transfer items; B8-B12 items are the prototype items of Set Variations I and B8-E12 are the prototype items of Set Variations II. An analysis of variance (ANOVA) of Initial Performance Level by Teaching Condition by Type of School (6 × 2 × 2) was carried out on the Set Variations I (grades 4 to 6) score. The same ANOVA procedure was used for the Set Variations II score except that the number of values for Initial Performance Level was 5. The results are presented in Table 7.6.

As can be seen from Table 7.6 all main effects for both analyses were significant. These findings indicate that (a) initially lower performing subjects achieved lower scores than did higher performing subjects, (b) subjects in HT conditions achieved higher scores than did subjects in LT condition, and (c) regular schoolchildren achieved higher scores than did disadvantaged schoolchildren. The triadic interactions of Initial Performance Level by Teaching Condition by Type of School was ignored because in some cells there were only 4 to 5 cases, not enough to rely on in making any inferences. The interaction of Teaching Condition by Type of School found for Set Variations II (See Figure 7.3) indicates that whereas among regular schoolchildren the difference between conditions

TABLE 7.6. Analyses of variance of Set Variations I (Grades 4–6) and Set Variations II (Grades 7–9) Scores by Initial Performance Level, Teaching Condition, and Type of School.

	Set Variations I			Set Variations II		
Source of Variation	df	MS	F	df	MS	F
Initial Performance Level (A)	5	812.29	26.01***	4	2906.68	29.90***
Teaching Condition (B)	1	245.04	7.85**	1	2229.08	22.93***
Type of School (C)	1	229.32	7.34**	1	1192.75	12.27***
A × B	5	36.70	1.18	4	83.52	0.86
A × C	5	44.73	1.43	4	118.09	1.21
B × C	1	79.72	2.55	1	505.04	5.19*
A × B × C	5	75.77	1.43*	4	178.74	.46
Error	415	31.23		500	97.23	

Note: Initial Performance Level in analysis of Set Variation I is based on six score intervals (0–5) of items B8-B12. In analysis of Set Variations II, Initial Performance Level is based on five score intervals (0–1, 2–3, 4–5, 6–7, 8–10) of items B8-B12 and items C7, C8, C12, D12, and E12.

*$p < .05$. **$p < .01$. ***$p < .001$.

TABLE 7.7. Analysis of covariance of total RSPM gain scores by Initial Performance Level, Teaching Condition, and Type of School (Total Sample).

Source of variation	df	MS	F
Initial Performance Level (A)	2	41.74	1.44
Teaching Condition (B)	2	521.24	18.02***
Type of School (C)	4	26.46	.91
A × B	2	83.89	2.90
A × C	2	63.69	2.20
B × C	2	76.28	2.64
A × B × C	4	24.07	.83
Initial RPM score (covariate)	1	2038.32	70.45***
Error	1375	28.93	

***$p < .001$.

was minute, among disadvantaged schoolchildren the HT condition was drastically more effective than was the LT condition. This interaction is already presented in Figure 7.3 above.

Analyses of Gain Scores on the RSPM

Three types of gain scores were analyzed: (a) gain on total RSPM, (b) gain on B8-B12, and (c) gain on B8-E12. Whenever total RSPM gain score was analyzed, the concomitant Initial Performance Level variable was composed of three levels (low, medium, and high) based on the total RSPM score, and the whole sample was included. Whenever gains on B8-B12 or B8-E12 items were analyzed, the Initial Performance Level was the same score derived from the preteaching RSPM and only grades 4 to 6 or 7 to 9 were included, respectively. Unlike the analyses on the Set Variations, which contained only two teaching conditions, the analyses of gain scores included a third no-teaching condition. An analysis of covariance was employed on total RSPM score, using the whole sample (N = 1,394). Initial Performance Level, Teaching Condition, and Type of School (3 × 2 × 2) were the independent variables, the RSPM initial score was introduced as a covariate, and the total gain score was the dependent variable. The summary of the analysis is presented in Table 7.7.

As can be seen in Table 7.7, both the main effect of Teaching Condition and the interaction of Teaching Condition × Initial Performance Level, were statistically significant. Both findings are depicted in Figure 7.5.

In general, initially low-performing subjects achieved higher gains in all conditions, even in the NT condition. However, the most dramatic result revealed in the analysis of total RSPM gain score was that the highest gap

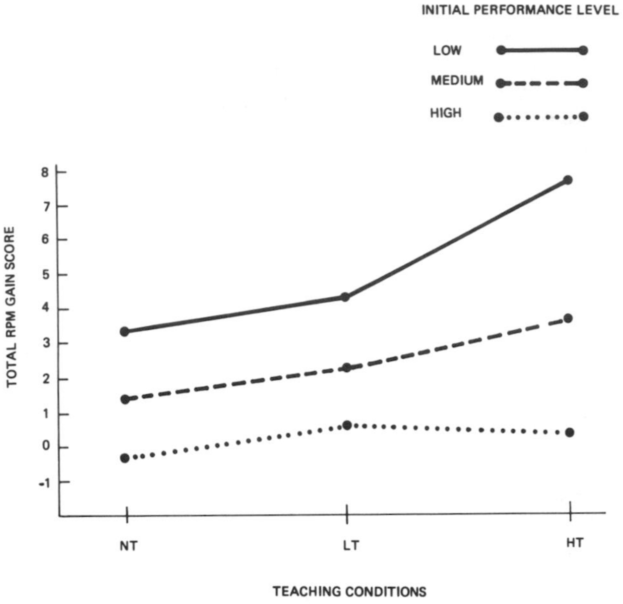

FIGURE 7.5. Total gain on Raven's Standard Progressive Matrices as a function of initial (preteaching) performance level and teaching condition (high or low).

between the initially low performers and other performance groups was in the HT condition.

It should be mentioned here that the effects of Teaching Condition and Initial Performance Level were significant after the effect of the initial RSPM score was "washed out" by taking this variable as a covariate.

Analysis of Gain Scores on B8-B12 and B8-E12 Items

Two ANOVA were carried out, one for B8-B12 gain score in grades 4 to 6 and the second for B8-E12 gain score in grades 7 to 9 (Table 7.8). In both analyses, Initial Performance Level was taken as the actual score on the same items before the intervention. Because the B8-E12 variable contains 10 items (values), thus enlarging the cell numbers, only a few cases (4 to 5) have entered some cells. To solve this problem interval scores of 0–1, 2–3, 4–5, 6–7, and 8–10, rather than the whole range of scores, were taken to maximize the number of subjects in each cell. The other independent variables were Teaching Condition and Type of School.

The results for both variables indicate in general that initially low-performing subjects had higher gain scores than did initially higher per-

TABLE 7.8. Analysis of covariance of B8-B12 (Grades 4–6) and B8-E12 (Grades 7–9) scores as a function of Initial Performance Level, Teaching Condition and Type of School.

	B8-B12			B8-E12		
Source of variation	df	MS	F	df	MS	F
Initial Performance Level (A)	5	154.61	91.96***	4	59.24	21.88***
Teaching Condition (B)	2	11.08	6.59***	2	46.16	17.05***
Type of School (C)	1	.01	.01	1	17.26	6.38***
A × B	10	1.12	.67	8	3.18	1.18
A × C	5	2.31	1.38	4	1.73	.64
B × C	2	.45	.27	2	7.03	2.60
A × B × C	10	1.97	1.17	5	.80	.30
Error	608	1.68		588	2.71	

***$p < .001$.

forming subjects and that subjects in HT condition achieved the highest gain scores followed in descending order by subjects in the LT condition and NT condition (see also Tables 7.4 and 7.5). The variable of Type of School was significant only for the B8-E12 score, indicating that disadvantaged children had higher gain scores than did regular schoolchildren. It should be emphasized that the results of gain scores on the specific items were much more drastic than total Raven's Standard Progressive Matrices (RSPM) gains, reaching peaks of 60% on B8-B12 and 38.9% on B8-E12 among initially low-performing subjects.

Discussion

The main findings of this study indicate the importance of teaching in the assessment of cognitive performance. In almost all analyses, children who were exposed to the HT condition performed better than did children who were exposed to the LT or NT condition. Cognitive modifiability, as defined by children's cognitive performance following a learning process, was affected not only by teaching but also by initial performance level and the type of school (regular vs. disadvantaged).

In general, cognitive performance on the various measures increased with increasing teaching intensity. Teaching effects were particularly large for the initially low-performing children. Significant main effects of Initial Performance Level were found in five out of seven analyses of Set Variations and RSPM gain scores. On Set Variations I, however, only the medium performance-level group showed improvement from LT to HT condition. It seems that the initially low-performing group was too low to benefit from the standard group teaching, whereas the initially high-performing group was too high to show effects of additional help over what they already knew. By contrast, on Set Variations II all groups, especially the low- and high-performing groups, showed improvement from LT to HT conditions. A possible explanation might be that items on Set Variations II are much more difficult than are items on Set Variations I, thus requiring intensive teaching even for the higher grades.

The analysis of total RSPM gain scores revealed that the initially low-performing group benefitted from the HT condition more than did the other groups (see Figure 7.5). The most dramatic results were found on items B8-B12 (grades 4 to 6) and items B8-E12 (grades 7 to 9) of the RSPM. These items require various abstract operations: some of the problems require the discovery of a complex relationship among components of the problem (e.g., positive and negative numbers), systematic and active exploration of principles, and deduction of rules contained within the same problem. These items clearly tap the Level II type of thinking considered by Jensen (1969) as essentially untrainable. Our findings indicate that the first two low groups of initial performance in grades 4 to 6 achieved a mean gain score equivalent of 54% and 60% on items B8-B12. One might argue that these high gains were the result of a statistical regression phenomenon. Although the statistical regression factor might contribute partially to the high gains, there are reasons to believe that most of the variance accounting for the gain scores in the HT condition was due to the teaching itself. The first evidence is the high performance on the Set Variations, which is a different test given before administration of the RSPM the second time (see Tables 7.3 and 7.4). The lowest performing group in grades 4 to 6, for example, made a remarkable improvement (48.7%) on Set Variations I when compared to their zero score on B8-B12 items. Their performance of 54.6% correct items on the second RSPM only validates the durability of their achievement. In the same way the lowest group in grades 7 to 9 achieved 35.3% in the HT condition as compared to 3.9% correct answers on the RSPM preteaching scores. This group improved their performance on the second administration of RSPM to 42.7% correct answers. In both examples the scores on postteaching RSPM improved, compared to the Set Variations scores.

Other evidence for the effects of the HT condition in the low-performing group is the interaction found between the two factors ($p < .05$) even after controlling the initial performance on RSPM by taking the scores as a covariate. We might infer that also in analyses of B8-B12 and B8-E12 scores the contribution of the HT condition was above and beyond what was contributed by a statistical regression factor. As mentioned above, the B8-B12 and B8-E12 items are more similar to the examples used in the intervention (HT condition) than to many RSPM items, especially those that are based on operations of identity (Set B) and construction of a Gestalt (Set A). If the HT condition was especially effective for the low-performing group on the total RSPM score, how much more then was it effective for items B8-B12 and B8-E12?

It should be noted that even in the NT condition there was an increase of 47% on B8-B12 (grades 4 to 6) and 24% on B8-E12 (grades 7 to 9) for the initially low-performing group. High gains, though less dramatic, were found for the initially low-performing children in the NT condition on the total RSPM score. It seems that even the mere fact of a second administration of the RSPM had significantly increased performance. This last finding confirms what we have already recognized in clinical work, namely that mediated learning experience can sometimes be of a very simple nature (e.g., non verbal focusing, repeating, ordering, naming). In many cases a simple repetition of a task by itself causes significant changes.

Type of School was found to to be significantly related in 10 out of 11 analyses to various measures of performance. In all main effects, regular schoolchildren performed at a higher level than did disadvantaged schoolchildren. The interaction of Type of School with Teaching Condition found for Set Variations II indicates that the disadvantaged children benefited more from the HT than from LT condition as compared to the regular schoolchildren, who showed little improvement. On Set Variations I given for grades 4 to 6 it seems that the disadvantaged schoolchildren could benefit from the HT condition more than the disadvantaged children, as compared to the LT condition in which the differences between the two groups were smaller (see Figure 7.3). However, on Set Variations II, which contains more difficult items, a reverse trend was evident: whereas the regular children were much higher than the disadvantaged children in LT condition, no significant differences were found in the HT condition. Thus, we may conclude that when dealing with more abstract and complex problems the HT condition might be more important for children who function on a low level.

The results thus far address an important question: To what degree can we trust conventional-static test scores for assessment of cognitive level, if just administration of the same test twice can bring about an increase of performance? Furthermore, teaching of principles and strategies for solving problems has been shown to be critical, as evidenced by the gains of 13% (total RSPM), 51% (Set Variations I), 41% (Set Variations II), 60% (B8-B12), and 39% (B8-E12), for initially low-performing children. The vast majority of patients sent to clinics for educational assessment are those who can be described as low functioning. Our results are even more critical when taking into account the fact that the assessment was carried out in a group situation with all the interfering factors of class teaching. We would expect much higher performance should the intervention take place individually. From our clinical experience in individual dynamic testing we have found much higher improvements in cognitive performance than what was found in the present study carried out in groups. It should be noted that the gains in our groups were found 2 weeks after the intervention so that we can be sure that the teaching effects are durable, at least for the investigated time period.

The educational implications for teaching are clear. Children at a low functioning level in school can benefit most from mediated learning experience (MLE, Feuerstein & Rand, 1974). Rather than bombarding children with concrete information exposing them to perceptual-sensory experiences to establish schemata before moving to the abstract, we suggest "attacking" the mental functioning directly by teaching abstract rules and relations. Low-functioning children can benefit most from the learning of abstract ideas. Of course this would depend on the specific teaching strategies used by the teacher to address the learning difficulties. Another educational implication is related to the belief that objective test scores point to the true capacities of children. A vicious circle is built when test scores are believed to validate school achievements, and vice versa. Appropriate teaching can "shake up" the static and docile situation in which children are living and turn upside down their strategies and approaches toward learning. Test scores as well as academic level of achievement should not be taken as static points on a continuum of an ontogenetic development but rather as an opportunity or even a request of change and modification.

Acknowledgment. This study was supported by the Schnitzer Foundation for Research on the Israeli Society and Economy.

References

Feuerstein, R., Haywood, H. C., Rand, Y., Hoffman, M. B., & Jensen, M. R. (1986). *Learning potential assessment device: Examiner manual.* Jerusalem: Hadassah-WIZO-Canada Research Institute.

Feuerstein, R., & Rand, Y. (1974). Mediated learning experience: an outline of the proximal etiology for differential development of cognitive functions. *International Understanding*, *9–10*, 7–37.

Feuerstein, R., Rand, Y., & Hoffman, M. (1979). *The dynamic assessment of retarded performers*. Baltimore: University Park Press.

Feuerstein, R., Rand, Y., Hoffman, M., & Miller, R. (1980). *Instrumental Enrichment: an intervention program for cognitive modifiability*. Baltimore: University Park Press.

Jensen, A. R., (1969). How much can we boost I.Q. and scholastic achievement? *Harvard Educational Review*, *37*, 1–123.

Raven, J. C. (1947). *Progressive Matrices, Sets I and II*. Dumfries: The Crichton Royal.

8
Assessment of Attention, Simultaneous-Successive Coding, and Planning

J. P. DAS and JACK NAGLIERI

Present trends suggest a receding of the term intelligence concurrent with a shift of research emphasis from the goal of refining the definitions of abilities in order to further their measurement. (Estes, 1976, p. 304)

There has been a significant shift away from the definition of abilities toward an interest in understanding cognitive processes (Glaser, 1972; Messick, 1973). In response to this shift from ability to process, some psychologists have turned to information processing (e.g., Hunt, 1980; Simon, 1981) because the broad framework that information processing provides can accommodate disparate approaches to intelligence such as computer-based and neuropsychological models. Understanding how information is processed requires some attempt to comprehend how it occurs in the brain. This intention to understand the proverbial "black box" is shared by intelligence theorists such as Eysenck (1981) and Jensen (1981), especially evidenced through their attempts to discover a biological foundation for intelligence.

The information-integration model developed by Das (1972, 1973, 1984a, 1984b) and recently expanded by Ashman, Kirby, and Naglieri (see Naglieri & Das, 1988; Das & Varnhagen, 1986) is an attempt to understand human functioning that is based upon the desire to know how information is processed in the brain. The model follows the neuropsychological research of Luria (1966a, 1966b, 1973). It expands on Luria by operationalizing his notions of the organization of cognitive functions, and it incorporates concepts from research in cognitive psychology (e.g., Atkinson & Shiffrin, 1968; Broadbent, 1981; Hunt, 1980).

A theory of intelligence such as ours has a base jointly in cognitive psychology as well as neuropsychology. By choosing this combined foundation, we hope we have moved away from another trend that currently engulfs some theories of intelligence. This trend is (a) toward formalizing intelligence without a reference to the realities of brain functions, and (b) an unintended disregard for metaphysical implications by positing such "explanatory" concepts as "executive" processes and "componential analysis" of mental functions. The notion of an "executive" is so reminiscent of the homunculus sitting in the mind or whispering in the ear that it should be rejected. If we agree with this, then the foundations of cognitive strategy training aimed at strengthening the powers of an executive need rebuilding. Likewise, although mental operations need to be broken down into components, and these in turn into numerous subcomponents, we should not lose sight of the unity of mental functions. If there is no underlying *structure* that unifies the various components that have been logically derived by analyzing the performance of an individual, then a study of these components will not advance our understanding of intelligence.

Perhaps because of the past history of intelligence research, which is associated with the development of IQ tests, it is desirable to refocus our efforts and understand cognitive processes rather than intelligence. This will be attempted in the first part of the chapter. The tasks for assessing cognitive processes will be discussed next. Finally, in keeping with the overall theme of the book, the assessment procedure will be discussed in the context of interactive assessment.

The Model and the Measures

Although cognitive processes have a structural base in the central nervous system, it is the aim of cognitive psychology to examine how "knowledge is organized and accessed in the memory system, and with the mental operations by means of which intellectual tasks are actually accomplished" (Estes, 1981, p. 7). Therefore, we will begin this chapter with a discussion of Luria's neuropsychological model and the contribution it has made to the understanding of intelligence.

Luria's Organization of the Brain

The influence of neuropsychology on intelligence must be attributed largely to the clinical work of Luria (1966a, 1966b), who observed behavioral dysfunctions that resulted from lesions in the brain. His observations, which spanned some 40 years of research, led him to divide the brain into three functional units. The word *functional* is very important here because Luria makes a distinction between a dynamic functional organization and a static anatomical location for a mental function. In this section, we will present Luria's views on the three functional units and provide a discussion of the cognitive activities that characterize these units, with examples specifically related to operationalization of the model.

Three Functional Units

According to Luria (1966a, 1966b, 1973, 1980) there are three functional units, which he examined through his neuropsychological investigations, responsible for human cognitive processing. These mental processes are complex functional systems that are not localized in narrow areas of the brain, but take place through the interaction of brain structures that work in concert. Luria (1973) states that all three functional units participate in any type of mental activity. The first functional unit is responsible for regulating tone or waking (arousal), the second unit receives, processes, and stores information (simultaneous and successive coding), and the third unit programs, regulates, and verifies mental activity (planning).

Three Zones

In addition to the three functional units, Luria further describes three hierarchically structured zones within each unit: the primary, secondary, and tertiary zones. The primary, or projection area, receives impulses from and sends impulses to the peripheral parts of the nervous system. The secondary, or projection-association area, receives impulses from the primary area and processes the information for output. The tertiary zone receives input from both the primary and secondary zones and acts to translate the sensory information into symbolic processes so that concrete perceptions can be transformed into abstract thinking at this level. There are three principles that describe the functioning of the brain's three zones. The first principle states that the three zones are hierarchical. The line of control is from the tertiary to the secondary and onto the primary zones, although there are reciprocal connections among the three zones. The second principle describes the diminishing modality character of the information processing in the three zones. That is, the primary zone retains modality characteristics of the information that it has received.

Although modality information diminishes in the secondary zone, there remains some information on the specific receptor through which the message was received. The secondary zone also synthesizes information that has been received from different sense modalities. In contrast, the tertiary zone is completely free of modality information, which is important in facilitating the integration of information from all sensory sources. This allows for the integration of what we hear in a lecture with what we read in a book, for example.

The third principle states that there is progressive lateralization of function with the brain. At the level of the primary zone, there is essentially no difference in the function between the right and left hemispheres. On the other hand, at the level of the tertiary zone, many functions are lateralized. For example, speech is lateralized in the left hemisphere in the majority of right-handed people.

A Closer Look at the Three Functional Units

The First Functional Unit

Luria's first unit is a prerequisite for human mental processes because it maintains a proper state of cortical tone. Anatomically, this unit is found in the brain stem, diencephalon, and medial regions of the hemispheres. The principal structure in this unit is the reticular formation, the integrity of which is crucial for the maintenance of cortical tone and determination of levels of consciousness. The reticular formation can be subdivided into ascending and descending systems that activate and regulate cortical tone, and control impulses from higher cortical centers, respectively.

Only when a proper waking condition is achieved can an individual receive and analyze information and regulate mental activity. An appropriate level of arousal not only maintains cortical tone but provides the opportunity for other cortical activity, and in turn experiences "the differentiating influence of the cortex" (Luria, 1973, p. 67). Maintaining an appropriate level of arousal is also important for effective performance because too much or too little interferes with proper processing of information and with making effective plans of action. According to Das (1984b), too much arousal (for example, when a child is anxious or impulsive), interferes with the determination of relevant and irrelevant details and thus blocks learning. The individual whose cortical system is not sufficiently aroused will experience difficulty with coding and planning tasks due to an understimulation of the second and third functional units.

Arousal is much more than the maintenance of wakefulness and the general energy level of mental activity. The neurophysiological relationships between the reticular formation and the frontal lobes are complex and intimate and involve a host of cognitive processes such as the orienting response, expectancy, and intentions, which blend with the processes of planning. Arousal, as manifested in attention, interacts with learning and memory, which are included in coding (acquisition, analyses, synthesis, storage, and retrieval of information).

The Second Functional Unit

The purpose of the second functional unit is to code information, that is, receive, analyze, and store information. Luria (1966b) stated that "there is strong evidence for distinguishing two basic forms of integrative activity of the cerebral cortex, by which different aspects of the outside world may be reflected" (p. 74). These two forms of information processing are simultaneous (integration of stimuli into synchronous and primarily interrelated groups), a function located in the occipital-parietal lobes, and successive (integration of stimuli into temporally organized serial order), located in the temporal lobe. Simultaneous processing involves the integration of stimuli into groups (or the ability to see a number of elements as a single whole). An important aspect of simultaneous processing is that each element of the task is interrelated to every other element (i.e., is surveyable). Simultaneous processing tasks are said to be surveyable because all the components included in the task are interrelated and accessible to inspection either through examination of the actual stimuli during the activity (as in the case of copying a design) or through memory of the stimuli (as in the case of reproduction of a design from memory). Luria stressed the importance of surveyability by stating that "the grasping of any system or relationships, whether the grammatical system of a language or a system of arithmetic concepts, is impossible without arrangement of the elements into a simultaneously surveyable scheme" (Luria, 1966b, p. 76).

Simultaneous processing is involved in its simplest form when a person is required to copy geometric figures (or draw the figure from memory) and in more complex form when a person examines logical grammatical relations (for example "the father's brother" and "the brother's father" or "a circle above a square" and "a square above a circle") or solves nonverbal figural matrices (e.g., Raven, 1958; Naglieri, 1985). These examples illustrate that simultaneous processing may take place during direct perception (design copying), during retention of information (drawing the design from memory), or at conceptual levels (logical, grammatical, verbal statements and solving matrices).

Successive processing involves the integration of stimuli into a specific series, in which each element is related only to the next. The essential feature of this kind of processing is that the components of the task are not surveyable (interrelated) and, more importantly, that each part consecutively, activates the next.

During successive synthesis, each stimulus is arranged in a specific series so that the elements form a specific chain-like progression. The relationship among stimuli in successive tasks is mainly an ordered one without surveyability (in contrast to simultaneous tasks, in which the elements are all interrelated). Successive synthesis is important for skilled movements such as writing because such activity requires "a series of movements which follow each other in a strictly defined order . . . without surveyability" (Luria, 1966b, p. 78). In the early stages of the formation of a skilled movement, each stimulus link exists as a separate unit and may be taught as a specific step in a behavior. Only when each action becomes automatic can the initial stimulus in the chain become the signal that leads to the automatic execution of the complete successive action. Luria (1966a, 1966b) also stated that the synthesis of musical elements into rhythmic or tonal melodies requires successive processing just as serial recall of words does. As with simultaneous processing, successive processing may be involved in tasks of various modalities (auditory, visual, kinesthetic) and involve different types of stimuli (verbal or nonverbal).

Both simultaneous and successive processing are involved with the acquisition, storage, and retrieval of knowledge, according to the demands of the task rather than to its modality, presentation, or content. Das, Kirby, and Jarman (1979) demonstrated how tasks of different modalities, such as an auditory (Wechsler Intelligence Scale for Children-Revised [WISC-R] Digit Span) and visual (Visual Short-Term Memory) task, both involve successive processing. Similarly, although the methods of presentation for the Figure Copying and Memory-For-Designs tasks employed by Das et al. (1979) are very different, they both have been shown to measure simultaneous processing. Finally, research summarized by Luria (1966a, 1966b) and Jarman (1980) reveals that both forms of coding (simultaneous and successive processes) are involved with language but that each type of coding contributes a different component. For example, understanding the syntax of a sentence involves the appreciation of the serial relation of one word to the next and successive processing, whereas the comprehension of the meaning of a sentence involves simultaneous processing.

Simultaneous processing is directly related to understanding the meaning of grammatical statements, which allow us to obtain the meaning of words combined into groups. For example, in the item "point to the pencil with the key," the child must analyze the logical arrangement of the words and, at the same time, must suppress following the order of the actions corresponding directly from the order of the words in the command; that is, pointing with the pencil, because it came first, to the key, because it came second (Luria, 1980, p. 500).

The syntactic relationships among words, however, involves successive processing. Lashley (1951) regarded the organization of speech as one of the most obvious examples of serial organization. The successive nature of speech is involved in development of the "order of vocal movements in pronouncing the word, the order of words in the sentence, (and) the order of sentences in the paragraph" (Lashley, 1951, p. 515).

Although these examples illustrate that simultaneous and successive coding is involved in the use and comprehension of language, coding is not the only type of activity involved. Planning is an important process required for effective use of language as well as for other generative activities.

The Third Functional Unit

Luria's third unit is responsible for programming, regulation, and verification of activity. This unit acts to organize the individual's conscious activity once information has been received, coded, and stored so that the individual can form plans of action, regulate behavior so that it conforms to these plans, and then compare the effects of these actions with the original intention so that correction of mistakes is possible. The third functional unit is responsible for such activities as regulation of voluntary actions, impulse control, and linguistic functions such as spontaneous speech (Luria, 1980, p. 517). This unit also entails the aptitude for asking new questions, solving problems, and self-monitoring, which as Arlin (1977) and Das (1984a) suggest, may represent one of the most complex forms of human behavior. The third functional unit is located in the frontal lobes, especially the prefrontal areas. This area was not studied by neurologists for a long time because it has no sensory areas, and damage to the frontal lobes does not always result in obvious decrements in ability as measured by standardized IQ tests. It is, however, the most important functional unit, the last neurological area to develop over the evolution of the species, and constitutes one third of the entire human brain. Moreover, the tertiary zone in the prefrontal area has a massive system of neural connections with almost all parts of the brain. For example, the frontal lobes interact extensively with the reticular formation (in the first functional unit) in discriminating between relevant and irrelevant information for the purpose of allocating attention (Pribram & Luria, 1973).

The application of coding processes is an important function of planning, which may be efficient, resulting in good performance, or inefficient, resulting in poor performance. For example, although Digit Span is usually a task that involves recalling numbers one by one in a linear fashion, some people use a strategy such as chunking the digits into groups of two or three to facilitate recall. The digits within the chunks are treated as one unit, thereby processing a string of discrete digits in simultaneous units, and the order of the chunks involves successive processing.

Typically, successive processing is used only when simultaneous units become so long that they cannot be held together as a whole. What determines the individual's choice of one or the other process depends on the demands of the task, the person's habitual mode of solving that type of problem, the level of proficiency, and his/her knowledge base. This is how the three functional units interact to make an individual unique.

Relationships Among the Units

Luria's functional systems respond to the experiences of the individual, are subject to developmental changes, and form an interrelated system. Examination of Figure 8.1 shows that the three units are interactive and influence one another while at the same time they maintain independence by having distinct functions. These units also rely on and influence a base of knowledge. Plans operate on information (knowledge) that has been coded or properly analyzed. Without the base of coded information, planning becomes empty, and in the absence of a plan, information coding is blind. Coding and planning interact to facilitate acquisition of knowledge, but at the same time these higher functions depend on a

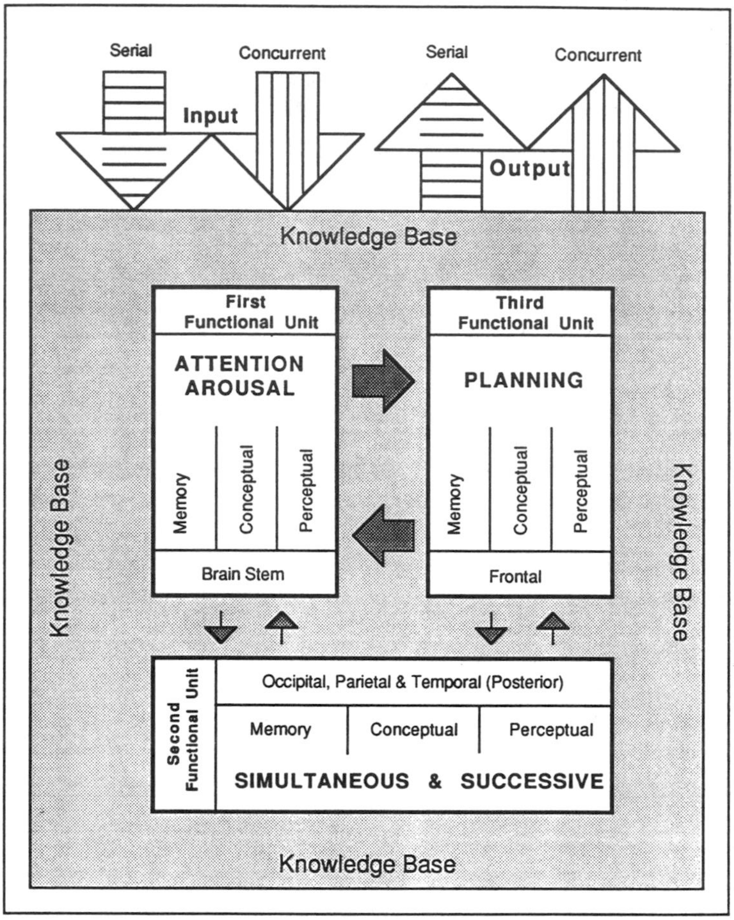

FIGURE 8.1. PASS cognitive processing model.

proper state of arousal to provide the opportunity for learning. These four interactive processes, Planning, Arousal-Attention, Simultaneous and Successive coding are given the acronym PASS.

The knowledge base is the sum total of a person's experiences. Formal and informal educational background, and habits and predispositions, which may be either conscious or unconscious, make up the knowledge base. This base involves memories, attitudes and orientations, inborn capacities, and energy level, which interactively intervene in the interpretation of reality as well as the structure and content of the thoughts of a person. The knowledge base should resemble *image*, conceptualized by Miller, Galanter and Pribram (1960) as the accumulated knowledge that the organism has about itself and its world. It is also very close to the

Buddhist notion of the self as the aggregate of memories, knowledge, and experience, which is impermanent and ever changing (Murti, 1980). The base of knowledge, therefore, influences in a dynamic manner all of our attentional, coding, and planning activities.

Planning and structuring activities require an adequate state of arousal so that attention can be focused. Only when an appropriate level of activation, attention, and arousal exist can we begin to plan our behavior to fulfill a predetermined activity. Planning, therefore, depends on an appropriately aroused state as well as the inhibition of an inappropriate level of arousal. Selectively inhibiting arousal is one of the important functions of the third functional unit, which is associated with planning. Without selection of priorities and plans to fulfill, and without an appropriate level of arousal, overarousal and disorganization (as in the case of the hyperactive child) will characterize an individual's behavior. There appears to be a direct relationship, therefore, between planning and arousal, just as a similar relationship exists between coding and planning. Plans can influence the way information is sorted before it is coded. Because the same information could be coded in many different ways, how one manages the information is a planning function that influences the coding approach used. These plans are also influenced by coded information in the form of a person's past learning experiences. Although much of our planning uses information that has been coded, new information may be incorporated into a novel problem solving situation to arrive at a particular plan of action.

Measurement of the Three Functional Units

Measurement of Arousal and Attention

Arousal is a reflexive response to a stimulus input and can be described as the orienting reaction involving a set of physiological and behavioral changes occurring to a novel stimulus (e.g., head turning). This aspect of the first functional unit is essentially involuntary, in contrast to attention, which is more under voluntary control. The distinction between voluntary and involuntary attention does not preclude the interaction of the two types and is described by Eysenck (1982). High arousal leads to attentional selectivity. The level of arousal could also be manipulated by instructions that assign high and low priority to tasks, and by requiring performance under noisy or quiet conditions. Arousal levels also influence *sustained attention* as in prolonged execution of some activity. During periods of low alertness caused by sleep deprivation and monotony, our attention is low, and our ability to react with accuracy and swiftness decreases substantially. Performance on vigilance tasks is a conventional method of demonstrating this (Parasuraman & Davies, 1984).

In a classic paper on components of attention, Posner and Boies (1971) identified three major components: alertness, selectivity, and processing capacity. The component of alterness is perhaps most easily understood in terms of the basic notion of arousal. It certainly is the central concept in vigilance. The *selectivity aspect of attention* borders on planning but also relates to the intentional discrimination between stimuli. For example, in the Posner name-match versus physical-match letter paradigm, the problem of selective attention is tested quite effectively. Processing capacity is implied in all tasks of selective attention.

Both arousal and attention constructs have face validity as components of intelligence because a weakness in either one of them should be expected to result in reduced cognitive competence. Geschwind (1982) showed how failure to comprehend, learn, or memorize may be due to a lack of attention. He further implied that selective attention has to be maintained over a period of time in order to achieve coherence in thought and action.

Geschwind suggested that selective attention is a prerequisite for sustained attention because the only way attention can be successfully maintained over a period of time is to develop and maintain a selective plan for attention. In other words, if the subject is actively discriminating the relevant from irrelevant stimuli in a selective attention task, then attention can be maintained for a relatively long time. Geschwind also stated that an important characteristic of attention is distractibility, or the necessity to shift attention. We constantly monitor and shift our attention in order to be sensitive to environmental changes, and therefore, distractibility can be used in a good sense as a mechanism for paying attention to environmental changes.

Several other researchers have considered attention as an important measure of cognitive capacity. Furby (1974) reviewed a number of research studies in this context as it relates to the problem-solving behavior of mentally retarded children. She suggested that the major difference between nonretarded and retarded children lies in problem-solving behavior and that the reasons for poor performance of retarded children are (a) the slower habituation of the orienting response, and (b) the greater difficulty on the part of retarded children in inhibiting positive approach responses. The speed at which the orienting response habituation proceeds is suggested as an index of cognitive development.

It is not only the habituation of orienting responses that separates retarded from nonretarded children matched on mental age (MA), but also the frequency of anticipating orienting responses. Das and Bower (1971) showed that, whereas retarded subjects gave more frequent responses to a stimulus than did nonretarded subjects, the latter gave more frequent responses to a warning signal anticipating the stimulus.

To conclude, these observations on attention and arousal imply that a comprehensive assessment of cognitive functions must include measures of attention (see Hunt, 1980). In assessing nonretarded as well as special children such as the mentally retarded, the learning disabled, and those who are suffering from attentional deficits, both sustained and selective attention should be measured.

Measurement of Coding

Measurement of coding, in the two forms of simultaneous and successive processing, has been examined by Das since the early 1970s and Luria (1966a, 1966b) prior to that time. The major difference between two researchers' approaches to evaluation of these constructs has been that Luria used the method of syndrome analysis (Luria & Artem'eva, 1970), whereas Das (1972, 1973; Das et al., 1979; Naglieri & Das, 1988) used factor analytic techniques. These factor analytic studies have uncovered planning, simultaneous, and successive factors for exceptional children (mentally retarded and learning disabled) and individuals from different age groups and cultures. Factor analytic studies on simultaneous and successive processing provide strong evidence for the existence of these two types of information processing. The relative invariance of the two modes of coding across age was established by Das and Molloy (1975) and more recently by Naglieri and Das (1988). The two processes were also identified in factor analytic studies by Das (1972), Jarman and Das (1977), and across different IQ groups, which showed that mentally retarded children and children of average intelligence appear to have similar factor loadings (Das et al., 1979).

The tests used to measure simultaneous and successive processing have been varied in terms of form and content. For example, simultaneous processing factors have been found to emerge from such tasks as Raven (1958) matrix problems, which involve nonverbal analogical reasoning; Figure Copying, which requires drawing a design; Graham & Kendall's (1960) Memory for Design task; which requires recall and reproduction of a figure exposed for a brief period of time, a verbal test such as the Token Test (Naglieri & Das, 1988), WISC-R Block Design (Wachs & Harris, 1984), the Embedded Figures test (Ryckman, 1981), and Concrete Paired Associates (Das, Kirby & Jarman, 1975), all have been shown to load on a simultaneous factor. Similarly, successive processing factors have been found using tasks of serial recall of words and digits (Das et al., 1979), successive hand movements (Naglieri & Das, 1988), a test of syntax involving sentences presented orally (Naglieri & Das, 1988), Wepman's auditory discrimination tests (Ryckman, 1981), and sound-blending (Wachs & Harris, 1986).

Measurement of Planning

Planful behavior is the most difficult of the three functions to measure for two reasons. First, since all behavior must involve plans, conscious or unconscious, how can planning be measured apart from coding? The answer must be found in designing tasks in such a manner as to highlight planning by using tasks with minimal coding requirements. A second difficulty is to measure planning in a relatively brief amount of time without making the task appear to be simply a test of speed. This problem has been addressed by the careful selection of planning tasks and the use of tests that illustrate efficient performance not necessarily involving speedy performance.

The tasks used to measure planning, and which have been shown to load on a planning factor, as with tests of coding, have been varied on the basis of form and content. These have included a verbal test requiring the writing of a composition about a picture, a modified version of the game Mastermind (Das & Heemsbergen, 1983), as well as trail making, visual search, and verbal syllogisms (Das, 1984b). Additionally, other tasks such as matching numbers (Naglieri & Das, 1988) and clustering (Schofield & Ashman, 1986), have loaded on a planning factor. These tasks vary sufficiently on the basis of the amount of speed required to demonstrate that planning involves organization, direction of actions, and in general, efficient solutions of problems, not simply speed, and are examples of how tasks with minimal coding requirements can be used to measure planning processes. Further evidence of this is presented below.

Evidence for Planning, Attention, and Coding

To present some evidence of construct validity of the PASS model, such as the separation of coding from speed and the relative independence of planning from coding, two investigations will be discussed. The first illustrates how planning and speed can be distinguished, and the second focuses on the relationship between planning and coding using a variety of tasks.

Experiment 1

A group of 70 third-grade children who attended regular class were administered a battery of the standard cognitive tasks used by Das to measure planning, simultaneous, and successive processes and speed. These were: planning (Visual Search and Trail Making); simultaneous (Figure Copying & Memory for Designs); successive (Auditory Serial Recall and Digit Span Forward); and speed (Word Reading and Color Naming). The Word Reading speed was obtained by timing the child when he/she read 40 words (red, green, yellow, and blue) each written 10 times in random order on a page. Color Naming speed was measured by the child's naming of colored patches arranged in rows as the words were. These two tasks, formerly described by Das, Kirby, and Jarman (1975),

TABLE 8.1. Principal components analysis of measures for simultaneous, successive, planning, and speed (varimax rotation).[a]

Measure	Factors 1 Successive	 2 Simultaneous	 3 Speed	 4 Planning	h^2
Figure Copying		−884			823
Memory-for-Designs (errors)[b]		865			806
Auditory Serial Recall	891				839
Digit Span	891				812
Color Reading[b]			810		735
Color Naming[b]			835		706
Trail Making (A)[b]				801	736
Visual Search				802	727
Variance	1.713	1.599	1.550	1.319	
Percentage of total variance	21.418	19.992	19.374	16.489	

[a] Decimals omitted in loadings. Loadings below 300 have been omitted.
[b] A high score indicates poor performance.

were included in this battery of tests to show that a planning factor defined by the timed tasks of Visual Search and Trail Making is distinct from measures of speed (Word Reading and Color Naming). That is, although response time is the measure for the four tasks, the tasks represent two different cognitive processes—planning and speed. Word Reading and Color Naming represent lexical access speed whereas Visual Search and Trail Making measure planning (search) processes. Results of the four-factor principal components analysis (varimax rotation) presented in Table 8.1 illustrate this relationship between speed processing tasks. The planning, simultaneous, and successive factors emerged as anticipated, and speed formed a distinct and separate factor. These results illustrate that, although response time is the unit of measure for both planning and speed tests, the tests are distinctive enough to load on separate factors (Das & Dash, 1983).

These data were further subjected to a hierarchical factor analysis, which is presented in Table 8.2. The results of this analysis support the existence of two independent higher order factors at the level 2 factoring. The emergence of two second factors is due to the inclusion of planning tasks in that there is a relative independence of coding and planning.

The relative independence of coding and planning also affects the relationship between the cognitive processing tasks and standardized IQ tests, which was further examined using this sample of third-grade children. Correlations were obtained between the factor scores for each of the processing measures and the Verbal, Quantitative, and Nonverbal Ability scales of the Canadian Cognitive Abilities Test (CCAT). The correlations were as follows: planning (−.08, .09, −.12), simultaneous (.44, .56, .59), and successive (.30, .27, .30), with Verbal, Quantitative, and Nonverbal scores, respectively. These results illustrate that the

TABLE 8.2. Schmid-Leiman hierarchical orthogonalization of simultaneous, successive, and planning tasks for grade 3 children.

	Factor						
	Second Order			First Order			
	G_1	G_2		Succ.	Simult.	Speed	Plan.
Figure Copying	.420	−.056		−.104	.675	.031	−.023
Memory for Designs	.378	.135		.116	.638	−.065	.027
Serial Recall	.433	−.029		.741	−.043	.074	−.017
Digit Span	.346	.068		.687	.046	−.024	.006
Word Reading	.593	−.099		.067	−.031	.559	.023
Color Naming	.395	−.172		−.014	.039	.345	−.022
Trail Making	−.196	.537		.025	−.091	−.051	.175
Visual Search	.026	.522		−.075	.075	.113	.187
	R_1^a				R^b		
	1.000	−.094	Succ.	1.000	.241	.305	.011
	−.094	1.000	Simult.	.241	1.000	.366	−.013
			Speed	.305	.366	1.000	−.251
			Plan	.011	−.013	−.251	1.000

[a] R_1: Correlations among second-order factors.
[b] R : Correlations among primary oblique factors.

CCAT is mainly a measure of coding processes and that planning process is not a major part of the abilities being measured by the CCAT (Das & Dash, 1983).

Experiment 2

The second investigation involved several aspects of construct validity for the planning, simultaneous, and successive tasks for three samples of intellectually average subjects: grade 2 (N = 149), grade 6 (N = 160), and grade 10 (N = 125). In this study, the cognitive processing tasks used were planning (Trails, Visual Search, and Matching Numbers), simultaneous (Figure Recognition, Tokens, and Matrices), and successive (Word Recall, Successive Ordering, and Hand Movements). Although many of these tasks are revised versions of those previously used by Das, some are additions. Matching Numbers, which requires the child to find the two out of six numbers (ranging from one to six digits in length) in each row that are the same, had not been used before. Tokens (Lezak, 1976) and Matrices (Naglieri, 1985) are variations of tests developed and used in other settings. Similarly, Successive Ordering, which requires the child to touch a series of objects in the same order as demonstrated by the examiner, and Hand Movements, which requires the subject to reproduce a series of two to six hand movements (six different movements are used), are also variations on tests already in use. These tasks were developed as part of the experimental battery called the Cognitive Assessment System (Das & Naglieri, in preparation). This experiment was designed

TABLE 8.3. Varimax and promax factor loadings of cognitive processing tasks ($N = 434$).

Tasks	Varimax			Promax		
Tokens	−.16	.42*	.20	−.20	.42*	.08
Figure Recognition	−.14	.40*	.13	−.03	.42*	.01
Matrices	−.14	.51*	.15	.00	.56*	.00
Hand Movements	−.08	.15	.44*	.02	.04	.47*
Successive Ordering	−.28	.18	.44*	−.19	.01	.42*
Word Recall	−.03	.11	.43*	.07	.00	.48*
Matching Numbers	.51*	−.18	−.19	.51*	−.02	−.07
Visual Search	.54*	−.11	−.04	.61*	.03	.08
Trails	.53*	−.21	−.12	.55*	−.07	.01

* Loadings greater than .4 are noted.

to examine the factor structure of this largely new battery of planning and coding tasks. There are two factor analyses presented in Table 8.3, varimax and promax solutions using the total sample ($N = 434$). To gain greater stability, the subjects' scores were combined across ages by converting the raw score obtained on each task by subject to a standard score to control for age effects. The three factors that emerged formed factors that clearly can be labeled planning, simultaneous, and successive. Both the varimax and promax solutions illustrate that the factors representing the processes are diverse. For example, the tasks loading on planning were verbal (Matching Numbers) and nonverbal (Visual Search). Similarly, the simultaneous factor comprised verbal (Tokens) and nonverbal (Figure Recognition and Matrices) tasks, and the successive factor involved verbal (Word Recall) and nonverbal (Successive Ordering and Hand Movements) tasks. Additionally, these results provide support for Das' (1984b) statement that coding processes may occur at perceptual (Figure Recognition, Matching Numbers), memory (Word Recall, Trails), and conceptual (Tokens, Matrices) levels (Naglieri & Das, 1988).

Evaluation of the Model

The information provided in this chapter presents one possible approach to understanding the multiple and complex intellectual processes of man. We will now evaluate the model of information processing from the perspective suggested by Sternberg (1985, pp. 20–24). Sternberg lists eight points by which to evaluate various theories of information processing:

1. Does the theory provide detailed specificatin of mental structures and processes? The structure for this model may be understood in terms of its neuropsychological roots. The reference to neuropsychology may be discarded by the reader. But what it does is provide us with an

analogy of mental functions substantiated by a reasonable amount of clinical research and knowledge. The model identifies processes that are commonly studied in experiments in cognition and psychopathology. These processes are reflected as factors in studies that were carried out on regular and special samples of schoolchildren. The model recognizes the multiple and unique forms of intellectual activity, and relates them to three specific groups of functions. The underlying neurological structures of the processes are described in some detail in this chapter.

2. Does the view of intelligence go beyond operational definitions? The view of cognitive processes certainly does; it is not atheoretical. Theories from cognitive psychology of attention-arousal, perception-memory, problem solving, and planning on the one hand, and neuropsychology on the other, provide the background as discussed in this chapter. Broadbent, Miller, and Posner, together with Pavlov, Vygotsky, Luria, and Pribram, have influenced this model for assessing cognitive processes.
3. Does the model have heuristic value? The theory has heuristic value in that it provides an approach for understanding and measurement of cognitive processes and suggests that any comprehensive measure of intelligence should have the triple functions of normative measurement, specification of processes, and prescription for remedial training.
4. Does it have practical value? The model provides a framework for a complete assessment of different intellectual abilities. Additionally, according to Das (1984a, 1985a), the theory provides an understanding of normal and exceptional (such as retarded, learning disabled and disadvantaged) children's intellectual performance, and has implications for remedial training.
5. Is the theory difficult to falsify? Theories about general intellectual functions are hard to falsify because most often they contain a core of truth and they are judged in terms of how economical they are in explaining a large amount of empirical data. The present model is open to verification on the basis of testable hypotheses. Two examples are given below: (a) Factor analytic replications should show the emergence of two separate coding and planning factors. (b) Experiments based on the suggested processes should validate the major processes derived from factor analysis; for example, "good planners" should show better organization and planning in comprehension of text than "poor planners."
6. Does the theory have relevance to the real world? The model presented above is related to the real world in that it is derived from the neuropsychological investigations of Luria involving persons with real difficulty in functioning on a daily basis. Clearly, the theory is based on findings from experimental psychology of attention, memory, and higher cognitive processes that are tied to real-world behavior.

7. Does the theory attend to contexts in which intelligent behavior occurs? Previous research with different cultural samples, such as the Canadian natives and high castes from India, shows that the processing tasks are approached differently by cross-cultural groups (see Das et al., 1979). However, it is assumed that the cognitive framework proposed in the model is a universal one, inherent in the human brain.
8. Does the theory provide an explicit basis for selection of tasks? The tasks included in the assessment of the cognitive processes were intentionally selected to incorporate samples of behavior that were, on the basis of both rational and empirical evidence, consistent with the model. Task selection was not arbitrary or atheoretical. We did not select a task simply because it was similar to school learning or loaded on some factor without theoretical justification or rationale.

Interactive Assessment and Alternatives

A child's score on an ability test such as the WISC-R is to be considered as an initial score only; it may improve following the child's interactions with an adult who helps him/her with the test. The wording of the above statement may not exactly reflect "dynamic assessment," but the spirit does. Essentially, dynamic or interactive assessment follows from Vygotsky's observation that "what children can do with the assistance of others might be in some sense even more indicative of their mental development than what they can do alone" (Vygotsky, 1978, p. 85). But Vygotsky was interested in the process of development, not in normative ability. The primary objectives of the ability testers such as school psychologists who administer the WISC-R or other IQ tests do not include a study of processes or the antecedents of improved performance on the tests. Therefore, for them, the repeated application of a standardized test is not a legitimate practice. Contrary to their practice, interactive assessment requires that between two testing sessions, there should be interleaved sessions of tester-child interactions. Such a procedure is not standardized and objective because it will allow improvisations, and the personal style of the tester's interactions to influence the product, which is the test score.

Interactive assessment or dynamic assessment will be tolerated by school psychologists and others who provide ability testing only as long as the improvised procedures are a small part of the standard administrative procedures of the test. These examiners will also need to be assured that the interactive assessment (a) will not invalidate the use of standard procedure, and (b) will do some good to the child (such as lead to an appropriate program placement or help in designing remedial training for the child).

This delicate balance can be expressed as follows:

$$P = \mathrm{f}(st, ia)$$

where P is test performance, st is standardized procedure, and ia is interactive assessment procedure, with the proviso that it requires only a small part of the test administration (e.g., $Pia = KPst$, where $0 < K < .10$).

Standard and interactive procedures must be multiplicative, or better still, transactional, and not additive in terms of their effect on performance (P).

P is acceptable for normative samples as long as its value (subjects' score) is not significantly different when $ia = 0$, that is, when interactive assessment is not given. It is also acceptable when it is different, but only when special subject samples are assessed.

There are at least two alternatives to improvised interactive assessment. Because the study of *processes* is the overall objective of *Pia*, with a minor interest in facilitation of remedial training, one alternative is to build various *processing requirements* into a test. To clarify, a test of visual search can have (a) an automatic and (b) a controlled search variation by manipulating the target and nontarget stimulus characteristics. The target can be a single digit embedded in a display of pictures of common objects or vice versa; this is given in the automatic condition. On the other hand, a target digit presented in a background of other digits will require controlled search. To further test the automaticity of processing, the number of background items may be increased by 50% in a second form of the test, the expectation being a minimal slowing down in search speed for automatic processing but a significant slowness in the controlled condition. Comparing mentally retarded children with nonretarded children, however, may show that the search process is not automatic because the retarded children, unlike nonretarded children, require a longer search time when the density of the background items is increased in automatic forms of the test. Differential practice effects on search speed can also be examined by giving several trials in each condition.

Another process variable is examined by varying the stimulus type in visual search test, such as pictures, numbers, and letters. Pictorial stimuli are processed differently than letter stimuli; the latter require phonological recoding, and this difference can be studied for special children (i.e., reading disabled versus fluent readers) by selecting pictures, and letters as stimuli for visual research.

The combination of processes is simply expressed as

$$P = \mathrm{f}(\sum_{a}^{n} p)$$

where $pa \ldots pn$ represent distinct cognitive processes (e.g. pattern recognition in case of pictures, phonological coding for letters).

Therefore, whereas *P*, the test score, is expressed as a function of the total score of process-related subtests, the identity of *pa–n* is available for use in comparing *P* in different populations. Note that *P* is *not* necessarily the sum of the scores on the subtests as it may be a transformed score (e.g., log, subtraction).

In the interactive assessment procedure, the first few trials will provide a learning experience for the subject; in fact, the use of a few trials for teaching how to handle the test should be standard procedure in any cognitive assessment.

The above may be named as the *process alternative*. It does lead to a formulation of remedial training because of its power to locate processing failure far more precisely than an ability score, such as verbal or performance IQ, or a test score, such as Similarities or Arithmetic (in WISC-R) can do.

When interactive assessment is unacceptable because of its improvisations, which will have to vary from one examiner to the other, another alternative procedure is the observation of overt strategies. This alternative includes strategy assessment and retest improvement, as elaborated below.

Strategy assessment is an aspect of dynamic assessment that can easily and effectively be incorporated into our test battery. We suggest that strategy assessment be accomplished by direct observation and interviewing of the subject.

1. Direct observation of the subject as he/she is performing the subtest provides the examiner with behavioral observations relevant to the approach the child has used to solve the task. This does not necessarily tell the examiner the "process" that has been used, but it reveals the strategies used by the subject to solve the subtest. For example, during visual search, the examiner may notice the subject looks at the entire field by moving away from the stimulus in an attempt to view the entire field at one time. This approach may work well for automatic search and yet be an inefficient style on controlled search items. In another example, the child may verbally mediate during Trails as a means of keeping track of which number or letter is next.
2. Interviewing the subject following the completion of each planning subtest provides additional information; it is assumed here that the child has the communication skills needed to explain how he/she did the task. The child's explanation need not be verbal; that is, it may be in the form of a demonstration, as long as the method used by the child is communicated to the examiner.
3. An empirical approach to strategy assessment will first involve the collection of strategies used by subjects in the standardization sample of the cognitive tasks. This will include both the observational and interview data. The various strategies used on each subtest will then be

rated according to their effectiveness on the basis of which strategies were used by those who scored high on each subtest. For example, assuming that there were 10 strategies used for the visual search subtest planning, those used by the higher scoring subjects would be rated as more desirable than those used by the lower scoring subjects. These 10 strategies would then be rank-ordered in terms of efficiency. Additionally, an actuarial approach should be used; the percentage of subjects who adopted each type of strategy, by subtest, should be determined. This will be especially important when differences between good and poor planners are examined, as well as when normal and exceptional subjects are compared.

4. A qualitative component of strategy assessment will include things such as the interaction between the particular strategy selected by the subject and the way in which it was applied—efficiently or inefficiently. For example, if a child used a good strategy to solve Trails, but did so without regard to performing the task as fast as possible, we could say that he/she had a good planning strategy but failed to conform to the demands of the task, perhaps due to poor attention to the instructions (a low selective attention score could support this). Additionally, a child may be using a particular *planning* strategy to solve a *coding* task, as in the case of using chunking to remember a series of words, or using verbal mediation to solve matrices, in order to compensate for less-than-adequate simultaneous and/or successive processing capacity. In such a case, the evaluation of the results by the examiner will indicate that, for a particular *coding* subtest in which the child used a *planning* strategy to solve the coding task, planning may be a relative strength of the subject. It will have implications for remediation.

Retest improvement is another important aspect of the strategy option. A retest condition should be included during standardization of our assessment battery. We suggest that the retest improvement assessment be standardized so that the examiner knows the amount of regression or improvement due to a second exposure to the materials following a standardized interactive condition and over a specified interval. These aspects of strategy assessment have been illustrated by using the tests of planning but are not limited to the planning scale. It will be most likely that strategies will be used and observed for the other process tasks as well.

Concluding Remarks: Intelligence and Cognitive Processes Reconsidered

Where does the above discussion leave us in understanding and assessing intelligence? We started out by rejecting an ability view of intelligence because of the implication of regarding intelligence as an immutable and fixed capacity. The score on an intelligence test neither gives us an idea of the processes underlying the level of performance nor reflects the extent to which the intelligence score of an individual is depressed due to the absence of mediated experience. The processes were identified under the broad functional organizations of cognition as planning, simultaneous-successive processing, and attention-arousal.

Neuropsychological findings support the above system of viewing cognitive functions. Each of these has been investigated extensively in experimental psychology. Thus the view of cognitive processing proposed by Das following Luria's clinical research and insight can bring together the knowledge from the two sources, neuro- and cognitive psychology, to understand intelligence.

However, three problems remain to be resolved. (a) How does one view intelligence vis-à-vis cognitive processes? Are these to be regarded as one and the same? (b) How does one assess processes in contrast to abilities? (c) Lastly, is interactive or dynamic assessment a prelude to remedial training or an integral part of assessment?; If it is the latter, then it creates its own paradox by recommending that each interactive assessment score must replace the previous one.

In answer to the first question, we think intelligence and cognitive processes have substantial if not total overlap. What we call intelligence or intelligent behavior must be the result of intellectual processes. A contemporary name for intellectual processes is simply cognitive processes. We include within this global category such broad mental activities as perception, memory, and thinking. Across all of these broad mental activities, and specifically cutting across them, are varieties of cognitive processes. For example, simultaneous and successive processes were shown to be involved in solving tasks that are usually described as perceptual, mnestic (concerning memory), and conceptual.

However, there might be a reason for distinguishing between intelligence and cognitive processes. The reason has to do with the controversial history of intelligence and the pejorative connotation the word might have acquired in some circles. But for those of us who wish to do research in the area of intelligent behavior, the identification of processes on the one hand, and interaction between them in determining intelligent behavior on the other, is a common agenda.

A certain agenda holds for most of the contemporary researchers of intelligence, such as the ones we have referred to before, (e.g., Hunt, Jensen, Sternberg). The difficulty arises when some researchers in the field of education and psychology wish to improve cognitive processes and demonstrate improvements due to a variety of procedures including what is nowadays labeled as cognitive strategy training. The difficulty arises because intelligence is not malleable; IQ scores have not been significantly improved by remedial training except when the training is similar to the methods and content represented in IQ tests. Under those conditions it may be useful to distinguish between intelligence as measured by a standardized psychometric instrument and cognitive processes.

Responding to the second question, processes cannot be directly assessed; they have to be inferred from performance. The tests suggested in this chapter for measuring the different processes in attention, coding, and planning essentially result in performance scores. How can we attempt to measure processes as distinguished from the measurement of abilities? It can be distinguished in terms of (a) the purpose of measurement, and (b) the utilization of the results of measurement.

Basically, the purpose of measuring abilities is to categorize and classify individuals. In contrast, process measures aim at separating the cognitive aspects that may underlie performance on a test. For instance, in measuring planning, we include a visual search task which has an automatic and a control search subtest, and further, within each of those subtests, the density of the background items is either high or low. There would be no rationale for doing this if one were motivated by measuring the capacity of an individual for visual scanning. Such a capacity could be useful as a general indicator for an occupation in which scanning is necessary. However, the reason we varied the density of the background items was to examine if search time was insensitive to the increment in the number of background stimuli in automatic form, whereas it became sensitive to increment in the control form.

The usefulness of the *results* from a process measure is linked as well with the *objective* of process measures. A process measure is particulrly required if we are engaged in improving the cognitive processing of special children. An ability measure does not lead to suggestions for adopting procedures for improving performance. These points are made quite clearly in Chapter 4 on remediation.

Lastly, interactive or dynamic assessment deserves some rethinking. The movement toward dynamic assessment appears as a reaction against the static assessment procedures in standardized tests. This is welcome progress in the field of intelligence testing. However, as we have pointed out in the discussion, dynamic assessment can be tolerated only if it does not lead to a substantial revision of the assessment score obtained for a majority of the normative samples. We think that dynamic assessment is a precursor to remedial training or treatment. It is essential for formulating remedial or instructional procedures for cognitive retraining. However, it is difficult to fit interactive assessment within the notion of assessment that is carried out by schools for education and training, simply because with true mediated learning, as Feuerstein calls it, the performance of the individual is expected to improve, and his/her approach to the task should change. The problem here is this: A continuous revision of previous assessment on the individual must occur. This may go on in a long spiral, if not an endless one. Thus, the alternative we have suggested calls for a two-phase approach. First one must distinguish those individuals who need special education, e.g. culturally deprived, emotionally disturbed, learning disabled, or mentally retarded, from those who are normal, that is, who have no special problems. The assessment of the normal sample should be carried out within those procedures. Subsequently, the special individual should be given the benefit of interactive assessment only because such assessment is expected to lead to remediation.

References

Arlin, P. K. (1977). Piagetian operations in problem finding. *Developmental Psychology*, *13*, 297–298.

Armitage, S. F. (1946). An analysis of certain psychological traits used for the evaluation of brain damage. *Psychological Monographs*, *60* (Whole No. 277).

Ashman, A. (1978). *The relationship between planning and simultaneous and successive synthesis*. Unpublished doctoral dissertation, Department of Educational Psychology, University of Alberta, Edmonton, Alberta.

Atkinson, R. C., & Shiffrin, R. M. (1968). Human memory. In K. W. Spence & J. T. Spence (Eds.), *Advances in the psychology of learning and motivation research and theory* (Vol. 2). New York: Academic Press.

Broadbent, D. E. (1981). From the percept to the cognitive structure. In J. Long & A. Baddeley (Eds.), *Attention and performance* (Vol. 9, pp. 1–26). Hillsdale, NJ: Erlbaum.

Christensen, A. (1974). *Luria's neuropsychological investigation*. Copenhagen, Denmark: Munksgaard.

Cowalt, C. A., & McCallum, R. S. (1984). Simultaneous-successive processing across the life-span: A cross-sectional examination of stability and proficiency. *Experimental Aging Research*, *10(4)*, 225–229.

Das, J. P. (1972). Patterns of cognitive ability in nonretarded and retarded children. *American Journal of Mental Deficiency*, *77*, 6–12.

Das, J. P. (1973). Cultural deprivation and cognitive competence. In N. R. Ellis (Ed.), *International review of research in mental retardation* (Vol. 6). New York: Academic Press.

Das, J. P. (1980). Planning: Theoretical considerations and empirical evidence. *Psychological Research* (W. Germany), *41*, 141–151.

Das, J. P. (1984a). Intelligence and information integration. In J. Kirby (Ed.), *Cognitive strategies and educational performance*. New York: Academic Press.

Das, J. P. (1984b). Aspects of planning. In J. Kirby (Ed.), *Cognitive strategies and educational performance*. New York: Academic Press.

Das, J. P. (1984c). Simultaneous and successive processes and K-ABC. *Journal of Special Education*, *18*, 229–238.

Das, J. P. (1985a). Remedial training for the amelioration of cognitive deficits in children. In A. F. Ashman & R. S. Laura (Eds.), *The Education and training of the mentally retarded* (pp. 215–244). London: Croom Helm.

Das, J. P. (1985b). Aspects of digit span performance: Naming time and order memory. *American Journal of mental Deficiency*, *89*, 627–634.

Das, J. P., & Bower, A. C. (1971). Originating responses of mentally retarded and normal children to work signals. *British Journal of Psychology*, *62*, 89–96.

Das, J. P., & Dash, U. N. (1983). Hierarchical factor solution of coding and planning processes: Any new insights. *Intelligence*, *7*, 27–38.

Das, J. P., & Heemsbergen, D. B. (1983). Planning as a factor in the assessment of cognitive processes. *Journal of Psychoeducational Assessment*, *1*, 1–15.

Das, J. P., Kirby, J., & Jarman, R. F. (1975). Simultaneous and successive synthesis: An alternative model for cognitive abilities. *Psychological Bulletin*, *82*(1), 87–103.

Das, J. P., Kirby, J. E., & Jarman, R. (1979). *Simultaneous and successive cognitive processes*. New York: Academic Press.

Das, J. P., & Molloy, G. N. (1975). Varieties of simultaneous and successive processing in children. *Journal of Educational Psychology*, *67*, 213–230.

Das, J. P., & Naglieri, J. A. (in preparation). *Cognitive assessment system*.

Das, J. P., & Varnhagen, C. K. (1986). Neuropsychological functioning and cognitive processing. *Child Neuropsychology*, *1*, 117–140.

Estes, W. K. (1976). Intelligence and cognitive psychology. In L. B. Resnick (Ed.), *The Nature of intelligence* (pp. 295–306). Hillsdale, NJ: Erlbaum.

Estes, W. K. (1981). Intelligence and learning. In M. Friedman, J. P. Das, & N. O'Connor (Eds.), *Intelligence and learning*, New York: Plenum.

Eysenck, H. J. (1982). *A model for intelligence*. Berlin: Springer-Verlag.

Furby, L. (1974). Attentional habituation and mental retardation. In *Human Development*, *17*, 118–138.

Gardner, H. (1983). *Frames of mind*. New York: Basic Books.

Garofalo, J. (1986). Simultaneous synthesis, regulation, and arithmetical performance. *Journal of Psychoeducational Assessment*, *4*, 229–238.

Geschwind, N. (1982). Disorders of attention: a frontier in neuropsychology. In D. E. Broadbent & L. Weiskrantz (Eds.), *The Neuropsychology of cognitive function*. Philosophical transaction of the Royal Society of London (pp. 173–185).

Gibson, E., & Rader, N. (1979). Attention. In G. A. Hale & Lewis M. (Eds.), *Attention and cognitive development* (pp. 1–22). New York: Plenum.

Glaser, R. (1972). The new aptitudes. *Educational Researcher*, *1*, 5–13.

Graham, F. K., & Kendall, B. S. (1960). Memory-for-designs test: Revised general manual. *Perceptual and Motor Skills*, *11*, 147–188.

Heemsbergen, D. S. (1980). *Planning as a cognitive process*. Unpublished doctoral dissertation, University of Alberta, Edmonton, Alberta.

Hess, W. R. (1967). Casulty, consciousness and cerebral organization. *Science*, *158*, 1279–1283.

Hunt, D., & Randhawa, B. S. (1983). Cognitive processes and achievement. *The Alberta Journal of Educational Research*, *29*(3), 206–215.

Hunt, E. B. (1980). Intelligence as an information processing concept. *British Journal of Psychology*, *71*, 449–474.

Jarman, R. F., & Das, J. P. (1977). Simultaneous and successive synthesis and intelligence. *Intelligence*, *1*, 151–169.

Jarman, R. F. (1980). Cognitive processes and syntactic structure: Analyses of syntagmatic and paradigmatic associations. *Psychological Research*, *41*, 153–169.

Jensen, A. R. (1981). Reaction time and intelligence. In M. P. Friedman, J. P. Das, & N. O'Connor (Eds.), *Intelligence and learning* (pp. 39–50). New York: Plenum.

Karrer, R. (Ed.). (1976). *Developmental psychophysiology of mental retardation*. Springfield, Il: Charles C. Thomas.
Lashley, K. S. (1951). The problem of serial order in behaviour. In J. A. Jeffreys (Ed.), *Cerebral mechanisms in behavior: The Hixon symposium*. New York: Wiley.
Leong, C. K. (1974). *Spatial-temporal information processing in disabled readers*. Unpublished doctoral dissertation, University of Alberta, Edmonton, Alberta.
Lezak, M. D. (1976). *Neuropsychological assessment*. New York: Oxford University Press.
Luria, A. R. (1966a). *Higher cortical functions in man*. New York: Basic Books.
Luria, A. R. (1966b). *Human brain and psychological processes*. New York: Harper & Row.
Luria, A. R. (1969). *The origin and cerebral organization of man's conscious action*. A lecture given to the XIX International Congress of Psychology, London.
Luria, A. R. (1970). The functional organization of the brain. *Scientific American*, *222*, 66–78.
Luria, A. R. (1973). *The working brain*. Middlesex, England: Penguin Books.
Luria, A. R. (1980). *Higher cortical functions in man* (2nd ed). New York: Basic Books.
Luria, A. R., & Artem'eva, E. Y. (1970). Two approaches to an evaluation of the reliability of psychological investigations. *Soviet Psychology*, *8*, 271–282.
Luria, A. R., & Vinogradova, O. S. (1959). An objective investigation of the dynamics of semantic system. *British Journal of Psychology*, *50*, 89–105.
McCallum R. S., & Merritt, F. M. (1983). Simultaneous and successive processing among college students. *Journal of Psychoeducational Research*, *1*, 85–93.
Messick, S. (1973). Multivariate models of cognitive and personality: The need for both process and structure in psychological theory and measurement. In J. Royce (Ed.), *Contributions of multivariate analysis to theoretical psychology*. New York: Academic Press.
Miller, G. A., Galanter, E. & Pribram, K. H. (1960). *Plans and the structure of Behavior*. New York: Holt, Rinehart, and Winston.
Murti, T. R. V. (1980). *The central philosophy of Buddhism*. London: Unwin Paperbacks.
Naglieri, J. A. (1985). *Matrix Analogies Test-Short Form*. San Antonio: The Psychological Corporation.
Naglieri, J. A., & Das, J. P. (1988). Planning-Arousal-Simultaneous-Successive (PASS): A model for assessment. *Journal of School Psychology*, *26*, 35–48.
Parasuraman, R. (1983). Vigilance, arousal and the brain. In A. Gale & J. Edwards (Eds). *Physiological correlates of human behavior* (pp. 35–55). London: Academic Press.
Parasuraman, R., & Davies, D. R. (Eds.). (1984). *Varieties of attention*. New York: Academic Press.
Pavlov, I. P. (1928). *Lectures on conditioned reflex* (W. H. Gantt, Trans). New York: International Publishers.
Popper, K. R., & Eccles, J. C. (1978). *The self and its brain*. New York: Springer-Verlag.
Posner, M. I. (1978). *Chronometric exploration of mind*. Hillsdale, NJ: Erlbaum.

Posner, M. I., & Boies, S. J. (1971). Components of attention. *Psychological Review*, *78*, 391–408.
Pribram, K. H., & Luria, A. R. (1973). The frontal lobes and the regulation of behavior. In R. H. Pribram & A. R. Luria (Eds.), *Psychology and the frontal lobes*. New York: Academic Press.
Pribram, K. H., & McGuinness, D. (1975). Arousal, activation and effort in the control of attention. *Psychological Review*, *82*, 116–149.
Randhawa, B. S., & Hunt, D. (1979). Some further evidence on successive and simultaneous integration and individual differences. *Canadian Journal of Behavioral Science*, *11*(4), 340–355.
Raven, J. C. (1955). *Coloured Progressive Matrices Sets A, AB, B*. London: H. K. Lewis.
Raven, J. C. (1958). *Standard Progressive Matrices Sets A, B, C, D and E*. London: H. K. Lewis.
Reitan, R. M. (1956). The relation of the trail making test to organic brain damage. *Journal of Consulting Psychology*, *19*, 393–394.
Ryckman, D. B. (1981). Reading achievement, IQ, and simultaneous-successive processing among normal and learning disabled children. *Alberta Journal of Educational Research*, *27*, 74–83.
Schofield, N. J., & Ashman, A. F. (1986). The relationship between digit span and cognitive processing across ability groups. *Intelligence*, *10*, 1–8.
Shallice, T., & Evans, M. E. (1978). The involvement of the frontal lobes in cognitive estimation. *Cortex*, *14*, 294–303.
Simon, H. A. (1981). Studying human intelligence by creating artificial intelligence. *American Scientist*, *69*(3), 300–309.
Spreen, O., & Gaddes, W. H. (1969). Developmental norms for 15 neuropsychological tests age 5 to 15. *Cortex*, *5*, 171–191.
Sternberg, R. J. (Ed.). (1985). *Human abilities*. New York: Freeman.
Stuss, D. T., & Benson, D. F. (1984). Neuropsychological studies of the frontal lobes. *Psychological Bulletin*, *95*(1), 3–28.
Vygotsky, L. S. (1978). *Mind in society—the development of higher psychological processes*. Cambridge, MA: Harvard University Press.
Wachs, M. C., & Harris, M. (1986). Simultaneous and successive processing in university students: Contribution to academic performance. *Journal of Psychoeducational Assessment*, *4*, 103–112.

9
Assessing Cognitive Modifiability of Infants and Toddlers: Observations Based on Mediated Learning Experience

PNINA S. KLEIN

Background

Conventional testing focuses on the child as he/she appears to perform on various test items in the present time. The dynamic assessment model (Feuerstein, Rand, & Hoffman, 1979) taps the individual's performance before, during, and after a learning situation. I suggest in this chapter the application of the theory of cognitive modifiability, which serves as the basis for dynamic assessment, to the evaluation of the adult-child interactions occurring in the homes of infants and young children. The basic assumption behind this approach is that, because the major agents of change in children's development are their primary caregivers, assessing the quality of the interaction between children and their caregivers is necessary for the construction of a valid basis for the evaluation of children's chances for cognitive development. Many previous attempts have been made to evaluate the characteristics of the environment that contribute to children's development. Of all these variables the ones most commonly used during testing are demographics such as parental education or IQ, parental occupation, and number of siblings. Variables such as these have been found to correlate significantly with measures of cognitive performance, but this does not explain the process of cause and effect that may serve as a basis for intervention geared to promote growth and development.

Despite the abundance of research data on the relationship between early environment and later cognitive performance, this relationship is still a matter of considerable speculation. Many attempts have been made to identify patterns of continuity in child development over time in relation to caregivers' behavior. In the domain of socioemotional development, for example, the significance of a socially responsive early environment has been demonstrated repeatedly, e.g., Boulby's and Ainsworth's theories of attachment suggest that maternal responsiveness is crucial for the development of attachment. Erikson presents a similar argument for the development of basic trust. More recently, Sroufe

(1983) emphasized caregivers' role in helping infants to maintain organized behavior in the face of novelty-produced excitation.

Maternal behavior variables such as attentiveness, warmth, responsiveness, nonrestrictiveness, and provision of appropriate play objects have been found to correlate significantly with measures of children's cognitive performance (e.g., Beckwith, 1971a, 1971b; Beckwith, Cohen, Kopp, Parmelee, & Marcy, 1976; Belsky, Good, & Most, 1980; Bradley, Caldwell, & Elardo, 1979; Clarke-Stewart, 1973; Yarrow, Rubenstein, & Pedersen, 1975).

Beyond the attempts to find possible links between general maternal characteristics and infants' developmental measures, Stern (1977a, 1977b) has identified a number of components of maternal behavior during face-to-face interaction that affect the frequency and duration of selected infant behavior and that have been suggested to have a long-lasting effect on infants' social development (Stern, 1977a, 1977b; Tronick, Ricks, & Cohn, 1982; Weissman & Paykel, 1974).

It has also been demonstrated that, as behavioral domains diverge, specific patterns of parental behavior may be more directly related to some domains than to others (Bradley & Caldwell, 1984). Thus, numerous attempts have been made to delineate children's special needs at different developmental phases with desired characteristics of caregivers' behavior during each of these phases (i.e., Greenspan & Porges, 1984; Sroufe, 1983).

Although relationships between caregivers' characteristics or behavior and developmental outcomes were demonstrated in each of the studies cited, none has defined as yet the necessary and sufficient conditions inherent in any adult-child interaction in order for that interaction, regardless of its content, to be considered a mediated learning experience for the child.

The Theory of Mediated Learning Experience

Feuerstein's theory of cognitive modifiability and mediated learning experience (MLE)has been in use in special education for over 30 years and its clinical value has already been demonstrated. (For summaries of the theory and related research, see Feuerstein, et al., 1979, 1980). The theory has only recently been applied in studies of early childhood and infancy (Klein & Feuerstein, 1984; Klein et al., 1987, 1988). The basic assumptions behind this theory are that human cognition is modifiable and that the primary factor affecting variability in modifiability of individuals can be traced back to the kind and amount of MLE they have experienced.

The process of mediated learning, as distinct from direct learning through the senses, is the process of learning that occurs when the environment is mediated to the child by another person who understands the child's needs, interests, and capacities, and who takes an active role in making components of that environment, as well as of the past and future experiences, compatible with the child. The mediator consciously schedules, selects, accentuates, frames, or groups the stimulus in time and space. The mediation affects the individual's present learning and may improve his or her opportunity to learn from future experiences.

The concept "culturally deprived," or "culturally disadvantaged," according to Feuerstein's theoretical framework, reflects a condition characterized by the low ability of individuals to be modified through direct exposure to stimuli, a condition caused by lack of, or deficient, MLE. Furthermore, the theory describes limited modifiability as manifested in a series of restrictions on information processing. These may include a lack of systematic ways of obtaining accurate information through the senses, sweeping exploration, lack of need for precision, inappropriate use of temporal and spatial dimensions, lack of perception and projection of sequences, lack of spontaneous comparative behavior, and the lack of need for logical evidence. If one manifests these difficulties, how is one going to benefit from direct exposure to stimuli? According to the theory of MLE, a person acquires the need for adequate functioning of these processes, and others, through mediated learning experiences.

MLE begins with interactions on a preverbal level and is not specifically related to a modality, language, or content. It is a universal phenomenon and is found in every culture. There are two basic components of MLE. One relates to contents that were it not for MLE, could never have reached the consciousness of a person. The other component relates to structures, to the form of information processing.

Through MLE, children can benefit from experiences that they have not perceived directly: the transmission of the past is made possible through mediational processes. The awareness of the past and mediated anticipation of the future enables children to expand their understanding of time and space.

A child who receives MLE develops a need for more mediation (i.e., a need for events or objects to have meaning) and a need to search for relations beyond the information provided by the senses at any given moment.

MLE is one of the two basic modes of learning from experience. It is universal, not specific to one culture or content. It enables further change of the individual through direct exposure to stimuli, and allows a child to acquire basic structures that prepare him/her for future learning.

In line with the theory of MLE, adult-child interactions can be considered as mediated learning experiences if they are intentional and reciprocal, if they transcend the satisfaction of an immediate need, and if they mediate meaning. These three components are necessary and sufficient for behavior to be considered MLE. Mediated feelings of competence, and mediated regulation of behavior, which are both presented as criteria of MLE in Feuerstein's theory, are necessary for MLE but cannot be considered as sufficient conditions for the definition of any specific behavior as MLE.

Forms of Observation

In the research outlined below, the model for observation of MLE with infants and young children was applied in two basic forms: (a) an assessment of mediation provided under naturalistic conditions at home, and (b) an assessment of MLE in a structured "free play" situation at a clinic, school, or other setting. Both forms of observation will be discussed; it should be noted, however, that the same criteria were used in both forms of observation with minor variations, i.e., correction for variables or time, if cross-situational or cross-time comparisons were called for. Both forms of observation were based on the ferquency of appearance of specific adult behavior in relation to child behavior.

In contrast to microanalytic, sequential procedures of observation, which commonly result in an overwhelming amount of detailed behavior codes requiring some form of data reduction (e.g., Belsky, Taylor, & Rovine, 1984; Farran & Ramey, 1980), the assessment method presented below is an observation of molar maternal behavior based on MLE (Klein, 1984b). The guidelines for observation include definitions of the five basic characteristics of MLE and descriptions of possible patterns of behavior that may reflect these experiences in everyday mother-child interactions, e.g., in feeding, bathing, and play situations.

Empirical Definitions of MLE Criteria

The categories of mother-infant interaction based on the MLE characteristics used in the construction of the assessment manual were empirically defined as follows:

Intentionality and Reciprocity

This category represents any act or sequence of acts on the part of an adult that appears to be directed toward achieving a change in the child's perception, processing, or response; e.g., selecting, exaggerating, accentuating, scheduling, grouping, sequencing, or pacing stimuli. Behavior that is intentional is considered reciprocal when the infant or child in the interaction responds vocally, verbally, or nonverbally, even by visual focusing, to adults' behavior.

Mediation of Meaning

This category represents adults' behavior that expresses verbal or nonverbal appreciation or affect toward objects, animals, or concepts and values. This behavior may include facial gestures, sounds, verbal expressions of affect, classification or labeling, and identification of value in relation to the child's or adult's past and future experiences; e.g., "Look at this beautiful flower," or "This cup is special; it belonged to Grandfather."

Transcendence

Adults' behavior that is directed toward the expansion of a child's cognitive awareness, beyond what is necessary to satisfy the immediate need that triggered the interaction, may be considered as transcendence; e.g., talking to a child about the food during feeding is beyond what is necessary to assure provision of nutrition. Exploring body parts or characteristics of water during bathing is not necessary for bathing and thus may be considered as transcendence. Transcendence can be expressed, for example, through inductive and deductive reasoning, spontaneous comparisons, clarifying spatial and temporal orientation, and pointing out strategies for short- and long-term memory and for memory search and recall.

Mediated Feelings of Competence

This category includes any behavior of an adult expressing, verbally or nonverbally, satisfaction with a child's behavior and including an identification of the specific component or components of the child's behavior that were considered by the adult as a success. This process of identification can be carried out, for example, through timing of the verbal or gestural expression of satisfaction, through repetition of the desired behavior, or through its verbal identification.

Mediated Regulation of Behavior

This category represents adult behavior that models, demonstrates, and/or verbally suggests to the child regulation of behavior in relation to the nature of the task, or to any other cognitive process prior to overt action. Mediated regulation of behavior may be expressed, for example, through processes in which matching the task requirements with the child's capacity and interests, as well as organization and sequencing of steps, is expressed: for example, "Slowly, not so hard; it is delicate, do it softly," or "First, turn all the pieces over then search for the right piece." Mediated regulation of behavior may be related to processes of perception, (e.g., systemactic exploration), to the process of elaboration (e.g., planning behavior), or to processes of expressive behavior (e.g., reducing egocentric expressions and regulating intensity and speed of behavior).

Observation Procedures

Rather than rating every behavior occurring during situations in which parents and infants are found in the same physical setting, the observation used in this research required noting only the behavior that fell within the defined characteristics of MLE; other behavior was ignored. Behavior of either parents or infants was not coded as unrelated units, but rather, in relation to each other's verbal or nonverbal behavior. For example, observing a parent hand a toy to a child could have been coded as reflecting intentionality and reciprocity only if this behavior was met by a response suggesting reciprocity on the part of the child. If one uses observations in which parents' and children's behavior is coded separately, the sum of such behavior may not necessarily convey the occurrence of reciprocity. Similarly in the case of transcendence, a mother may present an elaborate explanation in relation to an observed event but her behavior will not be considered as an MLE if her child did not seem to listen. Thus, behavior was considered to be MLE only if there was observable evidence that the child attended to it.

Home Observation

For this form of observation it is crucial that observers be well trained, because observations are usually not videotaped and cannot be reviewed. Observers were thus trained using live and videotaped sessions over a period ranging from 6 to 8 weeks. Interrater reliability of the home observation was established using a sample of 75 mother-child dyads, 25 for each of the three age groups studied: 6, 12, and 24 months.

Interrater reliability measured by Pearson's product moment correlation coefficients comparing frequencies of MLE across all three situations and age groups observed ranges between .72 and .91 ($\bar{x}$ = .77) for intentionality and reciprocity, .59- and .84 ($\bar{x}$ = .80) for transcendence, .92- and .71 ($\bar{x}$ = .81) for mediated feelings of competence, and .55- and .87 ($\bar{x}$ = .74) for mediated control of behavior.

Every infant was visited at home. At each of these visits, an observation of $2\frac{1}{2}$ to 3 hours was carried out. The objective of the visit was to assess mother-child interactions during feeding, bathing, and a play session with the child. Because the units of analysis were frequencies, these were corrected for temporal variations in the length of observation periods.

Although participating mothers agreed to take part in the assessment, most of them expressed some concern over being observed at home. To relieve that concern, the observers arrived at the home about 10 minutes prior to the onset of the observation and assured the mothers that they were not focusing on any home variables such as cleanliness or household organization. The observers asked mothers to go on doing what they normally did at home while they fed, bathed or played with the infants and to ignore the observer. The home observations were carried out mostly during one visit. In a few exceptional cases it was necessary to visit a home twice in order to assure inclusion of a feeding, a bathing, and a play situation in the observation. The majority of the observations were carried out in the morning hours during weekdays. All observers were female to assure that mothers would feel comfortable during breast feeding. To improve observer objectivity, attempts were made to avoid consecutive visits of the same observer in any of the homes.

Structured Observation

For the free-play session, mothers were left with their infants in a carpeted playroom approximately 3 × 4 m, furnished in a home-like manner with a couch, a desk, some chairs, and a box of toys. The toy box contained a ball, an egg carton with multicolored, plastic eggs, some toy animals, dolls, hand puppets, household utensils (a pot and cover and measuring spoons), and three children's books.

Mothers were instructed to be with their children "as you usually are at home" for 10 to 15 minutes, until the examiner returned. Videotaping took place through a one-way mirror and mothers were informed of the videotaping. The first 10-minute segments of these tapes were coded, using the criteria for observation of MLE. Every behavior that was identified as an MLE was coded. Behavior that continued for more than 15 seconds was coded again; a 15-second audio tone was introduced for that purpose. (A variation of this form of observation found to be particularly effective with 2- and 3-year-old children is described by the author elsewhere; Klein, 1985).

Interrater reliability of the observation used in the current study was established using a sample of 40 mother-child dyads; 10 for each of the following age groups: 6, 12, 24, and 36 months. One-half of the infants were boys. This sample was drawn from a low socioeconomic status (SES) Israeli population. Interrater reliability across all age groups observed ranged between correlations of .76 and .85 for intentionality and reciprocity, .62 and .83 for transcendence, .65 and .80 for mediation of meaning, .92 and .74 for mediated feelings of competence, and .68 and .81 for mediated control of behavior. No significant differences were found in interrater reliability of observations for boys and girls.

Predictability and Stability of the Observation

In a recent 4-year follow-up study of low-SES American children and their high-risk mothers (Klein, Wieder, & Greenspan, 1987), mothers' free-play sessions with their infants were videotaped when infants reached 4, 8, 12, 24, and 36 months. These tapes were analyzed using the criteria for observation of MLE (Klein, 1984b). The predictability of the observed variables was examined in relation to the children's Bayley Mental Development Scale (MDI) scores at 4, 8, 12, and 24 months and to the McCarthy Scales of Children's Abilities scores at 36, 42, and 48 months (Klein, Wieder, & Greenspan, 1987). One of the most interesting findings of this study relates to the fact that 10-minute observation of mother-child interactions in infancy and up to 2-years of age, using criteria of observation based on MLE, predicted cognitive performance of the same children at 4 years of age—with the 12-month observation being the most predictive of long-term performance. Significant and high stability over time was reported in the above-mentioned study as well as in another longitudinal study (Klein, 1988) of middle-class Israeli infants and their mothers. In the latter study, 40 infants were observed at home for approximately 2½ to 3 hours when infants were 6, 12, and 24 months old. Observations at each age included a feeding, bathing, and play interaction with the child. Significant cross-age and cross-situation stability were found for each of the MLE criteria observed using the method for home observation described in this chapter. Based on the findings of the latter study it was concluded that the amount and type of MLE provided by mothers is fairly stable across various situations of child care. However, when their children were around the age of 2 years, mothers in my longitudinal study were found to provide significantly more MLE during play sessions as compared with other interactions in caregiving situations, e.g., feeding and bathing. It appears that around that time mothers begin to differentiate between their role as caregivers and their role as "educators." The latter is perceived as more directly "boxed" into play sessions with the child and having very little to do with other situations of everyday living. This approach curtails the children's chances of getting MLE on many other occasions when they are most interested in events occurring around them and when they are most susceptible to cognitive modifiability.

Assessment of MLE with Toddlers

Provision of appropriate MLE early in a child's life is expected, in line with the theory of cognitive modifiability, to bring about changes in a child's need system. One can expect changes such as an increase in the need for information beyond what is perceived by means of direct learning through the senses. More specifically, such needs may be expressed, for example, through the following behavior: a child's attempts to inquire about information linking the immediate experience with past and future experiences, with information that transcends the satisfaction of the immediate goals of a behavior or experience, and with the affect associated with it; and with attempts to seek awareness of the kind of processes and the temporal or spatial order necessary for efficient performance on specific tasks. Toddlers who have had sufficient MLE can hardly be expected to spend periods of time (even as short as 10 or 15 minutes) without expressing their needs, e.g., asking questions, demanding information, and verbalizing awareness of cognitive processes related to planning, meaning, feelings of competence, or even regulation of behavior. Such toddlers are likely to reflect the MLE they have experienced by mediating to their parents. In other words, it may be the children now who are providing the parents with mediated feelings of competence, mediation of meaning, transcendence, and so forth. It is thus clear that an observation of MLE focusing only on parental mediation is missing a good part of the picture of MLE provided in a particular home if children's mediation and requests for mediation are not taken into consideration. All these variables are included in the assessment of MLE and can be seen in the sample observation sheet for evaluation of MLE with toddlers (Figure 9.1). Frequencies of appearance of each designated behavior are marked during the observation. The sum of frequencies for each category indicates the category score and serves as a basis for the construction of a profile of MLE provided to a particular child.

For a specific child two or more different profiles of mediation may be obtained depending upon the adult mediating to that child. These profiles should be presented separately rather than in a combined form because it has not been empirically tested whether mediation provided by different people, e.g., mothers and fathers, functions in a cumulative manner or whether various criteria within the MLE profile are more effective when provided by one person as compared to another or to others.

Mediation of Other Children

Based on an ongoing study in which home observations were carried out, it was suggested that children (3 to 6 years) make special efforts to "teach" or mediate to their younger siblings. In this study, several aims of children's mediation to infants and toddlers where identified:

1. to draw the younger child's attention to an object so that the mediator can have another desired object to him/herself;

MLE criteria	Provision of MLE by mother	Provision of MLE by child	Request for MLE by mother	Request for MLE by child	Total mother	Total child
Intentionality and						
Reciprocity						
Verbal						
Nonverbal						
Combined verbal and nonverbal						
Mediation of Meaning						
Expression of Affect (nonverbal)						
Naming						
Naming and Affect						
Relating to Past or Future						
Transcendence						
In relation to content of specific experience						
Clarifying processes (insight)						
General rules						
Other						
Mediated Feelings of Competence						
"Good," "Great," "Fine" (statement only) but with good timing						
Reinforcement + explanation						
Modification of situation to allow success						
Mediated Regulation of Behavior						
In relation to time						
In relation to space						
Sequencing of steps						
Matching ability & task requirements						
Other						

FIGURE 9.1. Partial sample of observation sheet for the assessment of MLE with toddlers.

2. to gain parental approval when the younger sibling demonstrates newly learned behavior that was acquired following his/her teaching;
3. to prepare the younger sibling to be a playmate in a specific game;
4. to exercise his/her newly learned skill, with the younger sibling serving as audience.

Of the basic criteria necessary and sufficient for MLE, intentionality and reciprocity and mediation of meaning were quite frequent, but transcendence was relatively low.

Styles of Mediation

The cross-cultural study of mother-child interactions applying MLE criteria (Klein, 1988) yielded interesting information regarding the styles of mediation used by different mothers. It became relatively clear that certain patterns of mother-child interaction were frequently observed for mothers who showed high frequencies of MLE (high mediators) as opposed to mothers who showed low frequencies of MLE (low mediators), and vice versa for other patterns or styles of mediation. Some of these interactions are presented in Table 9.1. In addition to the construction of a profile of MLE based on the observation previously described, the identification of the style of mediation provides insight into the qualitative nature of this mediation.

Modifiability of Mediation

The findings regarding the predictive power of the criteria of MLE observed in infancy and early childhood as well as their stability over time should not be interpreted as indicators of permanence and unmodifiability of these criteria. It should be understood that if no attempt is made to

TABLE 9.1. Comparing mediation styles of low and high mediators (mothers of 8- to 12-month-old infants)

High MLE	Low MLE
Mothers use frequent verbalization to mediate their thinking about the child. It sounds almost like reporting to another adult. "You are too busy, you don't know what to choose."	Almost no "reporting" behavior. Little verbalization. Frequent substitution of sounds, e.g., "oh oh" for words to express disagreement, anger, concern. No differentiation.
If one form of calling an infant's attention does not bring about the desired response, mothers tend to combine a number of techniques, e.g., calling infant's name and making sounds with a toy and movement, changing body position to improve possibility of eye contact.	Tend to repeat same form of calling child's attention (also true for attempts to get the child to comply).
Only 10% of the mothers engaged in encouraging motor activity, e.g., walking during the play session rather than exploring the offered toys.	70% of the mothers encouraged their infant's gross motor activities.
Mothers sat on the carpet with the baby attempting to achieve eye-to-eye contact or at least to see the infant's face.	30% of the mothers did not attempt to achieve eye contact with their infant and remained seated on the couch throughout the entire play session.

TABLE 9.1. cont.

High MLE	Low MLE
Most intentional acts are met by reciprocity. Intentionality without reciprocity is primarily of a verbal nature, e.g., many rhetorical questions building expectations for need to reply.	Intentionality without reciprocity primarily of motor and visual perceptual nature.
Much of the mother's behavior is orgasnized in sequences of behavior, each expanding on the previous ones, e.g., starting with calling the infant's attention, followed by manipulating and naming objects, repeating actions, or pointing out salient characteristics of the target behavior.	Many fragmented behaviors, e.g., mothers call the infant by name or use other methods of capturing attention, but when they have that attention they do not proceed to use it. Any reciprocity that is achieved is short-lived.
Mothers rarely label objects or actions using one single word. Labeling frequently appears with an age-appropriate expansion of information, not necessarily verbal, related to the labeled object or action.	Most frequently, labeling occurs with only word labels, stated once.
Mothers express verbally their own learning from the play session at the center (spontaneously), e.g., "I see you like that toy more than the others; we'll have to get you one like that."	No expression of learning from the play session.
Mothers repeat building-up of expectations for meaning, e.g., "What is in there?", "What is that?", or opening boxes, pots, containers, putting things inside. Mothers answer the questions as they arise.	No systematic repeated experience of mediated request for mediation. In several cases when questions were posed by mothers, e.g., "What is in there?", these were left unanswered or answered in a manner unsynchronized with child's attention.
Many verbal statements of praise expressed together with nonverbal indications of excitement and positive affect, e.g., smiles, clapping hands, changes in tone of voice.	Show almost no clear expression of praise following infant's behavior.
Few and brief episodes of rough physical play or tickling.	Many rather prolonged episodes of tickling and rough physical play. The use of tickling as a means of quieting the baby.
Few commands. Any instructions given, e.g., "get the ball," are preceded by attempts to assure that the infant focuses and by repeated attempts to model the desired behavior, and to reinforce approximation of it.	Many commands stated with no or little nonverbal elaboration, direction, or attempt to model the desired behavior. Hardly any reinforcement for approximations of the target behavior.

TABLE 9.1. cont.

High MLE	Low MLE
Demonstrate little physical rough and tumble play but express physical pleasure in the relationship.	Demonstrate much physical pleasure in the relationship and much rough and tumble play. Repeated request for the infant to kiss or hug mother.
Goal-setting behavior is present but there is a reinforcing episode of goal reaching following infant's efforts to reach it.	"Teasing" the child in order to teach goal reaching, e.g., showing the child a desired object then moving it away, out of reach repeatedly following infant's attempts to reach it.
Cause-and-effect sequences are intentionally modified by mothers to bring about more dramatic effects, e.g., when the infant bangs on the carpet with a set of metal measuring spoons and moves it up to meet the child's arm. Repeated.	Few sequences of cause and effect are repeated or modified to mediate the cause-and-effect relationship.
Mediated competitive behavior present in combination with mediated feelings of competence, e.g., mother makes the ball roll slightly and crawls together with the baby to get it.	What appears to be mediated competitive behavior most frequently turns into episodes of teasing the child.

affect parent-child interaction with regard to these criteria, they may remain quite stable and predictable across time.

Dynamic assessment includes the following three phases: testing, teaching, and retesting. The change occurring between the initial testing and the postintervention testing reflects the individual's cognitive modifiability.

The assumption behind the assessment-intervention approach described in this chapter is that every parent can become a good mediator to his child. The time and amount of effort required to achieve this goal may vary depending on variables related to the parent (e.g., level of education, age, personality, cultural values and needs, living conditions, and SES), to the child (e.g., variables related to pregnancy, delivery, parity, nutrition, general health, and temperament), and to the type and intensity of the intervention (e.g., individual vs. group sessions, time of onset, and length of intervention).

An attempt to examine modifiability of the MLE criteria was carried out by this author in a small primarily low-SES community in the north of Israel. Forty families within this community received a special program called "more intelligent and sensitive children" (MISC). Twenty other families served as a control group.

The objective of the MISC program was to raise parental awareness of the five basic MLE criteria operationally defined in this chapter. The basic underlying assumption of the program was that once parents become aware of what it is in what they do with their child that affects cognitive development, they will tend to increase and improve the mediation they provide.

Mediation to the parents was provided weekly at their homes by trained local paraprofessionals who observed parental behavior and reinforced and modeled expressions of MLE.

The intervention model used incorporated one or more of the following strategies:

1. Mediation of the MLE criteria to the adult caregivers, in most cases to the mother, using situations from *adult* daily life. Following this initial stage, the criteria were identified as they appear in daily activities ongoing in the home, and expanded to demonstrate other possible ways of expressing the same criteria in different interactions with the *child*.
2. Role playing; mediating to the mother the possibility of understanding the child's behavior if placed in his/her position.
3. Identification with feelings similar to those felt by the child as they may appear in the adult life experiences, e.g., "How would it feel if your boss told you . . . ?"
4. Sharing, verbal or nonverbal demonstrations of the thinking processes, and overt behavior sequences or methods one uses in different situations, e.g., "When I look at this kind of question I feel confused and so I ask myself first . . . and then. . . ."

An assessment of preintervention and postintervention conditions in the homes and an assessment of the children were carried out, following 1 and 2 years of intervention. Significant differences in parental mediation and in the children's cognitive performance were found between the pre- and postintervention conditions, in favor of the experimental group.

Based on the MLE observation, a profile of MLE may be constructed for each adult-child dyad. The most common types of profiles found in both the American and the Israeli populations studied were as follows:

1. High, flat profile: a profile indicating relatively high frequency of mediation for each of the basic criteria of MLE observed.
2. Low, flat profile: a profile of low frequencies distributed relatively equally among all MLE criteria.
3. Uneven profile: a profile reflecting significantly more or less of one characteristic of MLE as compared to others.

The most common characteristic of MLE profiles found for middle-class families was a high frequency of maternal intentionality unbalanced by reciprocity on the infants' part. It was found also that all families could modify the MLE they provided. Families with high, flat profiles and families with uneven profiles of MLE frequently showed more rapid modifiability as compared to families with low, flat profiles.

It is interesting to note that, of the two criteria selected as indicators of change—parental verbal ability to recite the basic MLE criteria, and an observed increase in the frequency of these criteria in parent-child interactions—it was found that parental behavior changed before there was a parallel change in the parents' verbal capacity to recite the criteria.

The length of time it took a family to modify significantly the MLE provided to their children depended on a number of variables, some of which are commonly reported in literature in relation to changes of attitude. However, in this case, parental motivation to improve their child's cognitive development was clearly present in all homes and was unrelated to parental level of education, income, or ethnic background. It must be noted that there was significant variability between parents with regard to their own belief in the medifiability of their child and in their self-perception as agents of this desired change. Assessing these parental attitudes and beliefs may serve as an indicator of the need to spend more time mediating to the parents about their power in shaping the child's mind and about their child's potential to change. Parental attitudes or beliefs should not be perceived as indicators that MLE cannot be practiced in some homes.

Summary

Dynamic assessment focuses on the potential of an individual to change as a result of an encounter with experiences of new learning. In infancy and early childhood, one cannot expect to evaluate a child's capacity to change without assessing the type of preparation for learning he/she experiences, i.e., the amount and type of MLE provided to him/her. A method of assessment of these experiences has been presented in this chapter.

Bloom (1964) has suggested that the effects of early environment may be particularly salient and lasting, provided no major changes occur in a child's environment. Contrary to that notion, Kagan, Kearsley, and Zelazo (1978) suggested that the effects of early experiences are exaggerated, that later environmental variables explain more of the variability in cognitive performance, and that high correlations between early environment and later cognitive performance reflect more of the stability in the child's environment than the isolated effects of the early environment. Based on the theory of MLE, an additional explanation may be offered: According to this theoretical approach, MLE at any age affects later cognitive performance. Changes occurring in the environment are potentially effective if these changes include MLE experiences. Children who have not experienced MLE are less likely to benefit from future direct exposure-type learning, and thus may remain unchanged, despite major changes in their environment. The theory postulates that cognitive modification can occur at any age, provided appropriate mediation is made available to the individual (Feuerstein 1979; Feuerstein et al., 1979, 1980).

Infancy and early childhood are periods in which children are particularly sensitive and ready for cognitive modifiability. Thus, assessment of the potential for modifiability during this age is of special interest.

Many predictors of cognitive development other than direct measures can be found in the literature; among the most commonly used, for example, are material IQ, education or other criteria of SES (Bayley & Schaefer, 1964; Ramey & Gowen, 1984), or even family interaction variables independent of SES (Sameroff, Seifer, Barocas, & Greenspan, 1985). What could clearly have added explanatory power to the trends suggested by these studies is a model such as the one presented in this chapter, that helps to identify some of the key interactional variables that are predictive of later cognitive performance, and that should be considered in assessment or in planning early intervention programs.

References

Bayley, N., & Schaefer, E. S. (1964). Correlations of maternal and child behaviors with the development of mental abilities: Data from the Berkeley growth study. *Monographs of the Society for Research in Child Development*, *29*(6).

Beckwith, L. (1971a). Relationships between attributes of mothers and their infants' I.Q. scores. *Child Development*, *42*, 1083–1097.

Beckwith, L. (1971b). Relationships between infants; vocalizations and their mother's behaviors. *Merrill-Palmer Quarterly*, *17*, 221–226.

Beckwith, L., Cohen, S. E., Kopp, C. B., Parmelee, A. H., & Marcy, T. C. (1976). Caregiver-infant interaction and early cognitive development in preterm infants. *Child Development*, *47*, 579–587.

Belsky, J., Good, M. K., & Most, R. K. (1980). Maternal stimulation and infant exploratory competence: Cross-sectional, correlational, and experimental analysis. *Child Development*, *51*, 1163–1178.

Belsky, J., Taylor, D. G., & Rovine, M. (1984). The Pennsylvania infant and family development. II: The development of reciprocal interaction in the mother-infant dyad. *Child Development*, *55*, 706–717.

Bloom, B. S. (1964). *Stability and change in human characteristics*. New York: Wiley.

Bradley, R., & Caldwell, B. M. (1984). The relation of infants' home environments to achievement test performance in first grade: A follow-up study. *Child Development*, *55*, 803–809.

Bradley, R., Caldwell, B., & Elardo, R. (1979). Home environment and cognitive development in the first two years: A cross-lag panel analysis. *Developmental Psychology*, *15*, 246–250.

Clarke-Stewart, K. A. (1973). Interactions between mothers and their young children: Characteristics and consequences. *Monographs of the Society for Research in Child Development*, *38*(6–7, Serial No. 153).

Farran, D. C., & Ramey, C. T. (1980). Social class differences in dyadic involvement during infancy. *Child Development*, *51*, 254–257.

Feuerstein, R., Rand, Y., & Haffman, M. B. (1979). *The dynamic assessment of retarded performers*. Baltimore: University Park Press.

Feuerstein, R. (1979). Ontogeny of learning in man. In M. A. B. Brazier (Ed.), *Brain mechanisms in memory and learning* (pp. 361–372). New York: Raven Press.

Feuerstein, R., Rand, Y., Hoffman, M. B. & Miller, R. (1980). *Instrumental enrichment*. Baltimore: University Park Press.

Greenspan, S. I., & Porges, W. (1984). Psychopathology in infancy and early childhood: Clinical perspectives on the organization of sensory and affective-thematic experience. *Child Development*, *55*, 49–70.

Kagan, J., Kearsley, R., & Zelazo, P. (1978). *Infancy: Its place in human development*. Cambridge, MA: Harvard University Press.

Klein, P. S. (1984a). Behavior of Israeli mothers toward infants in relation to infants' perceived temperament. *Child Development*, *55*, 1212–1218.

Klein, P. S. (1984b). *Criteria for observation of mediated learning experience*. Unpublished manuscript, Bar-Ilan University, Ramat Gan, Israel.

Klein, P. S. (1985). *Developing intelligence in infants and young children*. Ramat Gan: Bar-Ilan University Press.

Klein, P. S. (1988). Stability and change in interaetion of Israeli mothers and infants. *Infant Behavior and Development*, *11*, 55–70.

Klein, P. S., & Feuerstein, R. (1984) Environmental variables and cognitive development: Identification of potent factors in adult-child interaction. In S. Harel & W. N. Anastasio (Eds.), *The at-risk infant: Psycho-socio medical aspects* (pp. 369–377). Baltimore: Paul H. Brookes.

Klein, P. S., Weider, S., & Greenspan, S. I. (1987). A theoretical overview and empirical study of mediated learning experience: Prediction of preschool performance from mother-infant interaction patterns. *Infant Mental Health Journal*, *8*(2), 110–129.

Ramey, C. T., & Gowen, J. W. (1984). A general systems approach to modifying risk for retarded development. *Early Child Development and Care*, *16*, 9–26.

Sameroff, A. J., Seifer, R., Barocas, R., & Greenspan, S. I. (1985). *The probability of childhood developmental morbidity as a function of early cumulative environmental risk*. In press.

Sroufe, L. A. (1983). The coherence of individual development. *American Psychologist*, *34*, 834–841.

Stern, D. (1977a). *The first relationship*. London: Open Books.

Stern, D. (1977b). *The first relationship: infant and mother*. Cambridge, MA: Harvard University Press.

Tronick, E. A., Ricks, M., & Cohn, J. F. (1982). Maternal and infant affective exchange: patterns of adaptation. In T. Field & A. Fogel (Eds.), *Emotion and interaction: normal and high risk infants* (pp. 241–268). Hillside, NJ: Erlbaum.

Weissman, M. M., & Paykel, E. S. (1974). *The depressed woman: a study of social relationship*. Chicago: University of Chicago Press.

Yarrow, L. J., Rubenstein, J. L., & Pedersen, F. A. (1975). *Infant and environment*. New York: Wiley.

10 Evaluating Preschool Programs: The Role of Dynamic Assessment

MARILYN T. SAMUELS, STEVE M. KILLIP, HEATHER MACKENZIE, and JOEL FAGAN

Over the past few years, dynamic assessment approaches have been used with increasing frequency to assess children and adults experiencing learning difficulties. Research on dynamic assessment has focused primarily on their use with particular groups: children with learning disabilities (Samuels, Tzuriel, & Malloy-Miller, 1989), with cultural deprivation (Feuerstein, Rand, & Hoffman, 1979) and hearing impairment (Keane, 1987). Dynamic assessment has also been used to evaluate the outcome of intervention programs, such as Feuerstein, Rand, Hoffman, & Miller's (1980) Instrumental Enrichment, for teaching thinking to adolescents (Arbitman-Smith, Haywood, & Bransford, 1984; Narrol, Silverman, & Waksman, 1982; Samuels, Roadhouse, Conte, & Zirk, 1984). However, little research has examined the use of dynamic assessment for evaluating the outcome of preschool intervention programs. The purpose of this chapter is to discuss the use of dynamic assessment for evaluating the effectiveness of preschool programs for children with learning difficulties. A project evaluating two approaches to programming for preschool children with special needs will be described to illustrate the use of dynamic assessment.

Two vignettes of children placed in a specialized program for children with learning difficulties illustrate typical profiles and predicted outcomes from static assessment and the additional information provided by dynamic assessment. A pilot study using both dynamic and static assessment is then reported and suggestions are made about the type of information gained from dynamic assessment including its usefulness in predicting responsiveness to programming and future school success.

John—A Slow Learner with High Modifiability

John was 5 years, 6 months of age when we first met him. He had a history of mild cognitive delay and moderate delays in speech, language, and fine motor development. In addition, there were behavioral concerns which included impulsiveness, distractibility, and aggressiveness toward other children.

John attended a preschool program for normally achieving children between the ages of $4\frac{1}{2}$ and $5\frac{1}{2}$. During that time he also received individual speech-language therapy and consultative input from an occupational therapist. During the following year, John attended a program for developmentally delayed preschoolers (described later in the chapter) where he continued to receive therapy.

On standardized measures of receptive and expressive vocabulary development, John exhibited consistent 1-year delays during the period from $4\frac{1}{2}$ through 7 years of age. Standardized cognitive testing indicated similarly consistent 10- to 16-month delays over the 3-year period. These results suggested that John was developmentally "keeping pace with time" but that he was functioning in the borderline to mildly mentally handicapped range. This history and developmental profile would typically identify a child like John for placement in a special education class on reaching school age.

Dynamic assessment results obtained on several occasions during the same period of time, indicated greater learning potential than was suggested by the standardized measures. On each administration of a test-teach-test instrument, the Children's Analogical Thinking Modifiability Test (CATM; Tzuriel & Klein, 1985), John exhibited high degrees of modifiability (i.e., 6- to 7-point gain out of a maximum 16 points) between the pretest and the posttest, which followed brief mediation to curb impulsiveness and teach rules and strategies.

John's programming and placement were assumed completely by the local school board after leaving the special needs preschool program. Two years have now passed and John, in keeping with the learning potential observed, is enrolled and achieving in a regular education program. This placement would not have been predicted by standardized test scores.

Michael—A Slow Learner with Low Modifiability

Michael presents a slightly different story. He had a similar background of developmental delay but few behavioral concerns. He had the benefit of early placement in preschool programs and individual speech-language therapy.

On standardized measures of receptive and expressive vocabulary, Michael exhibited consistent 1-year delays during the period from $4\frac{1}{2}$ to 7 years of age. Standardized cognitive assessment results indicated relatively consistent $2\frac{1}{2}$-year delays over the same time span. Like John, Michael showed that his development was "keeping pace with time" and the standardized test results would identify him for special education placement.

Dynamic assessment results from the same period of time showed that the change in Michael's performance following brief intervention was substantially less than John's. On each administration of the dynamic assessment instrument, Michael exhibited either minimal (i.e., 1-point) increases or slight decrements between pretest and posttest scores. These findings would suggest that Michael needed more intensive mediation than John to learn effectively.

The local school system has independently determined Michael's educational needs over the last 2 years, since he left our preschool program. Unlike John, who exhibited good modifiability in dynamic assessment, Michael is enrolled in a special education program.

These vignettes illustrate that, based on conventional static assessment, both of these boys would be predicted to need intensive educational support. These scores indicated below average functioning both before and after preschool intervention. Michael's cognitive assessment scores were somewhat lower than John's, but for both children special education placement would normally be prescribed. The gain scores on the dynamic assessment measure, both prior to and following the preschool program, were markedly different for the two boys and appeared to relate to their later academic attainment.

Issues in the Assessment of Preschool Children

A goal of all intervention programs is to produce meaningful change in targeted areas of functioning. Standardized testing prior to and following a program has generally been used to evaluate effectiveness. The tests measure the child's level of functioning upon entry to the program and are assumed to predict his or her future academic success, if no specialized intervention is provided. Significant deviations from the prediction (i.e., greater than expected change as compared to a control group) are then assumed to be due to the intervention. There are, however, a number of difficulties in using standardized tests with preschool-aged children.

The first major difficulty lies in the assessment process itself. Preschool children present special challenges in an assessment situation, which make understanding their difficulties and future learning needs particularly difficult. The young child's short attention span, distractibility, low verbal skills, and transient responsiveness make the assessment process difficult and the results often unreliable (Bagnato & Neisworth, 1981; Lerner, Mardell-Czudnowski, & Goldenberg, 1981; Lidz, 1983). Standardized assessment instruments, by their nature, constrain the examiner from intervening in these areas. Yet, for the child with special needs, understanding the factors impeding learning and an assessment of learning potential are essential for determining appropriate educational interventions.

The second major difficulty is the assumption that standardized test results can predict future performance. A guiding principle in educational practice for many years has been the stability of individual performance. The idea that a child who does poorly on psychoeducational assessment in preschool will have difficulties in later years has led to the questionable practice of preschool screening and labeling. Some studies have demonstrated a relationship between performance on standardized tests and later academic success in preschool children (Funk, Sturner & Green, 1986; Schmidt & Perino, 1985) but many other studies have not (Badian & Serwer, 1975; Goodman & Cameron, 1978; Keogh & Becker, 1973). Of greater interest is the emphasis on assessment of the child's current areas of difficulties, regardless of whether they are associated with future disabilities (Lidz, 1983). The only real justification for an assessment at any age is to gain information that will assist in anticipating and remediating current problems as soon as possible (Keogh & Becker, 1973; Paget & Nagle, 1986).

This same justification can be applied to evaluations of children that will be used to measure success of a program. Given that the program has been chosen because it is believed to be effective in remediating the difficulties of the participants, assessment measures need to focus on the current difficulties and what will be needed to overcome them. In other words, assessment should seek not merely to predict future performance but to establish the conditions under which it is possible to promote positive change. The type of information needed to produce change and, hence, defeat the predictions is of primary interest.

This brings us to a third major difficulty with standardized assessment. Standardized assessment approaches, traditionally used to identify, plan, and evaluate educational interventions, have been criticized by many as attributing too much importance to performance and insufficient emphasis on the processes of learning (Feuerstein et al., 1979; Lidz, 1983; Sigel & Brodzinski, 1977; Tzuriel & Klein, 1985). These assessments can provide an underestimation of intellectual performance and only indirect inferences can be made about learning potential (Baumeister, 1984; Bryant, Brown, & Campione, 1983; Campione, Brown, Ferrara, & Bryant, 1984; Mercer, 1973). It is recognized that although normative assessment may be useful for purposes of identification and for arriving at specific diagnoses (Reynolds & Clark, 1983), dynamic, or clinical, assessment approaches provide more accurate and useful information about a child's learning potential. Dynamic assessment permits the examiner to directly assess the learning process and the factors impeding it by producing change during assessment (Feuerstein, Miller, Rand, & Jensen, 1981). The amount any type of intervention required to produce change can be used as evidence of the modifiability of the child's performance, given appropriate intervention.

Dynamic Assessment: Rationale and Research

Feuerstein and his colleagues have developed a dynamic approach to assessment that is based on the theories of structural cognitive modifiability (SCM) and mediated learning experience (Feuerstein et al., 1980). The basic assumption underlying SCM is that human beings throughout their lives have a unique capacity to change or modify the structure of their cognitive functioning in adaptation to changing demands. The mode of interaction between the individual and the environment accounts for most of the structural changes that occur in human cognition. This mode of interaction, termed mediated learning experience (MLE), is contrasted with direct exposure modes in which individuals register and respond to stimuli or actively interact with stimuli to which they are exposed. Jensen and Feuerstein (1987) suggest 10 criteria for an interaction to be considered a mediated learning experience. The first five will be discussed here as they are most relevant to dynamic assessment at the preschool level. The first three criteria, intentionality, transcendence and meaningfulness, are always present, whereas a fourth and fifth, regulation of behavior and mediation of competence, are often present. Intentionality refers to an intent on the part of a more experienced person to interpose him/herself between the stimulus and the child in order to modify the stimulus in some way. The mediator attempts to focus the child's attention, organize the information, and transform the stimuli so that the child is able to perceive the environment in a more meaningful way. A mediated learning experience also transcends the moment so that what is learned can be applied in other similar situations. Third, the mediator ensures that the child understands the meaning and purpose of the learning experience. Regulation of behavior, (i.e., curbing impulsiveness, stopping trial-and-error responses) is a precursor to efficient gathering of information and careful responding. Mediation of feelings of competence as a learner is extremely important for children used to experiencing failure. Reinforcement of process (not just product) and specific feedback about what was "good" about a response increase feelings of competence.

Inadequate mediated learning experiences due to conditions inherent in the child (e.g., brain damage) or conditions in the environment (e.g., severe deprivation), may lead to cognitive functions that are poorly developed, arrested, impaired, seldom used, and/or inefficient. The locus of the deficiencies may be at one or more of three phases: input, or information gathering phase; elaboration, or thinking phase; and output, or communication of information phase. Deficient functioning may reflect cognitive deficits as well as attitudinal and motivational deficiencies.

The Learning Potential Assessment Device (LPAD) (Feuerstein et al., 1979) is based on the theories of structural cognitive modifiability and mediated learning experience. In the LPAD, the examiner engages the individual in mediated learning experiences by regulating behavior, teaching concepts, operations, rules and strategies, and producing insight in order to promote and assess the examinee's capacity for structural change. The amount and type of mediation needed to produce change is the variable of interest in dynamic assessment.

Research on the LPAD has focused primarily on older school-aged, adolescent, and adult populations (reviewed in Feuerstein et al., 1979; Feuerstein et al., 1981; Missiuna & Samuels, 1988). More recently, dynamic assessment procedures have been developed and evaluated for use with preschool children.

Tzuriel and Klein (1985) developed a test for preschoolers, the Children's Analogical Thinking Modifiability Test (CATM). This test, described in detail later in this chapter, assesses analogical reasoning using manipulable objects that vary in shape, size, and color. The validation study included kindergarten children aged 4 to 6, from three criterion groups (normal, economically and culturally disadvantaged, and special needs) and older children in institutions for the mentally handicapped. The older mentally handicapped group consisted of children, aged 10 to 16, with mental ages of 5 to 6 years as determined by standardized intelligence tests. The special needs group was a heterogeneous group of children enrolled in special education classes and included children identified as having learning difficulties, social maladjustment, and/or emotional problems.

All children were assessed using a pretest-teach-posttest approach. During the teaching phase, intervention was provided to teach rules and strategies needed for successful performance on the task. The intervention was not, however, specifically contingent upon each child's performance. Although this intervention was termed "mediated learning," it was provided in a preestablished manner and thus, did not meet Feuerstein's criteria for a mediated learning experience.

Results of the study showed that there were significant changes from pre- to posttest performance for the normal and disadvantaged children. Change in the special education and older mentally retarded groups was not significant when responses were scored as either completely correct or incorrect. However, when partial credit was given for each correct variable (e.g., color and size correct, shape incorrect), the mentally handicapped group also showed significant improvement on the posttest. Children in the special education group actually exhibited a decrement in performance when the partial-credit scoring procedure was applied.

It has been suggested (Missiuna & Samuels, 1989; Tzuriel & Klein, 1985) that the special needs group showed little change from pre- to posttesting because the instruction provided was not appropriate for their needs. There is some support for this contention from an earlier study by

Burns (1983) in which a graduated prompt method (i.e., prescripted, noncontingent intervention) was compared to a mediational procedure. Four- to six-year-old children determined to be mentally handicapped or at-academic-risk by standardized measures were administered an adaptation of the Stencil Design Test (Arthur, 1947) in a test-teach-test format. Children in both groups showed pre- to posttest improvement. However, children who received mediation scored significantly higher on the posttest and on a transfer task (Animal House subtest of the Wechsler Preschool Primary Scales of Intelligence; Wechsler, 1967).

Missiuna and Samuels (1989) further investigated if the type of intervention provided during dynamic assessment influenced the amount of change. They compared performance on the CATM using two methods of intervention, an instructional approach and a mediational approach. Children who were functioning with approximately a 1-year delay in language, behavior, and/or fine or gross motor areas, were assessed using either scripted intervention similar to that used by Tzuriel and Klein (1985) (termed "instructional" in this study) or a mediational intervention based on Feuerstein et al.'s (1979) criteria for mediated learning experiences. The performance of the two groups did not differ on the pretest, but significant differences were found on the posttest. The mediation group performed significantly better, whereas the performance of the instructional group remained unchanged.

These studies suggest that mediation during dynamic assessment can indicate a child's responsiveness to teaching and, hence, may be a good indicator of the degree to which children will benefit from education programs. When used as part of a battery of pre- and posttest measures for evaluating a program, an important question is how the information from dynamic assessment relates to information derived from standardized assessment. What do we learn from the former that we do not know from the latter?

The Use of Dynamic Assessment to Evaluate Preschool Programs

A dynamic assessment, the Children's Analogical Thinking Modifiability Test (Tzuriel & Klein, 1985) was used as part of a larger battery of assessment instruments during a 2-year research/treatment project in which the effects of intensive therapeutic and educational interventions were examined (Samuels, Fagan, MacKenzie, & Killip, 1988). Employed as both a research tool and, to a lesser extent, as an aid to programming for special needs children, the dynamic assessment was seen to have considerable promise.

Description of the Project

During year 1 of the project, children participated in either of two preschool programs. Year 2 was a follow-up year during which the children attended a variety of classrooms within the regular school system. In year 1, the project was conducted at two different sites, each operating two classes of between 7 and 10 children. The program implemented at one site was a skills- or activity-based approach to education in which the acquisition of basic motor, social, language, and preacademic skills was emphasized. The rationale for this approach is that learning these basic skills is assumed to be a necessary prerequisite to the future acquisition of more complex cognitive skills. Using this approach, explicit attempts to directly teach or introduce "thinking skills" or problem solving skills is deemphasized, with the hope that they will develop coincidentally with the content.

At the other site, the classroom program was based on a cognitive education model. The program incorporated a mediational interaction style with specific activities developed from the Cognitive Curriculum for Young Children (Haywood, Brooks, & Burns, 1986). Like the skills-based approach, it takes into account the principles of normal child development and the introduction of preacademic skills and concepts, but it also strongly emphasizes the processes of learning. By this we mean that children are explicitly taught the rules for perceiving, analyzing, understanding, and solving problems.

All children enrolled in the project were exhibiting at least a 1-year delay in two or more major areas of functioning (e.g., language and fine motor), as determined through the administration of standardized assessment devices. The children also typically displayed some area or areas of relative strength. All children were between the ages of 4 and $5\frac{1}{2}$ years at the beginning of the project. Each child attended one of the two preschool programs for $2\frac{1}{2}$ hours per day, 5 days per week for a 10-month period. Following a summer break, children entered a variety of full- or half-day programs in their neighborhood schools.

Numerous assessments, behavioral observations, parent questionnaires, and teacher questionnaires were administered or sampled over the 2 years. Of interest here is the dynamic assessment. Children were given the CATM (Tzuriel & Klein, 1985) on three separate occasions: at the beginning of the project, at the end of the preschool year, and at the end of the follow-up year. Also administered on these three occasions, but during a separate session, was the Peabody Picture Vocabulary Test–Revised (PPVT-R), a standardized measure of receptive vocabulary that correlates significantly with a number of standardized tests of cognitive ability (Dunn & Dunn, 1981). Children were seen individually by a trained assessor using standard procedures prescribed in the manual. This assessor was not the person who administered the CATM.

The CATM Administration

The CATM instrument is comprised of 18 colored flat wooden blocks. The blocks vary in terms of shape (square, circle, triangle), size (3 inches across, 1 inch across), and color (red, yellow, blue). Also included are three sets of parallel items (sets A, B, and L), each set containing 13 analogical reasoning problems of increasing difficulty. Four levels of difficulty are included within each set: level I (items 1 and 2), one dimension changes while two are held constant; level II (items 3 to 7), two dimensions change while one remains constant; level III (items 8 to 10), all three dimensions change; level IV (items 11 to 13), three additional small blocks are placed on three large blocks and, for both sets of blocks (small and large), the other two dimensions change.

The dynamic assessment process consisted of four phases: (a) baseline, (b) pretest, (c) mediation, and (d) posttest. The total assessment was approximately $1\frac{1}{2}$ hours in length. For the first and second administrations the baseline and pretesting were administered in one session and the mediation and posttesting were administered in a second session within 1 week. For the third administration, all phases occurred on the same day with a short break between the mediation phase and the posttest. In addition, during the first administration a second pretest set was administered immediately after the first to determine the stability of performance prior to mediation. Performance on the second pretest set did not differ significantly from the first pretest set, so this set was not administered subsequently. Results of the first administration of the CATM, which compared the performance of all the children in this study with another group of children who received scripted "instructional" intervention rather than mediation, are reported elsewhere (Missiuna & Samuels, 1989).

Three sets of problems, two developed by Tzuriel and Klein (1985) and one by Missiuna and Samuels (1989) were used in the pretest 1, pretest 2, and posttest phases. The order of administration of sets was counterbalanced to eliminate any bias if one set was easier than another. A fourth set, the learning set, was used in the mediation phase. It was reduced from 13 to 9 items to decrease the time required in this phase.

Procedures for the baseline, pretest,and posttest phases were scripted to ensure examiner reliability. Mediation procedures were outlined but not scripted because the teaching varied depending upon the individual performance and behavior of each child. The assessment procedure was as follows:

1. Baseline: The assessment began with a phase during which a baseline level of competence was established. The child's knowledge of specific labels and concepts was determined. Unlike in the Tzuriel and Klein (1985) study, children were not required to have receptive or expressive knowledge of the labels for all subordinate and superordinate

terms in order to proceed with testing. The minimum level of competence required to pass this phase was defined as the ability to visually match identical blocks. In the latter part of this phase, task-specific rules and strategies (e.g., make a pattern, search for and turn over blocks, etc.) were also taught. Two practice items were included which allowed examiners to ensure that each child comprehended the task.

2. Pretest: During the second phase, the child's initial response to analogical thinking problems was assessed. A set of 13 problems was presented to the child. On each item, the child was required to compare the attributes of three blocks, and to determine, by analogy, what attributes a fourth block would have. The child's verbatim response, if given, (e.g., "red, little") as well as his actual selection of a block from a set of 18 were noted.
3. Mediation: The teaching phase involved the examiner working with the child on nine analogical problems similar to those used in the pretest phase. Mediated learning was provided by the examiner in a manner that was individualized and directly contingent upon the perceived needs of the child. At the beginning of this phase, the examiner's intentions and the purpose of the session were conveyed clearly to the child. The emphasis throughout the session was on the teaching of general rules and strategies that could transcend the specific learning situation. For example, efforts were directed toward verbally or nonverbally assisting the child to focus on the problem, gather information, compare relevant features, summate and integrate the information, systematically explore the choices, and then make a single selection. The learning strategies selected for teaching as well as the techniques used to teach varied depending upon the behaviors and learning difficulties of each child. Children might be encouraged to

TABLE 10.1. CATM and PPVT-R results for children in cognitive and skills-based class.

		Cognitive-based (N = 13)		Skills-based (N = 7)	
Administration		$\bar{x}$	s.d.	$\bar{x}$	s.d.
Prior to preschool program	CATM Pre	1.42	.71	2.07	1.06
	CATM Post	4.77	2.71	6.43	1.72
	PPVT-R[a]	40.62	6.68	50.57	6.02
End of preschool program	CATM Pre	2.23	1.36	1.43	.79
	CATM Post	4.85	2.67	5.57	2.37
	PPVT-R	49.62	7.87	60.00	11.21
One year following preschool program	CATM Pre	3.00	2.27	3.71	2.29
	CATM Post	8.15	3.16	7.00	2.31
	PPVT-R	61.46	13.48	65.29	10.42

[a] PPVT-R scores are age-equivalents in months.

focus their attention by pointing to each block or stating the verbal descriptors (e.g., small yellow circle). In the case of impulsive responders, the examiners sometimes increased the latency period before permitting the child to respond. A board was used to cover the array of blocks so that children were not able to choose an answer until they had looked at and considered the task. A final component of the mediation procedure was the inclusion of a justification process at the end of each item, during which time the examiner gave the child specific feedback regarding his solution, and also assisted the child to review the process he had used in deriving that answer.

4. Posttest: The final phase of assessment included the administration of a third set of 13 analogical problems. This phase, as with the pretest, was performed in a standardized fashion with no additional intervention given by the examiner.

Scoring

The number of correct responses that a child gave on both the pretest and the posttest were documented. The scores could range from zero correct choices to 16 correct choices from each phase. Although there were only 13 items in a phase, the final three sequences contained both a large and a small block and thus the child could score two points for each of the last three problems.

Results

The data presented here are from those children who received all three administrations of both the CATM and the PPVT-R. For the cognitive-based program, 13 children had complete data, whereas 7 children from the skills-based program had complete data. Although the small sample size is limiting, the results nevertheless offer an interesting starting point for discussion of the utility of dynamic assessment.

The mean scores and standard deviations obtained by children in each of the two preschool programs on the three administrations of the CATM are presented in Table 10.1. Utilizing an analysis of covariance with the pretest scores as the covariate revealed no significant effects for program type. Paired *t* tests were utilized to examine the changes from one administration to the next. As might be expected there was a steady increase in the pretest scores across the 2-year time period, with the exception of the slight decrement seen at Administration Two for the skills-based group. However, only the Administration One to Administration Three change in pretest score for the cognitive-based group was significant ($t_{12} = 2.32$, $p < .05$). For the posttest scores, only the cognitive-based group exhibited a significant increase over the 2 years, with the Administration One to Administration Three and the Administration Two to Administration Three changes being significant ($t_{12} = 5.70$, $p < .001$ and $t_{12} = 4.12$, $p < .001$, respectively).

The pretest to posttest change and the change by program interaction, at all three administrations, were examined. After collapsing across program type, significant pre- to post- changes following mediation were evident ($t_{19} = 6.50$, $p < .001$; $t_{19} = 6.31$, $p < .001$; $t_{19} = 8.11$, $p < .001$; Administrations One, Two and Three, respectively).

Also presented in Table 10.1 are the mean age equivalents from the Peabody Picture Vocabulary Test–Revised at all three administrations. As expected, the age-equivalent score increased significantly from Administration One through Three for both groups ($F_{1,19} = 7.58$, $p < .001$). There was a significant difference between the cognitive-based versus skills-based groups at Administration One ($F_{1,18} = 10.78$, $p < .01$) and at Administration Two ($F_{1,18} = 5.90$, $p < .05$), with the skills-based group achieving higher age-equivalent scores. However, at Administration Three this difference had narrowed considerably and was not significant. The cognitive-based group continued to make large gains (12 months), whereas the rate of increase for the skills-based group had slowed from 10 months to 5 months in the year following the preschool project.

In summary, the dynamic assessment (CATM) and the static, standardized test of receptive language (PPVT-R) failed to consistently and significantly differentiate between the children from the two preschool programs. Other standardized measures reported elsewhere (Samuels et al., 1988) also failed to differentiate the groups. Given that both programs were intensive treatment-oriented programs, these results would not be surprising immediately following the program. However, we had hoped that if the cognitive education program had, in fact, increased the child's modifiability, changes would continue to occur in the following year. The PPVT-R data at Administration Three support the notion of modifiability in that the children from the cognitive education program appear to be closing the gap between groups. The significant increase in CATM posttest scores at Administration Three also suggest that the cognitive education group is demonstrating greater modifiability. However, the lack of a significant difference between programs leaves any hypotheses tentative at best.

As part of our follow-up program, we obtained information from each child's school about plans for future placement. We wanted to know if the

TABLE 10.2. Placements for year 3.

	Regular ed.	Special ed.[a]	Other[b]	Total
Cognitive classroom	9	5	1	15
Skills-based classroom	2	7	4	13

[a] Special education placements were primarily for children categorized as slow learners.
[b] Other classes were primarily for children with severe behavior or emotional difficulties.

focus on thinking and learning processes versus skills and content would affect how children later fared in school. Would this earlier focus be reflected in school placements? One of the goals of the Cognitive Curriculm for Young Children (Haywood et al., 1986) is "to prevent future special education placement." Did the cognitive curriculum have this effect in spite of the fact that test scores showed few differences between the two groups?

Table 10.2 presents placement plans for children from both project classrooms. These placements were determined by school personnel with no input from staff involved in the research project. They were based on the year-2 teacher's recommendations in May, almost 1 year after the children left our project classes. Of the 28 children with known placements, two from the skills-based program were to enter regular classrooms, whereas seven were to enter various special placements the following September. From the cognitive education program, nine children were to be placed in regular programs and five in special education programs. The remaining children, four from the skills-based and one from the cognitive education programs, were to enter other classes, primarily for children with severe behavior and emotional difficulties. Chi-square analyses indicate a significant interaction of placement with program ($\chi_2^2 = 6.48$, $p < .05$).

This marked difference in proposed placement caused us to reexamine the data from a different perspective. We wanted to know if the placement outcomes related to or could have been predicted by either the standardized or dynamic assessment test scores. The data were reanalyzed according to the type of program the child would enter 1 year after leaving the preschool program. Only those children with complete CATM and PPVT-R data were included in this analysis. Children entering a "regular" stream classroom ($N = 10$) were contrasted to those entering a "special needs" class ($N = 9$) for children classified as slow learners. Children placed in "other" settings, such as behavior classes, were not included in this analysis.

Means and standard deviations obtained from children grouped according to placement in special education and regular education, for the CATM and PPVT-R, are presented in Table 10.3.

As was done previously, we examined the pattern of change in the pre- and post- scores acorss the three administrations. Consistent increases are most evident for the regular-stream children. Analyses of covariance were performed for each of the three administrations on the CATM and analyses of variance on the PPVT-R scores. No significant differences were found between the two placement groups on PPVT-R scores. In fact, the group placed in the "special needs" classrooms scored about 7 months higher at Administration One than did the regular-stream children. However, at Administration Two there was little difference between these two groups.

TABLE 10.3. CATM and PPVT-R results for children in regular vs. special education class.

Administration		Regular (N = 10)		Special education (N = 9)	
		$\bar{x}$	s.d.	$\bar{x}$	s.d.
Start of year 1 program	CATM Pre	1.70	.79	1.61	1.05
	CATM Post	6.10	2.13	4.33	2.74
	PPVT-R[a]	40.60	7.55	47.33	7.42
End of year 1 program	CATM Pre	2.30	1.34	1.33	.71
	CATM Post	6.00	2.36	4.11	2.62
	PPVT-R	51.60	10.52	53.00	8.75
End of year 2 program	CATM Pre	4.30	2.50	2.00	1.32
	CATM Post	9.70	2.11	5.44	1.94
	PPTV-R	60.70	10.25	61.33	9.47

[a] PPVT-R scores are age = equivalent in months.

Examination of the CATM scores reveals a different picture. The mean posttest dynamic assessment scores were consistently higher for the regular-stream children than for the special needs–stream children (6.10 vs. 4.33; 6.00 vs. 4.11; 9.70 vs. 5.44). This was most evident at Administration Three. Analysis of covariance, using the pretest score as the covariate, revealed a significant group effect at Administration Three ($F_{1,16} = 11.10$, $p < .01$) with the regular-stream children scoring higher than special-stream children with the effects of pretesting covaried out.

This data supports the suggestion that by simply examining results from static assessment measures, one does not get a complete picture of the potential of the child. The dynamic assessment data suggested that, indeed, modifiability on this instrument was relevant to placement and programming issues.

In summary, the results of this project indicate a number of points. First, a widely used standardized measure, the PPVT-R, failed to show consistent differences between the children in the two programs and did not differentiate between those who went on to regular (versus special) stream classes. Second, on both the CATM and the PPVT-R, children showed increases in performance over the 2 years. On the CATM, significant positive changes were observed following mediation. Finally, these changes appeared to be indicators of which children later entered regular-stream placements. In other words, high modifiability on the CATM was related to school success, albeit, only as measured on the third administration.

What Did We Learn From Using Dynamic Assessment?

Like many previous studies comparing cognitive education programs to more traditional programs, unequivocal data in favor of the cognitive education program have not been observed (Chance, 1986; Samuels &

Conte, 1987). Neither the CATM results nor the PPVT-R scores clearly differentiate between the two programs. In both programs, children appeared to make similar gains, but other indicators suggested that there were differences between the two groups. The finding that significantly more children from the cognitive education program were later placed in regular education programs suggests that perhaps the tests used to evaluate the two programs were not sensitive to the process changes that were occurring. This concern over lack of sensitivity of pre- and post-measures has been raised previously in research on cognitive education programs in adolescents (Arbitman-Smith & Haywood, 1980; Bradley, 1983; Samuels & Conte, 1987).

One could argue that it is not surprising that few differences were found between groups on the PPVT-R results given that both programs stressed language and all children received speech/language therapy. However, the dynamic assessment results are harder to explain. If, in fact, the children in the cognitive education classes were becoming more modifiable, and hence better able to benefit from their learning experiences, why is this not clearly evident on the CATM? One explanation is that this particular test sampled only one domain of functioning. The CATM tests analogical reasoning in a nonverbal, concrete modality, and may not have been sensitive to other changes resulting from the cognitive education program. Other dynamic assessment studies (Vye, Burns, Delclos & Bransford, 1987) have not found spontaneous transfer of processes or strategies learned across domains. This suggests that in future studies, dynamic assessment approaches that sample several domains or modalities (e.g., verbal, numerical, serial, logical) should be used. Lidz and Thomas (1987) discuss ways of taking standardized measures and administering them in a dynamic format so that one can look at learning potential in several areas. Other researchers are developing versions of Feuerstein's Learning Potential Assessment Device that are suitable for younger children (Mearig, 1987) or new assessment devices (Tzuriel, personal communication; Lidz, in press; Vye et al., 1987) that tap several domains.

The dynamic assessment results proved interesting in terms of their relationship to placement in regular versus special education programs. Children who were independently placed in programs based on their school performance were found to have benefited more from mediation provided during dynamic assessment than were children placed in special education. This finding was significant only at the third administration but there are indications of this difference in the data at Administrations One and Two. Perhaps with a larger sample size, the study would have had more power to detect a true difference, if one existed.

The suggestions from this data, that children who are responsive to the CATM were later placed in regular education classes, raises important questions regarding the use of dynamic assessment to predict how children will do in preschool programs. If, in fact, children who show high modifiability during dynamic assessment regardless of standardized scores to the contrary, also do better in school, what does this say about assessment practice? It points to the need to use a continuum of assessment services model as suggested by Vye et al. (1987), who argue for a model in which one starts with standardized assessment. Children who perform below average on standardized assessments are then given a "graduated prompt" type of dynamic assessment (Brown & Ferrara, 1985) which is a prescripted form of dynamic assessment in which children are provided with a series of increasingly explicit cues to assist them in solving the task. It has been shown that this form of assessment is beneficial for some children but not others (Burns, 1983; Vye et al., 1987). For those who do not show improvement with graduated prompt assessment, mediational dynamic assessment may be beneficial. This is a more costly procedure than either standardized assessment or graduated prompt procedures as it requires highly trained clinicians to administer. For those children who do not benefit from a brief mediational dynamic assessment, a more intense series of mediational assessments is indicated. This model assumes that the purpose of assessment is to discover what a child will need in order to learn. It is very different from static assessment models which categorize and predict but do not discover the type and intensity of teaching required to produce change in this child. This model raises a question about the use of dynamic assessment in our study. Many children showed little change from pre- to posttesting. These children were later observed to have continuing difficulties in school. One might argue that they did not benefit from their preschool experience to the same degree as the children showing high modifiability. Perhaps the mediation in the dynamic assessment procedure was not sufficiently intensive, or of the right nature, to produce change. In the future, we would recommend adding additional mediation sessions as suggested by Vye et al. (1987) until change is produced and the examiner has a better understanding of what will be required to produce change. The prescriptive information gained from this assessment will provide valuable insights for the teacher and parents.

Dynamic assessment also has the promise of providing important information about effective teaching of preschoolers that will be critical in the design and implementation of programs. Research on preschool dynamic assessment approaches suggests that the type of intervention provided during testing is critical for obtaining change. Mediation appears to be a more effective intervention strategy than prescripted interventions that are not contingent upon the child's specific difficulties (Burns, 1983; Missiuna, 1986; Vye et al., 1987). Children who respond well to prescripted interventions will likely profit from traditional programs in which teachers analyze tasks and teach the necessary skills. Children who require mediational intervention will likely require more specialized programs in which teachers use a mediational teaching style (Haywood, 1987). Haywood et al. (1986) and our own experience using mediational teaching argue strongly for this approach. However, careful studies are needed to define the critical aspects of good mediational teaching and to ascertain how much mediational teaching is required to produce lasting change. Longitudinal studies of children who have been in mediational classrooms will begin to provide some answers.

Our own experience with both dynamic assessment and mediational teaching also suggests that parents have an important role to play in their child's education. Klein and Feuerstein (1985) discuss the importance of parents and caregivers using a mediational style in cognitive development generally. Weatherford and Goodroe (1987) emphasize the importance of training parents to be effective mediators outside the educational setting so that they can complement and reinforce the approach being taught in classes using the Cognitive Curriculum for Young Children (Haywood et al., 1986). Marshman (1986) found in interviews with parents of children enrolled in our project that those with children in the cognitive education class reported being more involved in the program. They felt they personally learned more about their child than was reported by the parents of children in the skills-based program. Typical of comments from this group was one by a parent who suggested that "the improvement in their child was not due to the child's involvement in the CCYC program as much as it was due to the knowledge they had gained on how to handle their child's behavior" (Marshman, 1986). These comments support the importance of parents, as well as teachers, understanding the potential of mediated learning experiences for promoting significant changes in children.

Opportunities to view dynamic assessment can be an excellent starting point for both parents and teachers to observe the effectiveness of mediation. Delclos, Burns and Kulewicz (1985) have demonstrated that an important role for dynamic assessment can be to change the attitude of teachers. Teachers appeared to have a more accurate appreciation of the learning potential of children who were observed during dynamic assessment than during static assessment. We would argue that it is equally important for parents to view dynamic assessment and observe change during a condensed time period, so that they can obtain a glimpse of the type of performance that is possible with effective mediation.

Many questions remain. What specifically were teachers observing about the children from the cognitive education program that made them think these children would profit from regular programs? Was modifiability or teachability a factor, and behaviorally, what does that mean? Comparison of behavioral observation data from children in each program may begin to shed some light on this question.

The relationships among present performance, indications of high and low modifiability, and later school success remain unclear. Of interest is the type of intervention that will be needed to improve performance in line with indications of high modifiability and the amount and types of intervention required to increase modifiability in those who initially show little change. With this type of information we can begin to defeat the predictions from initial performance and provide effective education for all children.

Concluding Comments

This chapter has attempted to illustrate the usefulness of dynamic assessment in evaluating preschool programs. Our research has shown that dynamic assessment, when used as a pre-post measure, did not distinguish between children who had participated in a cognitive education program, the Cognitive Curriculum for Young Children (Haywood et al., 1986), and those in a skills-based program. However, it did distinguish between children who were later placed in regular education programs versus those placed in special education programs.

The potential of dynamic assessment as a tool for evaluating the potential of preschool children is promising. When used in a more standardized way, as in this study, it may be a good predictor of which children will benefit from preschool programs, but will probably not provide the information needed by teachers to defeat those predictions. Dynamic assessment procedures that are truly clinical (i.e., those that provide mediation until change occurs as opposed to those that provide relatively set amounts of mediation) are necessary for an understanding of the intensity and nature of educational intervention required in order that pessimistic predictions be defeated. It is evident however, that much research remains to be done.

References

Arbitman-Smith, R., & Haywood, H. C. (1980). Cognitive education for learning disabled adolescents. *Journal of Abnormal Child Psychology*, *8*, 61–64.

Arbitman-Smith, R., Haywood, H. C., & Bransford, J. D. (1984). Assessing cognitive change. In M. McCauley, R. Sperber, & P. Brooks (Eds.), *Learning and cognition in the mentally retarded*. Baltimore: University Park Press.

Arthur, C. (1947). *A point scale of performance tests*. New York: Psychological Corporation.

Badian, N. A., & Serwer, B. L. (1975). The identification of high-risk children: A retrospective look at selection criteria. *Journal of Learning Disabilities*, *8*(5), 283–287.

Bagnato, S. J. & Neisworth, J. T. (1981). *Linking developmental assessment and curricula: Prescriptions for early intervention*. Rockville, MD: Aspen.

Baumeister, A. A. (1984). Some methodological and conceptual issues in the study of cognitive processes with retarded people. In P. H. Brooks, R. Sperber,

& C. McCauley (Eds.), *Learning and cognition in the mentally retarded*. Hillsdale, NJ: Erlbaum.

Bradley, T. (1983). Remediation of cognitive deficits: A critical appraisal of the Feuerstein model. *Journal of Mental Deficiency*, *27*, 79–92.

Brown, A. L., & Ferrara, R. A. (1985). Diagnosing zones of proximal development. In J. Wersch (Ed.), *Culture, communication and cognition: Vygotskian perspectives*. Cambridge, MA: Cambridge University Press.

Bryant, N. R., Brown, A. L., & Campione, J. C. (1983, April). *Preschool children's learning and transfer of matrices problems: Potential for improvement*. Paper presented at the Society for Research in Child Development Meeting, Detroit.

Burns, M. S. (1983). *Comparison of graduated prompt and mediational dynamic assessment and static assessment with young children*. Unpublished doctoral dissertation, Vanderbilt University, Nashville.

Campione, J. C., Brown, A. L., Ferrara, R. A., & Bryant, N. R. (1984). The zone of proximal development: Implications for individual differences and learning. In B. Rogoff & J. Wertsch (Eds.), *New directions for child development: Children's learning in the "zone of proximal development"* (Vol. 23). San Francisco: Jossey-Bass.

Chance, P. (1986). *Thinking in the classroom: A survey of programs*. New York: Teachers College Press.

Delclos, V. R., Burns, S., & Kulewicz, S. J. (1985). *Effects of dynamic assessment on teacher's expectations of handicapped children* (*Technical Report No. 3*). Vanderbilt University, Nashville.

Dunn, L. M., & Dunn, L. M. (1981). *Peabody Picture Vocabulary Test–Revised*. Circle Pines, MN: American Guidance Service.

Feuerstein, R., Miller, R., Rand, Y., & Jensen, M. R. (1981). Can evolving techniques better measure cognitive change? *The Journal of Special Education*, *15*(2), 201–219.

Feuerstein, R., Rand, Y., & Hoffman, M. B. (1979). *The dynamic assessment of retarded performers: The Learning Potential Assessment Device; theory, instruments and techniques*. Baltimore: University Park Press.

Feuerstein, R., Rand, Y., Hoffman, M. B., & Miller, R. (1980). *Instrumental enrichment: An intervention program for cognitive modifiability*. Baltimore: University Park Press.

Funk, S. G., Sturnen, R. A., & Green, J. A. (1986). Preschool prediction of early school performance: Relationship of McCarthy Scales of Children's Abilities prior to school entry to achievement in kindergarten, first and second grades. *Journal of School Psychology*, *24*, 181–194.

Goodman, J. F., & Cameron, J. (1978). The meaning of IQ constancy in young retarded children. *Journal of Genetic Psychology*, *132*, 109–119.

Haywood, H. C. (1987). A mediational teaching style. *The Thinking Teacher, 4*, 1–6.

Haywood, H. C., Brooks, P., & Burns, S. (1986). Stimulating cognitive development at developmental level: A tested, non-remedial preschool curriculum for preschoolers and older retarded children. *Special Services in the Schools*, *2*(3), 127–147.

Jensen, M. R., & Feuerstein, R. (1987). The Learning Potential Assessment Device: From philosophy to practice. In C. S. Lidz (Ed.), *Dynamic assessment*. 379–402, New York: Guilford.

Keane, K. J. (1987). Assessing deaf children. In C. S. Lidz (Ed.), *Dynamic assessment*. 360–376, New York: Guilford.

Keogh, B. K., & Becker, L. D. (1973). Early detection of learning problems: Questions, cautions and guidelines. *Exceptional Children*, *40*, 5–10.

Klein, P., & Feuerstein, R. (1985). Environmental variables and cognitive development. In S. Harel & N. Anastastow (Eds.) *The at risk infant: Psychosocial-medical aspects*. 369–377. Baltimore, MD: Brooks.

Lerner, J., Mardell-Czudnowski, C., & Goldenberg, D. (1981). *Special education for the early childhood years*. Englewood cliffs, NJ: Prentice-Hall.

Lidz, C. S. (1983). Issues in assessing preschool children. In K. D. Paget & B. A. Bracken (Eds.), *The psychoeducational assessment of preschool children*. New York: Grune & Stratton.

Lidz, C. S. (in press) *Practitioner's guide to dynamic assessment*. New York: Guilford.

Lidz, C. S., & Thomas, C. (1987). The preschool learning assessment device: Extension of a static approach. In C. S. Lidz (Ed.), *Dynamic assessment*. 288–326, New York: Guilford.

Marshman, M. E. (1986). *Parental perception of generalization in preschool children with special needs*. Unpublished master's thesis, University of Calgary, Calgary, Alberta.

Mearig, J. S. (1987). Assessing the learning potential of kindergarten and primary-age children. In C. S. Lidz (Ed.), *Dynamic assessment*. 237–267, New York: Guilford.

Mercer, J. R. (1973). *Labelling the mentally retarded*. Berkley, CA: University of California Press.

Missiuna, C. (1986). *Dynamic assessment of preschool children with special needs: Comparison of mediation and in struction*. Unpublished masters thesis, Calgary: University of Calgary.

Missiuna, C., & Samuels, M. (1989). Dynamic assessment of preschool children with special needs: Comparison of mediation and instruction. *Remedial and Special Education*, *10*(2), 53–62.

Missiuna, C., & Samuels, M. (1988). Dynamic assessment: Review and critique. *Special Services in the Schools*, *5*(1 & 2), 1–22.

Narrol, H., Silverman, H., & Waksman, M. (1982). Developing cognitive potential in vocational high school students. *Journal of Educational Research*, *76*(2), 107–112.

Paget, K. D., & Nagle, R. J. (1986). A conceptual model of preschool assessment. *School Psychology Review*, *15*(2), 154–165.

Reynolds, C. R., & Clark, J. H. (1983). Assessment of cognitive abilities. In K. D. Paget & B. A. Bracken (Eds.), *The psychoeducational assessment of preschool children*. New York: Grune & Stratton.

Samuels, M., & Conte, R. (1987). Instrumental enrichment with learning disabled adolescents: Is it effective? *Journal of Practical Approaches to Developmental Handicap*, *11*(2), 4–6.

Samuels, M., Fagan, J., MacKenzie, H., & Killip, S. M. (1988). *Cognitive education for preschool children with severe learning difficulties. Final report*. The Learning Centre, 3930 20th St. S.W., Calgary, Alta, T2T 4Z9.

Samuels, M., Roadhouse, A., Conte, R., & Zirk, H. (1984). *Instrumental enrichment with low-achieving adolescents*. Edmonton: Alberta Education Technical Report.

Samuels, M., Tzuriel, D., & Malloy-Miller, T. (1989). Dynamic assessment of children with learning difficulties. In R. Brown and M. Chazan (Eds.), *Learning difficulties and emotional problems*, 145–165, Calgary: Detselig.

Schmidt, S., & Perino, J. (1985). Kindergarten screening results as predictors of academic achievement, potential and placement in second grade. *Psychology in the Schools*, *22*, 146–151.

Sigel, I., & Brodzinsky, D. M. (1977). Individual differences: A perspective for understanding intellectual development. In H. L. Hom, Jr. & P. A. Robinson (Eds.), *Psychological processes in early education*, 295–329, New York: Academic.

Tzuriel, D., & Klein, P. S. (1985). The assessment of analogical thinking modifiability among regular, special education, disadvantaged and mentally retarded children. *Journal of Abnormal Child Psychology*, *13*(4), 539–553.

Vye, N. J., Burns, M. S., Delclos, V. R., & Bransford, J. D. (1987). A comprehensive approach to assessing intellectually handicapped children. In C. S. Lidz (Ed.), *Dynamic assessment*. 327–359, New York: Guilford.

Weatherford, D. L., & Goodroe, P. (1987). Manual on parent participation in the cognitive education of their young children. In H. C. Haywood, P. Brooks, & S. Burns (Eds.), *Cognitive curriculum for young children*. Nashville: Vanderbilt University.

Wechsler, D. (1967). *Manual for the Wechsler Preschool and Primary Scale of Intelligence*. New York: Psychological Corporation.

Part 3 Applications of Interactive Assessment

Diversity is once again the major theme. In this section, chapters are devoted to illustrations of diverse application of interactive assessment. One large dimension of variation is that of populations. These chapters represent the use of interactive assessment with adults with learning disabilities (Samuels, Lamb, & Oberholtzer, Chapter 11), deaf persons (Keane, Tannenbaum, & Krapf, Chapter 12), young children with learning problems (Delclos, Vye, Burns, Bransford, & Hasselbring, Chapter 13), university applicants from a nondominant ethnic group (Shochet, Chapter 14), penitentiary inmates (Silverman & Waksman, Chapter 15), and public school children (Ashman, Chapter 16). Many other applications are possible, but there is sufficient diversity here to suggest that these procedures would also be useful with still other groups of persons.

There is great diversity as well in these applications from the standpoint of different uses of interactive assessment. As a means of examining the learning potential of deaf persons, interactive assessment is one good way of separating assessment of learning processes from assessment of achievement levels, and of specifying what teaching can be done to improve performance. Two of the chapters (Ashman and Delclos et al.) deal directly with the quite close relation between interactive assessment and some technologies of instruction. Samuels et al. use interactive assessment to identify cognitive barriers to vocational and social functioning of adults, and then use the data from their assessments to plan programs that may include cognitive remediation, academic remediation, vocational training, or social intervention. Shochet uses interactive assessment to learn what is wrong with the predictions made from standardized, normative assessment, and to find out what to do to defeat pessimistic predictions. Silverman and Waksman show us how to look for undiscovered—and perhaps unsuspected—learning potential in penitentiary inmates, a process that could lead to rehabilitation prescriptions and postincarceration planning.

Just as in the preceding section, this group of applications should not be seen as exhaustive but rather as suggestive of the wide variety of possible applications of interactive assessment. Some investigators have begun to explore the utility of interactive assessment in the clinical diagnosis and treatment of persons with major psychiatric disorders and with mental retardation. Others have reported uses with immigrant and language-different persons. Although we know of no research on it at this moment, it would almost certainly be useful to employ these procedures to discover specific cognitive barriers in an aging population, including persons with Alzheimer's syndrome and other degenerative nervous system conditions. Research on interactive assessment with diverse clinical groups, and for a variety of investigative purposes, should produce a rich fund of literature over the next few years.

11
Dynamic Assessment of Adults with Learning Difficulties

Marilyn T. Samuels, Carol H. Lamb, and Lorna Oberholtzer

The nature of learning disabilities,[1] their diagnosis, and treatment have been well described for school-aged children (Alley & Deshler, 1979; Reid & Hresko, 1981). Recently, growing evidence has demonstrated that children do not outgrow their learning disabilities as they reach adulthood (Blalock, 1981; Faford & Haubrich, 1981; White, et al., 1983). An estimated 7 to 10% of the adult population have learning problems such that reading, written and spoken language, attention, memory, and/or organization are deficient (Buchanan & Wolf, 1986; Kronick, 1985). Often having experienced years of repeated failure, they also present as individuals with low self-esteem, who lack appropriate problem-solving skills as well as adequate social skills (Blalock, 1981). Adults with learning disabilities, who are of normal intelligence, experience difficulties that not only continue to interfere with their academic pursuits (Fravenheim, 1978; Hartzell & Compton, 1984) but affect their employability (Brown, 1984) and their social development (Hartzell & Compton, 1984). Longitudinal and follow-up studies of students who experienced learning difficulties in school indicate that as adults, this group is disproportionately represented in low job classifications and that they tend to be less satisfied with their jobs than are their normally achieving peers (Howell, 1986; Lehtinen & Dumas, 1976).

Despite growing recognition of the difficulties experienced by adults with learning disabilities, there is a paucity of information related to the identification and assessment of this population. Generally, the same approaches that have been used to assess children suspected of learning

[1] The term *learning disability* generally refers to individuals of normal intelligence who have difficulties in the process of learning (presumably neurologically based) that are not due to primary emotional disorders or sensory impairment. In this chapter, we have used the term *learning disability* when referring to past research that has used that term. Otherwise, we have used the more generic term *learning difficulties* to reflect our belief that the focus should be on the presenting problem and remedial needs and not on the etiological basis.

disabilities have been used with adults. Heavy reliance has been placed on the results of psychological and educational examinations using standardized psychometric approaches to gather information on intelligence, academic achievement and personality functioning (Buchanan & Wolf, 1986; Newell, Goyette, & Fogarty, 1984). Standardized assessment has been criticized extensively when used to predict future success for children whose environmental and educational background differ from the norm (Ginsburg, 1972; Ysseldyke & Algozzine, 1982). Similarly, standardized assessment raises some alarming concerns when used with adults, as it does not take into account the learning history and often underestimates the client's level of functioning. Hershenson (1984, p. 40) notes that with adults with learning difficulties, standardized tests "must be used with caution because of the client's difficulties with reading directions, following instructions, understanding items, recording responses, working within time limits, and/or maintaining attention to the task." In addition, years of failure in learning situations lead to a limited knowledge base which affects performance on standardized tests. Repeated failure also results in poor test-taking strategies and an extrinsic motivational orientation. Low self-esteem, which is characteristic of adults who have experienced repeated failure, may also create anxiety and interfere with cognitive functioning (Tzuriel, Samuels, & Feuerstein, 1988). Identification of adults with learning difficulties can also be problematic because the social/emotional ramifications of long-standing learning failure may mask or interact with the primary learning disability.

The complexity of learning problems in adults necessitates a transdisciplinary approach to assessment that goes beyond traditional assessment instruments and conventional testing. Currently, there exists a dearth of diagnostic instruments for determining the presence and nature of a learning problem in adults (Crimando, 1984) and the traditional assessment instruments are inadequate for diagnosing the factors impeding learning ability and for providing information for planning appropriate interventions (Salvia & Ysseldyke, 1978; Short & Mueller, 1985). Haywood (1977) has suggested that when the goal of assessment is to ascertain effective intervention strategies, as it must be with adults with learning difficulties, rather than identifying the "disease," the processes of assessment and intervention must be intertwined in a dynamic way.

The Learning Potential Assessment Device (LPAD; Feuerstein, Rand, & Hoffman, 1979) is one dynamic approach that meshes assessment and intervention through a teach-test model to assess modifiability or learning potential. For a discussion of the theory underlying this approach, see Chapter 1.

The LPAD has been used extensively with culturally disadvantaged children (Feuerstein et al., 1979), with deaf children (Keane, 1983, 1987), and with learning disabled, educably mentally handicapped, and other populations of special needs children (Delclos, 1983; Feuerstein et al.,

1979; Lidz, 1987; Missiuna & Samuels, 1988; Samuels, Tzuriel, & Malloy-Miller, 1989).

Little has been reported about the use of dynamic assessment approaches with adults. Waksman, Silverman, and Weber (1983) found significant changes in performance on the LPAD following intervention with low-achieving penitentiary inmates. Barr and Samuels (1988) report on three cases in which the LPAD was helpful for prescribing treatment as it separated the effects of emotional from cognitive factors in clients with severe learning difficulties. They noted that with the increasing awareness of learning difficulties in adults, many clients are being diagnosed on the basis of standardized tests as learning disabled when in fact the primary problem is an emotional one. This inaccurate diagnosis impedes the provision of appropriate counseling interventions and promotes inappropriate vocational placement.

Several characteristics that distinguish dynamic assessment from standardized assessment (Feuerstein, Miller, Rand, & Jensen, 1981) are keys to its usefulness with adults. These characteristics are (a) the focus on the process rather than the product of problem solving, (b) the dynamic interactional assessment process, (c) the structure of the tests that permit learning and generalization to occur, and (d) the interpretation of the results in terms of the amount and type of intervention needed for learning rather than through a comparison to norms. In addition, the relatively content-free nature of the tasks militates against the clients' usual counterproductive reactions to "school-like" material on which they expect to fail (Barr & Samuels, 1988).

The purpose of this chapter is to illustrate the benefits of using a dynamic assessment approach, the LPAD (Feuerstein et al., 1979) with adults with learning difficulties. Over the past few years, the LPAD has been administered, along with more traditional assessment of academic skills, to adults referred to our center because of persistent employment problems thought to be due to learning difficulties.

The Learning Centre Study

Assessment results from 12 women and 10 men (mean age = 26.4 years) referred to the Learning Centre, an applied research and demonstration center for the diagnosis and treatment of learning difficulties, were analyzed. Clients in this sample were all referred by vocational counselors from a federal employment agency. These counselors deal specifically with clients who are having difficulty obtaining and maintaining employment due to varying handicapping conditions. The slight preponderance of females in this sample, in an area of disability usually dominated by males, is likely due in part to the referral sources, one being a special unit for women with employment difficulties.

All clients referred to the Learning Centre were first interviewed by a social worker (psychosocial interview) and then administered a standardized battery of academic tests prior to receiving the LPAD. Clients included in the sample were all considered of normal intelligence based on past testing, observations, or present assessment.

Social and Academic Characteristics

There was wide variability in both reading achievement and psychosocial factors in the clients in this sample. Nine clients (8 females, 1 male) were categorized as literate on the basis of scores above the sixth-grade level on the Jerry Johns Basic Reading Inventory and/or Jerry Johns Advanced Reading Inventory (Johns, 1981, 1985) (mean score = gr. 8.9, range gr. 7–12). Thirteen clients (4 females, 9 males) scored at or below sixth-grade level (mean score = gr. 1.9, range gr. 0–6).

Sixteen clients (9 females, 7 males) were categorized as having poor psychosocial adjustment based on the information from the psychosocial interview. Those clients who lacked appropriate social skills, showed low self-esteem, and who reported being isolated in the community were placed in this category. This compares to only six clients (3 females, 3 males) who were considered to have good psychosocial adjustment.

Using both criteria, literacy and social adjustment, four groups emerged: (a) literate, poorly adjusted ($N = 6$, 6 females; reading mean = 8.5); (b) literate, well adjusted ($N = 3$, 2 females, 1 male; reading mean = 9.7); (c) nonliterate, poorly adjusted ($N = 10$, 3 females, 7 males; reading mean = 1.9); and (d) nonliterate, well adjusted ($N = 3$, 1 female, 2 males; reading mean = 2.0). As the number of clients considered well adjusted was very small and equally distributed between the literate and nonliterate groups, the two literate and two nonliterate groups were combined for further analysis.

Dynamic Assessment

Dynamic assessment of cognitive and affective factors affecting the client's learning was performed using various tests from the LPAD (Feuerstein et al., 1979; Feuerstein, Haywood, Rand, Hoffman, & Jensen, 1986). The LPAD consists of 15 tests, each designed to tap different areas of cognitive functioning. The tests contain relatively novel content that the clients reported not having encountered in this exact form in past testing. Tests are structured so that in the first phase the client is taught the content, strategies, and rules necessary for task solution and has opportunities to apply this learning in increasingly complex tasks of a similar nature with examiner assistance. In the second phase, his ability to apply independently what he has been taught is evaluated. The examiner intervenes extensively in the first teaching phase and as necessary in the test phase to insure that the client is functioning optimally and to give the client feedback. Of interest on the LPAD is the amount and type of intervention necessary to achieve optimal performance rather than the absolute number of correct responses. Assessment results are presented in terms of cognitive strengths, the type of deficient cognitive functions and affective factors observed, and the amount and type of intervention needed to overcome the observed difficulties.

The particular tests used with each client in this study were determined by the examiner based on information from the psychosocial interview, academic testing, and general clinical impressions. Two matrices tests, Raven's Coloured Progressive Matrices (Raven, 1965) and Set Variations I and II (Feuerstein et al., 1986) were used with virtually all the clients as these tests provided opportunities to observe many areas of deficient functioning and are of sufficient difficulty to challenge even higher functioning clients. Other tests such as Organization of Dots (Feuerstein et al., 1986) were used with a few very low-functioning clients because the task requirements are less demanding and hence "to easy" for many adults. The Organizer, a highly verbal, abstract task requiring some reading was used selectively, primarily with clients in the literate group.

Assessment results collapsed across all tests administered were analyzed for the frequency of particular deficient cognitive functions and non-intellective factors observed, and for the amount and type of mediation strategies used to improve performance.

Deficient Cognitive Functions

Feuerstein et al. (1979) propose that learning, or the mental act, can be divided into three phases: input or gathering of information; elaboration or processing of information; and output, communication of the information, verbally or nonverbally. Deficient cognitive functioning may occur at any or all of these phases. Deficiencies at the input and output phases often obscure well-developed elaborational capacities and must be mediated during assessment in order to gain an accurate picture of the client's intellectual functioning. For example, if data gathering is incomplete or inaccurate, the elaboration and output phases may appear deficient as the client attempts to solve the task with only partial information. The client may appear to be unable to recall several instructions when, in fact he did not even read or hear all of the instructions. The client's response to the intervention provided by the examiner is the key to determining whether the deficiencies are predominantly at the input, elaborational, or output phases. A complete list and description of the deficient functions is available elsewhere (Feuerstein et al., 1979; Feuerstein et al., 1986).

Only 12 of the 24 deficient cognitive functions described by Feuerstein et al. (1986) were observed frequently enough in this sample to be discussed here. Table 11.1 presents the proportion of clients in each group rated as exhibiting the deficient cognitive function with high frequency. Differences between groups for each deficient function were analyzed using a Fisher Exact Probability Test (Siegel, 1957). It should be noted that the sample size in this study is small so application of these results must be made with caution.

The clients in the literate group appeared to exhibit more difficulty at the output or response phase than at the input phase with the exception of unsystematic exploratory behavior. They had significantly more difficulty than clients in the nonliterate group applying rules learned on one problem to other similar problems. Many also exhibited blocking. Blocking refers to a client's seeming inability to give a response, possibly due to a fear of failure, even though there are indications that he or she knows the answer.

The clients in the nonliterate group exhibited difficulties across all three phases. Over half the clients in the nonliterate group were rated as having difficulty with unsystematic exploratory behavior, and planning and organization. They also exhibited significantly more difficulty than the literate group on precision and accuracy, considering two or more sources of information simultaneously, using spontaneous comparative behavior, and with expressive language.

Of interest in an LPAD is not just the fact that a client exhibits various deficient cognitive functions. This information is available from standardized assessment. The focus of the LPAD is on how these deficits interfere

TABLE 11.1. Deficient cognitive functions observed with high frequency.

Function	Literate (N = 9)	Nonliterate (N = 13)
Input PHASE		
1. Unsystematic exploratory behavior	.44 (4)	.54 (7)
2. Receptive language	0	.07 (1)
3. Need for precision and accuracy	0	.38 (5)*
4. Considering two or more sources of information simultaneously	0	.54 (7)**
Elaboration PHASE		
5. Definition of the problem	.22 (2)	.38 (5)
6. Relevant vs. nonrelevant cues	.33 (3)	0
7. Spontaneous comparative behavior	0	.54 (7)**
8. Interiorization	.33 (3)	.23 (3)
9. Planning/organization	.22 (2)	.62 (8)
Output PHASE		
10. Applying rules	.44 (4)	0**
11. Blocking	.44 (4)	.08 (1)
12. Expressive language	.22 (2)	100% (13)**

*$p < .05$. **$p < .025$.

with cognitive performance and the amount of intervention needed to modify them. For example, two clients in the literate group and all the clients in the nonliterate group were rated as having severe expressive language problems. For the clients in the literate group, simply providing the labels or assisting the client to realize that labeling is an effective strategy in problem solving was sufficient to improve performance. For others in the nonliterate group, more intensive language remediation appeared warranted as basic syntactic and semantic structures were deficient. When expressive language was identified as a factor in poor performance, the examiner intervened so that cognitive functioning could be assessed as much as possible independent of language. This was done by allowing clients to demonstrate knowledge in nonverbal ways or by having the examiner provide the necessary language. Assessment of intellectual or learning potential independent of language is critical for understanding adults with learning difficulties.

Nonintellective Factors

Nonintellective factors refer to affective and motivational factors that often interfere with learning and may obscure effective cognitive functioning. Such factors have long been considered critical for understanding scholastic achievement in children and recently have been discussed in the testing context (Scarr, 1981). Tzuriel et al. (1988) review the literature on effects of nonintellective factors on assessment of children and discuss various nonintellective factors that can be observed in dynamic assessment such as the need for mastery, confidence in correct responses, and fear of failure that affect learning and test performance. For the adult with learning difficulties, these factors are as critical to the prognosis as are cognitive or intellective factors because they will be indicative of the client's responsiveness to future learning and his ability to accept feedback from instructors and employers. They are also important in making appropriate recommendations for vocational placement and remediation.

Nonintellective factors observed in this sample were summarized into nine categories. Table 11.2 presents the proportion of ratings in each category. One client may have been rated in several categories. As with the deficient cognitive functions, a greater proportion of clients in the nonliterate group exhibit nonintellective factors that interfere with performance than in the literate group. However, a Fisher Exact Probability Test (Siegel, 1957) revealed that only one factor, external locus of control, differed significantly ($p < .025$) between the two groups.

A lack of need for mastery, defined as the client's not striving to cope effectively with the task, was observed in over half the nonliterate clients. Lack of persistence on a task, lack of willingness to continue working, and difficulty working independently were some of the behaviors observed.

TABLE 11.2. NonIntellective factors observed.

Factor	Literate (N = 9)	Nonliterate (N = 13)
No need for mastery	.22 (2)	.54 (7)
High frustration tolerance	.33 (3)	.54 (7)
External locus of control	.11 (1)	.62 (8)**
Fear of failure	.44 (4)	.38 (5)
Lacks confidence in correct response	.78 (7)	.77 (10)
High defensiveness	.33 (3)	.38 (5)
Lack of receptiveness to mediation	.33 (3)	.23 (3)
High anxiety	.33 (3)	.31 (4)
Depressed affect	.22 (2)	0

** $p < .025$.

Frustration tolerance refers to the client's reaction as tasks become difficult or he/she encounters tasks requiring extra effort. Low frustration tolerance is observed during assessment when the client becomes impatient, angry or disappointed when he/she has to keep working to solve a task. It was observed in over half the nonliterate clients and in one third of the literate clients.

Locus of control refers to the individual's perception of himself or herself as responsible for the outcome of his/her behavior and having some control over life events (Lefcourt, 1976). Individuals with an external locus of control believe that things outside of themselves are responsible for their difficulties and often blame others or bad luck for their lack of success. Sixty-two percent of the nonliterate clients exhibited an external locus of control as compared to 11% (one client) in the literate group ($p < .025$).

Fear of failure is observed when clients are afraid to risk, hesitant to respond, or need confirmation before responding. Both groups showed equal numbers of clients experiencing fear of failure.

Lack of confidence in a correct response refers to situations in which the client has solved a problem correctly but has little confidence in it. Without immediate confirmation, such clients will change their response, assuming it must be incorrect. They may also make self-derogatory remarks such as, "It's probably wrong. I'm no good at this." This was the most frequently rated category for both the literate and nonliterate groups, observed in 17 of 22 clients (77%). This finding is perhaps not surprising as adults with learning difficulties generally exhibit low self-esteem (Patton & Polloway, 1982). Further analysis, regrouping the clients according to social adjustment, found that a significantly greater percentage of poorly adjusted (87.5%) than well-adjusted clients (50%) were rated in this category ($p < .01$). To increase the client's confidence during the assessment, the examiner gave feedback on whether a response was correct and also on exactly what part of their response or the process used to arrive at that response was correct. Clients were also assisted to review why they were successful on one problem and less so on another.

Defensiveness is observed when the client remarks that the task is easy and he/she does not need help when in fact he/she is having difficulty. It was observed in approximately one third of our sample.

Lack of receptiveness to mediation refers to clients who reject attempts by the examiner to assist them. Often such clients will rigidly maintain that their way of responding is best for them.

High anxiety and depressed affect refer to a more general affective state in which the client appeared particularly anxious or depressed in the test situation. These were observed in both the literate and nonliterate clients. Further analysis revealed that all the clients so rated were considered to have poor social adjustment.

Mediation During Assessment

The amount and type of mediation provided by the examiner during the assessment was summarized. Five categories were used to describe the examiner's behavior (Feuerstein et al., 1986):

1. Regulation of behavior: this refers to interventions to help the client control his behavior during task solution. Four subcategories describe the nature and intent of the intervention: (a) using verbal and nonverbal means for restraining impulsivity, (b) using verbal and nonverbal (i.e., pointing) means to focus the client's attention, (c) using various techniques to help the client begin the task (overcome blocking), and (d) prompting the client to help him continue solving the task once started.
2. Production of reflective-analytic thought: this refers to interventions designed to encourage the client to use analytic thought processes and to reflect on the thinking processes necessary for task solution (metacognition).
3. Establishment of prerequisite behavior: this refers to examiner interventions to provide clients with necessary content, concepts, and language, and to teach necessary rules and strategies for task solution. This type of intervention was provided primarily during the training phase to insure that poor performance was not due simply to lack of knowledge. It was also provided as needed during the test phase so that cognitive processes could be evaluated independently of content knowledge.
4. Mediation of competence: this is a category of intervention, perhaps unique to the LPAD, that refers to specific intervention by the examiner to give feedback regarding competence in a way that pro-

vides the client with direct evidence of his or her ability to solve these tasks. Barr and Samuels (1988) indicate it is a critical factor in the usefulness of the LPAD with adults lacking in self-esteem.

5. Crystallization of learning: this refers to interventions such as summarizing and discussing overall principles or rules designed to assist the client to clearly understand what he has been learning.

The proportion of clients rated as requiring no, moderate, or intense mediation, is presented in Table 11.3.

A Mann-Whitney nonparametric test (Siegel, 1957) was used to ascertain differences in the amount of mediation required by the two

TABLE 11.3. Summary of mediation.

	Amount	Literate ($N = 9$)	Nonliterate ($N = 13$)	U
1. Regulation of Behavior				
(a) Restraint of impulsivity (verbal and nonverbal)	None	.55	.70	62.50
	Moderate	.33	.08	
	Intense	.11	.22	
(b) Focusing (verbal and nonverbal)	None	0	0	72.00
	Moderate	100	.62	
	Intense	0	.38	
(c) Overcoming blocking	None	.55	.77	71.00
	Moderate	.22	.23	
	Intense	.22	0	
(d) Prompting and probing	None	.22	0	42.00
	Moderate	.77	.46	
	Intense	0	.54	
2. Production of Reflective-analytical thinking				
(a) Hypothetical thinking	None	.44	0	0.00**
	Moderate	.55	.46	
	Intense	0	.54	
(b) Awareness of own thinking	None	.22	0	24.50*
	Moderate	.77	.54	
	Intense	0	.46	
3. Establishment of prerequisite behavior				
(a) Teaching prerequisite concepts and language	None	.66	0	3.00**
	Moderate	.33	.08	
	Intense	0	.92	
(b) Teaching of rules and strategies	None	.11	0	8.00**
	Moderate	.88	.54	
	Intense	0	.46	
4. Mediation of competence	None	.22	0	8.00**
	Moderate	.33	.69	
	Intense	.44	.31	
5. Crystallization of learning	None	.33	0	0.00**
	Moderate	.55	0	
	Intense	.11	100	

*$p < .01$. **$p < .001$.

groups. There were no significant differences between groups in the regulation of behavior categories. It can be seen that restraining impulsivity was seldom needed for either group but that all clients needed either some focusing or intensive focusing of their attention during test performance. This latter finding supports the concerns regarding attention deficits cited earlier (Hershenson, 1984) with respect to the need for caution in interpreting standardized test data of adults with learning difficulties. Few clients were rated as requiring mediation to overcome blocking. However, both groups received prompting and probing mediation.

Significant differences were found between groups on the remaining categories, with the nonliterate clients consistently requiring more mediation. Particularly striking but not surprising was the intense mediation required by the nonliterate group to teach prerequisite concepts and language, and to crystallize learning.

The results regarding the amount and type of mediation needed for clients to perform optimally represents a major departure from the type of information generated from standardized assessment. It is this information, in conjunction with the results concerning areas of deficient cognitive functioning and nonintellective factors, that leads to determination of recommendations to assist the client.

Recommendations

The types of recommendations made on the basis of the psychosocial interview, the academic testing, and the LPAD are summarized in Table 11.4 for each group. As might be predicted from both the standardized and the LPAD results, the nonliterate group had the broadest range of recommendations. In the literate group, academic upgrading and personal counseling were recommended for virtually all clients. In the nonliterate

TABLE 11.4. Type of recommendations.

	Literate ($N = 9$)	Nonliterate ($N = 13$)
Academic upgrading	.88	.85
Cognitive training	.22	.69*
Vocational Counseling	.33	.23
On-job training	.33	.54
Personal counseling	.88	.46
Language remediation	0	.31
Audiology assessment	0	.15
Leisure activities	0	.15

*$p < .05$.

group, academic upgrading was also recommended frequently. The two clients for whom it was not recommended were nonliterate but had good social skills. Their past histories indicated that academic upgrading had not been successful. Indicators of modifiability on the LPAD suggested that these clients would be more successful with specific training on the job. The examiner was able to make specific suggestions to the vocational counselor or employer based on the client's performance during dynamic assessment. Cognitive training was frequently recommended in the nonliterate group based on the finding that these clients needed to learn thinking and problem solving strategies in order to improve performance during the assessment. Language remediation and audiology were also recommended only for clients in this group based on the observed language difficulties and the lack of modifiability of language during the assessment.

Summary of Group Results

The two groups differed in the number and type of deficient cognitive functions observed during testing, the nonliterate group demonstrating the greatest number and diversity.

There were few differences between groups in the nonintellective factors observed. Clients in the nonliterate group were rated as having an external locus of control more often than clients in the literate group. A lack of confidence in correct responses was the most frequently observed nonintellective factor occuring in both groups.

The amount and type of mediation for the most part appeared related to the number and type of deficient cognitive functions. The nonliterate group required more intensive mediation to correct deficient cognitive functioning than did the literate group. There were no differences between groups on the "regulation of behavior" items.

The nonliterate group had a broader range and greater number of recommendations than the literate group. Academic upgrading was the most frequently recommended course of action for both groups. In virtually all cases, it was recommended in conjunction with other activities, personal counseling in the literate group, and cognitive education in the nonliterate group.

The results presented thus far indicate the types of difficulties observed and the mediation required generally for each group. However, the group data does not present a clear picture of how mediation during assessment provides evidence of a specific deficient cognitive function or nonintellective factor and their modifiability. Four cases will be presented to illustrate the integration of testing and teaching in dynamic assessment. Two of the cases are clients considered literate, one with poor social adjustment and one with good social adjustment. The other two cases are nonliterate clients, again, with poor and good social adjustment.

Case Vignettes[2]

Anna: A Literate Adult with Poor Social Adjustment

Anna, age 35, is a single woman living at home with her mother. She reported tremendous conflicts within her family as a child, indicated that her father was very hard on her because of her school difficulties and that she received very little emotional support from her family. Academically, Anna reported completing high school although she remembers school with much displeasure. She experienced great difficulty making friends and today remains an isolated woman with no social network available to her other than her mother. She has few leisure interests. Vocationally, Anna has been employed in a number of unskilled jobs but due to academic and social difficulties she has been unsuccessful in maintaining gainful employment.

Anna's functioning level in reading, spelling, written language, and mathematics was ascertained using standardized tests. Her independent reading level was at a grade seven to eight level. Vocabulary weaknesses were evident. Spelling and written expressive skills were at the junior high level. Math skills varied but overall were estimated to be in the upper elementary range.

Results of the Wechsler Adult Intelligence Scale-Revised (WAIS-R) indicated low-average intellectual functioning with wide variability on subtests. The examiner reported that because Anna was extremely anxious during testing and approached the tasks in a very disorganized manner, the results were probably a low estimate of her intellectual functioning.

Throughout both the achievement testing and the WAIS-R, the examiners noted that Anna was anxious, appeared to lack confidence, and made many derogatory comments about herself. During the reading assessment, for example, when asked to express the main idea of a paragraph she had just read, Anna responded "I can't remember. My brain just doesn't work." It was noted that Anna appeared to distract herself by her own verbalizations and to have limited systematic work strategies but due to the constraints of standardized testing, the examiners could only speculate on the effect of these factors on her performance.

Several tests from the LPAD were administered to Anna to assess if the affective factors noted during the standardized assessment and other cognitive factors were in fact limiting Anna's performance, and to assess the degree of modifiability of the factors following mediation. Three major areas of deficient cognitive functioning were observed throughout the subtests. Anna had a great deal of difficulty defining what she had to do on each new task or variation of the task. She appeared to focus on

---

[2] Identifying information has been changed in the case vignettes that follow.

only part of the information or on irrelevant information in attempting to understand what was required. Thus, on Set Variations I and II, an analogical reasoning task, she needed assistance to focus on what information was relevant in order to abstract the rules for each new type of problem. She was then able to apply these rules on subsequent similar problems.

A second area of difficulty was expressive language. Anna had problems labeling figures (e.g., triangle) and communicating precisely. She used terms vaguely. For example, she could identify a square but could not define the characteristics of a square and often referred to rectangles as squares. She also had poorly developed concepts for commonly used terms (e.g., opposite). Her poor language resulted in incorrect responding even though elaboration was good. For example, on the Organizer, after working out a correct solution, she would state the answer incorrectly and then write down what she had said rather than what she had figured out. Mediation to raise her awareness and insistence on using precise language resulted in improved performance.

Unsystematic search strategies for gathering information was another area of difficulty that resulted in poor performance and obscured good elaborational capacities. Anna was able to solve tasks with two or three variables with little assistance. As the complexity of the tasks increased, Anna's approach became unsystematic and impulsive. With assistance from the examiner to use an organized approach and with statements such as "What do you need to do first?" and "What do you do now?", Anna was able to solve tasks with six and seven variables. Without this assistance, Anna's successful performance would have been limited to the easy items and one might have concluded that she did not have the ability to solve the more difficult ones.

Nonintellective factors such as low self-esteem, fear of failure, and anxiety compounded Anna's difficulties on the LPAD tasks as they had for the standardized assessment. A major difference, when these factors were observed on the LPAD compared with the standardized tests, was that the examiner intervened to modify their effect on performance. Continual encouragement as Anna worked through the tasks was given. Derogatory self-statements were directly discouraged. Throughout the testing Anna was very concerned about how she was doing. On the LPAD this anxiety was allayed to some degree by immediate feedback as to correctness of a response and opportunities to continue working on a task with assistance, if necessary, until it was solved successfully. Discussion of the processes Anna used when she was successful provided her with direct evidence that she could be in control.

On the standardized intelligence testing the examiner had noted an increase in anxiety, particularly as items became difficult. Anna referred to herself as "dumb" when she could not solve a problem, and showed a decrease in confidence and greater fear of risking on subsequent items. In contrast, on the LPAD Anna's performance improved on more difficult items as a result of receiving specific feedback and mediation of competence. As Anna saw that she could solve difficult problems, her confidence increased and she was willing to take greater risks. Anxiety lessened due to the interactive nature of the test situation.

Two major recommendations arose from this assessment. Anna's difficulties in defining new tasks correctly but her observed ability to solve subsequent similar problems effectively after minor intervention suggested that her employer should take extra time initially to insure that Anna clearly understood what she was to do and that she had focused on the relevant variables. Specific feedback regarding her performance was also recommended to allay Anna's anxiety. A second recommendation was that Anna attend a combined cognitive education-counseling program. It was apparent from the LPAD that Anna responded well to intervention and that many of her cognitive deficiencies were due to inefficient gathering of information and poor response strategies compounded by affective factors. Menal and Haywood have reported on the effectiveness of cognitive psychotherapy, a combination of Feuerstein's (1980) Instrumental Enrichment and psychotherapy with a client similar to Anna.

In summary, the LPAD demonstrated that both cognitive and affective factors were interfering with Anna's learning. Her intellectual potential was much higher than indicated by a standardized intelligence test. Anna's responsiveness to intervention during the assessment indicated that with some modifications in the work place and a combined program of cognitive education and counseling, Anna would likely be capable of a more challenging job and improved social functioning.

Mary: A Case of a Literate Well-Adjusted Client

Mary was referred for assessment to evaluate the extent and modifiability of long-standing learning difficulties, as she wants to pursue academic upgrading in preparation for a new career as a dental hygienist. Mary is a 27-year-old single woman who left home at 21 years of age to attend postsecondary school in the city. She completed a diploma in early childhood education and is currently employed in a day-care facility. Mary presents as a well-adjusted woman with a good support network. She is one of five children born to middle-class parents with whom she continues to have a close relationship. She showed good social skills and a good sense of humor. Avocationally, she is very involved in her community and volunteers with a youth group affiliated with her church.

Mary reported that she disliked school because of her difficulties with reading. Though she had strengths in maths and science, she believes she was perceived as "dumb" by the other students at school.

Academic testing ascertained Mary's general functioning level in reading, spelling, written language, and mathematics. Independent reading was estimated to be at the grade-seven level. With assistance she was able to read grade-nine–level material. Semantic and syntactic cues were used to compensate for inadequate sight word knowledge and weak word analysis skills. Spelling and written language skills were estimated to be at an upper elementary level and were the most problematic of the academic areas assessed. Mispronunciation ("probley"/probably) and difficulties with sequence ("unqueal"/unequal) were evident. Content in written expression was relatively adequate but form (i.e., writing mechanics) was weak. General functioning in mathematics appeared to be in the high-school range.

The LPAD was administered following the academic assessment to uncover cognitive deficits and affective factors related to the academic difficulties noted and to ascertain the amount and type of mediation necessary for Mary to perform more effectively.

Mary demonstrated sophisticated thinking skills on the LPAD. She was reflective, worked easily with analogous relationships and defined problems efficiently. Her adept problem-solving skills were evident on the Raven's Coloured Progressive Matrices and Set Variations I and II. Although Mary made a few errors with some problem types (usually multiple variables), she corrected these errors with minimal intervention. Precise language was used to explain her responses. The verbally based Organizer, one of the most difficult tests of the LPAD battery was enjoyable and challenging for Mary. She applied the strategies learned on the first few training items to later problems. Mary worked systematically, spontaneously comparing information in the statements given. She used inferential thinking and rquired only minimal examiner assistance in the completion of the problems.

One area of difficulty evident on both the Rey's Complex Figure, a figure drawing task, and the Word Memory Test was Mary's failure to fully grasp organizational principles. On the former test, the examiner's mediation focused on the need for labeling and a strategy for reproduction. Mary was then able to reproduce and execute a drawing from memory with complete accuracy. On the Word Memory Test, Mary did not spontaneously organize words by categories. Once categorization was suggested, recall improved significantly. Memory was enhanced when associative cues were used to trigger items for recall.

LPAD testing indicated that deficient cognitive functioning was not a major factor underlying Mary's difficulties with reading, spelling, and written language. Mary's adept performance on tasks requiring abstract formal operational thought was beneficial in convincing Mary that she was not "stupid" and that she could learn. High-motivational factors combined with her cognitive strengths resulted in the recommendation that Mary pursue academic upgrading, as a first step in achieving her goal of a new career.

Tom: A Case of a Nonliterate, Poorly Adjusted Client

Tom, age 24, is a single male who was raised in a rural working-class family. He attended school but met with tremendous frustration from an early age. He reports repeating grade one over and over with little success despite good effort on his part. He was in a vocational program through high school and then placed in a vocational training institute for mentally handicapped adults. After several years of trying to succeed, Tom gave up in frustration. Tom has held a variety of laboring jobs but has been unable to maintain permanent employment. He believes that this is due to his illiteracy.

During the psychosocial interview, Tom reported that he was living in a common-law relationship but was very unhappy. He had few friends in the community and his isolation exacerbated his feelings of low self-esteem. Tom believed he was incapable of learning, showed very poor social skills, and indicated that anger management has been an ongoing struggle for him. His counselor reported that he often interpreted sincerely positive feedback from employers as patronizing. Tom was referred for assessment because his vocational counselor believed he had more potential than his present performance indicated and the counselor wanted more in-depth information to assist Tom in finding an appropriate job.

Tom's reading was at a preprimer level. He had limited sight vocabulary and poor word attack skills, and he needed a great deal of assistance to decode and comprehend beginning material. He knew few sound-symbol correspondences. Arithmetic skills were also low, at an age 7 level. However, Tom reported being able to manage money well and he showed excellent temporal organization with a good understanding of time and the calendar.

There were indications throughout both the reading and math assessment that Tom's auditory discrimination and his general language skills were deficient. Further language testing indicated difficulties discriminating sounds, categorizing words, giving definitions, and generally being able to express himself. Receptive language was a relative strength but still somewhat deficient.

It appeared from the standardized tests that expressive language was likely a major factor underlying Tom's severe academic difficulties. However, the degree of modifiability of his language functioning and the level of Tom's general intellectual functioning were still unclear. Test scores to this point were consistent with someone of low intellect, as Tom was assumed to be.

On the LPAD, Tom had difficulties initially in defining the problem and using task-appropriate strategies. He did not attend to several variables simultaneously, had difficulty deciding what information was relevant and what was irrelevant for a particular problem, was impulsive, and tended to use trial-and-error responding. Language was also deficient. He referred to a triangle as "reptangle," could not use labels consistently (e.g., top, middle, bottom) did not know many labels (e.g., horizontal and vertical) and was unable to express reasons for choices.

Tom was very amenable to instruction and immediately tried to apply what he learned during the assessment. With minimal intervention from the examiner, he understood what he was expected to do on each subtest, and spontaneously applied the strategies taught. He began to attend to several variables simultaneously, to focus on the relevent ones and to work in a thoughtful, systematic way.

Language functioning proved less modifiable. After considerable examiner intervention, Tom learned some new labels. For example, on each problem where the terms *horizontal* and *vertical* were applicable, the examiner pointed to the horizontal and vertical lines and asked Tom to label them. It took, at least, 10 such repetitions but when Tom finally learned the terms he retained them and began to use them spontaneously. A month later he had still retained these terms.

The use of labels to aid in problem solving remained severely deficient even after intensive mediation. On Set Variations II, the examinee is required to choose the correct location for a hexagon after studying the locations of eight other hexagons and abstracting the rule governing position in the rows and columns. Problem solution is aided by labeling locations as "top right," "top middle," "top left," etc. Tom could not use these terms consistently even though he gave evidence of having the concepts. Very little improvement was seen in labeling after extensive mediation. This was in marked contrast to Tom's performance on later items in Set Variations II that involved more difficult rule abstraction principles but less language demands.

Although it was already evident from the achievement and language testing that language was a major area of difficulty, the LPAD testing provided several pieces of information not available previously. First, it was noted that although Tom had many initial difficulties in solving the tasks, he was able to quickly learn and apply more effective problem solving approaches. Second, where language was not a factor in task solution, Tom was able to function effectively giving evidence of the ability for abstract formal operational thinking (Piaget, 1958). Third, although language for the most part remained a severe problem, Tom was able to learn new terms with great effort and, once learned, retained them. Lastly, Tom's success on solving difficult problems (e.g., Set Variations II) had the effect of boosting his self-concept, albeit temporarily, and convincing him that he was capable of learning.

Recommendations included a program of language therapy combined if possible with cognitive eduation (e.g., Instrumental Enrichment; Feuerstein, 1980). In addition, information was given to his employer regarding the effect of his language difficulties on performance and effective strategies to assist Tom.

George: A Case of a Nonliterate Well-Adjusted Client

George, age 25, was adopted at age 5, by parents with whom he presently resides. His mother reports that he was born prematurely and encountered developmental delays particularly in the areas of motor and language development. George experienced tremendous difficulty academically despite continual support and advocacy for special education programs by his parents. He completed high school through a work-study program and went to an employment preparation program before taking a menial labor job. George has had a variety of unskilled jobs that he has had difficulty maintaining because of his literacy problems.

George has a good relationship with his parents and many friends in the community. He participates in a variety of leisure activities and presents as a well-adjusted young man. His career aspirations are to work as a pipe fitter. George was referred for an in-depth assessment of academic and cognitive functioning to provide direction for career planning.

Achievement testing indicated that George is nonliterate. He was unable to read even the most basic informal reading selection, spelled only the word "up" correctly on the spelling test administered and was unable to express himself in the written mode. Problems with auditory and visual discrimination and memory were evident. Receptive language was stronger than expressive language. Listening comprehension was a relative strength (upper elementary). Math skills were at a lower elementary level. George was pleasant but difficult to engage in the academic testing. He articulated years of frustration with school which manifested itself in his passive, detached approach to tasks presented by the examiner.

The LPAD was administered following the academic battery to ascertain what cognitive deficits if any related to the academic difficulties, the type and amount of mediation required for learning to occur, and to what extent emotional and motivational factors were affecting learning. As well, the relatively content-free nature of the LPAD subtests were perceived as tasks in which George would more readily engage.

George's attitude toward the LPAD tasks and his ability to concentrate were inconsistent initially. With continuous examiner support and assistance, George became noticeably more confident in his ability to think and to solve subsequent problems. Fear of failure decreased with success but resurfaced when tasks became more complex and novel. George did not appear to have a need for mastery of the tasks.

Cognitive deficiencies affecting learning were evident at the input, elaboration, and output phases. Language problems (particularly expressive) were most pronounced. The examiner had to invest considerable time and effort in teaching George language required for efficient problem solving. For example, the examiner had to teach and reteach the labels "square" and "rectangle" and their distinguishing characteristics. Initially, George was very unsystematic in the manner in which he explored problems. Trial-and-error behavior was apparent. With intensive mediation, George was able to use self-talk strategies to assist himself in planning and organizing information more effectively. His impulsivity was restrained by covering answers and modeling step-by-step strategies for problem solution. George was able to apply these techniques to similar problems but reverted back to trial-and-error behavior when problems became more complex and novel. Blocking, a lack of willingness of attempt a problem perceived as difficult, was reduced by reassuring George that he had completed similar problems correctly and by providing him with step-by-step assistance on the current problem.

The changes in George's performance on the LPAD led to the conclusion that with considerable intervention, he has the potential to learn and apply new content and strategies. It was suggested that George would learn best when placed in a supportive environment where information was organized and presented in small segments and sufficient repetition was available. At the same time, it was considered imperative that George have opportunities to develop effective organizational and learning skills so that he could become an independent learner and thinker. These findings were shared with the referral agency. Long-term assessment of vocational interests through a community program was recommended. The possibility of apprenticeship as a pipe fitter was also discussed.

Discussion of Case Vignettes

These four case vignettes further illustrate the nature of the problems encountered by clients with learning difficulties and the type of information forthcoming from an LPAD to assist the clinician in better understanding their client's needs. The characteristic difficulties of this population are such that a dynamic interactional approach with an emphasis on process rather than product and the use of relatively content-free, unschool-like tasks is necessary to obtain a full picture of the client's skills and abilities.

One characteristic in common for all the clients in the sample was a lack of success in school. Although the degree of school difficulties varied from extreme to moderate, virtually all the clients viewed themselves as failures in learning situations and were anxious in a test situation. Several aspects of the LPAD were critical for obtaining a more accurate picture of the client and his needs given this history of past failure. Most important was the interaction between the examiner and the client. On the LPAD, the examiner assisted the client as necessary so that he or she would perform successfully, gave precise feedback, and questioned the client about his performance to increase self-awareness.

The importance of this interaction was illustrated in the case of Anna, where it could be seen that her lack of confidence and low self-esteem led to increased anxiety and poor performance on standardized measures. On the LPAD, it was evident that affective factors, such as fear of failure and diffuse anxiety, were major impediments to her learning, but she was capable of normal intellectual functioning when these adverse factors were controlled. With continual specific feedback on the correctness of her responses and the processes used to reach an answer, Anna gained the confidence to risk in the test situation. Her ability to solve complex abstract problems with assistance was not only important information for the examiner's understanding of Anna but for Anna's understanding of her difficulties. Before Anna could pursue help, whether counseling or academic upgrading, she needed to believe that she was capable of learning.

Similarly, in the case of Mary who, in contrast to Anna, exhibited few areas of deficient cognitive or affective functioning, self-esteem regarding her ability to be successful in an academic setting was low. Successful completion of complex abstract tasks provided her with concrete evidence of her ability to think and learn effectively and helped increase her self-confidence.

Tom, who was both nonliterate and had social difficulties, required intensive mediation from the examiner to teach him the prerequisite knowledge and strategies needed for task solution. Equally as important, he needed support from the examiner to increase his feelings of competence. The dynamic interaction between Tom and the examiner provided the necessary encouragement and positive feedback so that Tom had the confidence to learn in the test situation. He began to understand his difficulties in terms of cognitive and emotional factors rather than simply focusing on his ability to master the particular skill—reading. Barr and Samuels (1988) suggest this promotion of self-understanding is a major asset of the dynamic interactional approach.

George, whose past failures in school and on tests led to a lack of engagement in the academic tasks also benefited from the examiner's assistance and feedback. Again the dynamic interactional approach was instrumental in his willingness to engage in the tasks and persist even as the tasks increased in difficulty.

The nature of the tasks was also instrumental in the usefulness of the LPAD with this population. The tasks, which are often referred to as content-free, in fact, require some prior knowledge but for the most part are relatively novel and unrelated to school curriculum content. This novelty helps circumvent the traditional resistance or passivity seen in clients such as George and Tom who have encountered years of failure in school. George appeared passive and uninterested during the academic assessment, whereas Tom had a totally defeated attitude. Both were willing to invest significant time and effort on the LPAD subtests. Tom, in fact became so involved that he asked to continue working on one of the subtests alone when the examiner had to end the session.

The structure of the tests provide opportunities for clients to apply newly learned rules and strategies in increasingly complex and novel situations. In the case of Anna, this structure provided opportunities for the examiner to give feedback about successful approaches Anna was using and to encourage her to apply these as the tasks appeared more difficult and hence, her anxiety increased. Similarly, George had difficulty applying previously learned rules and strategies as complexity increased but was encouraged to do so. The realization that he could be successful increased his feelings of competence and his willingness to persist. In Tom's case, having multiple items based on the same general rules and strategies, allowed for intensive mediation on early items to teach prerequisite knowledge and skills, and then application of this learning with increasing independence on similar but more complex later items or on items differing slightly in form or the rule required.

Adults with learning difficulties who were not identified as such in school may be, in essence, uneducated and hence exhibit many cognitive deficiencies due to a lack of mediated learning experiences. This lack of mediated learning experiences according to Feuerstein et al. (1979) leads to lower levels of intellectual functioning or retarded performance. The case of Tom illustrates how his early undiagnosed difficulties led to inappropriate educational placement and eventually the classification of borderline intellectual functioning. This classification, in turn, led to inappropriate job training and placement. Because Tom lacks the knowledge base upon which standardized tests are based and has poor learning and test-taking strategies, his performance, even on nonverbal standardized tests, is likely to be poor. As noted earlier, his performance is consistent with the classification of borderline intellectual functioning but standardized test results give no indication of his intellectual potential or the remedial help needed to reach that potential. The amount and type of mediation needed to produce change on the LPAD provided this information. Tom's language difficulties, the major underlying factor in his illiteracy were diagnosed from the standardized tests but the effect of language factors on overall intellectual functioning and learning potential only became apparent in the teach-test situation.

Overall, the LPAD was least useful in the case of Mary. Her specific difficulties were evident from the standardized assessment, and other than serving to increase Mary's confidence regarding her thinking skills little new information was gained. In clients with reasonable literacy skills and good psychosocial functioning, the LPAD may not be warranted.

In summary, the four clients discussed in this section, considered representative of clients with learning difficulties, benefited from the dynamic interaction during testing with its focus on process and affective factors, the content-free nature of the tasks, the structure of tasks that allows application of learning, and the teach-test approach. The LPAD information contributed least in the case of the literate client with good social adjustment.

Conclusion

In conclusion, this chapter illustrates the use of the LPAD with adults with learning difficulties. The results from the LPAD indicated that the population sampled showed the typical difficulties associated with adults with learning disabilities, such as disorganization, attention deficits, poor learning strategies, language difficulties, and low self-esteem. Hence, it was particularly useful as an alternative or adjunct to standardized assessment in those cases in which poor social adjustment, low literacy, and associated factors render comparison to the norms meaningless.

The LPAD identified specific areas of deficient cognitive functioning and assessed the effect of affective or nonintellective factors on performance. It also indicated the amount and type of mediation needed to overcome the factors impeding performance. This latter information was critical for prescribing appropriate courses of action to assist the client to function better in the workplace and in general. The LPAD was also useful in highlighting areas of efficient cognitive functioning, which served the dual purpose of giving the examiner information on the clients' areas of strength and of demonstrating these strengths to the clients themselves, who often believed they were incapable of learning and thinking.

The dynamic interactional nature of the assessment was the most critical factor in the tests' usefulness with this population. The supportive, examiner-client relationship helped allay clients' test anxiety, encouraged them to try, and made them aware of their abilities to process information. It also allowed for teaching of prerequisite content, rules, and strategies. The relatively content-free nature of the materials and the increasingly complex structure of the tasks with their focus on use of rules and cognitive strategies provided opportunities to observe the process of learning, unencumbered by past experiences with school failure. This permitted direct observation by the examiner of learning potential and areas of modifiability that were most useful in making recommendations for change.

Acknowledgements. The authors would like to thank Mary Hodges and Gillian Hutton for assistance with the data analysis and staff at the Learning Centre for comments on earlier drafts of this paper.

References

Alley, G. R., & Deshler, D. D. (1979). *Teaching the learning disabled adolescent: Strategies and methods*. Denver: Love Publishing Ltd.

Barr, P., & Samuels, M. (1988). Dynamic assessment of cognitive and affective factors contributing to learning difficulties with adults. *Professional Psychology: Research and Practice*, *19*(1), 6–13.

Blalock, J. W. (1981). Persistent problems and concerns of young adults with learning disabilities. In W. Cruikshank & A. Silver (Eds.), *Bridges to tomorrow—The best of ACLD* (Vol. 2, pp. 35–55). Syracuse, NY: Syracuse University Press.

Brown, D. (1984). Employment considerations for learning disabled adults. *Journal of Rehabilitation*, *50*, 74–77,88.

Buchanan, M., & Wolf, J. (1986). A comprehensive study of learning disabled adults. *Journal of Learning Disabilities*, *14*, 404–407.

Crimando, W. (1984). A review of placement-related issues for clients with learning disabilities. *Journal of Rehabilitation*, *50*, 78–81.

Delclos, V. (1983). *Differential error analysis in the group administration of the Representational Stencil Design Test*. Unpublished doctoral dissertation, Vanderbilt University.

Faford, M., & Haubrich, P. (1981). Vocational and social adjustment of learning disabled young adults: A follow-up study. *Learning Disability Quarterly*, *4*, 122–130.

Feuerstein, R. (1980). *Instrumental Enrichment*. Baltimore: University Park Press.

Feuerstein, R., Miller, R., Rand, Y., & Jensen, M. R. (1981). Can evolving techniques better measure cognitive change? *Journal of Special Education*, *15*(2), 201–219.

Feuerstein, R., Haywood, H. C., Rand, Y., Hoffman, M., & Jensen, M. R. (1986). *Learning Potential Assessment Device Manual, experimental version*. Jerusalem: Hadassah-Wizo Canada Research Institute.

Feuerstein, R., Rand, Y., & Hoffman, M. B. (1979). *The dynamic assessment of retarded performers*. Baltimore: University Park Press.

Fravenheim, J. (1978). Academic achievement characteristic of adult males who were diagnosed as dyslexic in childhood. *Journal of Learning Disabilities*, *11*, 476–483.

Ginsburg, H. (1972). *The myth of the deprived child*. Englewood Cliffs, NJ: Prentice Hall.

Hartzell, H., & Compton, C. (1984). Learning disability: 10 year follow-up. *Pediatrics*, *74*, 1058–1064.

Haywood, H. C. (1977). Alternatives to normative assessment. In P. Mittler (Ed.), *Research to practice in mental retardation: Education and training* (Vol. 2, pp. 11–18). Baltimore: University Park Press.

Hershenson, D. (1984). Vocational counselling with learning disabled adults. *Journal of Rehabilitation*, *50*, 40–44.

Howell, K. W. (1986). Direct assessment of academic performance. *School Psychology Review*, *15*(3), 324–335.

Johns, J. L. (1981). *Advanced reading inventory: Grade seven through college*. Dubuque, IA: Wm. C. Brown.

Johns, J. L. (1985). *Basic reading inventory: Pre-primer-grade eight*. Dubuque, IA: Kendall/Hunt.

Keane, K. (1983). *Application of mediated learning theory to a deaf population: A study in cognitive modifiability*. Unpublished doctoral dissertation, Columbia University, New York.

Keane, K. (1987). Assessing deaf children. In C. S. Lidz, (Ed.), *Dynamic assessment* (pp. 360–376). New York: Guilford.

Kronick, D. (1985). Learning disabilities—vocational and employment implications. *Canadian Association for Children and Adults with Learning Disabilities National News*, *22*(4), 6–8.

Lefcourt, H. (1976). *Locus of control: Current trends in theory and research*. Hillsdale, NJ: Erlbaum.

Lehtinen, L., & Dumas, L. (1976). *A follow-up study of learning disabled children as adults: A final report*. Evanston, Il: Cove School Research Office.

Lidz, C. S. (1987). *Dynamic assessment: An interactional approach to evaluating learning potential*. New York: Guilford.

Menal, C., & Haywood, H. C. *Cognitive-developmental psychotherapy: A case study*. Unpublished manuscript, Vanderbilt University, Nashville.

Missiuna, C., & Samuels, M. (1988). Dynamic assessment: Review and Critique, *Special Services in the Schools*, *5*(12), 1–22.

Newell, B. H., Goyette, C. H., & Fogarty, T. W. (1984). Diagnosis and assessment of the adult with specific learning disabilities. *Journal of Rehabilitation*, *50*, 34–39.

Patton, J., & Polloway, E. (1982). Learning disabilities: The adult years. *Topics in Learning and Learning Disabilities*, *2*, 79–88.

Piaget, J. (1958). *The growth of logical thinking from childhood to adolescence* (A. Parsons & S. Seagrin, Trans.). New York: Basic Books.

Raven, J. C. (1965). *Guide to using the coloured progressive matrices: Sets A, AB, and B*. London: Lewis.

Reid, K., & Hresko, W. P. (1981). *A cognitive approach to learning disabilities*. New York: McGraw Hill.

Salvia, J., & Ysseldyke, J. (1978). *Assessment in special and remedial education*. Dallas: Houghton Mifflin.

Samuels, M. T., Tzuriel, D., & Malloy-Miller, T. (1989). Dynamic assessment of children with learning disabilities. In R. I. Brown & M. Chazan (Eds.), *Learning Difficulties and Emotional Problems*. Calgary: Detselig Press, 147–164.

Scarr, S. (1981). Testing for children: Assessment and the many determinants of intellectual competence. *American Psychologist*, *36*(10), 1159–1166.

Short, R. H., & Mueller, H. H. (1985). Analysis and meta-analysis of the WISC-R. *Alberta Psychology*, *14*, 5–7.

Siegel, S. (1957). *Nonparametric statistics for the behavioral sciences*. New York: McGraw-Hill.

Tzuriel, D., Samuels, M., & Feuerstein, R. (1988). Nonintellective factors in dynamic assessment. In R. M. Gupta & P. Coxhead (Eds.), *Cultural diversity and learning efficiency* (pp. 141–163). London: Macmillan.

Waksman, M., Silverman, H., & Weber, K. (1983). Assessing the learning potential of penitentiary inmates: An application of Feuerstein's Learning Potential Assessment Device. *Journal of Correctional Education*, *34*(2), 63–69.

Ysseldyke, J., & Algozzine, R. (1982). *Critical issues in special and remedial education*. Boston: Houghton Mifflin.

12
Cognitive Competence: Reality and Potential in the Deaf

KEVIN J. KEANE, ABRAHAM J. TANNENBAUM, and GARY F. KRAPF

How we come to know the world around us and our place in it is a question that has baffled philosophers and fools alike from the earliest days of philosophy and foolishness. Nevertheless, educators are duty-bound to produce some kinds of operational answers in order to shape school policy, programs, curricula, and even classroom lessons which impact all learners. In the twentieth century, especially in post industrial Western cultures, a corollary pragmatic investigation has centered on ways to assess individual capacities for consuming and producing knowledge.

At present, psychometric practice has become an integral part of our educational system and thought, especially as it pertains to handicapped learners. Mental ability tests are still administered widely with distorted assumptions about their meaning and importance. These instruments are designed to measure a child's learning status, which is highly changeable, but too many educators confuse learning status with learning capacity, or the fixed upper limits of a child's potential, as if each mind were a different-size receptacle for knowledge and the test score were a permanent indicator of that size. Luckily, physicians do not fall into a similar trap of regarding blood pressure readings as unalterable, for if they did, it could prove disastrous to some patients suffering from extreme hypertension. The fact is that test scores say nothing about a mind's absorptive power because they fail to show how modifiable a child's level of accomplishment can be; they only denote what the child has already learned in a far-from-perfect learning environment. Allowing that environment to retain its imperfections helps make the test score a good forecaster of how much the child *will* achieve, leaving in the realm of mystery how much (s)he *might have* achieved under enriched circumstances. It is out of such stuff that self-fulfilling prophesies are made, all in support of educational fatalism and inertia.

Although disenchantment with the use of static measures of cognitive competence has grown, traditional testing practices still predominate in research and education pertaining to deaf children. Prior investigations into the cognitive/intellective functioning of the deaf has primarily utilized the psychometric model or concept to explain similarities and differences between the deaf and hearing populations. However, the translation of findings into general explanations of performance with this population has not been simple for a variety of reasons. The history of the education of deaf persons has been marked by controversy with highly charged emotional overtones. A case in point, the issue of the preferred method of communication for instruction, oral versus manual, is referred to as the "Hundred Years War." Likewise, research into the cognitive functioning of this population has been influenced by a number of forces, among them social and even political.

A review of twentieth century research regarding the cognitive competence of the deaf as a group conjures, at times, the story of the three blind men trying to describe an elephant. Their positions around the elephant shaped their perspective, resulting in three very different conclusions as to the physical nature of the animal. Their singular perspectives also inhibited communication of the parts to describe the whole. Similarly, researchers with psychometric, linguistic, social, or behavioral orientations have arrived at different conclusions at different times concerning the cognitive characteristics of the deaf.

Over 70 years of research into the intellectual functioning of the deaf, as measured by standard tests, has led to conflicting conclusions that, compared to their hearing counterparts, the deaf are cognitively inferior (Pintner, Eisenson, & Stanton, 1941), intellectually normal but cognitively different (Myklebust, 1960), and finally that no real difference exists between the hearing and deaf (Moores, 1978). These interpretations, although different, rely on a traditional psychometric model with its implied concept of intelligence to render their explanations. From a pragmatic viewpoint, the value of standard performance measures as tools for intervention on behalf of the deaf has been questioned as they have been for other populations (Lambert, 1981; Newland, 1972). More important, however, is whether this conventional conceptual framework inhibits the deaf from realizing a greater potential.

At present, most researchers agree that there is not a specific "psychology of deafness," that the deaf population is part of the general population, although they may have a somewhat different acculturation. For this reason, general theories of human development and knowledge acquisition have been applied to this population. However, applying any theory of knowledge acquisition to a specific population assumes comparable learner characteristics between the specific and the general population for which it was generated. Take for example, the theory of structural cognitive modifiability, with its integral component of mediated learning experience (MLE), which was developed by Feuerstein and his associates (1979, 1980) through their work with low-functioning or educationally retarded populations. Feuerstein's (1979) concept of both the nature of intelligence and the forces that affect its development in individuals clearly departs from the conventional psychometric concept (Arbitman-Smith, Haywood, & Bransford, 1984). According to this theory, individuals represent open systems and are thus capable of change. To produce needed changes, Feuerstein (1979) has indicated that, in approaching low-functioning individuals, changes in the nature of the surrounding environment, assessment practices, and intervention procedures are necessary. The Learning Potential Assessment Device (LPAD) model was developed from this theory.

Some have already rejected out of hand the application of this theory to the deaf. For example, Braden (1985) argues that the theoretical assumptions of MLE could not be used to explain cognitive deficiencies in deaf children. He bases this contention on a factor analytic study that showed that "deaf children perform much better than minority children on nonverbal IQ tests" (p. 125). According to Braden, this finding challenges Feuerstein's (1979) notion that lack of mediated learning experience was the proximal etiology in deficiencies in the deaf because the deaf did not demonstrate these deficiencies on a performance measure.

It is true that the deaf, as a group, depart from Feuerstein's (1979) population by virtue of their sensory loss and the fact that they perform within the normal ranges of cognitive/intellective ability on standard performance intelligence measures (Levine, 1981; Tomlinson-Keasey & Kelly, 1978). However, traditional psychometric measures do not reflect this population's adaptation to education or to life in general. Levine states that even though the average deaf group manifests normal or even better than normal mental endowment, the bulk of them represent "education's failures" (p. 157). This group leaves the educational system with "scholastic retardations, linguistic deficiencies, and related conceptual gaps and limitations" (p. 157).

With regard to social and behavioral functioning, research shows that, as a group, the deaf manifest higher degrees of impulsivity, egocentricity, dependency, lack of reflectivity, and rigidity than the population at large (Altshuler, Deming, Vollenweider, Rainer, & Tender, 1976; Harris, 1978; Levine, 1976, 1981; Myklebust, 1960). In a cross-national study, Meadow and Dyssegard (1983) reported that teachers of deaf children in the United States and in Denmark tended "to see their students (at both young and older age levels) to be lacking in motivation, independence, and initiative" (p. 347). In another study that asked educators of the hearing impaired from elementary to postsecondary programs to prioritize the personal and social needs of their hearing impaired students, results indicated that acceptance of responsibility for one's actions was the most deficient competency (White, 1982). This behavior is related to locus of control and concurs with other studies (Dillon, 1980; Harris, 1978) that indicate that the deaf manifest a more external locus of control in their adaptation to life.

The gap between the findings on conventional yardsticks and manifest performance characteristics attests to a potential that is not actualized for a large segment of the deaf population. Documentation of this underachievement is evident in research with explanations from diverse points of view (Furth, 1966; Levine, 1981; Myklebust, 1960; Tomlinson-Keasey & Kelly, 1978). Braden's (1985) use of a standard performance measure as a gauge to reject the application of MLE theory to the deaf population is questionable in light of the manifest performance characteristics of the "average" deaf group. Contrary to Braden's contention, the present authors argue that Feuerstein's (1979) theory presents a reasonable framework for understanding the manifest characteristics of the deaf and, further, tools exist to test this hypothesis with such a population.

Defining Characteristics of the Deaf Population

Although sensory loss is the common denominator for a deaf population, those suffering from it represent as much a heterogeneous group as the hearing population (Levine, 1981). Deafness refers to the degree of auditory loss. Educationally, deaf persons are defined as individuals whose hearing impairment is so severe that it is nonfunctional for purposes of educational performance (Federal statute, PL 94–142). Audiometrically, individuals manifesting a hearing loss greater than 90 dB (profound) are considered deaf; those in the range above (70 dB) (severe) are classified as being in a "transitory category between hard-of hearing and deaf" (Quigley & Kretschmer, 1982, p. 3).

Consideration of other major impacting conditions are also necessary to understand the unique nature of this group. One variable is the age of onset of hearing loss; prelingual deafness refers to a loss encountered prior to the establishment of language (usually 2 or 3 years of age). A second variable is the etiology of the loss. Deafness may be caused by either endogenous or exogenous factors. Heredity, syndromes, and blood incompatibilities are examples of endogenous etiologies, whereas accident, drugs, and bacterial infections are examples of exogenous etiologies (Quigley & Kretschmer, 1982). Many of these causative factors may impart other handicapping conditions along with deafness. Quigley and Kretschmer considered a third intervening variable, the hearing status of the parents. Deaf children with hearing parents comprise 90% of the deaf population. Research concerning performance characteristics of deaf children with deaf parents compared with deaf children of hearing parents indicates significant group differences along a number of academic, behavioral, and cognitive parameters (Brill, 1969; Conrad, 1979; Meadow,

1980; Ray, 1979; Schlesinger & Meadow, 1972; Vernon & Koh, 1970). It is important to clarify as many of these intervening variables as possible when engaging in research with a deaf population.

Conventional Cognitive Testing with the Deaf

Because of the concomitant English linguistic deficit accompanying deafness, performance-type intelligence tests are the preferred measures used to assess the intellectual abilities of deaf persons (Brill, 1962; Levine, 1974; Sullivan, 1982) with the Wechsler Intelligence Scale for Children (WISC; now the revised WISC-R) Performance scale being the most frequently administered (Levine, 1974). Along with the Hiskey-Nebraska Test of Learning Aptitude, which was standardized on deaf children, the WISC-R also has deaf norms (Anderson & Sisco, 1977). Other performance tests that are used frequently, such as the Leiter International Performance Scale, were not standardized on the deaf and, thus, are not normed for this population. As noted, at present a number of researchers have questioned the utility and even validity of standard intelligence measures with populations whose cultural, linguistic, or social background differs from that of the mainstream society (Garcia, 1981; Olmedo, 1981). Likewise, Gerweck and Ysseldyke (1975) have questioned the validity of using many of these popular performance measures with deaf populations because of a difference in the acculturation of the deaf from that of the hearing groups on which the tests were standardized and because the instructional communication for the tasks vary so widely among psychologists serving the deaf.

Just as verbal intelligence assessments are used for hearing special education populations, performance tests are used for important decisions concerning programming and placement of deaf children. However, even from a psychometric viewpoint, the utility of these measures for purposes other than classification is questionable. Generally, correlations between these tests of intelligence and achievement have not been high for this population (Childers, Lao, & Lingerfelt, 1979; Joiner, Erikson, Crittenden, & Stevenson, 1969). According to Levine (1974) the predicatability of cognitive performance on standarzied scales with school achievement is not generalizable to the deaf population. Brill (1962) observed that a mean IQ of 118 on the WISC Performance scale predicted a ninth grade achievement test level for deaf children at age 18. A Performance IQ of 101 predicted a fifth grade achievement and a Performance IQ of 90 indicated little chance of successfully completing even a vocational school program.

Besides the low correlation to school performance, traditional psychometric approaches, as product-oriented ability measures, are further limited in their implications for pedagogical or habilitative intervention

(Feuerstein, 1979; Glaser, 1981). This limitation greatly impacts the deaf because, as noted, academic retardation, linguistic deficiencies, and conceptual limitations are realities within this population (Bonvillian, Charrow, & Nelson, 1973; Lane, 1976; Levine, 1981; Meadow, 1980; Tomlinson-Keasey & Kelly, 1978; Trybus & Karchmer, 1977). It must be noted, however, that a large percentage of deaf individuals perform well in comparison with their hearing age peers on a variety of cognitive and achievement measures and attainments (Levine, 1981), which would preclude the notion that the sensory loss alone is the causative element in poor performance. Presently, researchers stress the heterogeneity within the deaf population and indicate that the variables affecting the performance of deaf individuals are of a complex nature (Levine, 1981).

In light of the manifest performance of deaf individuals, Quigley and Kretschmer (1982) noted that present assessment and educational practices are limited in their ability "to fully help deaf people develop and use their abilities" (p. 63). Such recognition has led some researchers to investigate alternative assessment approaches with deaf populations, including "testing the limits" procedures (Carlson & Dillon, 1978; Dillon, 1979, 1980) and a learning-potential format (Koehler, 1977). However, the findings of these studies, even when positive, have been generally interpreted from a conventional psychometric framework. This interpretive approach has been altered by degrees in studies using the LPAD.

LPAD Practice with the Deaf

The LPAD is an approach to clinical assessment that departs from traditional psychometric procedures theoretically and procedurally. Traditional psychometric measures assess past environmentally learned abilities; the LPAD, on the other hand, consists of a battery of instruments that assess the ability of an individual to learn. Learning in this context refers to the ability of the individual to modify existing cognitive structures through exposure to mediated intervention. The LPAD permits the investigation of deficiencies that may impede performance, classifies them according to specific information-processing concepts, and seeks to mediate them in the testing situation itself. In this way, the cognitive potential of an individual may be measured more directly. In practice, the LPAD attempts to rectify the mismatch between the nature of the cognitive deficits in culturally deprived individuals and the nature of instruments used in assessing these deficits.

Applications of LPAD to handicapped learners show evidence of its promise as a tool for testing the theoretical hypothesis of mediated learning with deaf populations as well. Feuerstein (1979) noted in his studies that mediational intervention through LPAD results in higher gains for low achievers than for high achievers. Huberty and Koller

(1984) investigated this premise in a study comparing deaf and hearing subjects, the sample consisting of 40 hearing subjects with a mean age of 12.11 and 28 deaf subjects with a mean age of 13.6. For the hearing group, those who scored in the top 25% of the Stanford Achievement Test were classified as high achievers and those in the bottom 25% as low achievers. For the deaf group, those who scored in the 65% percentile or better on the Stanford hearing-impaired version were designated as high achievers, and those at the 35th percentile or lower were grouped as low achievers. Subjects in each group were randomly assigned to either training or nontraining groups.

One LPAD instrument, the Representational Stencil Design Test (RSDT) was used in this study. The RSDT is a variation of the Grace Arthur Stencil Design Test in that the same stencil designs are used; however, they are not manipulated by hand. In the RSDT the subjects must project the stencils mentally in the appropriate order for completion of a design. Because of the complexity of this task, the training and nontraining samples were further broken down into input and noninput subgroups. Those receiving input were informed as to the number of stencils needed to complete a design; the noninput group did not receive this information.

Results indicated that (a) low achievers performed as well as high achievers with training regardless of hearing ability; (b) input manipulation had a powerful effect on the ability of hearing and deaf students to solve a cognitive task; (c) there were no differences in the ability of hearing and deaf students to learn complex problem solving skills with proper training, input, and control of language variables; and (d) learning-potential procedures could be used effectively with the deaf (Huberty & Koller, 1984, p. 27). They concluded that, although there were practical limitations, learning potential approaches are amenable to research and application for both deaf and hearing persons. However, they also cautioned that "at present, learning potential procedures appear best considered as supplementary to traditional measures" (p. 27).

Katz and Bucholz (1984), in a single case study design, administered seven instruments from the LPAD battery to a 14-year-old deaf girl with a WISC-R Performance score of 85. They found the LPAD to be a useful tool in delineating cognitive deficiencies, strengths, and potential. Further, they stated that their observations seem "to support the notion that mediational deprivation is contributory or causally related to poor performance of some deaf children on many achievement and intelligence measures" (p. 105). Katz and Bucholz also supported the value of the LPAD process-oriented approach in that it provided the examiner with more of an opportunity to generate prescriptive recommendations for instructional planning.

Keane (1983, 1987) and Keane and Kretschmer (1987) suggested that beyond the practical utility of the LPAD for deaf persons, Feuerstein's

(1979) mediated learning construct may provide a framework for understanding the manifest functioning of this population. Over 90% of deaf children are born to hearing parents. For a majority of these parents, it is their first direct encounter with the handicap of deafness (Schlesinger & Meadow, 1972). Mindel and Vernon (1971) cited guilt, anger, grief, and repression as stages through which parents normally pass in coping with the reality of having a hearing impaired child. As the nurturing agents in the environment of the deaf child, the nature of the parents' coping mechanisms may cause a significant disruption or reduction in the mediational learning process, that is, a situation where the organization of environmental stimuli is not adequately interpreted for the child.

As the deaf child's world expands into the realm of schooling, the causative factors of cultural (mediational) deprivation may persist. Levine (1981) stated that deaf children were more dependent upon formal schooling than hearing children because they had less access to informal out-of-school input. However, she criticized formal education of the deaf for its limitations "in opportunities for independent thinking and for developing mental initiatives and controls" (p. 142). Meadow (1980) indicated that teachers tended to lower their expectations for their deaf students and, according to Liben (1978), restricted the levels of experience available to them. Such an environment may serve to reinforce such behaviors as passive acceptance of certain kinds of information, dependency, and lack of responsibility for one's own behavior, which are associated with the syndrome of cultural (mediational) deprivation.

Based on the contention that mediated learning may be a powerful factor in the ontology of development in the deaf child, and that impoverishment in mediated learning experience masks cognitive potential, Keane (1983) investigated the cognitive modifiability of a sample of deaf children when exposed to mediated intervention through the LPAD. Using a multigroup pretest-posttest design, 45 prelingually deaf subjects between the ages of 9 and 13, with hearing parents, were randomly assigned to one of three test-treatment conditions prior to testing. These test-treatment conditions consisted of one experimental group and two comparison groups: a standard and an elaboration condition. The mean WISC-R Performance score for each group was 91.3, 94.6, and 99.8, respectively. The three conditions varied in the nature of the examiner-examinee interaction in each and in the alteration of one set of stimulus materials. All groups received both the training and the assessment sections of each LPAD instrument.

In the experimental condition, 15 subjects received the of LPAD battery as designed by Feuerstein (1979). In the standard condition, 15 subjects received the same instruments as the experimental group, except for one of the tasks in which a motor-manipulative form of the test was administered. However, the distinctive feature of this condition was the use of standard psychometric practice in which the examiner was an objective assessor rather than a participant observer, as in the experimental condition. In the second comparison group, the elaboration condition, 15 subjects received the same test instruments as the standard group; however, the examiner-examinee relationship was altered in still another way. Because Dillon (1979, 1980) and Carlson and Dillon (1978) demonstrated that elaborated feedback (testing-the-limits procedure) during testing improved performance of deaf subjects on certain cognitive/intellective tasks, this group served to compare the effect of a "testing-the-limits" procedure with mediated exposure and standard practice. Using Dillon's (1979) format, the examiner provided feedback to the examinee as to the correctness or incorrectness of response, requested the examinee to articulate a rationale for each response, and, if the response was incorrect, explained the underlying premise of the task item. However, the alternate correct response was not provided.

The instruments in the LPAD battery can be roughly grouped into three major categories. These involve visual-motor organization, higher mental processes, and memory with a learning component. The instruments in this study were selected from all three of these categories. Following is a description of six instruments that were administered to each group:

1. and 2. Raven's Coloured Progressive Matrices (RCPM) and LPAD Set Variations I involving figural analogies. The LPAD Set Variations I is similar in construct to the latter portion of the Raven's CPM; however, the subject chooses from eight alternatives to solve a 2 × 2 matrix problem. The Set Variations consist of five sets of analogies: each set contains seven analogies, the first of which is used for training; the other six analogies are variations of that training analogy (see Figure 12.1 for an example of a Set Variation problem).
3. The Organization of Dots consisting of amorphous arrangements of dots that have to be organized according to an imposed geometric structure.
4. The Plateaux Test, a positional learning task which involves a projection from a three-dimensional to a one-dimensional frame of reference and a mental transformation of learned positions through various rotations.
5. The Associated Recall Test, an associative memory task that taps the ability of an individual to use increasingly reduced visual cues to remember 20 figures. Because of the nature of this task, all subjects received the test under the same format.
6. The Representational Stencil Design Test (RSDT), as previously noted, is a procedural variation of the Grace Arthur Stencil Design Test (GASDT) in that the motoric manipulation of the stencils is removed. The experimental group received the RSDT and the two comparison groups received the GASDT form. All groups received the same set of training/practice stencils and set of test stencil designs.

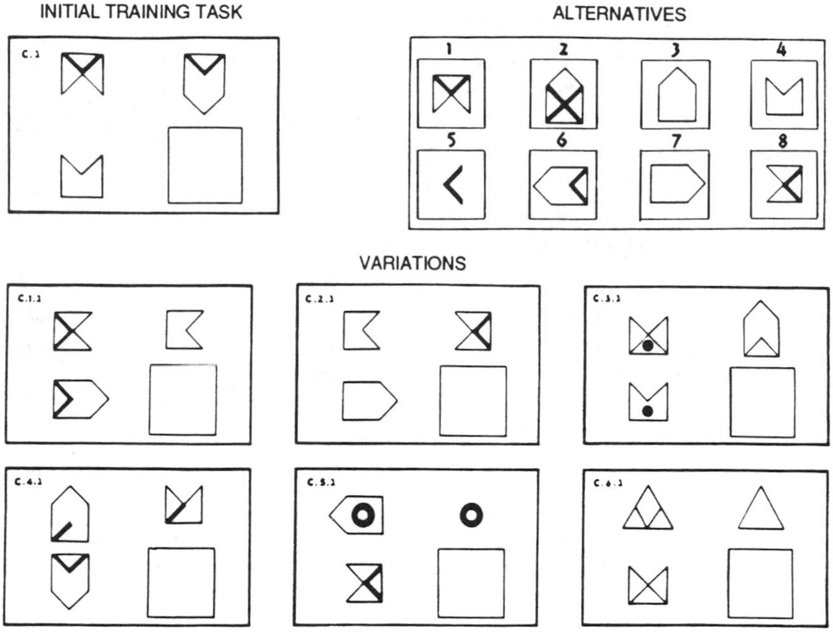

FIGURE 12.1. Example of a Set Variation I problem. The initial task is used for training. The examinee is then given six variations of that problem to assess the effect of training. The pool of alternative responses is the same for all problems.

The nonverbal battery of the Cognitive Abilities Test (CAT) (Thorndike & Hagen, 1979), which consists of three subtests (Figure Classification, Figure Analogies, and Figure Synthesis), served as a pre-post measure and was administered to all three groups under standard psychometric conditions. The Kohs Block Design (Kohs, 1923) was also administered as a pretest-posttest measure. Because impulsive responding was overtly treated in the experimental condition where necessary, the block design served as a device to measure change in "planning" behavior, that is, the number of trials attempted to successfully complete a given design on the test. The purpose of administering both measures was to observe transfer effect along cognitive and/or behavioral dimensions that might occur from treatment.

Results of the experiment indicated a significant main effect for treatment for five of the treatment instruments. Post hoc analysis for contrasts showed that the experimental group had performed significantly better ($p < .01$) than the two comparison groups. The subjects in the elaboration group performed significantly better ($p < .05$) than those in the standard group on two of the five tasks. The only task that did not indicate a significant main effect was the Associated Recall Test. Because of the nature of this instrument, all three groups were administered the task in the same way. Therefore, this instrument served as an internal check with regard to interaction effect.

Post hoc analysis for contrasts on the CAT showed a significant difference ($p < .001$) between the experimental condition and the standard, and a significant difference between the two comparison groups ($p < .01$) in favor of the elaboration group but no significant difference between the experimental and elaborative conditions.

For the Kohs Block Design, a nonparametric sign test was performed on (a) the pre- to posttest increase in the number of designs successfully completed by each individual in each group, and (b) the number of trials from those designs successfully completed on the pretest versus the same designs completed on the posttest. The results of the sign test for design completion indicated a significant increase in the number of designs successfully completed for the experimental group ($p < .01$, $N = 14$) but no significant increase for the other two groups. In terms of number of trials, the sign test indicated a significant decrease in the number of trials used for the experimental group ($p < .05$, $N = 13$) but no significant decrease in trial performance for the other two groups. Keane (1983) noted that a significant limitation of this study was that only one examiner provided treatment across all three groups. This was a necessary limitation because of an absence of examiners who were (a) trained on the theory and practice of the LPAD and (b) conversant in manual communication. To adjust for this, the pretest and posttest measures were counterbalanced as well as internally checked for reliability by two examiners. Keane (1983) noted that the posttest results mitigate examiner bias in the treatment conditions.

Krapf (1985), cognizant of the possible limitations in Keane's (1983) research, attempted to verify and extend the findings of the previous studies with the LPAD. In his study, he focused on one complex cognitive process, figural analogic reasoning. This process was chosen because (a) previous research with deaf individuals on figural analogic and other formal operational tasks indicated negative or conflicting findings when compared with hearing peers (Canabal, 1970; Dicker, 1970; Farrant, 1964; Gupta, 1965), (b) Raven's (1938) contention that problem solving of this nature is "irrespective of previously acquired information" (p. 12), and (c) Raven's (1962) and Jensen's (1969) belief that the level of cognitive abilities inherent in the solution of true analogic problems were not amenable to training. In a pretest-posttest control group design, 45 prelingually deaf subjects between the ages of 12 to 18, with hearing parents, were randomly assigned to one of two treatment conditions or to a control group. The two treatment conditions consisted of an experimental group and a comparison group. In the experimental group, 15 subjects received figural analogic instruments from the LPAD battery as designed by Feuerstein (1979). In the comparison condition, 15 subjects received the same instruments; however, the interaction between the examiner and examinee followed standard psychometric practice. The WISC-R Performance scores for these two groups were 102.7 and 101.8, respectively; the score for the control group was 101.8. The control group received only the pre- and posttest instruments.

Three instruments from the LPAD battery were administered to the two treatment groups. Following is a description of the instruments used:

1. LPAD B8-B12 Variations, consisting of six variations on the last five items in the Raven's CPM. These variations comprise five sets of analogies, six in each set, the first analogy designated for training purposes and the other five functioning as variations of the training analogy.
2. LPAD Set Variations I, previously described.
3. LPAD Set Variations II involves 3×3 matrices with eight alternatives from which to choose. Set II consists of five series in which the initial task in each series contains 10 to 15 variations.

The Advanced Progressive Matrices Set I (APM I) and Set II (APM II) served as the pre-post measures and were administered to all three groups under standard psychometric conditions. The purpose of administering these instruments was to observe transfer of learning to comparable but novel tasks.

Statistical results from analyses of covariance (ANCOVAs) indicated a significant ($p < .001$) main effect for treatment favoring the experimental group on all LPAD treatment tasks. Further, the experimental group performed significantly better ($p < .01$) on the APM Set II than the comparison and control group. Behaviorally, the experimental group showed a 60-minute increase in time-on-task for the APM II from the pretest to posttest. Although the experimental group performed better than the other two groups on the APM I, the difference was not significant. However, this can be explained by the fact that this task contained relatively few (12) items.

Krapf (1985) used two counterbalanced examiners for the treatment conditions as well as the pre- and posttesting. Investigation showed that there was no examiner effect for treatment. This is an important finding because of the nonstandard format for administration of the LPAD and the altered communication interaction with this population.

Overall, the within-treatment and posttest results in Keane's (1983) and Krapf's (1985) research attest to the effect of mediated intervention on the cognitive performance of deaf individuals. Moreover, other indicators emerged from these two studies that also reinforce the effect. Both Keane and Krapf collected a number of demographic variables with the idea that they might impact performance. These variables included degree of hearing loss, age, sex, tested IQ, and academic performance as indicated by standardized reading and math scores. For both studies, age, sex, and degree of hearing loss did not correlate with the outcome variables. The finding that degree of hearing loss was not an impacting variable coincided with a number of other studies. However, the fact that age was not influential in either study contradicted a number of previous findings (Canabal, 1970; Hoemann & Briga, 1980).

In Keane's (1983) study, only IQ score demonstrated a high enough correlation to be used as a covariate in statistical procedures. However, Keane could not enter reading and math scores in a correlation procedure because too many subjects had not received formal testing in these areas as their manifest performance levels were deemed too low. For Krapf (1985), IQ and reading and math achievement scores correlated high enough with the outcome variables for use in statistical procedures. For the experimental, comparison, and control groups, the mean reading scores were 2.92, 3.58, and 3.64, respectively, whereas the mean math scores were 5.66, 5.38, in 6.88, respectively. Clearly, on the whole, the populations in the two studies do not represent high-achieving groups. Based on standard performance measures, Krapf's subjects represent an "average" group. The manifest performance characteristics of the groups in both studies contrast sharply with the demonstrated abilities of these subjects to perform efficiently on highly complex and abstract tasks and to transfer learning when exposed to mediated intervention.

Beyond Statistics

Product outcomes were used by Keane (1983) and Krapf (1985) as comparative measures to demonstrate the effect of mediated intervention on performance. In essence, stress on these product outcome scores is antithetical to the underlying theoretical foundations and actual process of the LPAD. For research, such static approaches are sometimes necessary. However, both Keane and Krapf maintained some anecdotal records regarding student performance. This information, although not empirically based, indicated that some cognitive deficiencies were more prominent that others and that they were pervasive across the range of ages in both studies. More importantly, however, these deficiencies, which inhibit the acquisition of information and knowledge, were highly modifiable. It is this modifiability that is reflected in the product outcome scores.

One other observation noted by both researchers, as well as Feuerstein (1979) in his case studies, is important to cite because of its implications for testing individuals in this population. The subjects in the experimental groups showed marked increases in task-intrinsic motivation during the assessment. At times, this motivation was also observed outside the assessment itself in that a number of students returned to their classes and shared some of their experiences not only with their peers but also with their teachers; this was then reported back to the examiners. The increase in motivation was further documented in Krapf's (1985) finding that the experimental group increased their time-on-task on one posttest resulting in significantly better performance. Further, the control group took more time and performed better (although neither measure was significant) than the standard group which had the availability of treatment as practice on performing analogies. In this study, practice without feedback on these complex tasks was not only ineffective but also detrimental because of a reduction in motivation.

In testing the deaf on standard measures, great care is taken to reduce certain conditions that may negatively influence performance (Hiskey, 1956). For example, researchers attempt to limit the communication requirements of the task. This is important from a conventional psychometric perspective. Conversely, however, the LPAD examiner-examinee relationship and demands of the tasks themselves, require a strong communicative interaction. Braden (1985) cited this as a drawback in implementing the LPAD with the deaf. In contrast, the studies cited above, from both procedural and theoretical positions with deaf populations, support the notion that increased examiner-examinee communication is a positive rather than negative factor impacting both intellective and nonintellective outcomes.

Future Considerations

Moores (1985) has argued that the last vestiges of the deficiency model should be discarded in research and educational practice with the deaf. Justifying poor performance because of deafness is neither appropriate nor useful. In the same sense, however, justifying a lack of difference in cognitive functioning between the deaf and the population-at-large through the evidence of standard performance measures is not realistic in light of the realities of the manifest performance of this population. To better enable the deaf population, an improved coordination between assessment and practice is necessary. The purpose of the LPAD is to provide insight into cognitive modifiability and to show how particular intervention procedures can facilitate learning.

Our society is highly complex, one that undergoes constant change and adaptation. It is not what we know, but how we can learn to know that promotes our ability to adjust to change. This is true for all individuals. Further research and practice with the deaf within the framework of mediated learning experience can provide insight into ways to shape the environment, assessment practices, and intervention procedures that will promote actualization of their evident potential.

References

Altshuler, K., Deming, W., Vollenweider, J., Rainer, J., & Tender, R. (1976). Impulsivity and profound early deafness: A cross cultural inquiry. *American Annals of the Deaf*, *121*, 331–339.

Anderson, R. D., & Sisco, F. H. (1977). *Standardization of the WISC-R for deaf children* (Series T, No 1). Washington, DC: Gallaudet College, Office of Demographic Studies.

Arbitman-Smith, R., Haywood, H. C., & Bransford, J. D. (1984). Assessing cognitive change. In C. M. McCauley, R. Sperber, & P. Brooks (Eds.), *Learning and cognition in the mentally retarded*. Baltimore, MD: University Park Press.

Bonvillian, J., Charrow, V., & Nelson, K. (1973). Psycholinguistic and educational implications of deafness. *Human Development*, *16*, 321–345.

Braden, J. (1985). LPAD aplications to deaf populations. In D. Martin (Ed.), *Cognition, education and deafness* (pp. 124–128). Washington, DC: Gallaudet College Press.

Brill, R. (1962). The relationship of Wechsler IQs to academic achievement among deaf students. *Exceptional Children*, *28*, 315–321.

Brill, R. (1969). The superior IQ's of deaf children of deaf parents. *The California Palms*, *15*, 1–4.

Canabal, J. V. (1970). *Comparison of deaf and normally hearing children on analogy items under different methods of instruction at different age levels*. Unpublished doctora dissertation, St. John's University, New York.

Carlson, J., & Dillon, R. (1978). Measuring intellectual capabilities of hearing impaired children: Effects of testing the limits procedures. *Volta Review*, *80*, 216–224.

Childers, J., Lao, R., & Lingerfelt, M. (1979) *A report of some non-traditional psychological and academic measures among hearing impaired residential students in three southeastern states*. Paper presented at the Southeastern Psychological Association Meeting, New Orleans.

Conrad, R. (1979). *The deaf school child*. London: Harper & Row.

Dicker, L. (1970). *Retardation of 9–14 year old deaf students on the 1938 Raven's Progressive Matrices*. Unpublished doctora dissertation, University of Kansas, Kansas.

Dillon, R. (1979). Improving validity by testing for competence: Refinement of a paradigm and its application to the hearing impaired. *Educational and Psychological Measurement*, *39*, 363–371.

Dillon, R. (1980). Cognitive style and elaboration of logical abilities in hearing impaired children. *Journal of Experimental Child Psychology*, *30*, 389–400.

Farrant, R. (1964). The intellective abilities of deaf and hearing children compared by factor analyses. *American Annals of the Deaf*, *109*, 306–325.

Feuerstein, R. (1979). *The dynamic assessment of retarded performers*. Baltimore, MD: University Park Press.

Feuerstein, R. (1980). *Instrumental Enrichment*. Baltimore, MD: University Park Press.

Furth , H. (1966). A comparison of reading test norms of deaf and hearing children. *American Annals of the Deaf*, *111*, 461–463.

Garcia, J. (1981). The logic and limits of mental testing. *American Psychologist*, *36*, 1172–1180.

Gerweck, S., & Ysseldyke, J. (1975). Limitations of current psychological practices for the intellectual assessment of the hearing impaired: A response to the Levine study. *Volta Review*, 243–248.

Glaser, R. (1981). Education and thinking: The role of knowledge. *American Psychologist*, *36*, 1103–1111.

Gupta, K. P. (1965). *A study of two non-language intelligence tests with deaf subjects in the intermediate and advanced departments of the Kansas School for the deaf*. Unpublished masters thesis, University of Kansas, Kansas.

Harris, R. (1978). The relation of impulse control to parent hearing status, manual communication, and academic achievement in deat children. *American Annals of the Deaf*, *123*, 52–67.

Hiskey, M. (1956). *Nebraska test of learning aptitude with separate standardizations for deaf children and for children with hearing from four to ten years of age*. Lincoln, NE: University of Nebraska.

Hoemann, H., & Briga, J. (1980). Hearing impairment. In J. Kaufmann & D. Hallahan (Eds.), *Handbook of special education* (pp. 222–248). Englwood Cliffs, NJ: Prentice Hall.

Huberty, T., & Koller, J. (1984). A test of the learning potential hypothesis with hearing and deaf students. *Journal of Educational Research*, *78*, 22–27.

Jensen, A. R. (1969). How much can we boost intelligence and academic achievement? *Harvard Educational Review*, *39*, 1–123.

Joiner, L., Erikson, E., Crittenden, J., & Stevenson, V. (1969). Predicting academic achievement of the acoustically-impaired using intelligence and self-concept of academic ability. *Journal of Special Education*, *3*, 425–431.

Katz, M., & Bucholz, E. (1984). Use of the LPAD for cognitive enrichment of a deaf child. *School Psychology Review*, *13*, 99–106.

Keane, K. (1983). *Application of mediated learning theory to a deaf population: A study in cognitive modifiability*. Unpublished doctoral dissertation, Columbia University, New York.

Keane, K. (1987). Assessing deaf children. In C. S. Lidz (Ed.), *Dynamic assessment* (pp. 360–376). New York: Guilford.

Keane, K., & Kretschmer, R. (1987). Effect of mediated learning intervention on cognitive task performance with deaf children. *Journal of Educational Psychology*, *79*, 49–53.

Koehler, L. (1977). *Learning potential assessment of a hearing impaired population*. Unpublished doctoral dissertation, University of Kansas, Kansas.

Kohs, S. C. (1923). *Intelligence measurement*. New York: Macmillan.

Krapf, G. (1985). *The effects of mediated intervention on advanced figural analogic problem solving with deaf adolescents: Implications for dynamic assessment*. Unpublished doctoral dissertation, Temple University, PA.

Lambert, N. M. (1981). Psychological evidence in Larry P. versus. Riles. *American Psychologist*, *36*, 927–952.

Lane, H. (1976). Academic achievement. In B. Bolton (Ed.), *Psychology of deafness for rehabilitation counselors*. Baltimore: University Park Press.

Levine, E. (1974). Psychological tests and practices with the deaf: A survey of the state of the art. *Volta Review*, *76*, 298–319.

Levine, E. (1976). Psycho-cultural determinants in personality development. *Volta Review*, *78*, 258–267.

Levine, E. (1981). *The ecology of early deafness*. New York: Columbia University Press.

Liben, L. (Ed.). (1978). *Deaf children: Developmental perspectives*. New York: Academic Press.

Meadow, K. (1980). *Deafness and child development*. Berkeley: University of California Press.

Meadow, K., & Dyssegard, B. (1983). Social-emotional adjustment of deaf students. Teachers' ratings of deaf children: An American-Danish comparison. *International Journal of Rehabilitation Research*, *6*(3), 345–348.

Mindel, E., & Vernon, M. (1971). *They grow in silence*. Silver Spring, MD: National Association of the Deaf.

Moores, D. (1978). *Educating the deaf: Psychology, principles, and practices*. Boston: Houghton Mifflin.

Moores, D. (1985). Reactions from a researcher's point of view. In D. Martin (Ed.), *Cogniton, education and deafness* (pp. 224–228). Washington, DC: Gallaudet College Press.

Myklebust, H. (1960). *The psychology of deafness*. New York: Grune & Stratton.

Newland, T. (1972). Assessing the cognitive capability of exceptional children *Selected papers from University of Virginia lecture series, 1970–71*. Charlottesville VA: University of Virginia Press.

Olmedo, E. (1981). Testing linguistic minorities. *American Psychologist*, *36*, 1078–1085.

Pintner, R., Eisenson, J., & Stanton, M. (1941). *The psychology of the physically handicapped*. New York: Crofts.

Quigely, S., & Kretschmer, R. (1982). *The education of deaf children: Issues, theory, and practice*. Baltimore: University Park Press.

Raven, J. C. (1938). *Progressive matrices: A perceptual test of Intelligence*. London: H. K. Lewis.

Raven, J. C. (1962). *Guide to the advanced progressive matrices—Sets I and II*. London: H. K. Lewis.

Ray, S. (1979). *An adaptation of "Wechsler Intelligence Scale for Children-Revised" for deaf children*. Unpublished doctoral dissertation, University of Tennessee, Knoxville, TN.

Schlesinger, H., & Meadow, K. (1972). *Sound and sign: Childhood deafness and mental health*. Berkeley: University of California Press.

Sullivan, P. (1982). Administration modifications on the WISC-R performance scale with different categories of deaf children. *American Annals of the Deaf*, *127*, 780–788.

Thorndike, R., & Hagen, E. (1979). *Cognitive abilities test*. Hopewell, NJ: Houghton Mifflin.

Tomlinson-Keasey, C., & Kelly, R. (1978). The deaf child's symbolic world. *American Annals of the Deaf*, *123*, 452–459.

Trybus, R., & Karchmer, M. (1977). School achievement scores of hearing impaired children: National data on achievement status and growth patterns. *American Annals of the Deaf*, *127*, 62–69.

Vernon, M., & Koh, S. (1970). Effect of manual communication on deaf children's educational achievement, linguistic competence, oral skills and psychological development. *American Annals of the Deaf*, *115*, 527–536.

White, K. (1982). Defining and prioritizing the personal and social competencies needed by hearing impaired students. *Volta Review*, *84*, 266–274.

13
Improving the Quality of Instruction: Roles for Dynamic Assessment

Victor R. Delclos, Nancy J. Vye, M. Susan Burns,
John D. Bransford, and Ted S. Hasselbring

Dynamic assessment is a relatively new and promising approach to educational evaluation. The term *dynamic assessment*, as defined in this discussion, refers to attempts to assess individuals' responsiveness to teaching (Feuerstein, Rand, & Hoffman, 1979) or "zone of sensitivity to instruction" (Vygotsky, 1978; Wood, 1980; Wood, Wood, & Middleton, 1978). The methods of assessment are different from those used in standardized, "static" assessments such as intelligence tests and achievement tests, where instruction on the part of the testor invalidates results. In dynamic assessment, instruction is essential. The critical components of dynamic assessment are systematic attempts (a) to change various components of tasks in order to assure that the examinee understands what is required, and (b) to experiment with different approaches to teaching the examinee how to complete the task. Both of these elements are included in order to determine specific instructional techniques that are most effective for each child.

The purpose of this chapter is to explore how dynamic approaches to assessment might help educators to improve students' learning by improving the quality of assessment, placement, and instruction that those students receive. Much of our discussion is based on data that were collected as part of the Dynamic Assessment of Young Handicapped Children research project at Vanderbilt University. We also consider issues that have been raised by the contributors to a book on dynamic assessment that includes chapters from a number of projects (Lidz, 1987a).

Our focus in this discussion is on dynamic approaches to assessment rather than on any specific application of dynamic assessment. This is an important point because there are many different ideas about what dynamic assessment is, when it should be used, and how its results should be interpreted. We will try to clarify some of these differences as we proceed.

We should also note that there are many claims about dynamic assessment that seem to be overblown and hence can discourage serious-minded scholars from examining its potentials. An illustration of this problem comes from a brochure we received announcing a workshop on dynamic assessment. The announcement claims that dynamic assessment is as profound and revolutionary as was the notion of the earth circling the sun, and the discovery of gravity, penicillin, and life on other planets. This would be an exciting claim if it were based on rigorous testing and strong data. Unfortunately, research in the area of dynamic assessment is in its infancy. In terms of analogies to history, we are closer to noticing that there are other planets and that their positions move than we are to discovering the Copernican theory. Nevertheless, even the initial level of insight about stars and planets had a great deal of potential for new avenues of thought in astronomy. We believe that the same is true of the general idea of dynamic assessment for the area of educational psychology. In the discussion below we consider some of this potential.

Most researchers do not argue that a dynamic form of assessment should necessarily replace more traditional forms of assessment. Instead, they assume that dynamic assessment provides information that is not available from static tests. In particular, whereas traditional tests focus primarily on the products of thought, dynamic assessments can provide information about (a) processes used to solve problems, (b) responsiveness to opportunities to learn new strategies and concepts, and (c) appropriate teaching activities for individual children.

Many people who discuss dynamic assessment emphasize the goal of identifying and correcting "deficient cognitive functions" on the part of the child—functions such as systematically searching for information, spontaneously making comparisons, and so forth. In our work, we have found it valuable to attempt to identify and change particular processes that may be hampering performance. However, we place special emphasis on the importance of finding teaching activities and task structures that are most appropriate for individual children. We will elaborate on this point later.

There are several ways in which dynamic assessment can contribute to the quality of instruction. One is directly related to a major argument made in the report of the Panel on Selection and Placement of Students in Programs for the Mentally Retarded of the National Research Council (Heller, Holtzman, & Messick, 1982). The report addresses the need to assess the quality of instruction that students receive in the classroom before deciding that academic difficulties are due to problems with the child. This is an important goal, but it is very difficult to achieve. First, the critical elements of "appropriate instruction" are not easy to define, particularly when we are discussing the needs of individual children. Dynamic assessment can help clarify this issue on a case by case basis. In addition, it is not an easy matter to evaluate instruction in a classroom setting. Again, dynamic assessment can play a role in determining the types of instructional conditions that are most appropriate for each child by varying instructional parameters during the assessment process.

In the discussion that follows we try to clarify how dynamic assessment might be used to improve (a) the validity of the referral and assessment procedures used to assign children to special education, and (b) the quality of the instruction that children receive. We rely on data as much as possible but, as noted earlier, the field is in its infancy and there is a need for more theoretical and empirical work. Later in the chapter, we suggest some important areas for future research.

Information About Responsiveness to Instruction

As an illustration of ways in which dynamic assessment can provide information that is not necessarily available from traditional assessments, consider some research we conducted with young (ages 4 to 8 years), handicapped children (Burns, Vye, Bransford, Delclos, & Ogan, 1986). In one of our first experiments we studied the relationship between static intelligence measures and measures of performance both during and after a session of the training that is included in dynamic assessment. The McCarthy Scales of Children's Abilities were used as the static measure of intelligence. The McCarthy gives a summary score, the General Cognitive Index (GCI), and scale scores in each of the Perceptual Performance, Quantitative, and Verbal areas. The dynamic assessment task was an adapted version of the Grace Arthur Stencil Design Test (Arthur, 1947; Burns, Haywood, & Delclos, 1987).

The instruction that was incorporated into the dynamic assessment using the stencil design task consisted of a series of hints or prompts. The hints were graduated in explicitness, with early hints being more general and subsequent hints being very specific (Campione, Brown, & Ferrara, 1982). After collecting static and dynamic testing performance on a number of children, we calculated two correlations. The first was between each of the McCarthy scores and unaided performance on the stencils following dynamic assessment. The second was between each of the McCarthy measures and the number of prompts needed by the child in order to answer four items correctly. In both sets of correlations we obtained a similar pattern of results (see Table 13.1).

TABLE 13.1. Correlations between McCarthy scores and scores on stencil design task during and after graduated promoting ($N = 44$)

	McCarthy scales			
	General Cognitive Index	Perceptual Performance	Verbal	Quantitative
Unaided performance	.18	.48*	−.05	−.15
Number of hints	−.40*	−.58*	−.20	−.02

*$p < .01$.

There was a moderate association between the Perceptual Performance measure and each of the dynamic assessment measures (one might expect to find the greatest degree of association here because both the static and dynamic measures were derived from tasks in the perceptual performance domain). As shown in Table 13.1, the correlations between GCI and the dynamic measures are less robust (the correlation was nonsignificant for the unaided performance measure, and significant for the number of prompts measure). These smaller correlations seem reasonable when one considers that GCI represents a more diverse set of cognitive skills than the Perceptual Performance scale. None of the other correlations are statistically reliable.

Consider some implications of the obtained correlations. Although it appears that there is a relationship between static and dynamic measures—indeed one would have cause to be suspicious if there was not—it is clear that a child's static score would not be a very reliable indicator of his or her response to instruction (see Lichtenstein, 1981, for further discussion). A slightly different breakdown of the data (plus some data from a subsequent study) makes the point more forcefully.

In Figure 13.1, 77 handicapped children are grouped according to GCI. Groups consisted of children whose GCIs were below 37, from 37 to 52, from 53 to 68, and from 69 to 108. The figure depicts the percentage of children in each group who reached a learning criterion of 75% correct on the stencil design task following dynamic assessment. A substantial number of children in each group reached the criterion after a brief session of instruction during dynamic assessment: 36% of the children with GCIs between 37 and 52 reached the criterion; 53% of the children with GCIs between 53 and 68; 82% of the children with GCIs between 69 and 108; and even in our lowest group, those children scoring below 37, 26% reached the criterion. In spite of the expectation of failure based on their performance on a traditional intelligence test, a sizable number of children in each group were responsive to instruction.

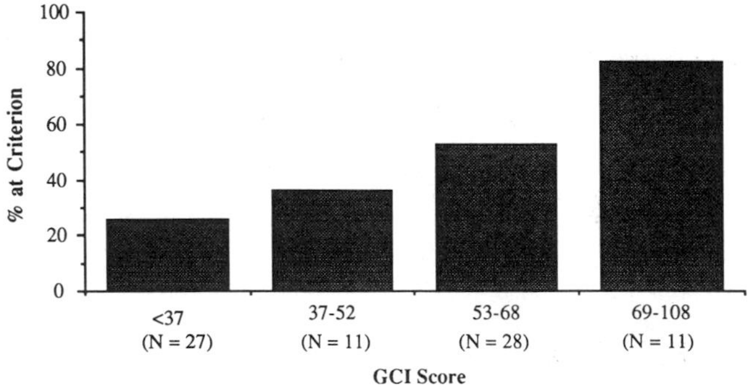

FIGURE 13.1. Percentage of children in each General Cognitive Index (GCI) group who reach the criterion of ≥75% correct on the stencil design task. (Adapted from Lidz, 1987a. Used with permission)

What we would suggest here is that dynamic measures, which allow us to evaluate responsiveness to instruction, provide information beyond that provided by static measures. We have presented correlational data showing at best a moderate relationship between learning and McCarthy scores, and have demonstrated by way of Figure 13.1 that classifying children on the basis of their static scores can provide an erroneous prediction of future performance.

A point about the validity of our dynamic measures should be made here. It has no doubt come to mind that dynamic measures might themselves bear little relationship to subsequent learning and performance. In response we can say that in our research thus far we have found a high degree of correspondence between dynamic assessment and near-transfer performance (Vye, Burns, Delclos, & Bransford, 1987).

Effects on Expectations

The preceding results raise a number of questions. For example, should we assume that students who learned in the context of our brief assessment can function in regular classrooms? If they were referred for assessment because of severe difficulties in the classroom, the answer would certainly be no. However, evidence that a child could learn quite effectively from teaching in a dynamic assessment context lends support to the hypothesis that one important problem was the nature of the instruction.

This shift in the conceptualization of the locus of failure, from the child to the instructional techniques, is an important first step toward changing the focus of the educational assessment and delivery system. For example, many who use dynamic assessment in clinical practice have advocated including parents and teachers as observers of the dynamic assessment session (Haywood, 1985; Jensen & Feuerstein, 1987; Lidz, 1987b). In this way they capitalize on the dramatic and unexpected performance changes that often occur during the assessment and convince the observers of the potential of the child. There are also data in the labeling effects literature that suggest information about children's abilities to learn has important effects on teachers' and parents' expectations about potential to learn (Aloia & MacMillan, 1983; Cooper, 1979).

In a study reported by Delclos, Burns, and Kulewicz (1987), we showed videotaped segments of assessment sessions conducted with moderately handicapped children to two groups of teachers. One group saw two segments of a child during static assessment. The second group saw one segment of static assessment and one segment of dynamic assessment. After viewing each segment, teachers completed a questionnaire in which they rated the child's task-specific performance, task involvement, and general competence. Teachers viewed the children as moderately involved in the assessment task under both static and dynamic condi-

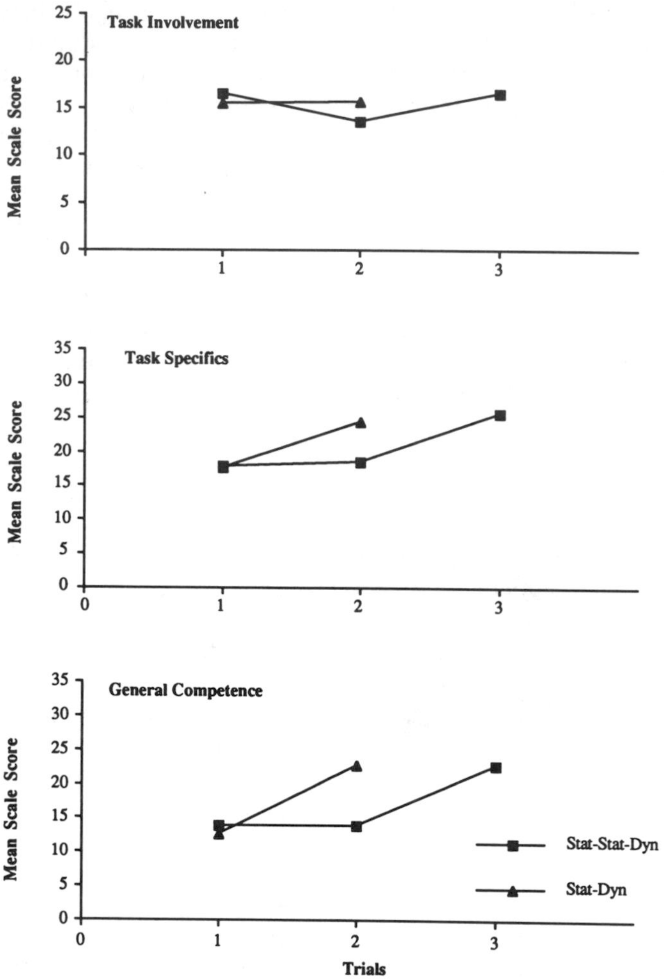

FIGURE 13.2. Teacher ratings of handicapped children viewed on videotaped assessment sessions. (Adapted from Lidz, 1987a. Used with permission)

tions. With regard to task-specific performance and general competence, teachers rated the children rather low after viewing the first segment of static assessment. Those who viewed more static assessment continued to rate the children low, whereas those who saw a dynamic assessment session rated the children much higher. Finally, when the static-static group was shown a third, dynamic segment of tape, their ratings increased to the level of the original static-dynamic group (see Figure 13.2).

The data suggest two conclusions. The first is that dynamic assessment can have a meaningful impact on teachers' expectations of the performance of handicapped children. The second is that the effect may depend on the actual experience of viewing the assessment session, either in person or on videotape. This second point is particularly strong when viewed in contrast to the results of a study by Hoy (1983) showing no such effects when *written* reports of dynamic and static assessments were compared.

The Importance of Different Types of Instruction

Although our data on changes in expectations are quite strong, we doubt that a mere change in expectations is sufficient to have a powerful impact on the quality of the instruction received by students. We suspect that teachers need more systematic information about the kinds of tasks and teaching strategies that seem most useful for individual students.

Earlier, we noted the recommendations of the National Research Council panel concerning the need to evaluate instructional quality (Heller et al., 1982). We argued that this recommendation seemed to be especially important yet could be difficult to implement because of different definitions of quality. Several studies we have conducted show that relatively subtle changes in quality can have strong impact on the degree to which learning and transfer occur.

Extended Work with Individual Students

One area in which we have encountered issues of instructional quality is with children who do *not* do well in the context of relatively brief dynamic assessments. A glance back at Figure 13.1 illustrates that there were a number of children who did not reach our learning criterion. It is also important to note that most research, including that of Brown and Campione (Campione et al., 1982) and our own research group (Vye et al., 1987), excludes these children from further participation in the training phase of the dynamic assessment. Should we conclude that these children have poor potential for learning, or should we look for better procedures for helping them learn? Answers to these questions involve an exploration of the quality of instruction and its effects on learning and transfer.

As an illustration of the importance of instructional quality, consider the results of a single subject design study (Delclos, Burns, & Vye, 1986). Three children (ages 5 to 6 years) took part in the study. All were multiply handicapped (mentally retarded and physically or emotionally handicapped), and none were able to perform the Stencil Design Test after many practice sessions (in one case after as many as 11 practice sessions), or after a brief session of mediational training. At this point we might well have stopped our study and concluded that these children do not profit from direct, one-on-one instruction. This begs the question, however, regarding the type of instruction that should be used. Therefore, we chose to look more closely at the type of instruction we were providing.

To standardize the experimental manipulation, our initial mediational dynamic assessment had been relatively scripted. Each child had been familiarized with the relevant dimensions of the stencils, explicitly taught the rules of the task, and given direct feedback about correct and incorrect responses. Nevertheless, in looking back at videotapes of the sessions, and at the results of the behavior coding scheme that was used (Burns et al., 1987), it became apparent that some aspects of our instruction could be better adapted to meet the individual needs of the children. Figure 13.3 summarizes the results of extended mediation tailored to meet the needs of three handicapped children over periods of up to 25 sessions. One of the children (see Bobby, Figure 13.3) needed careful regulation of motor behavior as part of his mediation, and once this was provided his performance on the stencil task improved considerably—indeed, performance on two uninstructed transfer tasks also improved. Another of the children was provided with guidance on using a model to self-check responses during his mediation (see Craig, Figure 13.3). Again, tailored instruction was followed by performance gains. Furthermore, the tailoring was accompanied by changes in the behaviors that were the focus of the instruction.

In summary, the results point to the importance of the quality of the instruction provided to children. The three handicapped children who initially had been unresponsive to our instruction showed significant improvements in criterion and transfer performance once the instruction was tailored to better meet their learning needs.

Prompting Versus Mediated Instruction

Several additional studies we conducted illustrate the importance of the nature of instruction on children's abilities to learn the stencil design task and to transfer their learning to other tasks. In this work we focused on two methods of instruction. The first involved graduated prompting, an approach developed by Campione and Brown (Campione et al., 1982); the second is an approach we call mediation, and is based on work by Feuerstein (Feuerstein et al., 1979). Our data suggest that mediation has somewhat more of an effect on transfer than the graduated prompting (Burns, 1985; Burns, Delclos, Bransford, & Sloan, 1986; Burns, Vye, et al., 1986), although both are equally effective for improving performance on the instructed task.

The data raise a question about which instructional approach is most appropriate to use, particularly since the choice has profound implications for our assessments of individual children. We suggest that the choice of approach is best made by considering the *purpose* of the assessment. We

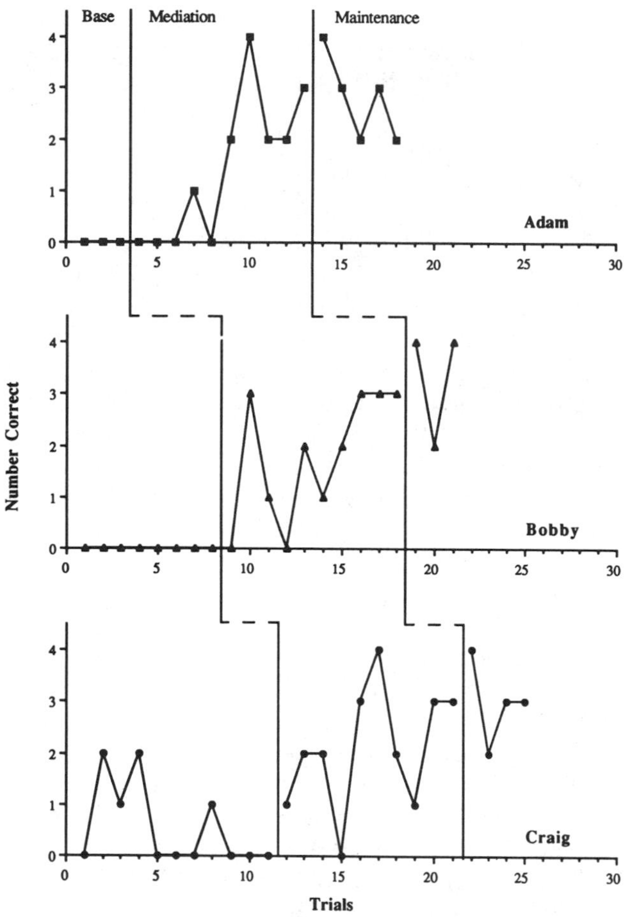

FIGURE 13.3. Results of extended mediation tailored to meet the needs of three handicapped children over periods of up to 25 sessions. Graphs show the number of stencils correct during baseline, mediation, and maintenance. Tailored mediation was introduced at the second mediation session. (Adapted from Lidz, 1987a. Used with permission)

have found that mediation is well suited for our purpose of discovering information about effective instructional strategies for individual children. Graduated prompting, on the other hand, may be better suited to address issues related to classification (Bryant, 1982).

Work on Basic Mathematics Facts

Issues about the quality of instruction have also surfaced in our work with fifth- and sixth-grade students who are math delayed (Hasselbring, Goin,

& Bransford, 1985). One area in which these students have special difficulty is in the ability to remember basic math facts such as 6 + 7 = 13 or 5 + 4 = 9. Difficulties with these facts have a number of ramifications. First, students seem embarrassed to be extremely slow or to have to count on their fingers in order to get answers. Second, students avoid a number of everyday problem-solving situations where knowledge of math facts is required.

Overall, we have found that math-delayed students are considerably slower and use less efficient strategies than students of the same age who are not math delayed. A straightforward way to handle this problem would be to recommend that students practice adding numbers. Although practice is certainly important for learning, our work suggests that it is not always sufficient for producing large gains. A major reason is that many students are using strategies that need to be changed rather than speeded up. By plotting response latency against minimum addends in a computerized test of math facts, we found that individual children may be very fast at providing answers to problems such as 3 + 1 = ? yet slow at other problems such as 8 + 6 = ?. Observations of children solving these problems suggest that the slow response times are due to the children using certain counting strategy to solve the problems.

The strategies students use to solve specific problems have important effects on their ability to learn from practice. Students who use a counting strategy (in most cases students count on their fingers) are not likely to significantly increase their solution speeds as a result of practice because it is difficult to increase the speed by which one can count to oneself. Students who *do* show across-the-board gains in speed and accuracy following extended practice are those who have already memorized the answers to simple addition problems. Drill and practice helps them become faster at retrieving correct answers from memory.

To produce qualitative shifts in strategies, we have been investigating the effectiveness of using a computer intervention. Three features of this intervention are noteworthy. First, it requires rapid responding; the student does not have time to finger count. Second, only a small number of unlearned facts are given to the student at any time. Third, the program uses an expanding retrieval system for presenting problems. That is, a particular problem is presented at increasingly greater lags. Thus, if a student is trying to learn the answer to 7 + 8 = ?, this problem may be presented and then reappear after a learned problem such as 2 + 0 = ?. It would appear next after three intervening problems, next after six intervening problems, and so forth—the lag for repetition keeps expanding. This instructional aspect seems ideally suited for providing practice at retrieving information from long-term memory.

The above research indicates that different children have different instructional needs. First, the effects of simple drill and practice vary considerably depending on the strategies that children are using initially (e.g., counting on their fingers versus retrieving—albeit slowly—from memory). Second, the ability to learn new facts is greatly facilitated by the use of the expanding recall paradigm. For many children, we may have been forced to postulate an inability to learn math facts if we had not attempted to produce qualitative changes in strategies and had not used the expanding retrieval system. The ability to learn can therefore depend heavily on relatively subtle differences in the instructional strategies that are used.

Solving Word Problems

Differences in instructional strategies are also having an effect on our math-delayed students' abilities to solve word problems. In our initial work with these students we presented a variety of word problems and tried to help students learn to solve them. Results were very discouraging, especially because students greatly disliked the task. In later work, we have used video sequences to create meaningful problems such as the need to determine the width of a pit that someone jumps in a movie. Could the students jump such a pit, and how could they accurately estimate its width (Bransford, Sherwood, & Hasselbring, 1986)?

In the problem described above, it is possible to use the actor as a standard of measurement. Thus, students can see that the pit is about two actors wide. In another problem students may see that the pontoons on an airplane are three actors long. By beginning with problems such as these we can focus on the conceptual aspects of problem representation and problem solving rather than immediately begin with difficult numbers. This helps eliminate the "number grabbing" that math-delayed students often exhibit and replace it with "concept driven" thinking. We have also been able to maintain the students' interest in learning to solve word problems. More complex numbers are introduced gradually. Given this procedure, our initial data indicate that the students' potentials to learn to think mathematically appear to be much greater than one would have assumed if only traditional word problems were used.

Theoretical Perspectives and Needs for Further Research

Studies such as those described above convince us that students may benefit considerably from new approaches to instruction. In addition, the results suggest that dynamic assessment procedures can play an important role in tailoring instruction to the needs of the individual child.

From a theoretical perspective, our results suggest that instructional quality will depend on at least two important factors. One involves the degree of "mediation" that is present during the instruction. We saw that mediation-based instruction that includes teaching of both task-specific and general strategies enhances task and transfer performance (Burns, 1985). These data are consistent with many other studies that illustrate the importance of "metacognitive" approaches to instruction (e.g., Bransford, Sherwood, Vye, & Reiser, 1986; Brown, Bransford, Ferrara, & Campione, 1983; Palincsar & Brown, 1984). It is important to note, however, that the success of these approaches requires a continual monitoring of children's processes. From this perspective, effective instruction involves a continual dynamic assessment and subsequent modification of instructional strategies that can help children learn.

The other factor involved in instructional quality involves decisions about the structure of the tasks that we give to children. Decisions about tasks are an important part of theories of dynamic assessment. For example, Feuerstein and colleagues' "cognitive map" provides important guidelines for deciding upon appropriate tasks (e.g., Feuerstein et al., 1979; Jensen & Feuerstein, 1987). In our work, we find that changes in the structure of various tasks have had an important effect on learning. In the stencil design task, for example, some of our tailored mediation required changes in task structure. Similarly, our work with math facts and the ability to solve word problems has involved some important changes in the nature of the tasks that children are asked to perform. Without these changes, a metacognitive approach to teaching seems to have much less of a positive effect.

An article by Burton, Brown, and Fischer (1984) provides an interesting illustration of the need to consider task structure as well as teaching style. They discuss the goal of helping people learn to ski effectively. The development of the "graduated length method" (GLM) of teaching skiing a number of years ago was a breakthrough that made successful and enjoyable skiing available to thousands of people who had not previously been considered candidates for participation in the sport.

In the GLM method, several elements of the task are carefully and systematically manipulated by a skillful coach so that the learner skis in a series of increasingly complex situations, each requiring an extension of the skills learned in the previous, less complex environment. So, a novice skier is given very short skis, no poles, and is put on a gentle slope. The short skis make turning easier and allow practice in developing rhythm, an essential component of successful control. The lack of poles helps the student to focus on balance and on the movement of the skis. The gentle terrain greatly reduces the frightening speed that novices often experience on steeper slopes and allows them to build confidence and to practice important movements that are critical for success on the more demanding slopes. In the course of training, the GLM coach analyzes the performance of the learner at each level of instruction and makes decisions about when and what to change based on the successes and failures of the student. Gradually, longer skis are introduced; wider, narrower, or steeper slopes are presented; the snow conditions are also varied; poles are added.

All of these changes are made at points when the coach decides they will help either to advance the student to the next level or to make the student aware of precisely what they are doing wrong. For example, the coach might have the student ski in soft, powdery snow so that a lack of rhythmic turning could be clearly visible in the tracks left by the skis, or, if the student was not using the skis properly in negotiating turns, the coach might move them to an icy area, where the proper use of the edges of the skis is critical in staying upright.

Many approaches to instruction emphasize the types of teaching or mediating activities required for effective learning. However, they often fail to address the need to analyze, and perhaps change, the structure of the task or the instructional context. These latter approaches are analogous to the method used to teach skiing before the development of the GLM method, when instructors attempted to teach in the context of long skis, steep slopes, etc. If one used the results of these efforts to estimate the people's potential to learn to ski, the conclusion would be that many people cannot succeed.

An analysis of skiing suggests that there must be an effective teaching strategy and a coach who understands the process of learning to ski. However, there is a need to consider task structures as well. The use of short skis, gentle slopes, and so forth helped coaches create a more effective environment within which their instructional strategies could be used. Similarly, we have found it useful to change the structure of tasks involving stencil design and math as we conduct dynamic assessments of children's abilities to learn from instruction.

The goal of creating effective instructional environments is a major challenge for education, but evidence suggests that it is possible to do so and certainly worth the effort (see also Bransford, Sherwood, Vye, & Reiser, 1986). Research on dynamic assessment can play an important role in helping us understand (a) the processes of mediation and (b) the structure of the environments in which this mediation may occur.

Acknowledgments. Preparation of this paper was supported by Grant No. G0083C0052 awarded to Vanderbilt University by the United States Department of Education. We wish to acknowledge the assistance of our research assistants, Brigid Barron, Ron Buen, Randi Glorski, Laura Goin, Rich Johnson, Stan Kulewicz, Kim Sloan, Deborah Stephens, and Julie Tapp, and the staff and children of Metropolitan Nashville Public School System. We would also like to thank other members of our research group, including H. Carl Haywood, Robert Sherwood, and Susan Williams.

References

Aloia, G. F., & MacMillan, D. L. (1983). Influence of the EMR label on initial expectations for regular-classroom teachers. *American Journal of Mental Deficiency*, *88*(3), 255–262.

Arthur, G. (1947). *A point scale of performance tests*. New York: Psychological Corporation.

Bransford, J. D., Sherwood, R. D., & Hasselbring, T. S. (1986). *Computers, videodiscs and the teaching of thinking*. (Technical Report No. 86.1.1). Nashville, TN: Peabody College of Vanderbilt University.

Bransford, J. D., Sherwood, R., Vye, N. J., & Reiser, J. R. (1986). Teaching thinking and problem solving: Suggestions from research. *American Psychologist*, *41*(10), 1078–1089.

Brown, A. L., Bransford, J. D., Ferrara, R. A., & Campione, J. C. (1983). Learning, remembering and understanding. In J. H. Flavell & E. M. Markham (Eds.), *Carmichael's manual of child psychology* (Vol. 1, pp. 77–166). New York: Wiley.

Bryant, N. R. (1982). *Preschool children's learning and transfer of matrices problems: A study of proximal development*. Unpublished master's thesis, University of Illinois.

Burns, M. S. (1985). Comparison of "graduated prompt" and "mediational" dynamic assessment and static assessment with young children. (Technical Report No. 2). In *Alternative assessments of handicapped children*. Nashville, TN: John F. Kennedy Center for Research on Education and Human Development, Vanderbilt University.

Burns, M. S., Delclos, V. R., Bransford, J. D., & Sloan, K. (1986). Performance and behavior of young children in different types of dynamic assessment. (Technical Report No. 7). *Alternative assessments of handicapped children*. Nashville, TN: John F. Kennedy Center for Research on Education and Human Development, Vanderbilt University.

Burns, M.S., Haywood, H. C., & Delclos, V. R. (1987). Young children's problem-solving strategies: An observational study. *Journal of Applied Developmental Psychology*, *8*(1), 113–121.

Burns, M. S., Vye, N. J., Bransford, J. D., Delclos, V. R., & Ogan, T. A. (1986). Static and dynamic measures of learning in young handicapped children. (Technical Report No. 8). *Alternative assessments of handicapped children*. Nashville, TN: John F. Kennedy Center for Research on Education and Human Development, Vanderbilt University.

Burton, R. R., Brown, J. S., & Fischer, G. (1984). Skiing as a model of instruction. In B. Rogoff & J. Lave (Eds.), *Everyday cognition: Its development in social context*. Cambridge, MA: Harvard University Press.

Campione, J. C., Brown, A. L., & Ferrara, R. A. (1982). Mental retardation and intelligence. In R. J. Sternberg (Ed.), *Handbook of human intelligence* (pp. 392–490). New York: Cambridge University Press.

Cooper, H. M. (1979). Pygmalion grows up: A model for teacher expectation communication and performance influence. *Review of Educational Research*, *61*(3), 389–410.

Delclos, V. R., Burns, S., & Kulewicz, S. J. (1987). Effects of dynamic assessment on teachers' expectations of handicapped children. *American Educational Research Journal*, *24*(3) 325–336.

Delclos, V. R., Burns, M. S., & Vye, N. J. (1986). Dynamic assessment of moderately handicapped children: A single subject design approach. Unpublished manuscript. Vanderbilt University, Nashville, TN.

Feuerstein, R., Rand, Y., & Hoffman, M. (1979). *The dynamic assessment of retarded performers: The learning potential assessment device: Theory, instruments, and techniques*. Baltimore: University Park Press.

Hasselbring, T., Goin, L., & Bransford, J. D. (1985). *Assessment and prescriptive teaching with elementary grade children*. Unpublished paper presented at annual meeting of American Association on Mental Deficiency, Philadelphia, PA.

Haywood, H. C. (1985). *The malleability of intelligence: Cognitive processes as a function of polygenic-experiential interaction*. Unpublished paper presented as keynote address to the National Association of School Psychologists, Las Vegas, NV.

Heller, K. A., Holtzman, W. H., & Messick, S. (Eds.) (1982). *Placing children in special education: A strategy for equity*. Washington, DC: National Academy Press.

Hoy, M. P. M. (1983). *The perceived value of the standard psychological report compared with the Learning Potential Assessment Device report*. Unpublished dissertation, University of Iowa.

Jensen, M. R., & Feuerstein, R. (1987). Dynamic assessment of retarded performers with the Learning Potential Assessment Device: From philosophy to practice. In C. S. Lidz (Ed.), *Dynamic assessment: Foundations and fundamentals*. New York: Guilford.

Lichtenstein, R. (1981). Comparative validity of two preschool screening tests: Correlational and classificational approaches. *Journal of Learning Disabilities*, *14*(2), 68–72.

Lidz, C. S. (Ed.) (1987a). *Dynamic assessment: Foundations and fundamentals*. New York: Guilford.

Lidz, C. S. (Ed.) (1987b). Introduction chapter. In C. S. Lidz (Ed.), *Dynamic assessment: Foundations and fundamentals*. New York: Guilford.

Palincsar, A. S., & Brown, A. L. (1984). Reciprocal teaching of comprehension-fostering and comprehension monitoring activities. *Cognition and Instruction*, *1*, 117–175.

Vye, N. J., Burns, M. S., Delclos, V. R., & Bransford, J. D. (1987). Dynamic assessment of intellectually handicapped children. In C. S. Lidz (Ed.), *Dynamic assessment: Foundations and fundamentals*. New York: Guilford.

Vygotsky, L. (1978). *Mind in society: The development of higher psychological processes*. Cambridge, MA: Harvard University Press.

Wood, D. (1980). Teaching the young child: Some relationships between social interaction, language, and thought. In D. Olson (Ed.), *The social foundations of language and thought*. New York: W. W. Norton.

Wood, D., Wood, H., & Middleton, D. (1978). An experimental evaluation of four face-to-face teaching strategies. *International Journal of Behavioral Development*, *1*, 131–147.

14
A Dynamic Assessment for Undergraduate Admission: The Inverse Relationship Between Modifiability and Predictability

Ian M. Shochet

This chapter[1] describes research on the use of a dynamic assessment technique as a possible aid in determining undergraduate admission for disadvantaged South African students. These are black students who have been severely educationally disadvantaged under the apartheid system of segregated schooling. Embedded within this research is the extension of dynamic assessment into two areas, namely (a) as a technique suitable and adaptable for a young adult undergraduate student population, and (b) as an assessment device that can shed light on the vexed problem of undergraduate academic prediction for disadvantaged students.

It will be shown in the course of this chapter that a dynamic assessment technique is certainly suitable and applicable even to an undergraduate population. In addition, although the assumptions underlying dynamic assessment and that of predictive research are clearly antithetical, this chapter demonstrates a possible role for dynamic assessment in the predictive process. It will provide a possible model whereby dynamic assessment can enhance an understanding of academic prediction in a way that does not undermine the central assumptions of dynamic assessment. Instead, it supports the basic critique of static predictors by showing that one can identify a subgroup of modifiable disadvantaged students for whom static predictors are specifically invalid, and that there is an inverse relationship between modifiability and predictability.

To introduce this research, it is necessary to describe the context of this study and the rationale for using dynamic assessment.

The Context of the Study

Education under the system of apartheid in South Africa has been rigidly segregated in the schools and the universities along racial grounds. After the nationalist government came to power in 1948, statutes were passed

[1] This chapter is based on work presented for a doctoral dissertation to the School of Psychology at the University of the Witwatersrand, Johannesburg, South Africa.

in the 1950s and early 1960s to explicitly divide school and university education into separate racial authorities.

More recently, however, there have been some developments with regard to university education. Changes in government policy have made it possible for the first time since 1959 for previously white universities to admit all students regardless of race. In South Africa there are a number of universities that refer to themselves as "open universities." These universities have been energetically resisting segregation since 1953 as a blatant infringement of academic freedom. One of these universities is the University of the Witwatersrand (Wits) situated in Johannesburg where this study was conducted. Wits University has welcomed (in principle) the opportunity to admit students of all race groups purely on merit.

The university, however, is now faced with the problem of appropriately discerning the merit of students who have matriculated from black schools. There has been a chronic and tremendous disparity in the allocation of resources between white schools and black schools.[2] Students from black schools in South Africa can unequivocally be considered to be disadvantaged in relation to their white counterparts, revealing a clear-cut division between advantaged and disadvantaged students. Therefore, it would be discriminatory to judge the relative merit of the two groups of students on scholastic criteria only. (This had been the criterion for admission when this study was conducted.) A brief look at the extent of the educational disparity will elucidate the above assertion.

From its inception, black education in the schools was deliberately and explicily designed to be both segregated and inferior. The following quotation from Verwoerd, the cabinet minister who was in charge of black education, encapsulates the early attitude toward black education.

> There is no place for him (the black man) in the European community above the level of certain forms of labour . . . for that reason it is of no avail for him to receive a training which has as its aim absorption in the European community, where he cannot be absorbed. Until now he has been subjected to a school system which drew him away from his own community and misled him by showing him the green pastures of European society in which he was not allowed to graze.
>
> Verwoerd (1954, p. 23)

Since then, black education has continued to be separate and inferior leading to an inevitable crisis of major proportions. In the year in which this research was conducted, it was estimated that close to 130,000 black scholars were boycotting classes in rejection of apartheid education (*Rand Daily Mail*, 1984).

---

[2] Black schools refer to schools governed by the Indian, "colored," and African education authorities.

In that same year, the government per capita expenditure for African education was only 11% of the amount spent on white education. (For "colored"[3] schools and Indian schools, the amount was 33% and 59%, respectively.)

It is not surprising, therefore, that according to recent statistics, for every 100 black pupils enrolling in grade 1, approximately 50 complete primary school (the equivalent of the seventh grade in the United States) and only ten reach standard 10 (the equivalent of the 12th grade). Of the ten who reach standard 10, only five pass and only one gains the matriculation exemption entitling him or her to go to university (*Weekly Mail*, 1987).

Under the circumstances, a very compelling moral argument can be made for not using the same scholastic criteria for the admission of white students and black students. What is the meaning of the word "merit" in the kind of system described above? It can be argued that it takes a scholar of such merit to jump over the hurdles of black education and complete 12 grades so as to warrant almost an automatic admission. Clearly, the school results of black students cannot be an indication of future academic potential.

However, even if one is a staunch antagonist of affirmative action, there are also strong technical or psychometric reasons for rejecting school results as the criterion for black admissions. Put very simply, the school results for black students (particularly those from African schools) have no predictive validity. In an unpublished study conducted by the present author, the correlation between school matriculation results and grade average for disadvantages students was .15 (as opposed to .55 for advantaged students). This means in essence that with regard to prediction the matriculation results following a disadvantaged education have the same value as a random number.

Thus, it can be seen that the open universities in South Africa (like Wits) are faced with the vexed question of finding alternative admissions criteria for disadvantaged students. At this juncture, let us examine the "wisdom" that has been handed down from countries like the United States that have been faced with a similar problem with regard to admission of minority students.

Undergraduate Academic Prediction—The Need for a New Paradigm

Countless studies have been conducted over the years linking cognitive and intellectual skills to academic success at undergraduate level. In essence, the rationale behind this body of research is that these tests

[3] "Colored" is the term used by the government in South Africa to designate people of mixed races.

measure intelligence or aptitude which, in turn, predicts academic success. This is an ostensibly simple rationale, yet this issue has been the focus of a long-standing intelligence debate.

Given that this rationale makes all kinds of assumptions about the static and stable nature of intelligence, it is not surprising that the field has been spinning in its own tracks. In fact, the field of "culture-fair" testing for university admissions is faced with the same anomolies and ad hoc hypotheses as it was 20 years ago. In the words of Kuhn (1962), it can be considered a paradigm in crisis and ripe for a "scientific revolution." A brief look at the state of the art will demonstrate the accuracy of this assertion.

By far the most extensively used aptitude test for undergraduate admission in the United States is the Scholastic Aptitude Test (SAT). The use of this test, though widespread, has been extremely controversial with regard to predictive, population, and construct validity.

There is some conflict about the overall predictive validity of the SAT but the sway of research is clearly uncovering a decline in its predictive validity over the past two decades (Aleamoni & Oboler, 1978; Dalton, 1976; Hartman & Bell, 1978; Hosseini, 1978; Houston, 1983; McDonald & Gawkoski, 1979; Slack & Porter, 1980). No one reason for the decline in the validity of the SAT can be isolated. Most suggestions put forward have invoked statistical arguments such as restriction of range or a lack of linearity (Hosseini, 1978). Surprisingly, the underlying assumptions of aptitude tests have never been cited as a possible problem.

With regard to the question of population validity, alternatively referred to as "test bias," the situation is even more bleak. The field is fraught with empirical and theoretical conflicts. Two fundamental questions have been raised. First, do the aptitude tests developed in the United States have the same predictive validity for black and white students? Second, can the same regression line be used for black and white students or would it represent an overprediction or an underprediction for black students?

No agreement has been reached in the literature on these issues. With regard to the strength of the predictive validity, at best we can say that the test predicts equally badly for white and black students (Breland, 1979; Flaugher, 1970). At worst, the test has little bearing for black students and sometimes even a negative relationship (Baggaley, 1974; Sedlacek, 1976; Sedlacek & Brooks, 1972).

With regard to the second question of whether the same regression line should be used for white and black students, the research is again conflicting. One body of research suggests that aptitude tests overpredict for black students and therefore if we used the same regression line, there would be a bias in favor of black students (Breland, 1979; Cleary, 1968; Kallingal, 1971; Zeidner, 1987). Other researchers have claimed that the tests underpredict for black students and to use the same equation would be unfair for black students (Baldwin, 1977; Davis & Temp, 1971; Farver, Sedlacek, & Brooks, 1975; Institute for Services to Education, 1983; Pfeifer & Sedlacek, 1971, 1974; Sedlacek, 1976).

Thus, on purely statistical grounds there is no agreement as to whether the SAT overpredicts, underpredicts, or simply does not predict for black students in the United States. In the 1970s, there was a desperate scramble to find statistical manipulations of regression coefficients to overcome test bias (e.g. Cleary, 1968; Darlington, 1971; Linn, 1973; Thorndike, 1971). These attempts, as Hunter and Schmidt (1976) point out, were simply statistical operations representing different ethical and political principles.

Some attempts have been made to look at alternative aptitude tests and other intelligence measures such as the Ammons Quick Test (Houston, 1983), the American College Test (Aleamoni & Oboler, 1978), or tests of abstract categorical reasoning (Leirer, Dawes, De Petris, & Furukawa, 1980). These attempts have not provided the magical solutions.

Thus, without even taking into account the assumptions of the fairness of static intellectual predictors, in purely statistical terms the field is in disarray. Incredibly, however, few people have questioned the assumptions underlying intellectual predictors or their construct validity. The assumptions are so deeply embedded that strict adherence to them seems quite illogical. For example, Sanford (1981) argues inexplicably that "an inability to predict who will graduate from college does not negate either the validity of the IQ model and its significance for college admission or the need for further research in the area" (p. 17).

Some researchers, however, are questioning the underlying assumptions of static intellectual predictors. Jencks and Crouse (1982) argued that the entire notion of "aptitude" testing in the SAT has to be reexamined. They pointed out that the SAT does not measure future performance but simply current levels of academic achievement and that the test ought to be relabeled an achievement test. They cynically suggested that the only reason why this cannot be done is that it would make too many people angry as they would feel as though they have been hoodwinked.

In addition, there is a body of research in higher education that recognizes the importance of cognitive process rather than product (Astin, 1979; Cloete & Shochet, 1986; Entwistle, 1984; Marton & Säljö, 1976; Nisbet, Ruble, & Schurr, 1982; Pask, 1976; Svensson, 1977; Watkins, 1984). These authors have been concerned with either isolating the important processes of thinking and problem-solving necessary for higher education or finding indices that would measure the capacity for growth. Astin (1979) sums up this argument:

> Most important is that there are probably no existing selection devices that adequately reflect the students' *potential* to benefit from the collegiate experience.

Lacking such measures, it might be argued that we should stick to traditional admissions tests until something better is found. The problem with this argument is that the negative effects of tests in college are not benign: they operate to the particular disadvantage of those minority groups who represent the most disadvantaged segment of our society . . . While I have no magical solution for this problem, selective institutions in the public sector might want to consider experimenting with alternative selection procedures identifying students with the greatest potential for *growth* and *learning*. (pp. 9, 14)

The present study is an attempt to take up precisely that challenge. The field of dynamic assessment, particularly Feuerstein, Rand, and Hoffman's (1979) work, provides the important theoretical model from which to proceed.

Dynamic Assessment and Undergraduate Prediction

The question now arises as to how the concept of dynamic assessment, as articulated by Feuerstein and his colleagues, could be used in the framework of prediction. Feuerstein et al. (1979) began their illuminating work on dynamic assessment by juxtaposing the concepts of "predictability" versus "modifiability." They specifically reject predictive approaches that imply a static view of intelligence in favor of educational modifiable approaches. (The theory underpinning dynamic assessment has been articulated in earlier chapters, especially chapters 1 to 4.) It is clear that dynamic assessment grew up as an antithesis to static predictive approaches. How then is this study proposing to synthesize the two approaches, as there are very few precedents on the use of dynamic assessment within the framework of prediction?

Dynamic assessment is clearly not neutral to the field of prediction. It has as part of its aim the deliberate attempt to show that intelligence is not static but modifiable, and that static intelligence measures will not predict future academic performance. Thus, dynamic assessment has a relationship with the field of prediction, albeit an inverse relationship. The relationship is one of demonstrating the unpredictability of future academic success by means of a static measure, wherever it can be shown that the static measure is not a reflection of the individual's intellectual potential. Therefore, it should be possible to show that the *more* modifiable the intellectual functioning, the *less* valid will be the predictiveness of the static measures.

No attempt has been made, to date, to empirically validate this claim on the part of dynamic assessment. In this section I will describe how this study tries to operationalize and demonstrate this relationship. This is a relationship that serves the dual purpose of extending dynamic assessment into prediction while also providing an important critique of static approaches to prediction.

Feuerstein et al. (1979) point out that one must distinguish between "manifest" and "potential" intellectual performance because they believe that cognition is modifiable at all ages of cognitive development.

This distinction and belief in modifiability stems from Feuerstein's view of the etiology of intellectual functioning. Feuerstein argues that the development of intellectual structures is a function of the quality and quantity of mediated learning experiences (MLE) received by the individual. This he considers to be the most immediate proximal etiology. Distal factors (such as poverty and poor parental education) can influence the amount of MLE people receive, but not determine it. In addition, the phenomenon of deficient functioning as a result of poor MLE is reversible through the provision of MLE at any age or stage of development.

Thus, for the disadvantaged students in the present study, the manifest level of intellectual functioning can be considered modifiable regardless of the severity of distal factors such as the formal educational disadvantage described earlier.

In agreement with Feuerstein, for the disadvantaged students a static measure would only indicate manifest functioning and not capacity, aptitude, potential, or modifiability. The way to assess potential or modifiability is through the use of a dynamic assessment technique. In the course of the dynamic assessment, the examiner would interact with the student and provide the appropriate mediation and teaching to help overcome weaknesses encountered in the static administration.

Thus, for the present study, students were assessed twice on the same cognitive test in order to derive three separate operational constructs. On the first occasion, students were given the test in the traditional static form. The result of this testing is known as the *traditional score* and the construct is called the *manifest intellectual function*.

On the second occasion (following immediately after the first), students were administered the same test in an enriched, dynamic way. The enrichment took the form of mediation and teaching (e.g., modeling, providing feedback) to help overcome difficulties encountered in the traditional administration. (See details in the next section.)

This condition of administration is known as the *enriched condition*. This is a term borrowed from Gordon (1972) and Haywood and Switzky (1974). These researchers enriched the standardized traditional form of the similarities subtest by adding three more exemplars (e.g., "In what way are a pear, peach, plum, apple, and banana alike?"). They found that there was an increase in score under the enriched testing condition which they interpreted as the "intellectual potential" for verbal abstraction once input deficits were overcome by the stimulus-enrichment procedure.

Thus, the score from the enriched condition is known as the *enriched score* and the construct is called *potential intellectual* functioning.

The difference between the traditional score and the enriched score represents the *modifiability* of the student. It is an assessment of the extent and ease with which the individual benefited from the mediation provided in the enriched condition of testing. Thus, the modifiability of the individual is estimated by the *difference score* (enriched score minus traditional score).

In sum, therefore, there are three separate constructs to serve as possible predictors in this study:

1. Manifest intellectual functioning—traditional score;
2. Potential intellectual functioning—enriched score;
3. Modifiability—difference score.

The question now arises as to how these constructs and scores interact to predict academic success and in which ways the dynamic measures (enriched score or difference score) can play a role.

In the first instance, it will have to be shown that the enriched condition significantly modified the students' functioning. Dynamic assessment has never been done before at the university level and therefore successful modifiability cannot be assumed. Thus, the first expectation of the present study was that the enriched condition of testing would enhance students' scores when compared to the traditional static condition. If this can be established, then the next step would be to determine whether the dynamic assessment scores could play a role in prediction. From both a conceptual and statistical standpoint, there are two possibilities by which dynamic assessment could inform the predictive process, namely either as a main effect or as a moderator effect.

For a main effect, one would have to show that the dynamic predictors of the enriched condition directly predicted university success. Thus, either the enriched score or the difference score would be directly correlated with university success. This kind of effect, however, would be inconsistent with the tenets of dynamic assessment, as it would imply that the results of the dynamic assessment are also immutable and static or stable enough to predict over time. It is probably for this reason that dynamic assessment has not been used in the context of prediction.

There is another way in which dynamic assessment could enhance prediction, namely through a moderator effect. In this instance, the scores from the dynamic assessment could indirectly enhance prediction by identifying those individuals for whom the static traditional scores are valid predictors and for whom they are not valid.

It is argued, therefore, that the academic success of disadvantaged students who are *more* modifiable (i.e., have a greater difference score) would be *less* predictable by the static traditional score. Conversely, the academic success of the less modifiable disadvantaged students should be more predictable by a static traditional measure.

Thus, the second expectation of this study was that the more modifiable the intellectual functioning of disadvantaged students, the less their manifest level of intellectual functioning would predict their university success.

This is precisely the inverse relationship to prediction that has been implied in dynamic theory but has never been shown empirically; namely, that intelligence is not static but mutable and, to the extent that it can be modified, the static measure will not indicate future success.

Method

Design

The present study consisted of subject variables, predictor variables, and criterion variables:

1. *Subject variables*. The sample consisted of 104 advantaged and 52 disadvantaged male and female first-year Bachelor of Arts students. The advantaged students were students who were schooled under the South African white education systems (or in private schools). The disadvantaged students were students schooled under the black education systems. The mean age of the sample was 19.6 years.
2. *Predictor variables*. The students were tested prior to the start of the academic year on a test known as the Deductive Reasoning Test. The test was first administered in its static traditional form and then immediately afterward the test was readministered in the dynamic enriched condition. *Thus, all of the students were exposed to both the traditional and enriched conditions*. This generated three predictor variables:
   (a) Deductive Reasoning, Traditional—DR/T (manifest intellectual functioning);
   (b) Deductive Reasoning, Enriched—DR/E (potential intellectual functioning);
   (c) Deductive Reasoning, Difference—DR/D (modifiability).
3. *Criterion variables*. The criterion for the above variables was prediction of academic success over a period of 1 year, i.e., at the end of their first year of study. Two alternative criteria were used, namely, the number of credits the students obtained (Credits), and the average grade obtained by students at the end of their first year (Average).

Testing Material

The important point of departure for the present study is the group dynamic assessment procedure of the enriched condition. The procedure adopted for the dynamic assessment was based on the concepts and techniques that Feuerstein uses in the Learning Potential Assessment Device (LPAD; Feuerstein et al., 1979). It must be emphasized, however, that the present study did not use any of Feuerstein's LPAD instruments or materials. Instead, a local test normed on South African students was used (namely, the Deductive Reasoning Test); this was then operationalized for dynamic assessment based on Feuerstein's constructs, techniques, and ideas (Feuerstein, et al., 1979; Feuerstein, Rand, Hoffman, & Miller, 1980).

The Deductive Reasoning Test is a test of deductive syllogistic reasoning designed by Verster (1973) of the National Institute for Personnel Research in Johannesburg. The test consists of 36 nonsense syllogisms consisting of two premises from which students have to draw the correct conclusion, e.g.,

All airplanes are huge.
Some people are airplanes.
∴ Some people are huge.

There were four reasons for choosing this test.

1. Feuerstein's LPAD model requires that tests or tasks must be constructed in such a way that the learning obtained on earlier items facilitates the individual's capacity to solve subsequent items. In other words, the mediation received must be generalizable to subsequent items. To facilitate this transfer of learning from one item to another, it is imperative that the test be internally consistent with regard to the requirements of the task. In terms of Feuerstein's cognitive map, this means that the test must not measure a mixture of "operations" in ever-changing "modalities." Instead, what is required is that the test measure the same basic operation within the same modalities while the "level of complexity" and the "level of abstaction" might vary. The Deductive Reasoning Test fits these requirements.
2. Feuerstein considers syllogistic reasoning to be an important cognitive operation and a prerequisite for academic success. In his intervention program for cognitive modifiability called Instrument Enrichment (IE), he has included a 60-page training "instrument" (consisting of pencil and paper problem solving tasks) designed to teach syllogistic reasoning (Feuerstein, et al., 1980, pp. 251–255). Embedded within syllogistic reasoning are other important operations for university success such as part-whole relationships and classifications. In addition, one needs to have a range of cognitive functions intact to perform these operations, such as systematic exploration, need for precision, receptive verbal tools, spontaneous comparative behavior, and hypothetical thinking. Thus, it would appear that the Deductive Reasoning Test calls upon a wide range of cognitive skills required for the synthesis of university material.
3. An important consideration was to choose a test that was at the appropriate level of complexity. This test had been normed on white graduate students. It was a fairly complex test that provided reassur-

ance that a ceiling effect would not be obtained in the enriched condition of testing.

4. The reliability of the test was high with a KR_{21} (with Tucker's correction) of .919 (Verster, 1973, p. 13). Thus, fluctuations in test scores as a result of the enriched condition could not simply be attributed to the unreliability of the test.

Procedures

Both the traditional and enriched form of the test were administered in a group format. The procedure for the traditional administration followed the standardized instructions outlined in the test manual.

The challenge for the present study was to determine the appropriate mediation in the enriched condition. Before this could be done, it was necessary to gain total familiarity with the test in order to understand the cognitive processes involved in solving the problems. The present author had previously administered the Deductive Reasoning Test to 18 disadvantaged students. An error analysis was conducted to determine the deficient cognitive functions students typically exhibited so that the mediation in the enriched condition could anticipate these difficulties and address them.

In the course of addressing these deficient functions, many of Feuerstein's criteria for the provision of mediated learning experiences (Feuerstein, et al., 1979, 1980; Feuerstein & Hoffman, 1982) were drawn upon. These included (a) an intention to mediate and to make the mediation transferable and transcendent from the immediate problem at hand, (b) the regulation of behavior through the inhibition of impulsivity (e.g., by providing an anticipation for the complexity of the task), and (c) the mediation of a sense of competence and challenge. For example, the introduction to the enriched condition was as follows:

Now you have all had an opportunity to do the deductive reasoning test. Some of you might have enjoyed it and some of you might have found it very difficult.

We are going to be doing this test again except this time we will be doing it quite differently; therefore, even if you found it difficult you will probably enjoy it this time around.

I am now going to be giving you some hints on how to do these problems. These hints will not only help you with these problems but will provide you with useful logic tools which will help you throughout your university years—especially in the Arts Faculty. One of the things that you are constantly asked to do is to discuss somebody else's theory or argument. As these theories can often be based on faulty logic, it is important that you understand something about the nature of logic and logical reasoning.

You might be wondering why it is that we are doing this test twice in a row. Essentially, what I am interested in in all these tests is your *potential*, in other words what you are capable of learning if taught properly. The previous test did not measure that at all. The reason I gave it to you though was because I want to compare how well you did in that test to how well you are capable of doing if given adequate teaching. So don't feel discouraged if you don't get all the items correct. All you need to try to do is to improve your previous score.

The procedure in this test is going to be very different from the previous test. You will not be doing this whole test at your own pace. In fact, we are going to be doing the first ten questions one question at a time.

After each of these questions, I will be telling you the correct answer and that will help you to solve subsequent questions. In addition, I will be giving general hints in the first few questions on how to do this type of problem. So the procedure will work like this: I will tell you when so start doing the first problem or question and, after a period of time, I will tell you to stop and mark down your answer, if you have not done so already.

The enriched condition was then divided into three phases: intensive mediation, minimal mediation, and nonmediation.

In the intensive mediation (items 1–5), students would attempt an item and commit themselves to an answer. At the end of each item, the mediator would provide the solution and model how the item should have been solved. The mediator would provide the students with a rudimentary use of the Venn diagram as a pictorial aid to representing and solving the syllogisms. In the course of the mediation, the mediator would examine alternative incorrect answers, anticipate the cognitive deficiencies that might result in errors, and address these. During the intensive mediation, there were two periods of repetition and summing up. Feuerstein places heavy stress on the importance of a repetitive experience in the formation of cognitive schemata.

In the minimal mediation phase (items 5–10), students were simply given the correct answer to the item after they had committed themselves and then time to reflect on where they went wrong (if they went wrong). In the nonmediation phase (items 11–36), students simply continued at their own pace without any mediation.

The traditional administration of the test lasted approximately 45 minutes. The enriched condition took approximately 2 hours.

The scoring procedure was to calculate the unweighted raw scores obtained by the student. Thus, a maximum score of 36 for the traditional or enriched score could be obtained.

Results and Discussion

Did the Enriched Condition Improve Performance

A large part of the study would have been rendered irrelevant if the mediation provided had had no effect on the students' scores. Therefore,

TABLE 14.1. The t test for paired differences between the traditional and enriched scores of the Deductive Reasoning Test.

Sample	Mean DR/T	Mean DR/E	Mean DR/D	t
All ($N = 156$)	16.89	20.93	4.13	10.96**
Disadvantaged ($N = 52$)	12.06	16.42	4.23	6.62**
Advantaged ($N = 104$)	19.31	23.18	4.07	8.69**

** $p < .01$.

it was important to determine whether there were significant differences between the scores on the traditional and enriched testing conditions.

To assess the effects of the enriched testing condition, a t test for paired differences for dependent samples was computed (Pfeiffer & Olson, 1981), comparing the differences in scores between the traditional (DR/T) and enriched (DR/E) conditions.

The enriched condition of administration succeeded in significantly improving students' performance (Table 14.1). It must be emphasized here that the mean DR/D score does not reflect how dramatic some of the improvements were. The DR/D scores ranged from −10 (one isolated individual) to 18, with a standard deviation of 4.7.

This finding, therefore, supports the first expectation of the study. The most immediate and important implication is that a dynamic assessment technique can be made operational for a young adult student population. This indicates that it is valid to make an assumption of modifiability of intellectual functioning for this age group regardless of the educational disadvantage that students have experienced.

It is important to point out that the enriched testing condition took less than 2 hours, yet significant and sometimes dramatic improvements were made. This test in its static form (with a high reliability) was thought to be measuring some immutable intellectual trait.

This evidence of modifiability is yet another study in a growing body of research (Feuerstein et al., 1980; Feuerstein et al., 1981; Messerer, Hunt, Meyers, & Lerner, 1984) to show the cognitive modifiability of individuals at all ages. Feuerstein et al. (1980) specifically rejects the concept of a "critical period" for cognitive development in favor of an "optimal period" (p. 69). Reversibility of deficient functioning can occur in Feuerstein's view because the immediate (proximal) etiology is a lack of mediated learning experiences and not the distal immutable factors over which one has little control (such as apartheid).

Did the Scores of the Enriched Condition Directly Predict Success (i.e., Main Effect)?

As mentioned, if the scores of the enriched condition predicted through a main effect, it would be inconsistent with the central assumption of

TABLE 14.2. Pearsons correlations between the Predictor and Criterion variables for the advantaged and disadvantaged students.

	Advantaged ($N = 92$)		Disadvantaged ($N = 49$)	
Predictor	Credits	Average	Credits	Average
DR/T	−.13	−.04	.25	.26
DR/E	−.19	−.08	.03	.03
DR/D	−.07	−.07	−.26	−.29*

* $p < .05$ (two-tailed).

dynamic assessment. Analyses were conducted to determine whether this was indeed the case.

The first part of the analysis was to assess any direct correlations between the predictor variables and the criterion. The correlations shown in Table 14.2 reveal a negative answer to the above question for both the advantaged and disadvantaged students. These results indicate that none of the predictors correlated positively with university success for either the advantaged or disadvantaged students. In fact, the only significance at this stage seems to be a weak negative correlation between DR/D and university success for disadvantaged students. If one ended the analyses at this point, one would have to conclude that the more modifiable the disadvantaged students, the poorer is the prognosis for success (albeit an extremely weak correlation)!

Multiple regression analyses were conducted to ascertain whether any of the predictors would predict if one partialed out or held constant the effect of other predictors. No linear combination altered the basic picture found in the zero-order correlations.

Did the Enriched Condition Indirectly Contribute to Predictions Through a Moderator Effect?

An important question is whether the modifiability (DR/D) of the students moderates the relationship between the static traditional predictor (DR/T) and university success. The second expectation was that the predictiveness of the manifest intellectual functioning would be moderated by the students' modifiability.

Zedeck (1971) and Zedeck, Cranny, and Vale (1971) described two possible statistical ways by which to examine a moderator effect. The first is by means of a moderated multiple regression analysis and the second is by means of subgrouping. In a moderated multiple regression analysis, the predictor variable (DR/T), whose predictiveness the researcher believes is likely to be moderated, is put into the equation, together with the variable the researcher thinks might moderate the predictor (DR/D)

TABLE 14.3. Moderated multiple regression to determine if the construct of "modifiability" moderates the predictiveness of the traditional intelligence measure for disadvantaged students. Model: Credits, Average = DR/T, DR/D, DR/T × DR/D.

	a Criterion = Credits			b Criterion = Average		
Predictor	beta	$F(1/45)$	p	beta	$F(1/45)$	p
DR/T	0.12	6.81	.012*	0.53	3.72	.060
DR/D	0.14	1.37	.248	0.16	0.05	.822
DR/T × DR/D	−0.02	3.47	.069	−0.05	0.85	.363
	Multiple $R^2 = 0.192$*			Multiple $R^2 = 0.165$*		

* $p < .05$.

and the cross products (DR/T × DR/D). All three possible combinations of these variables are then considered simultaneously.

Thus, the following moderated regression models were computed separately for advantaged and disadvantaged students: Criteria (Credits, Average) = DR/T; DR/D; DR/T × DR/D. The finding for the advantaged students was clear; the multiple R^2 of the moderated multiple regression model was nonsignificant.

The results for the disadvantaged students yielded very important features.

In Table 14.3, it can be seen that the multiple R^2 on both criteria was significant at the .05 level. Second, the moderator or interaction term (DR/T × DR/D) approached significance on the criterion of credits ($p = .069$). In addition, with the moderator term in place, DR/T had a significant beta weight against the criterion of Credits and approached significance against the criterion of Average ($p = .06$). This was only because the students for whom DR/T did not predict had been partialed out in the moderator/interaction term. Also, with the moderator term in place, DR/D no longer had a negative relationship with either of the criteria (it had a positive beta weight). In the zero-order correlation of Table 14.2, it appeared as if DR/D had a negative relationship with university success. Thus, it would seem that the real and more important function of the modifiability of the disadvantaged students was as a moderator of the relationship between DR/T and university success.

The subgrouping analysis demonstrates the result even more clearly. The disadvantaged student population was divided into two subgroups. Those who fell below the mean modifiability score (DR/D ≤ 4) were called the "less modifiable" students and those above were called the "more modifiable" students. The correlations between DR/T and the criteria for these subgroups are shown in Table 14.4, which very clearly demonstrates the moderator effect of DR/D uncovered in the moderated multiple regression. For the "less modifiable" subgroup (i.e., less than the mean on DR/D), there were significant positive correlations between DR/T and the criteria, explaining 30% of the variance in Credits. For the

TABLE 14.4. Correlations between DR/T and the criteria for the "more modifiable" and "less modifiable" disadvantaged students subgrouped on the DR/D mean score.

Level of modifiability	N	DR/T × Credits	DR/T × Average
Less modifiable (DR/D ≤ 4)	29	.55**	.50**
More modifiable (DR/D ≥ 5)	20	−.22	−.08

$^{**}p < .01$.

"more modifiable" students, there were small nonsignificant negative correlations.

Fischer's r–to–z transformations were computed to determine whether the differences in the correlations between the two subgroups were significant. The differences between the correlations for the "less modifiable" and "more modifiable" groups were significant at the .05 level on the criterion of Credits and on the criterion of Average.

This result supports the second espectation: *The more modifiable the intellectual functioning of disadvantaged students, the less their manifest level of intellectual functioning will predict university success, and vice versa.*

The theoretical and practical implications of these findings are discussed primarily with respect to the disadvantaged students in whom the effect was found. Some hypotheses about the advantaged students are presented at the end of the discussion.

Theoretical Implications

From a theoretical standpoint, these findings have demonstrated a role for dynamic assessment in the field of academic prediction for disadvantaged populations. The role is to identify those more modifiable disadvantaged students for whom a static intellectual assessment is specifically invalid. Notably, this role for dynamic assessment does not conflict with its central tenets, but provides critical empirical support for Feuerstein's critique of static assessment approaches.

Had a main effect occurred with any of the measures in the enriched condition, the educational modifiable underpinnings of dynamic assessment would have been undermined. Such a result would have implied that the measurements that were generated in the enriched conditions (the constructs of "potential intellectual functioning" and "modifiability") were measuring a static entity that could predict over a period of a year. Although this measure might have been fairer to certain individuals than the traditional test, it would still have meant that the students' intellectual potential was a stable quantity that could be measured and could predict performance in the future. Thus, hypothetically speaking, instead of the concept of general intelligence ("g"), one would have had the concept of "g potential." Such a static measure would imply that two students with the same enriched score have the same potential. This is certainly not the case. It is easy to see that exposing the two students to yet another period of teaching/enrichment/mediation and then retesting them would bring about differences in their scores.

At this point, the question arises as to whether it is at all possible to measure "potential intellectual functioning" and whether this is a valid construct. It is argued with hindsight that the construct of "potential intellectual functioning" as operationalized in the present study was not a valid construct. It is important to be reminded here that although Feuerstein has discussed the concept of potential, strictly speaking he has not written about the measurement of potential intellectual functioning but rather about the assessment of modifiability. Feuerstein equates intelligence with modifiability, and to have a separate construct called "potential intellectual functioning" may well have been a violation of his tenets.

It is proposed here that it is not helpful for future researchers to try to "measure potential." Potential implies something that is latent but has not yet emerged. It certainly takes one out of psychology and into metaphysics to determine whether or not one can measure something that is not yet manifest. Feuerstein's Learning Potential Assessment Device is probably a misnomer and would better be called an assessment of modifiability.

Modifiability was found in this study to be a crucial construct for the disadvantaged students. It played the important role of identifying two separate subgroups (more modifiable versus less modifiable) that behaved completely differently with regard to prediction. The more modifiable disadvantaged students behaved in the same way as the advantaged students in that none of the intellectual measures was valid for this subgroup.

The reason why the less modifiable disadvantaged students' university scores were predictable on the basis of the DR/T can be explained quite simply in Feuerstein's terms. The less modifiable students are less susceptible to being modified during a period of 1 year, either by direct exposure to stimuli or by mediated learning experiences. For those students, the test was measuring a range of cognitive skills that were stable enough to predict over a period of 1 year. Essentially this meant that less modifiable disadvantaged students who were initially high functioning on the traditional test did well, even though they were not readily modifiable; students who were low functioning and not readily modifiable did badly at the university.

Whether this traditional measure would have predicted over a longer period for the less modifiable disadvantaged students is a question unanswered by the study. It must be emphasized here that by referring to the students as "less modifiable" (rather than nonmodifiable) the implication is that these students are still modifiable but that more investment or a different type of MLE is necessary to elicit the modifiability.

The reason why the more modifiable students' performances did not predict to the criteria can also similarly be explained in Feuerstein's terms. Although DR/T was still measuring an important range of cognitive skills, its measurement of these skills in more modifiable students was not meaningful. Within a very short period, the more modifiable students demonstrated in the enriched condition that what was being measured in the traditional test was not a reflection of their skill in the range of cognitive areas being tested. This supports precisely what Feuerstein has been arguing for some time about traditional psychometry. Tests of manifest level of functioning are not meaningful predictors for individuals who have been mediationally deprived in some way or another but who are nevertheless modifiable. Not only are people modifiable, they can be shown to be modifiable and it can be shown that when they are modifiable, their manifest functioning does not predict future success.

Many critics of the proponents of dynamic assessment might have considered Feuerstein's assumption of modifiability and the distinction between manifest and potential performance as a misguided philanthropic gesture, to give mediationally deprived individuals a second chance. The results of the present study show that it is not only unfair to rely on static measures of intellectual functioning but also inaccurate in that the test was predictively invalid for the more modifiable disadvantaged students. One hopes that this channel of support is one that geneticists and classical psychometricians will not ignore because it relates to predictive validity, which is squarely in their own paradigm. It must create some concern about the possibility that traditional tests have been used as predictors on a global basis when for one-half of the sample (more modifiable individuals) they have been predictively invalid.

Is it not possible that this is the reason why the field of undergraduate academic prediction might be in such disarray? Population validity and test bias might need to be extended not only to gross population groups (such as white or black) but even to population subgroups (such as more modifiable versus less modifiable). The present research is consistent with the growing evidence that it is not possible to find predictors that are universally applicable. Perhaps it is time to admit students on the basis of different predictors, even if this is a problematic and complex political issue.

This study lends weight to the growing critique of the construct validity of the SAT and other intellective predictors. Jencks and Crouse (1982) argued that the SAT is not an aptitude test but an achievement test totally dependent on previous performance. If we extrapolate from the present study, it could be argued that in every intake of students sitting for the SAT, many of them are modifiable disadvantaged students for whom the SAT is an invalid predictor. Maybe if we could find a way to identify these students and treat them separately, the predictive validity of the SAT might improve. To do this we have to shift paradigms toward dynamic assessment techniques.

Some psychometricians may wish to argue that what is being demonstrated in the moderator effect of modifiability is nothing new but is simply the age-old issue of reliability. For those students who made significant gains in the enriched condition, the traditional test could simply be said to be unreliable. Psychometricians have known for years that unreliable measures do not predict.

This argument is a dangerous one for them to raise because it rebounds onto the weakness in their own paradigm. Psychometric principles do not distinguish between reliability and unreliability for individual examinees. This in fact is precisely what the present study has done. As a consequence, it raises a concern about the strength of psychometric claims that particular tests are considered reliable for populations or even subpopulations. There are modifiable individuals being tested within these populations for whom the test might be unreliable. (Possibly this study suggests that it might be necessary and appropriate to get an index of reliability for every individual examinee.)

Practical Implications

Wits University in South Africa has repeatedly confirmed its commitment to admitting all students of merit. The discerning of merit among students disadvantaged under the apartheid system is extremely difficult. The findings of the present study provide only a part of the solution to this problem, but in doing so suggest how not to proceed and possibly how to proceed in the future.

The moderator effect of "modifiability" on the predictability of DR/T means that the criterion performance of the less modifiable disadvantaged students is predictable on the basis of their DR/T scores. The clearest way to see this is to refer to the subgrouping analysis presented in Table 14.4.

The students who scored below the mean on DR/D (i.e., the less modifiable students) had a correlation between DR/T and Credits of .55. Thus, for these less modifiable disadvantaged students, 30% of their variance in success could be explained by DR/T. This is as high as the variance explained by school matriculation results for advantaged students. DR/T could legitimately have been used as an alternative admissions criterion for these students.

From this research there remains a category of more modifiable disadvantaged students for whom no predictors exist. What this research has shown is that it is all very well to diagnose disadvantaged students as "more modifiable," but their success or failure at university would then depend on whether this uncovered potential could be facilitated through educational intervention. Some of the "more modifiable" students did not do very well and some did extremely well.

From a practical admissions perspective, one could look at the modifiable students from two different paradigms: (a) from a classical predictive paradigm, and (b) from Feuerstein's educational modifiable paradigm. From a classical predictive paradigm, one could say that here is a subgroup of students for whom no predictors exist. Further research must be conducted to find alternative predictors for this group of students. In the interim, their admission to the university is a risk. It is worth selecting at random a few of these students in order to do the urgent research.

The classical predictive approach, therefore, involves searching for more factors inside of the modifiable disadvantaged students that will render them successful or unsuccessful. This is essentially a deficit model as it involves trying to isolate the deficits within the modifiable disadvantaged students who failed, and to ensure that similar students are not admitted in the future.

From educational modifiable perspective one would argue that here is a subgroup of disadvantaged students who have demonstrated their modifiability. Some of these students passed and others failed. The real question therefore is: What does the university need to do to ensure the success of modifiable disadvantaged students?

This latter approach, therefore, is not a deficit approach. It acknowledges the strengths of modifiable disadvantaged students and aligns itself with those strengths. It shifts the responsibility from the students to the institution.

Some might argue that it is unfair to place the burden of responsibility onto the university. It must be remembered that these students are a very special subgroup. They are grouped together because they have all demonstrated their learning potential or their modifiability in a range of cognitive skills. Thus, it is a subgroup categorized by learning potential rather than by some other descriptors such as race, sex, or age, which are no indication of the students' strengths.

The present author has done related research that showed that the single best "predictor" of university success for disadvantaged students was whether or not they received academic support (e.g., study skills, English for academic purposes, subject support). Wits University has a very good academic support program. It would have been far more useful if the enriched condition had yielded more sophisticated information about the modifiable students' processes of thinking so that one could tailor an intervention program accordingly, to respond to such questions as:

1. What were the students' profiles of efficient and deficient functioning?
2. What aspect of the mediation did the students respond to?

3. What needs to be done to fulfill the students' learning potential, and do the facilities to intervene currently exist?

These are questions that are not classically pursued in predictive research, but it was argued that it was necessary to bring prediction and education even closer together than was done in the present study.

Finally, one puzzle unsolved by the present study is why none of the intellectual measures predicted criterion scores for the advantaged students, and why "modifiability" did not serve as a moderator for this group. As mentioned, there is a growing body of research that shows that the overall predictiveness of intellectual measures is declining. Secondly, it could be argued that for people who have had adequate schooling their prior scholastic experience and achievement can offset (at least in the first year) some variations in "intellectual functioning." It is possible that these intellectual measures might distinguish between successful and unsuccessful advantaged students in later years of study. The advanced years require of students to draw more heavily on conceptual, abstract cognitive processes. If this is the case, then it may well be that this prediction could be moderated by the students' modifiability. Only further research could verify this assertion.

Conclusion

In the first instance, the present study has shown that a dynamic assessment technique can be made operational for young adult university students. Modifiability is a life-long phenomenon and should be assessed at all ages. In addition, the present study has brought together the seemingly antithetical paradigms of prediction and dynamic assessment. The advocates of the dynamic assessment paradigm, with its stress on education and modifiability, have rejected static predictive approaches and thus have not explicitly attempted research in the field of prediction.

I have argued that dynamic assessment and prediction are implicitly in a dialectical relationship. There is essentially an inverse relationship between modifiability and predictability. This relationship has never been tested or validated empirically. The present research provides the first step toward empirically evaluating this relationship, namely, the more modifiable, the less predictable.

The static paradigm of prediction for undergraduate admissions has not been successful. The failure of this paradigm can be considered to be its incapacity to interact with the field of education. In drawing the relationship between modifiability and predictive validity, the present study has shown that prediction and education are inseparable.

References

Aleamoni, L. M., & Oboler, L. (1978). ACT versus SAT in predicting first semester GPA. *Educational and Psychological Measurement*, *38*, 393–399.

Astin, A. W. (1979). *Testing in the post "Bakke" period*. San Francisco: Address presented at the Annual Meeting of the American Educational Research Association. (ERIC Document Reproduction Service No. ED 171 820.)

Baggaley, A. R. (1974). Academic prediction at Ivy League college moderated by demographic variables. *Measurement and Evaluation in Guidance*, *6*(4), 232–235.

Baldwin, A. Y. (1977). Tests can underpredict: A case study. *Phi Delta Kappan*, *58*(8), 620–621.

Breland, H. M. (1979). *Population validity and college entrance measures*. (Research Monograph No. 8). New York: College Entrance Examination Board. (ERIC Document Reproduction Service No. ED 177 999.)

Cleary, T. A. (1968). Test bias: Predictions of grades of Negro and white students in integrated colleges. *Journal of Educational Measurement*, *5*, 115–124.

Cloete, N., & Shochet, I. M. (1986). Alternatives to the behavioural technicist conceptions of study skills. *Higher Education*, *15*, 247–258.

Dalton, S. (1976). A decline in the predictive validity of the SAT and high school achievement. *Educational and Psychological Measurement*, *36*, 445–448.

Darlington, R. B. (1971). Another look at "culture-fairness." *Journal of Educational Measurement*, *8*, 71–82.

Davis, J. A., & Temp, G. (1971). Is the SAT biased against black students? *College Board Review*, *81*, 4–9.

Entwistle, N. (1984). Contrasting perspectives on learning. In F. Marton, D. Hounsell, & N. Entwistle (Eds.), *The experience of learning* (pp. 1–19). Edinburgh: Scottish Academic Press.

Farver, A. S., Sedlacek, W. E., & Brooks, G. C., Jr. (1975). Longitudinal predictions of university grades for blacks and whites. *Measurement & Evaluation in Guidance*, *7*(4), 243–250.

Feuerstein, R., Rand, Y., & Hoffman, M. B. (1979) *The Dynamic assessment of retarded performers: The Learning Potential Assessment Device, theory, instruments and techniques*. Baltimore: University Park Press.

Feuerstein, R., Rand, Y., Hoffman, M. B., & Miller, R. (1980). *Instrumental Enrichment: An intervention program for cognitive modifiability*. Baltimore: University Park Press.

Feuerstein, R., & Hoffman, M. B. (1982). Intergenerational conflict of rights: Cultural imposition and self-realization. *Journal of the School of Education/Indiana University*, *58*(1), 44–63.

Feuerstein, R., Miller, R., Hoffman, M. B., Rand, Y., Mintzker, Y., & Jensen, M. R. (1981). Cognitive modifiability in adolescents: Cognitive structure and the effects of intervention. *Journal of Special Education*, *15*(2), 269–287.

Flaugher, R. L. (1970). *Testing practices, minority groups, and higher education: A review and discussion of the research*. Princeton, NJ: Educational Testing Service. (ERIC Document Reproduction Service No. ED 063 324.)

Gordon, J. E. (1972). Intellectual potential in mentally retarded persons: Effects of stimulus enrichment in verbal abstraction and verbal learning. (Doctoral dissertation, George Peabody College for Teachers, 1972.) *Dissertation Abstracts International*, *33*, 1789b–1790b.

Hartman, W. T., & Bell, D. P. (1978). The predictive value of the Stanford University admission rating system. *College and University*, *53*(3), 289–290.

Haywood, H. C., & Switzky, H. N. (1974). Children's verbal abstracting: Effects of enriched input, age, and IQ. *American Journal of Mental Deficiency*, *78*, 556–565.

Hosseini, A. A. (1978). The predictive validity of the Scholastic Aptitude Test of the National Organization for Education Evaluation of the Iranian Ministry of Sciences and Higher Education for a group of Iranian students. *Educational and Psychological Measurement*, *38*, 1041–1047.

Houston, L. N. (1983). The comparative predictive validity of high school rank, the Ammons Quick Test, and two scholastic aptitude test measures for a sample of black female college students. *Educational and Psychological Measurement*, *43*, 1123–1126.

Hunter, J. E., & Schmidt, F. L. (1976). Critical analysis of the statistical and ethical implications of various definitions of "test bias." *Psychological Bulletin*, *83*, 1053–1071.

Institute for Services to Education. (1983). *Predicting the academic success of black students attending the historically black colleges. Part 2 of the research program on problems relating to the desegregation of higher education.* Wahsington, DC. (ERIC Document Reproduction Service No. ED 193 344.)

Jencks, C., & Crouse, J. (1982). Aptitude vs. achievement: Should we replace the SAT? *The Public Interest*, *67*, 21–35.

Kallingal, A. (1971). The prediction of grades for black and white students of Michigan State University. *Journal of Educational Measurement*, *8*, 263–265.

Kuhn, T. (1962). *The structure of scientific revolutions*. Chicago: University of Chicago Press.

Leirer, V. O., Dawes, R., De Petris, J., & Furukawa, K. (1980). *Grade point average and reasoning ability*. Montreal: Paper presented at the Annual Convention of the American Psychological Association. (ERIC Document Reproduction Service No. ED 198 457.)

Linn, R. L. (1973). Fair test use in selection. *Review of Educational Research*, *43*, 139–161.

Marton, F., & Säljö, R. (1976). On qualitative differences in learning: I—Outcome and process. *British Journal of Educational Psychology*, *46*, 4–11.

McDonald, R. T., & Gawkoski, R. S. (1979). Predictive value of SAT scores and high school achievement for success in a college honors program. *Educational and Psychological Measurement*, *39*, 411–414.

Messerer, J., Hunt, E., Meyers, G., & Lerner, J. (1984). Feuerstein's instrumental enrichment: A new approach for activating intellectual potential in learning disabled youth. *Journal of Learning Disabilities*, *17*(6), 322–325.

Nisbet, J., Ruble, V. E., & Schurr, K. T. (1982). Predictors of academic success with high risk college students. *Journal of College Student Personnel*, *23*(3), 227–235.

Pask, G. (1976). Styles and strategies of learning. *British Journal of Educational Psychology*, *46*, 218–248.

Pfeifer, C. M., Jr., & Sedlacek, W. E. (1971). The validity of academic predictors for black and white students at a predominantly white university. *Journal of Educational Measurement*, *8*(4), 253–261.

Pfeifer, C. M., Jr, & Sedlacek, W. E. (1974). Predicting black student grades with nonintellectual measures. *Journal of Negro Education*, *43*(1), 67–76.

Pfeiffer, K., & Olson, J. N. (1981). *Basic statistics for the behavioral sciences*. Chicago: Holt, Rinehart, and Winston.

Rand Daily Mail. (1984, September 19). Johannesburg: South African Associated Newspapers.

Sanford, T. R. (1981). *Predicting college graduation for black and white freshman applicants*. Washington D.C.: Paper presented at the Annual Meeting of the Association for the Study of Higher Education. (ERIC Document Reproduction Service No. ED 203 806.)

Sedlacek, W. E. (1976). *Should higher education students be admitted differentially by race and sex: The evidence*. (Research Report No. 5-75.) College Park, MD: Maryland University, Cultural Study Center. (ERIC Document Reproduction Service No. ED 119 558.)

Sedlacek W. E., & Brooks, G. C., Jr. (1972). *Predictors of academic success for university students in special programs*. College Park, MD: Maryland University, Cultural Study Center. (ERIC Document Reproduction Service No. ED 073 222.)

Slack, W. V., & Porter, D. (1980). The Scholastic Aptitude Test: A critical appraisal. *Harvard Educational Review, 50*, 154–175.

Svensson, L. (1977). Symposium: Learning processes and strategies. III—On qualitative differences in learning: Study skill and learning. *British Journal of Educational Psychology*, *47*, 233–243.

Thorndike, R. L. (1971). Concept of culture-fairness. *Journal of Educational Measurement*, *8*, 63–70.

Verster, J. M. (1973). *Test administrators manual for deductive reasoning test*. Johannesburg: National Institute for Personnel Research.

Verwoerd, H. F. (1954). *Bantu education policy for the immediate future*. (Report No. 7/6/1954). Pretoria: Government Press.

Watkins, D. (1984). Learning strategies as threshold variables in the prediction of tertiary grades. *Educational and Psychological Measurement*, *44*, 523–525.

Weekly Mail. (1987, October 16). Johannesburg: Weekly Mail Publishers.

Zedeck, S. (1971). Problems with the use of moderator variables. *Psychological Bulletin*, *26*(4), 295–310.

Zedeck, S., Cranny, C. J., & Vale, C. A. (1971). Comparison of "joint moderators" in three prediction techniques. *Journal of Applied Psychology*, *55*(2), 234–240.

Zeidner, M. (1987). Test of cultural bias hypothesis: Some Israeli findings. *Journal of Applied Psychology*, *72*, 38–48.

15
Assessing the Learning Potential of Penitentiary Inmates: An Application of Feuerstein's Learning Potential Assessment Device

HARRY SILVERMAN and MARY WAKSMAN

A wide variety of tests and assessments have been employed in efforts to examine the relationships between cognitive functioning and criminal behavior. In their review of the literature in this area, Ross and Fabiano (1985) identified four different philosophical frameworks, each of which generated a different assessment procedure. These assessment procedures fall into two categories: direct assessment and indirect assessment.

Direct Assessment

Direct assessment relies on individuals' self-reports of their thinking while viewing a motion picture or a videotape (Schwartz & Gottman, 1976) or while completing problem solving inventories (Heppner & Peterson, 1978). Such self-reports by prison inmates have often revealed such cognitive inefficiencies as distortion in perception, inaccuracies in output, overgeneralization, exclusions, and lack of need for logical evidence. Although the problems with self-reporting are obviorus, Mischel (1981) has expressed his faith in the reliability and validity of such measures, stating that they do not yield less information than do other, more sophisticated and objective, measures.

Indirect Assessment

Although there may be value in the data derived from self-report inventories, the procedure is addressed mostly to the content of the inmates' thinking and only indirectly deals with the processes of their thinking. Ross and Fabiano (1985) have produced a list of psychometric measures that they claim "will refine our knowledge of offenders' cognitive abilities" (p. 290). The criteria for inclusion in this list are (a) a sound psychometric component, (b) relevance to the inmates' cognitive functioning, and (c) the predictive validity of the instrument. The tests selected focused on such variables as self-control, abstract reasoning, locus of control, social perspective taking, cognitive flexibility, empathy, and critical thinking. Although the focus of most of the recommended tests seemed to indicate a need to examine the inmates' cognitive efficiency (as well as inefficiency), none of them dealt with the decision-making or thinking process itself. The results obtained from the majority of these tests would (at best) yield inferences about the products of past learning. In addition, these tests do not provide any information pertaining to the inmates' ability to modify their own cognitive structures as well as their specific cognitive strategies. The recommended group of tests would merely confirm (or refute) the presence of cognitive competence. They would not address the issue of modifiability, that is, the inmates' ability to improve and enhance (with the assistance of appropriate intervention) their cognitive competence. Any measure that lacks a dynamic component, i.e., the active probing of the individual's cognitive processes and the assessment of the extent and processes of cognitive modifiability, contributes only minimally to an understanding of the relationship between that persons's cognitive functioning and behavior. It also neglects the individual's potential to be modified cognitively. For these reasons the tests compiled by Ross and Fabiano (1985) for the detection of cognitive factors that could contribute to the execution of a criminal act are not seen as capable of yielding the type of information necessary for such a relationship to be drawn.

The dynamic, process-oriented component that is missing in most of these tests has been supplied in a direct assessment device developed by Feuerstein (Feuerstein et al., 1972; Feuerstein, Rand, & Hoffman, 1979): the Learning Potential Assessment Device (LPAD).

Feuerstein's Learning Potential Assessment Device

Feuerstein places very little faith in the reliability and validity of standardized, normative testing, which he terms "static testing." He asserts that conventional psychological tests are unsuitable for the assessment and prediction of cognitive potential because of their concern with the delineation of an individual's existing competencies or the products of that person's past learning. He suggests that it is the individual's potential for being modified by learning that should be the focus of psychological assessment.

Accordingly, Feuerstein (Feuerstein et al., 1972, 1979) developed an assessment procedure called the Learning Potential Assessment Device, which is focused on the assessment of the processes involved in learning as opposed to the products of prior learning, generally referred to as "dynamic assessment."

The essence of the LPAD is its combination of active teaching and testing-in-the-act-of-learning procedures. Modifiability of cognitive performance is assessed by measuring one's capacity to learn and then to apply a particular learned principle or skill in situations progressively more different from the initial one in which that principle was learned, and by measuring the amount of assistance, explanation, and direction required by the examiner to teach the individual the given principle.

This process of assessing a person in the act of learning provides considerable insight into the ways in which that person attempts to learn and to solve problems. The ability to modify the person's cognitive performance through this procedure then provides the basis for a prediction of cognitive potential. (See Tzuriel & Haywood, Chapter 1 in this volume, for a more detailed discussion of dynamic assessment generically and the Learning Potential Assessment Device in particular.)

The Study

The basic purpose of the study was to test the assumptions generated by Feuerstein's theoretical position on cognitive modifiability and the assessment of learning potential as they relate to adult prison inmates. That is, the research was designed to determine (a) to what extent, if any, educationally low-achieving inmates differ in their cognitive performance from high-achieving inmates, and (b) if such a difference exists, to what extent the level of cognitive performance in the former group can be improved by a specific learning experience. The vehicle for investigating these questions was Feuerstein's dynamic assessment procedure, the LPAD.

Our primary expectation was that inmates functioning at low levels of academic achievement, defined as grade 5 or below in reading and arithmetic, would exhibit potential for more effective cognitive performance than was apparent in their low academic achievement. Specifically, we expected that they would show improvement in their cognitive processes, as well as in their problem solving performance, as demonstrated on LPAD tasks, as a result of teaching or "mediation" between pretest and posttest. In fact, we expected that the "improved" performance of the low-achieving inmates (following mediation) would be up to the premediation level of the high achievers, defined as grade 8 or above.

Preliminary Procedures

Preliminary visits by members of the research team were made to each of the institutions participating in the research so that the nature of the project and the criteria for subject selection could be fully explained to the educational and administrative officials. The general purpose of the project was then communicated by school personnel to groups of inmates in preparation for their possible participation in the project.

Samples

The subjects for the project were selected by the educational personnel in each institution on the basis of two criteria: age 18 to 50 years, and academic achievement level of at least grade 8 or below grade 5. Because the only available information pertaining to level of academic achievement was that reported by the inmates themselves upon admission to the institution, the Tests of Adult Basic Education (TABE; Tiegs & Clark, 1976) was administered to corroborate this information. The results of the TABE indicated a mean grade level for the High group of 10.7 with range of 8.1 to 12.9. The mean grade level of the Low group was 3.9, with a range from illiteracy (nine inmates) to grade 5.5. These data confirmed the difference between the two groups and indicated that they met the criteria of selection. The mean difference in grade level between the two groups was approximately 7 years, with no overlap between the two groups. Subject selection was neither random nor representative, but involved inclusion of those inmates who met the age and educational criteria and who agreed to participate in the study. In institution A there were seven subjects whose achievement was at grade 5 or below, and 12 at grade 8 or above. In institution B there were 14 at grade 5 or below and 16 at grade 8 or above.

The Testing Program

In LPAD assessment, one attempts to assess cognitive modifiability, i.e., the extent to which an individual's approach to learning and the effectiveness of that learning can be modified by experience. Therefore, it involves a test-teach-test process. The initial test phase is intended to provide an objective baseline with which to compare performance during training and during the final test phase. All tests in the LPAD require active intervention by the examiner(s) in the form of assistance to the subject. This assistance takes the form of focusing the subject's attention on a salient feature of a problem when an incorrect answer is given, to determine whether the subject can then correct his response, or the form of "intervention" (Feuerstein et al., 1972, 1979) by which the subject is taken through a number of steps in the problem leading to its solution.

Test Instruments

Three LPAD instruments were used in this study in a pretest-training-posttest sequence in conjunction with the Lorge-Thorndike Nonverbal Intelligence Test, level 3, which was used as pretest and posttest for the LPAD experience as a whole. The Lorge-Thorndike was divided into two equivalent forms using a split-half technique. The LPAD instruments were (a) Organization of Dots, equivalent forms (Rey & Dupont, 1953); (b) Raven's Coloured Progressive Matrices (Raven, 1956, 1965) and

LPAD Variations I on Raven's Progressive Matrices (Feuerstein et al., 1972); and (c) the Representational Stencil Design Test (Feuerstein et al., 1972).

The Lorge-Thorndike was used as a measure of nonverbal reasoning and included in the study to determine whether and to what extent such cognitive mediation as exposure to and practice in reflection and planning, careful and systematic exploration of problem elements, hypothesis testing, and the determination of principles basic to the solution of problems would result in generalization to and improvement in performance on tests requiring the solution of different types of problems.

The Lorge-Thorndike Nonverbal Intelligence Test was divided into two equivalent forms using a split-half technique to avoid the effect of practice over a brief interval. The form consisting of even-numbered items was used as the very first test administered before the inmates had experienced the LPAD. The form containing the odd-numbered items was administered at the conclusion of the LPAD. A period of approximately 30 minutes was devoted to each of the Lorge-Thorndike testing sessions. Following are descriptions of the LPAD "instruments" used in this study.

Organization of Dots

Equivalent Forms

This test consists of a number of frames containing amorphous clouds of dots that have to be organized according to a completed model shown in a sample or "model" frame. The model frame in the first section contains a square and a triangle; in the second section it contains two squares, and in the third section it contains two squares and a triangle. The subject is required to organize the dots into the prescribed shapes in the model frame by connecting the discrete dots with straight lines. Successful completion of these tasks requires projection of "virtual" (projected) relationships, articulation of the visual field by means of analysis, capacity to plan ahead, and precision and accuracy both in data gathering and in expression.

Training Phase

The training requires explanation of salient principles underlying success on the task, pointing especially to preferential strategies for approaching the task. That is, the training involves interactive discussion between the teacher/examiner and the subjects with reference to the specific relationship of dots required by a particular model figure, the need to maintain constancy of shape despite changes in orientation and overlapping figures, induction of comparison of the model figures and the shapes drawn by the subjects in order to establish the required form and size and to check the accuracy of their productions, induction of a systematic and planful approach to each problem, use of summative behavior (e.g., counting the number of dots belonging to each shape), inhibition of impulsivity by hypothesis testing and consideration of alternative solutions before any lines were drawn. Following the training, the subjects were given five pages of Organization of Dots with which to practice these approaches and strategies. After a time, a parallel form of the Organization of Dots instrument was administered.

Raven's Progressive Matrices and its LPAD Variations (Subtests A, B, C)

Raven's Progressive Matrices (Raven 1956, 1965) was administered according to the instructions in the manual but with the examiner assisting the subject by focusing or by more active intervention as necessary. Each item on this test consists of a pattern in which a piece is missing. The subject is asked to select the missing piece from several (six or eight) alternatives presented below the pattern.

This test begins on a very simple level requiring the completion of the pattern on the basis of gestalt (perceptual) analysis and builds up to higher levels of functioning requiring more complex cognitive operations such as analogies, permutations, simultaneous use of two or more sources or information, and logical multiplication.

The Training Phase: LPAD Variations II

This material consisted of a set (up to 12) of variations of each of five items selected from Raven's Progressive Matrices sets C, D, and E. The training included teaching the strategies necessary to solve the matrix problems, such as analogical principles, systematic exploration of problem elements, and comparative behavior, using the original matrices from sets C, D, and E. Following this training, the subjects were given the LPAD variations on these matrix tasks, which reflect the previously elaborated principles. The problem tasks are varied progressively in each of the groups of problems by the placement of objects, by rows, by columns, then by rows and columns, by modification of figure content, modification of the figure itself, and finally by modification of the figure, its content, and the respective relationship. Thus, an individual confronted with this task who shows the capacity to master it can be considered to be able to use that acquired experience to adapt to new situations (Feuerstein et al., 1972, p. 76). After an appropriate interval, the Progressive Matrices test was once again administered.

The Representational Stencil Design Test (RSDT)

This test involves the examination of the effects of a structured task upon the individual's capacity to develop internalized problem solving behavior. Subjects are presented with a "poster" sheet of colored patterns representing stencils arranged in four rows. The bottom row contains squares of solid color—blue, green, black, yellow, red, white. Similar colored squares, out of which shapes (e.g., square, circle, cross, octagon) have been cut, are arranged in three rows above the solid colored squares.

During the introduction, the subjects are engaged in a discussion to ensure that they can label the colors and the cutout shapes. The stencil concept is discussed and care is taken that the subjects understand the stencil concept and can express the design results of placing a given stencil (cutout) on top of a solid colored square. Each element on the poster sheet is numbered. The subjects are then shown a sheet of 20 pictures of finished stencil designs. It is explained that each of the prescribed designs on the sheet can be produced by combining particular solid colors and particular stencils displayed on the "poster" sheet. It is also pointed out that the sequence of combination begins with a solid color at the bottom of the design and proceeds upward with subsequent colored stencils being superimposed on previous ones in an imaginary stack. For each prescribed design, each of the subjects is asked to write the numbers of the solid color and of the stencils in the order in which those elements would have to be superimposed to produce the design. The designs require from two to seven components. The task requires that subjects keep in mind, on a representational level, the outcome of their mental act of placing one stencil on top of another as they proceed to "build" each design.

The RSDT Training Phase

The training phase consists of guiding the subjects in the construction of 20 designs. Each design requires two or three stencil components and a solid colored square at the bottom of the imaginary stack. The subjects were instructed that the first step in the construction of each design is to "look down through" the imaginary stack of stencils to identify and select the solid colored square at the bottom, and then to identify the stencil(s) that must be superimposed on it.

Following the training, the subjects were presented with a test booklet of 20 designs and asked to indicate those elements on the poster that are represented in each design.

Sequence of LPAD Testing-Training-Testing

In *institution A*, the testing and training was done in the following sequence:

Lorge-Thorndike Nonverbal Intelligence Test (even-numbered items)
Organization of Dots—Test 1
Organization of Dots—Training Form
Organization of Dots—Test 2

RSDT—Test 1
RSDT—Training
RSDT—Test 2
Progressive Matrices—Test 1
LPAD Variations—Training
Progressive Matrices—Test 2
Lorge-Thorndike (odd-numbered items)

In *institution B*, the testing and training was done in the following sequence:

Lorge-Thorndike (even-numbered items)
Organization of Dots—Test 1
Organization of Dots—Training
RSDT—Test 1
Organization of Dots—Test 2
RSDT—Training
RSDT—Test 2
Progressive Matrices—Test 1
LPAD variations—Training
Progressive Matrices—Test 2
Lorge-Thorndike (odd-numbered items)

Testing Procedures

Testing occurred over 3 days in each institution and required approximately 12 hours per group. On the basis of the testing experience in institution A, it was decided to change the order of test items at institution B. This change was made in the interests of:

1. decreasing fatigue in the subjects over the course of testing that might be associated with the repetitive encountering of similar material in the test-teach-test procedure;
2. maintaining a high level of motivation and interest in the subjects, so they would continue with the testing program, by varying the nature of the materials presented to them;
3. allowing for the effects of teaching to become somewhat consolidated in the cognitive skill repertoire of the subjects before they were presented with the posttest on a particular test.

Analysis of the test results from the two institutions indicates that the difference in testing sequence did not differentially influence the performance on the LPAD of the two institutional groups.

Scoring the Group LPAD

The scoring of the LPAD differs considerably from scoring procedures and criteria used in conventional assessment approaches. As stated by

Feuerstein et al. (1972), "the essence of the LPAD is its focus upon the assessment of learning processes rather than the assessment of the products of prior learning." The process of scoring the LPAD focuses on determining the presence or absence of specific problem solving strategies that are prerequisite to successful completion of the given LPAD task. Thus, the "scores" that are derived from an LPAD assessment provide information pertaining not only to the amount of overall success achieved by the individual (or the group) on the task, but in addition provides a breakdown of the various types of thinking strategies employed in that process.

The following scoring categories were employed in the scoring of each of the three LPAD instruments used in this study.

The Organization of Dots

Total Number of Items Attempted: the total number of dot frames attempted by the subject in the course of the pre- and posttests. A total of 52 frames were presented on the five pages. The contents of each page increased in complexity, i.e., increased in the number of geometric shapes per frame and/or increased in the complexity of each of the geometric shapes.

Total Number of Items Correct: the number of frames successfully completed.

Total Time: the overall time used by the subject to complete the total of five pages of dot frames.

Total Number of Partially Correct Frames: dot frames that were (a) completed but were partially incorrect, or (b) only partially completed but that part done correctly. In these cases, partial scores were obtained for the parts of the frame that were successfully completed.

Spontaneous Corrections: instances in which one or both shapes in a frame were initially completed incorrectly, then erased and corrected without help from the instructors. Feuerstein et al. (1972) has elaborated on this particular cognitive strategy as being a critical ingredient of any problem solving strategies.

Total Number of Erasures: the number of erasures made while working on the task. Erasures in general suggest impulsive behavior.

Total Score: one point credited for each geometric shape correctly completed. For example, if a given frame contains three geometric shapes, the possible total score for that frame is 3. If only two out of the three shapes is reproduced correctly, the score for that frame is 2. The maximum score available for the 52 frames is 136 points.

Representational Stencil Design Test (RSDT)

Number Attempted: the number of items (stencil designs) that the subject tries, whether or not completed. Twenty designs are presented during the pretesting and posttesting procedures. The items become increasingly difficult, some designs requiring as many as seven stencils, and this scoring category (number attempted) is designed to indicate if the increase in difficulty deterred the individual from attempting the more complex items.

Number of Correct Designs: the total number of design items completed correctly and without errors.

Transpositions: the frequency of transposed position of stencils, or sequence errors, in solving the RSDT. Transpositions are common in this type of task (which requires arrangement of stencils in a given sequence).

Bottom Stencil Correct or Incorrect: the nature of the RSDT tasks requires a specific representational sequential arrangement of stencils in order to produce a final design. The understanding of the sequence of the stencils is necessary for the successful completion of the task. One of the basic strategies to be mastered while working on this task is that the bottom stencil—solid color—is the first one in a pile of stencils. This category allows one to examine any change in the frequency of use of this strategy, i.e., reduction in the number of incorrect bottom stencils, or increase in the number of incorrect bottom stencils, or increase in the number of correctly selected bottom stencils.

Top Stencil Correct or Incorrect: a related strategy that is helpful for the successful completion of this task is the understanding of which stencil must be on top of the stack of stencils in order to complete the design. The "top stencil correct or incorrect" scoring category permits examination of the frequency with which this strategy is used. In examining specific task-related strategies, e.g., "bottom stencil" or "top stencil," it is possible to determine the use of these problem solving strategies in an otherwise incorrectly completed task. In other words, although the sequential arrangement of the stencils on a given RSDT item may be generally incorrect, a correct top stencil and/or bottom stencil indicates a mastery of some of the task-related strategies.

Omitted Stencils: the number of instances in which essential stencils were left out of the design sequence. Due to the complexity of the task, many individuals fail to see all of the stencils in the sequence that would correctly complete each of the designs.

Spontaneous Corrections: when a subject corrects an error without assistance from the examiner.

Raven's Progressive Matrices Subtests A, B, C: number of correct responses on each subtest.

The scoring categories for the LPAD outlined here permitted us to look at any change in the frequency of use of certain problem solving strategies in our subjects. Whereas total scores on each of the LPAD instruments yield a general overall statement of achievement, the scores and information from the other categories yield important information as to the quality and type of the problem solving strategies used by the members of the group.

Results

Qualitative Data

As was indicated earlier, four groups of subjects (inmates) participated in this study: a High group (reading and mathematics achievement above grade 8), and a Low group (reading and mathematics achievement grade 5 or below) in each of two institutions. A test on the pretest scores of the two High groups indicated no significant difference between the two groups except on one variable, the RSDT total score ($p < .05$). Consequently, the data for the two High groups were collapsed, and the two High groups were treated as one group. A similar analysis examining the pretest scores of the two Low groups yielded no significant differences between the groups except on the total score of Organization of Dots ($p < .001$). Consequently, the two groups were treated as one.

Within-Group Comparisons

Organization of Dots

On the first three variables of the Organization of Dots (Number of Items Attempted, Total Correct, Total Time), nonsignificant differences were observed in the High group, but in the Low group there were significant differences ($p < .001$, $p < .001$, $p < .05$, respectively). Significant differences ($p < .001$) were observed in the High group on the Number of Items Partially Correct, whereas for the Low group, the mean scores remain unchanged. On the next three variables of Organization of Dots, (Spontaneous Correction, Total Erasures, and Total Score), the mean score of the High group remained relatively unchanged from the pretest to the posttest assessment. In the Low group, however, significant changes were observed on two of these variables: Total Erasures ($p < .001$) and Total Score. Although the pretest-posttest comparison on the Number of Spontaneous Corrections indicated that the differences were not significant for each group, examination of the raw mean scores indicated a slight increase in the Number of Spontaneous Corrections for the Low group and a decrease for the High group.

In summary, the comparison of the pretest scores with the posttest scores of both the High and Low groups on Organization of Dots yielded one significant change for the High group and five significant changes for the Low Group.

Representational Stencil Design Test (RSDT)

Examination of RSDT outcomes revealed that both groups had increased their mean scores significantly ($p < .001$) on the first two variables, Number of Items Attempted and Number of Correct Designs. Minimal changes from pre- and posttest were observed in the High group on the next six variables: Transpositions, Bottom Stencil Correct or Incorrect, Top Stencil Correct or Incorrect, and *Spontaneous Corrections*. The Low group, however, made significant gains (reduction in frequency of incorrect responses) on two of these variables: Bottom Stencil Incorrect ($p < .01$), Top Stencil Incorrect ($p < .05$). On the Transpositions category, an examination of the pretest-posttest mean scores for this group indicated a reduction in the number of Transposition errors, but this reduction was not significant.

In summary, the comparison of pretest and posttest scores of the High group and the Low group in the RSDT indicated that changes in the High group scores were relatively modest, but those for the Low group were large and statistically significant.

Raven's Progressive Matrices

Comparison (t test) of Raven's Progressive Matrices pretest and posttest scores (subtests A, B, and C) indicated that slight, nonsignificant gains were noted for the High group on subtests A and B, with a significant gain on subtest C ($p < .01$), but in the Low group the posttest mean scores were significantly higher on all three subtests ($p < .05$, $p < .01$, and $p < .001$, respectively).

Lorge-Thorndike Nonverbal Intelligence Test

On the Lorge-Thorndike, the mean score of the High group remained unchanged, but in the Low group the mean score increased significantly ($p < .001$) from pretest to posttest.

Between-Groups Comparisons

Organization of Dots

Although statistically significant differences were seen between the High and the Low groups on the first three variables of Organization of Dots (Total Attempted, $p < .001$; Total Items Correct, $p < .001$; and Total Partially Correct, $p < .05$), these differences disappeared on the posttest. In addition, the posttest mean scores for the Low group on the first two variables were higher than were those of the High group.

Significant differences between the High and the Low groups were observed for the Total Time variable on the pretest as well as on the posttest. Although the actual mean time (in minutes) for the Low group decreased (from 44.10 on the pretest to 36.35 on the posttest), the difference between the groups remained statistically significant ($p < .001$). On Spontaneous Corrections the differences between the groups remained nonsignificant, but an examination of the posttest mean scores indicated a slight increase for the Low group.

The differences between the High and the Low groups on the Erasures score remained nonsignificant on the pretest as well as on the posttest, although reduction in the number of erasures was seen in both groups.

The difference between the High and the Low groups ($p < .001$) on the pretest Total Score became nonsignificant on the posttest. This represented a dramatic gain for the Low group.

Representational Stencil Design Test

On the RSDT, the significant differences between the High and Low groups on the pretest on Number Attempted ($p < .05$) and on Number Correct ($p < .001$) disappeared on the posttest. A reduction in the mean scores on Transpositions from pretest to posttest was not significant.

Although the number of Top Stencil–Bottom Stencil errors was high for the Low group on the pretest, it decreased significantly on the posttest. Results from the pretest indicated that: (a) 23% of the High group sample made no errors at all; (b) 14.7% of the Low group sample made no errors; (c) a high percentage of the High group subjects made between 0 and 3 errors; (d) a high percentage of the Low group subjects made between 3 and 9 errors; (e) none of the High group subjects made more than 10 errors; (f) in the Low group, a few subjects made 12 to 14 errors. Results from the posttest indicated that: (a) 11.5% of the High group population made no errors, versus 29% of the Low group; (b) more subjects in the High group made no errors at all on the pretest than on the posttest; and (c) more subjects in the Low group made *no* errors on the posttest than on the pretest.

Although there were significant differences between the High and the Low groups on Number of Omitted Stencils at pretest, these differences disappeared on the posttest.

With respect to the Spontaneous Correction scoring category, there were no significant differences on pretest versus posttest comparisons between the High group and the Low group.

Raven's Progressive Matrices

Analysis of the Progressive Matrices pretest scores revealed significant differences between the High and Low groups: subtest A ($p < .05$); subtest B ($p < .001$); subtest C ($p < .001$). Analysis of the posttest scores indicated that some of the initial differences between the two groups had narrowed: there was no significant posttest difference between the two groups on subtest A; and there was a decrease in the difference on subtest B, although it was still significant ($p < .01$). The mean difference between the two groups on subtest C was relatively unchanged. The difference between the High and the Low groups on the pretest of the Lorge-Thorndike Nonverbal Intelligence test was somewhat reduced at posttest, but was still statistically significant ($p < .05$).

Another comparison was between the High group pretest scores and the Low group posttest scores. The primary objective of this comparison was to examine whether the intensive LPAD training had brought the Low group closer to the pretraining performance level of the High group. The data indicated that the two groups differed only on one of the seven categories of Organization of Dots (Total Time, $p < .01$).

On the Representational Stencil Design Test, the Low group's posttest mean was not significantly different from the pretest mean of the High group, except on the scoring category Number of Items Attempted ($p < .02$).

On Raven's Progressive Matrices, the Low group posttest mean differed from the High group pretest mean on only one of the three subtests used in the study (subtest B; $p < .05$).

Examination of the Low group posttest and the High group pretest mean scores on the Lorge-Thorndike Nonverbal Intelligence Test revealed that the High group mean was still higher ($p < .05$).

In summary, the results indicated that few significant differences existed between the High group pretest scores and the Low group posttest scores.

The results of the comparison between the High and Low groups' posttest scores indicated that, when the pretest differences were taken into account, there were no significant posttest differences between the groups on the following variables: Organization of Dots—Total Items Attempted, Total Items Correct, Total Score, and Total Number of Erasures. RSDT—Total Items Attempted, Total Number Correct, Transpositions, Bottom Incorrect, Omitted, Erasures, and Spontaneous Corrections. Raven's Progressive Matrices—subtest A, subtest B. Lorge-Thorndike—Total Score.

The two groups differed significantly on only three scoring categories: Organization of Dots—Total Time ($p < .005$); RSDT—Number of Top Incorrect ($p < .01$); Raven's Progressive Matrices—subtest C ($p < .02$).

Anecdotal Data

Informal observations are presented here, based primarily on informance gathered by the experimenters during the LPAD sessions. The group of four experimenters spent 3 days in each institution ($1\frac{1}{2}$ days per group, 7 hours per day). At the conclusion of each day, the experimenters met and reported their respective observations. These reports focused primarily on the inmates' attitudes, their behavior, and their general performance during the LPAD assessment procedure. The information gathered is summarized in the following subsections.

Inmates' Attitudes Toward the LPAD Procedures

Generally, the inmates who had achieved at least a grade 8 level of academic achievement responded positively to the call for volunteers to participate in the project. On the other hand, the inmates who achieved lower than a grade 5 academic level were generally anxious, reluctant, and skeptical. A few of them had to be coaxed into entering the classroom where the LPAD was being conducted. Others stated that they would stay for a short time and then leave as they pleased.

During a brief discussion preceding the LPAD assessment procedures, inmates in the Low group expressed a general dislike for school-related activities and recalled some of their own early experiences in school as being unhappy and frustrating. The members of the High group, however, expressed interest in the purpose of the study (which was discussed openly with them) and in obtaining the results of the various tests. Many of the inmates in this group were taking university courses and they became interested in the theory underlying the LPAD procedure.

During the LPAD assessment, as members of the Low group began to encounter difficulty their frustrations were expressed verbally in such comments as: "This is stupid," "I can't do it," "I'm going to leave," "I'm not coming back in the afternoon." Similar signs of frustration were evident in the High group, but they were not as extreme nor as frequent. The anxiety and frustration in both groups gradually decreased as many of the inmates began to find the tasks interesting as well as challenging. Moreover, they discovered their own potential for success as they continued to cope with the test items. Many inmates, especially in the Low group, shifted from their passive-reluctant role to a more active-interested one.

During the teaching sessions that occurred between the pretests and the posttests, the inmates had a chance to discuss some of the difficulties they had experienced in trying to solve the various LPAD problems, and to examine the various approaches and strategies that could be applied when working on similar problems.

As was indicated earlier, both groups stayed for a period of 7 hours a day (with a break for lunch) for a day and a half. Only one person in each group left prior to the conclusion of the assessment program and did not return. At the conclusion of the first few hours of assessment, inmates in both groups complained of fatigue and of excessive difficulty of particular tasks, especially the RSDT, which they found quite challenging. Nevertheless, all the inmates in both groups (except the two that had left earlier) returned the second day ready to complete the assessments tasks.

Inmates Problem Solving Behavior

Initially, the High group settled down and started working on the tasks with considerably fewer difficulties than did the Low group. Members of the Low group required additional instructions and clarifications on the first few items of Organization of Dots. In addition, most members of the High group generally worked faster than did those of the Low group, although a few members of the High group were very slow and inefficient in their approach to the test items. Impulsive behavior (erasures, working out of sequence) was evident in both groups, but was more prevalent in the Low group.

During the pretest period the Low group inmates were erratic, unsystematic, and careless in their approach. Following the teaching, the independently recorded notes of the experimenters showed an increased frequency of efficient problem solving strategies, including systematic search, comparative behavior, and hypothesis testing.

Relationship Between the Experimenters and the Inmates

The change in the quality of the relationship between the experimenters and the inmates was interesting. During the initial contact with each group, the atmosphere could be characterized as formal, cool, and reserved. It later changed to a very friendly and warm relationship, with the inmates conversing openly with the team of experimenters, discussing various topics that often included their own life stories. In addition, inmates in both groups showed interest in the outcome of this research project and indicated their interest in working with other LPAD or related materials.

Discussion

Generally, the results presented in the previous section support our expectations. Although the initial (pretest) cognitive performance of the Low group was significantly inferior to that of the High group, following a relatively short (although intensive), intellectually stimulating intervention, there was a marked improvement in the cognitive performance of inmates in the Low group. Members in this group (as well as members in the High group) demonstrated that they do have potential to learn, that they can benefit from help with learning, and consequently that they can improve their own cognitive performance. The extent of their modifiability is evident from the many gains made by the Low group from the pretest situation to the posttest situation as a result of mediation. In addition to increasing their scores on the LPAD tasks, there is clear evidence that members of the Low group developed a repertoire of efficient problem solving strategies that were not inferior to those of the

High group. The results in the various scoring categories point to a reduction in the number of trial-and-error responses, a reduction in the use of inefficient approaches to problem solving, and the internalization and application of more sophisticated and efficient strategies of problem solving.

Although there was a mean difference of approximately 7 years between the academic achievement levels of the High group and the Low group, there was only a minimal difference between the two groups with respect to their potential for learning, or in their use of cognitive strategies while solving problems.

The fact that the posttest scores of the Low group were quite similar to the pretest scores of the High group suggests that members of the Low group, once they had been given mediation on important cognitive functions, were able to perform at the same level of cognitive ability as did members of the High group. Equally encouraging results are available from the analysis of covariance with pretest differences between the two groups statistically controlled. Few significant differences between the two groups were identified. Except for these few differences, the performance level of the Low group was comparable to that of the High group.

The only difference between the learning patterns of the two achievement groups was in the length of time required for mastery of a skill or strategy. Generally, inmates in the Low group required significantly more time to complete some of the LPAD tasks; however, there was a general decrease in the amount of time required by members of this group, and one might suggest that with further training, there would be a further reduction in the time taken to achieve mastery. Further support for the learning potential of the inmates of the Low group comes from the pre-post comparisons on the Lorge-Thorndike Nonverbal Intelligence Test. The significant increase in the posttest score over the pretest score of the Low group could have been due to the development, internalization, and use of the more efficient cognitive strategies that were acquired by the inmates as a result of the mediation that was part of LPAD.

Implications and Conclusions

This study demonstrates the uniqueness and utility of the LPAD procedures in assessing cognitive potential and cognitive modifiability. Whereas conventional assessment procedures (IQ and various educational achievement tests) provide, at best, estimates of past learning, LPAD procedures are aimed at assessing the existence of a significant unused potential. With respect to the inmates who participated in this study, intelligence tests and educational attainment measures would provide a score or a grade level that would reveal little or no information as to the individual's ability to learn. Moreover, most of the conventional achievement tests are designed to assess acquired (through schooling) knowledge. Using these tests to assess the intellectual potential of penitentiary inmates who had only 3 to 5 years of formal education would seriously underestimate their intellectual potential. The information available from the LPAD, however, allowed us to shift the focus from the inferior academic performance of the inmates to their potential to be modified and to be changed through learning. Thus, the LPAD provides a measure of the inmates' abilities and not of their disabilities. This is a crucial factor and it should be seriously considered within the penitentiary rehabilitation framework. Rather than resorting to educational assessment procedures that are associated with academic failure and poor school grades, penitentiary inmates should be assessed with tests that can tap their ability to learn and that can allow for success.

In addition to the generally positive, success-producing nature of the LPAD, its assessment instruments are structured to yield information pertaining to task-specific behavior and problem solving strategies, information that is often unavailable from other assessment methods. An educational assessment procedure that fails to yield specific and relevant information that can be incorporated into or followed by a remedial instructional program has minimal utility and can often produce a negative, destructive effect.

Finally, the cooperation of the examinees was enhanced by their interest in the test materials, which are themselves intrinsically motivating and challenging. Uninteresting materials that fail to provoke the intellectual curiosity of the examinees will result in an attitude of indifference and consequently will produce a lower level of intellectual performance.

By demonstrating their ability to be modified through learning, most inmates, especially those in the Low group, showed that they can learn to perform complicated cognitive tasks with minimal instruction and training. In addition, the inmates in the Low group were able to solve complex problems after mediation with the same efficiency and success as did member of the higher achieving High group before mediation. This would tend to dispel any notion that their low school achievement was indicative of an inability to learn. It is quite possible that some of the inmates had not benefited from their earlier educational experiences because, in many instances, they required additional instructional time, alternative teaching methods, and the adaptation of educational procedures to meet their particular needs. These results have dramatic implications for the educational programs of penitentiary inmates, regardless of their educational background, suggesting that penal institutions have an obligation to mount educational programs for all levels of inmates; that one cannot and should not exclude some inmates from such programming on the basic of prior low academic achievement, low IQ, or a presumed learning disability. The results not only support the notion that education in penitentiaries has a role to play in personal reformation of inmates, but provides suggestions as to important components of educational programs that might contribute to the effectiveness of that role. Such educational programs should focus on the development and elaboration of basis cognitive processes and the strengthening of cognitive structures as well as development of general knowledge and competence in academic subjects.

References

Feuerstein, R., Shalom, H., Narrol, H., Hoffman, M., Kiram, L., Katz, O., Shachton, E., & Rand, Y. (1972). *Studies in cognitive modifiability: The dynamic assessment of retarded performers, Vol. 1., Clinical LPAD battery*. Jerusalem: Hadassah-WIZO-Canada Research Institute.

Feuerstein, R., Rand, Y., & Hoffman, M. B. (1979). *The dynamic assessment of retarded performers: The Learning Potential Assessment Device*. Baltimore: University Park Press.

Heppner, P. P., & Peterson, C. H. (1978). *The development, factor analysis, and initial validation of a problem solving instrument*. Paper presented at the meeting of the American Educational Research Association, Toronto.

Mischel, W. (1981). *A cognitive-social learning approach to assessment*. In T. Merluzzi, C. Glass, & M. Genest (Eds.). Cognitive Assessment. New York: Guilford Press.

Raven, J. C. (1956). *Coloured Progressive Matrices, Sets A, Ab and B*. London: H. K. Lewis.

Raven, J. C. (1965). *Guide to using the coloured matrices, sets A, Ab and B*. London: H. K. Lewis.

Rey, A., & Dupont, J. B. (1953). Organisation de groupes de points en figures géometriques simples. *Monographies de Psychologie Appliquée*, No. 3.

Ross, R., & Fabiano, E. A. (1985). *Time to think: A cognitive model of delinquency prevention and offender rehabilitation*. Johnson City, TN: Institute of Social Sciences and Art.

Schwartz, R., & Gottman, J. (1976). Toward a task analysis of assertive behavior. *Journal of Consulting and Clinical Psychology*, *99*, 910–920.

Tiegs, E. W., & Clark, W. W. (1976). *Tests of Adult Basic Education*. Monterey, CA: CTB/McGraw-Hill.

16
Process-Based Instruction: Integrating Assessment and Instruction

ADRIAN F. ASHMAN

The assessment and remediation of cognitive deficits have been two of the most perplexing problems for both researchers and practitioners in the field of educational psychology. Although there have been numerous and diverse attempts to clarify the nature of intellectual deficits and to train identifiable deficiencies, the transition from the theoretician's laboratory to the classroom has been slow in coming.

A major barrier limiting progress has been the achievement of generalization with educationally delayed students following what would appear otherwise to be successful interventions. Specifically, children can be taught to use information processing strategies appropriately within the training context, but fail to transfer them to other laboratory or classroom activities. This transfer barrier was recognized over 20 years ago, and with it came the realization that instruction needed to be specific, explicit, and intensive.

Initially, researchers concentrated upon teaching specific information processing strategies in isolation from both educational content and context. Later developments derived from research on metacognition linked strategy and metastrategy training in an effort to maintain and transfer learning (e.g., Kramer & Engle, 1981). Some writers began to examine other superordinate strategies using terms such as *planning*, *plans*, and *organizational strategies* (Belmont & Mitchell, 1987; Spitz, Minsky, & Bessellieu, 1985). Although the importance of both coding and organizational aspects of cognition has generally been accepted, few attempts have been made to develop an integrated intervention that reflects the synthesis of problem solving and information processing literature.

The growth of information processing theories and models was accompanied by a change in the methods of assessing cognitive competencies. However, although dynamic assessment and new test batteries may identify specific strengths and deficiencies in research subjects, assessment has typically been limited to pre- and posttests. It has not become part of the intervention itself.

Process-Based Instruction (PBI) was developed in response to three exigencies. First, there has been a demand for an instructional process that could find application in special and regular classrooms rather than just in the laboratory. Second, there has been a need to develop students' independent learning skills that can be maintained when the degree of control over what is taught (by the teacher to the students or by one child to another) is largely out of the researcher's hands. Third, there was a need to generate an ongoing assessment procedure during the instruction process that could identify learner characteristics and monitor changes as knowledge and skills improve.

PBI was developed as a systematic, integrated assessment-teaching procedure aimed at the enhancement of information processing competence in mildly disabled learners (Ashman, 1985). The rationale for including assessment and instruction components was based on the belief that teachers must determine initially what kind of help a student needs to overcome a learning problem, and secondly, how much aid is required by the student to succeed (see Brown & Campione, 1986).

The general purpose of this chapter is to present an overview of the PBI procedures and processes. In the first section, the foundations of PBI are outlined. In the second, the PBI process is described. Several excerpts from training sessions exemplify the various stages in the process. In the third section, I outline how PBI has been used up to the present time and review the results of two studies undertaken with mildly intellectually disabled adolescents.

The Foundations of Instruction

In the course of our daily lives, most humans are confronted with problems ranging from the most basic to the most complex of dilemmas. However, the successful, efficient resolution of problems appears to require essentially the same cognitive skills regardless of whether the problems are social, political, or arithmetic (Simon, 1978). As a conceptual framework for instruction, problem solving appears to have several advantages, not the least being the focus on knowledge, strategic and planful behavior, and the execution of appropriate goal-oriented actions (Anderson, Greeno, Kline, & Neves, 1981). Such a framework parallels the information processing literature dealing with coding, planning, and decision making.

Problem Solving

Although much of the research dealing with the nature and training of problem solving has used nondisabled subjects (see Fredericksen, 1984), the literature can be applied directly to the field of developmental disabilities. The problem solving difficulties of the intellectually disabled parallel those experienced by other developmentally young persons. They lack experience with real-life problems (Smith & Dutton, 1979), they fail to interpret task demands accurately (Sternberg, 1980), and they fail to identify goals correctly (Spitz et al., 1985) and isolate relevant variables and information (Siegler, 1976).

Furthermore, the study of problem solving behavior provides an indication as to why disabled children may be unable to generalize skills to tasks somewhat distantly related to the training activities. Most instruction deals with well-structured problems that are clearly presented, with all the information necessary for the solution available in the problem and/or long-term memory (Simon, 1980). However, generalization appears to demand application of skills to what would appear to be ill-structured tasks (i.e., relying primarily on long-term memory or external sources), or when a change in context is inolved.

For intellectually disabled learners to achieve transfer of learning, it may be necessary to increase the structure within the training program and teach explicit problem solving procedures, that is, planning and plan execution. Hence, the focus of attention would not simply be the individual's use of appropriate strategies, but ensuring that the learner understands how problems are solved and what the effect of strategic behavior will be. This approach seems consistent with the results of strategy training research, which has emphasized memory aids and goal-oriented activity.

Planning

Planning has been perceived as an important component of cognition since the late 1950s. It has been conceptualized as an intellectual ability (Berger, Guilford, & Christensen, 1957) and as an information processing mechanism (Das, Kirby, & Jarman, 1979; Hayes-Roth & Hayes-Roth, 1979; Miller, Galanter, & Pribram, 1960). Moreover, planning has been associated with information processing competence across ability groups (Brown, 1974; Schofield & Ashman, 1987).

The study of planning received impetus from the work of Luria (1973) and from the adaptation of Luria's functional organization of the brain into models of information processing. One such model (described by Das et al., 1979) incorporated interdependent processing systems including coding and planning components. The first empirical study of planning using the Das et al. model was reported by Ashman (1978). Since then, the multidimensional nature of planning and its relationship to academic achievement has been addressed in several studies (e.g., Kirby & Ashman, 1984; Kops & Belmont, 1985). Typically, planning activities enable the individual to make judgments about the goal of the activity being undertaken, task demands, available information, decisions made concerning the most expedient means of achieving the goal, the enactment of procedures, and the monitoring of performance.

Although problem solving and planning appear to be equivalent terms sharing a common purpose (goal-oriented behavior), planning might be conceived of as a "neurological" concept and problem solving as a behavioral concept. Planning is a process mediated by neurological activities that are common to human beings. For some activities, planning may involve explicit, conscious activity. For others, "unconscious" or "reflexive" responses may occur, for example, in simple search and monitoring tasks or even in some complex activities such as flying an aircraft (Ashman, 1986a). In brief, though the observed behavior may be different from task to task the same cognitive processes mediate the activity of problem solving.

Translating cognitive concepts into practice requires consideration of learner characteristics (knowledge, skills, ability) and the nature of instruction including ecological, content, and teaching variables (Marsh, Price, & Smith, 1983). In one sense, it necessitates consideration of how students engage in coding and planning for effective learning and problem solving. In another, the role of teachers in promoting the acquisition of knowledge, and interdependence in problem solving and learning, are important.

The stimulation of planful behavior through the use of effective teaching strategies is characteristic of another contemporary cognitive intervention, namely, Instrumental Enrichment. This is an approach that shares some common principles with PBI, although the instructional methods are quite different.

Teaching and Responsibility

Instrumental Enrichment is a broad, classroom-based intervention intended to improve the cognitive functioning of intellectually disabled adolescents (Feuerstein, Rand, Hoffman, & Miller, 1980). It was designed to encourage students to develop skills markedly different from those often encountered in regular classrooms, and as such provides a parallel to PBI. Within a structured instructional framework, teacher and students focus upon various problem solving processes such as evaluation, interpretation, planning, and comparison (processes involved in problem solving) rather than on school-based content.

Two related Instrumental Enrichment concepts seem particularly relevant to PBI, namely, cognitive modifiability and mediated learning experiences. Cognitive modifiability implies changes of a "structural" nature that relate to "the organism's manner of interacting with, . . . acting on and responding to, sources of information" (Feuerstein et al., 1980, p. 9). These changes may be realized through deliberate intervention that sensitizes students to both internal and external sources of stimulation. This awareness is achieved by concentrating on basic cognitive processes, problem solving tactics, and motivational considerations

(Rand, Tannenbaum, & Feuerstein, 1979). The principle of cognitive modifiability is consistent with the problem solving basis of PBI.

The second concept of Instrumental Enrichment related to PBI is called the mediated learning experience, and it was described as the theoretical basis for cognitive modifiability. The structure of an individual's cognition results from two modalities of interaction between the environment and the person. The first relates to the direct exposure to stimuli that leads to the development of a repertoire of skills. The second, mediated learning experiences, refers to the transformation and organization of stimuli by an agent (parent, sibling, or caregiver) so that the learner receives a culturally organized structure through which other stimuli may be understood.

Limited mediated learning experience may account for the learning difficulties of many low-ability students, suggesting inadequate instruction rather than poor learning ability. Indeed, Feuerstein et al. (1980) assigned responsibility to teachers for presenting information in a manner that would ensure that learning occurs. This principle is a tenet of PBI. If pupils have difficulty in grasping concepts or confront blocks to learning, it is the responsibility of teachers to discover the keys to comprehension. Identifying blocks and monitoring performance brings continuous assessment into the instructional process.

Assessment and Instruction

The link among competence, instruction, and performance is made explicit in PBI through on-going evaluation of strategic behavior and performance. Assessment activities not only cue teachers to the *what* and the *how* of instruction, but also orient students to the *why* and the *when* of learning.

Assessment is typically the first step in remediation: a teacher must determine a student's competence level before commencing instruction; however, assessment is both the antecedent of instruction and an essential component. Through the provision of an integrated program, assessment and instruction become the tools of a cooperative problem-solving activity that bonds teachers to students. Instruction becomes cyclic, involving the evaluation and development of stored information, strategies, plans, and activity. In other words, teachers and children become actively engaged in each facet of the problem solving process, regardless of the task being addressed.

What to teach and how to teach it become the essence of both assessment and instruction. What to teach has been documented in the processing, strategy, and metastrategy training literature, and depends upon the orientation of the teacher or the investigator. At what level instruction begins will depend upon the quality of the student's knowledge base (which contains facts, rules, principles, strategies, and plans). Some aspects of these schemata may be assessed using standardized intelligence tests or through processing measures such as the Kaufman and Kaufman (1983) or the Das et al. (1979) battery; however, each of these provides a static evaluation. Of more importance is the evaluation of how students' cognitive skills are being used during problem solving activities, and cataloging their use for consideration in later learning.

The goal of PBI is to enhance the cognitive competence of students experiencing learning difficulties by teaching effective problem solving practices. This involves teaching facts, strategies, plans, and the means of expanding one's knowledge base independently through challenge and instruction. The following section outlines the procedures of Process-Based Instruction, emphasizing the intimate relationship between assessment and instruction.

The Procedure of Process-Based Instruction

PBI focuses upon students' processing and learning styles by emphasizing the development of coding strategies and planful behavior. Two forms of coding have been identified by several investigators. One form relates to holistic, quasi-spatial processing, variously called simultaneous, synthetic-appositional, or parallel-multiple processing. The second relates to temporal, sequence-dependent processing, called successive, sequential, analytic-propositional, or serial processing (Das et al., 1979; Kaufman, 1984). Problem solving is introduced as a procedure containing several steps that are divided into task orientation and task performance components. They are described more fully below in the description of the PBI process.

How to teach strategic behavior also has been considered at length in the information processing literature. Many lists have been generated by writers identifying features considered essential for successful cognitive interventions (see Borkowski & Cavanaugh, 1979). Contemporary developments have moved toward a high degree of interaction between the teacher and the students, leading toward the establishment of peer-based support structures. Cooperative teaching, peer tutoring, and reciprocal teaching all promote the generation of questions by students to stimulate independence in learning (Manzo, 1968; Osguthorpe & Scruggs, 1986; Palincsar & Brown, 1984).

PBI parallels reciprocal teaching methods to the extent that the teacher provides support necessary to facilitate and extend skill in the early phases of instruction, then gradually transfers responsibility for learning to the students. Typically, the PBI teacher works with two children, one at a time while the second child watches. The role of pupil and observer alternates during the session. As teacher and students become familiar with the goals and the prescribed process and methods, the teacher interacts with the students only to stimulate the students' problem solving activities.

PBI involves four phases: task orientation and performance; instruction; impeded learning; and generalization. Each phase contains both assessment and instruction elements that are included in a 17-step sequence. The procedure is summarized in Figure 16.1 and described more fully below.

Task Orientation and Performance

This component represents a problem solving sequence. An explicit goal of PBI is to teach the student these eight steps so that they become automatic.

Provision of an Explicit Statement of Task Demands

The teacher's goal in this step is to introduce the exercise to be undertaken and to ensure that students have the prerequisite knowledge and

TASK ORIENTATION AND PERFORMANCE (Focus on problem solving sequence)		
	Task Orientation	State and review task demands, Demonstrate required behavior.
	Task Performance	Verbalize training activity, Identify relevant information, Initiate and monitor required behaviour (trial), Review performance.
INSTRUCTION (Focus on coding or memory strategies)		
	Strategy Acquisition	Identify and evaluate student's preferred strategy, Reinforce and/or extend preferred strategy.
	Task Performance	Verbalize training activity, Identify relevant information, Initiate and monitor required behaviour (trial), Review performance.
INTERVENTION (Focus on strategic behavior)		
	Learning Analysis	Identify blockages to progress, Recognize and evaluate blockages, Reinforce cooperative learning, Review strategic behavior.
	Task Performance	Verbalize training activity, Identify relevant information, Initiate and monitor required behaviour (trial), Review performance.
GENERALIZATION (Focus on adaptation of strategic behavior)		
	Transfer Activities	Introduce transfer activities, Evaluate strategic behavior for transfer tasks.
	Return to Task Orientation	

FIGURE 16.1. The four phases of the procedure for Process-Based Instruction (PBI).

skills. Performance will be reduced if a pupil is asked to manipulate materials that are unfamiliar, or to use words or to apply rules or principles that are unknown or unnecessarily complex. The teacher presents the materials to the students and explains what the task involves.

The extract below focuses upon two 12-year-old students attending a special education class. John is working with the teacher while Alex watches. As this is the second session, neither boy is familiar with the procedure, but they work cooperatively. This is their first introduction to rehearsal.

Teacher: John, we're now going to work at remembering some toys using this box here. You can see that it's got a lid with a space cut out so that we can look into the compartments, but only one at a time. Over here, I've got some toys. Can you name them for me? What's this?
John: It's a Transformer [a spaceman toy].
Teacher: That's right. What are the rest of them?
John: A car, poker chip, ring, . . . (pupil names ten objects).
Teacher: That's really good, John. Now I'm going to put four toys in the box, one in each compartment. Then I'll close the lid so you can't see them. Then I'll say, "Watch carefully" and slide the lid across so that you see each of the toys, but only one at a time. You have to look in each compartment, and try to remember each of the toys in the same order that you saw them. When I've shown you the toys, I'll look up and you then tell me in what order I showed you the toys. But remember, it has to be just the same way that I showed them to you.
Alex: I've never done this.
Teacher: No, we haven't learned how to remember things this way before.

Review of Task Demands by the Student

The pupil is asked to demonstrate comprehension by describing the task requirements. If confusion is found, the teacher clarifies or asks the observer (the second pupil of the training pair) to help interpret the requirements and objectives.

Teacher: John. Can you tell me what I want you to do?
John: I have to watch the box and remember the toys that you show me.
Teacher: Yes, that's almost it, but what's the important part of remembering?
John: Oh. I have to say 'em in the same way they came.
Teacher: Right, good work. You have to say them in the same *order*. The first one you saw first, then the second one, then the third one, then the last one you saw.

Demonstration by the Teacher of the Required Behavior

The students watch while the teacher demonstrates and describes how the task is to be performed.

Teacher: Alright. Both of you watch carefully while I show you what is going to happen. First, the toys will go in where you can't see them. (Teacher removes the box from the students' sight and inserts four toys, then brings it back above the table). Now I'm going to slide the lid across, showing the dollar coin first, then the horse, then the Transformer, then the racing car. You would be watching each of the compartments and trying to remember the toys in *order*. Then, I'll ask you to tell me the toys that you saw.

Verbalization of the Training Strategy by the Student

This step introduces the students to the idea of active learning; that they must "do something inside their heads" to recall the information correctly. During the impeded learning cycle, this step enables the teacher to check that the importance of using a memory strategy (in this case, rehearsal) is understood.

Teacher: John, how are you going to try to remember the toys? What are you going to do to help you remember them?

John: What do you mean?

Teacher: Well, you have to do something in your head to be able to remember the toys. What could you do?

John: I'd watch what they were and say them.

Teacher: That's a good idea, isn't it, Alex? To look at the toys one at a time a say them to yourself as you see them.

Identification of Task-Relevant Information

The teacher describes what information is needed from the task to ensure success, and questions the boys about what information must be gathered. This interaction focuses upon the important elements, thereby helping to reduce attention to task-irrelevant information.

Teacher: When I'm showing you the toys, you must watch only the compartment where the toy will be. You will be trying to remember what the toys are. So, you need to keep your mind on where the toys will be and what they're called. OK, just remind me. What are you trying to do?

John: Remember what the toys are called in the right order.

Teacher: Excellent. Let's try it. This time, say what's happening and what you're doing out aloud so that Alex and I can hear you.

The Student Attempts the Task

Students are encouraged to verbalize progress. In the early stages of the program, the teacher watches the student's behavior carefully. As training progresses, students learn to self-manage their behavior, either independently or through interaction between the students.

Teacher: (The teacher places four different toys in the box. Closes the lid and places it on the table.) John, watch carefully and remember to say what your doing out aloud so that we can hear you.

John: (As the lid is slid across to reveal each of the toys) There is a whistle . . . then the poker chip . . . then money . . . and the ring. Whistle, poker chip, money, ring.

Summary of Activity and Strategies

Following each trial, the teacher asks the student to summarize the performance and, as the program progresses, emphasizes and reinforces appropriate strategic behavior.

Teacher: John did very well then, didn't he, Alex? He remembered the toys just as they were shown to him. Can you tell us how you did it, John?

John: I said them out aloud.

Teacher: Yes, you did, and that's one way we can remember things when they come one at a time like that. Can you think of another way you could have helped yourself remember them?

Alex: He could've said them over and over again. I've seen my mum do that when she hears the Lotto numbers [lottery numbers given on TV].

Teacher: That's right, Alex. John could have said them over and over again until he learned them by heart. That's called rehearsing. Like actors who are trying to rehearse what they're to say in a movie.

Instruction

This phase links with the trial that has gone immediately before (e.g., the task described above). There are two major objectives in the instruction phase. The teacher must, first, identify and clarify the effectiveness of the strategies used by the student in the task (i.e., the student's preferred strategy), and second, enhance the student's strategic behavior by demonstrating an improved strategy (or an alternative). This phase draws on the teacher's observational skills and involves the generation and testing of hypotheses related to strategy use and effectiveness. It has four steps.

Identification of Student's Preferred Strategies

The first step involves clarification and evaluation of the student's behavior. The goal is to build upon the student's existing skills rather than impose unfamiliar procedures and strategies that may not facilitate performance (Turner & Bray, 1985). Moreover, the PBI process aims to evaluate how students attempt to problem solve and is designed to teach strategies only when students do not have an appropriate mechanism for dealing with the existing situation. Throughout PBI, the teacher must be mindful of the need to be active in collecting information about the student's knowledge and strategies based upon observation and clarification. For example, is the student rehearsing or chunking?

Recognition and Evaluation of Preferred Strategy

In this step, the teacher attempts to verify or reject the hypotheses made concerning the student's problem solving behavior. The interaction with the student promotes an awareness of strategic behavior. In later trials, the teacher emphasizes the pupil's selection of a preferred strategy for the particular task.

The interaction here was in the fourth session between the teacher and two girls attending a special class for students with mild intellectual disabilities in a large high school. The students were working on a task that had been introduced in the previous week. It was a serial processing task called "telephone dialing". In brief, the students were given telephone numbers of increasing length orally to be keyed into a push-button or dial-type telephone. Gabrielle understood the idea of rehearsal and chunking groups of numbers. Tanya had more difficulty with the task than Gabrielle.

Teacher: Tanya, I've been watching how you've been trying to remember the numbers. Can you tell how you've been trying to do it?
Tanya: I listen and try to remember them. Then I ring them.
Teacher: Can you tell me what you're doing to remember them?
Tanya: I hear you say them, and then remember them.
Teacher: Ok, Let me see if I've got it right. You tell me if this is what you do. Let's look at a telephone number. Gabrielle, why don't you give me a number? Write it down there. (Gabrielle writes "523154" on a small filing card provided by the teacher.)
Gabrielle: That's my phone number!
Teacher: Good. Now Tanya, if I say "5" (pointing to "5") would you say "5" to yourself? (Tanya nods affirmative.) If I say "2" (pointing) after the "5," would you say just the "2," or would you say "5, 2"?
Tanya: "2."
Teacher: OK. So when I say "5" you say "5." When I say "2," you'd say "2." When I say "3," you'd say "3." I say "1," you'd say "1," like that?
Tanya: Yeah.
Gabrielle: I do it different to that.

Reviewing the Student's Present strategy

The teacher now talks about the value of using effective coding strategies. In many cases at the beginning of training the pupil's strategic behavior (such as Tanya's), is rudimentary, but it is still more effective than just listening without undertaking any active coding behavior. At this stage, the teacher decided that it would be premature to discuss strategies in detail with Tanya but such a discussion may be appropriate with another child who uses a basic rehearsal strategy. In the latter case, the teacher might indicate that rehearsal can be improved by organizing the information further in units of two or three (e.g., 523, 154).

Teaching an Improved Strategy

This is the instructional step. The teacher demonstrates how the students may enhance their strategic behavior. If a pupil spontaneously uses an inefficient strategy (e.g., naming the elements only in a serial recall task), the teacher demonstrates how the strategy can be made more effective (e.g., by using rehearsal and/or chunking). If the strategy used by the pupil is effective, it is reinforced. Alternatively, if the pupil rehearses aloud, the teacher might suggest that subvocal rehearsal would help reduce the cognitive demands of the task.

In the transcript above, Tanya's strategy was not very successful. Introducing rehearsal would be the first step toward more efficient encoding. At this stage, the teacher talked about how Gabrielle used rehearsal to remember the words, and Gabrielle suggested that Tanya should try her way.

Teacher: Gabrielle's way of trying to remember numbers works because it means that instead of only hearing each number once, she gets to say them several times, and this helps her to remember them. The more times you say the numbers, the better chance you'll have of getting them into your mind just like as if I was putting this card into my brain. Do you understand what I mean? Do you think you can rehearse some numbers if I give you some?
Tanya: Yes.
Teacher: Ok, tell me how you'd do it. (Teacher loops back to task performance.)
Tanya: When you said a number, I'd say the number. When you say the next number, I say the first one then the second one. When you said the third one, I say the first one, then the second, then the last one . . .
Teacher: That's the way. Let's try one with just three numbers. Gabrielle, let's use part of your telephone number for this try.

Tanya then practiced the use of the strategy in a second trial using the same task. In the process, the teacher loops back to the task performance phase, verifying the use of the strategy, and identifying aspects of the student's problem solving behavior that may limit progress.

Intervention

During this phase, students attempt the task a second time using the amended strategy. The initial instructional steps are repeated to ensure that the pupil learns the procedure. The focus is not simply practice for the student, but provides the opportunity for the teacher to refine and reformulate hypotheses dealing with blockages that may affect the student's performance. The teacher's responsibility is to evaluate the performance and derive suggestions that will enhance the effectiveness of the training.

Identification of Blockages by Teacher

This steps links with the trial that has gone immediately before. After the child has attempted the task, the teacher evaluates the performance and draws attention to potential blockages that may inhibit progress. For example, the teacher may say: "It looks like we're having a problem here, let's see if we can find out what it is." The interaction then concentrates on how the student attempted the task.

The example involves two 13-year-old boys who were attending a remedial reading class in a rural high school. Both boys had problems with reading comprehension. In this example from their sixth session, they were using a scale drawing of the room in which they were working together with cardboard pieces (cut to scale) representing the furniture (see Figure 16.2). In this session, Kieran struggled with placement of the cardboard pieces.

Kieran: I can't find the right place for this (holding up a piece that represented a filing cabinet to the right of where Kieran was sitting). It should go there, but that's where the door is.
Teacher: Alright. Let's see how you're trying to work out where that piece goes. What piece is that there?
Kieran: The desk.
Teacher: How did you work out that it goes there (pointing to the desk)?
Kieran: 'Cause it's in the middle of the room.
Teacher: Fine, that's good Now what piece would you put in next?
Kieran: This piece [the filing cabinet].
Teacher: Why did you pick that one?
Kieran: 'Cause it's big.
Teacher: OK, now what? (Kieran looks at the cabinet, then puts the cutout in the doorway, looking puzzled.) Can you tell me what you're thinking?
Kieran: I'm trying to put the filing cabinet in.
Teacher: Yes, I can see that you looked at the filing cabinet and then took the cutout to put on the plan. Tell me some more.

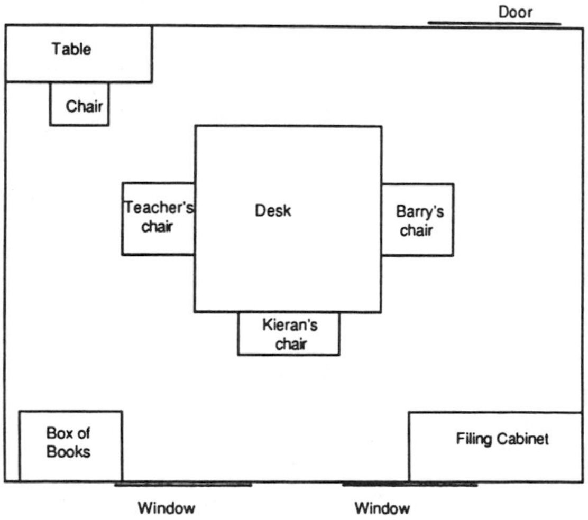

FIGURE 16.2. Diagram of a room and its furnishings used in the training task on spatial cues.

Kieran: Well, it won't go there (pointing to the doorway on the plan) because that's where the door is.
Teacher: And you think that that's where it should go on the plan?
Kieran: Umm. It can't go there.
Teacher: Where else could it go? (He picks up the piece and looks at the plan. The teacher watches Kieran's eyes and notices that they move from corner to corner on the plan of the room.) What are you looking at now, Kieran? Are you trying to decide if the cabinet should go in a different corner?
Kieran: Yes. The plan must be drawn wrong.
Teacher: I'm sure the plan is right . . . Here are the windows on the side away from the door, and here on the plan, the windows are on the opposite side to the door . . . and the filing cabinet is between . . .
Kieran: Yeah. Then the filing cabinet goes between the door and the windows.
Teacher: Yes, that's right, good thinking. Look at how the pieces go together.

The teacher discovered that Kieran's confusion came from disorientation. When he looked right, to the filing cabinet, he mentally transposed the position of the cabinet on the plan. When the position of the cabinet was resolved, the teacher had him place his chair on the plan, then established his orientation (looking at the door) on the plan. By pointing left and right, he was able to establish the relationships between the other items in the room.

Recognition and Evaluation of Blockages

Students are encouraged to suggest how the blockages may be overcome. These are evaluated and discussed.

Teacher: So, the first thing we need to do when we're making a plan like this one, is to look around and make sure we know where the fixed things are in the room, like the doors and the windows, and how they fit on the plan, if we already have one. What would be do next?
Kieran: Figure out where the big things go.
Teacher: Like what?
Kieran: The desk and where I am.
Teacher: Yes, that's a very good idea. You have to figure out which way you're looking so that you can work out whether the furniture is in front, or on the right or left side of you.

Use of Peers as Models and Tutors

PBI prescribes interactions between the teacher and students that are intended to develop problem solving behavior. In addition, the peer tutoring aspects provide the opportunity for students to reinforce knowledge and strategy use through the teaching-learning experience (Osguthorpe & Scruggs, 1986). Once students have learned a strategy, getting them to explain it to another student helps consolidate the skill and may lead to consideration of alternative problem solving methods. Kieran and Barry's session provided examples of both activities.

Teacher: Now let's pretend that Kieran has to teach this exercise to someone else in the class. Let's pretend that Barry doesn't know how to do it. First, let's take the furniture pieces off the plan and help Barry to get started. (Barry takes the pieces and starts to put them on the plan.) Hold on a minute, Barry. Remember, Kieran's going to explain to you how to go, step by step as if you haven't done this before. What you have to do is listen to him and do just the way he says. OK?

Barry: I know what to do.

Teacher: Yes, I'm sure you do because you've been watching very carefully, but remember how you had a turn last time, telling Kieran how to put the picture cards into a story? Well, it's his turn to show you how to do this one. And remember, you have to listen very carefully and follow his instructions, so that you can see if he's told you everything you need to know. (Barry nods agreement.) OK, go to it.

Kieran: You've got to put these pieces on the plan jus' the way they are here. Have a look to see where things are. I think you should look around and see how the plan is supposed to go. Like, there is the door there (points), and here it is on the plan, so it [the plan] has to be turned like that. Don't put any bits on yet. OK, you tell yourself that the desk has to go on first, then you . . . (Barry places the desk in the middle of the room but places it sideways). No, it has to go sideways. Look again. The long bit goes to the door. (Barry looks at the table and turns the card 90°, then positions the card correctly to represent his chair.) Is that your chair?

Barry: Yeah. (Barry completes the plan under Kieran's direction).

Teacher: Can you think of another way we could have tried to solve this problem? For instance, think about what you can see if you don't turn your head. Barry, can you see the cabinet without turning your head?

Barry: No, I have to turn around.

Teacher: That's right, so one way to see everything would be to stand somewhere where you can see where everything goes. Where would that be?

Kieran: If you were on the roof, like a cockroach.

Teacher: Yes, that'd be one way to get the whole picture. But think, when you first came into the room, would you see the whole room from the door? (The teacher emphasizes the essence of simultaneous processing, showing the relationship between all elements.)

Review and Reinforcement of Strategies

The strategies used during the trial are reviewed, and the student is encouraged to use the preferred strategy (if it is effective) or an improved version of the present strategy. Emphasis is given to metaprocessing, that is, ensuring that the students are aware of how successful they can become by using the newly acquired strategies.

Teacher: So, what have we learned about plans? Let's just think about it for a minute. Barry, what have we learned?
Barry: We need to put ourselves on the plan first.
Teacher: Yes, we must see everything in the room from our position, so we start to know how all the pieces fit together. Perhaps there's a step before putting ourself on the plan. Do you have any ideas, Kieran?
Kieran: We need to look around before we do anything.
Teacher: Yes, I think you're right, too. We need to look at what's in the room first, and where the pieces of furniture are in relation to other.

The teacher talked about the overall pattern on the plan giving information about relationships. The teacher rearranged the furniture pieces on the plan and asked each boy to point to where he would expect to find each piece if he was sitting in his seat in the newly arranged plan. This practices and reinforces the use of the newly acquired strategy.

Generalization Cycle

PBI provides the opportunity for students to consider appropriate uses for the newly acquired strategies as students can learn to use strategies without recognizing the importance of planful behavior in problem solving. Learning-how (to perform some complex activity) in contrast to learning-that (i.e., propositions about performance) is an important factor in the generalization of problem solving activities. Learning-how is achieved through induced performance, by modeling, practice, and feedback, whereas learning-that is accomplished by the presentation of rules and relationships that are consolidated by practice (Tharp & Gallimore, 1985).

The generalization cycle provides the opportunity for students to learn how strategies may be applied in new situations. Students learn that strategies can be transferred from one task and learning milieu to another. They have the opportunity to consider the effectiveness of strategic behavior in alternative situations. This exercise provides the opportunity for practice and feedback of strategic behavior in multiple contexts.

Identification of Generalization Activities

After the review of the pupil's performance in the intervention cycle, the teacher asks the students to suggest other problems in which the newly acquired skill and strategies could be used. With the furniture plan, for example, students might recognize the energy that is to be saved when rearranging their bedroom at home. Serial recall strategies could be applied to learning people's names at a party. In the early stage of training, the teacher may suggest a task for which the present strategy might be useful, but over the complete session, a list of activities or problem situations can be generated.

Recognition and Evaluation of Strategy Generalization

The students are encouraged to elaborate upon the use of strategies in new situations as this helps to establish the pupil's commitment to a strategy. In one sense, this step involves thinking through the use of the strategies in a variety of situations and contexts.

The teacher now changes the role of the active student to that of observer, and another activity is chosen. Throughout the intervention, the teacher discourages competition between the students and promotes cooperation. This may be achieved by suggesting that people can use many different techniques to solve the same problems and that one person's approach is not necessarily better than another. The teacher ensures that the input is consistent with the spirit of the training.

Implementing PBI: Two Studies

The examples presented above were drawn from training sessions in two studies undertaken to evaluate the efficacy of the PBI model as used by teachers with students experiencing learning difficulties. The first investigation was a pilot study designed to gauge the suitability of the procedures and materials for use with adolescent students. In the second study, attention was given to the effect of two forms of training tasks: (a) tasks using novel, laboratory-type materials that were unrelated to activities undertaken outside the schoolroom; and (b) tasks that used scenarios and materials that were analogous to activities or events commonly encountered by the students.

In both studies, PBI was introduced by two special education project teachers who were trained in the procedures over a period of 6 months. They were involved in developing the teaching materials and lesson plans. During the intervention, the PBI procedures were presented in a prescribed and systematic way using lesson plans that referred to each of the 18 steps. Probes were also generated for each session to evaluate the student performance. All sessions were tape recorded, and tapes were reviewed by the teachers and the author to ensure consistency of teaching approach and method. In addition, sessions were included during which the author and each of the teachers in turn observed a training session. These "reliability" sessions showed consistency in teachers' interactions with the students and in following the prescribed plan. Two intervention sessions were scheduled per week for 8 weeks, totaling 12 contact hours. Although a longer program would have been ideal, changes were expected after 8 weeks.

An Exploratory Study

The first study was undertaken with 34 mildly intellectually disabled teenagers attending regular high schools (Ashman, 1986b). The children were assigned to pairs by their class teachers on the basis on social compatibility and these pairs were randomly assigned to one of four groups. Group 1 received training in the use of simultaneous processing strategies and group 2 received sequential processing strategy training only. Group 3 received an intervention that dealt broadly with problem solving but without PBI or a strategy training component. Group 4 received no intervention.

A battery of processing tests and language tests (the latter from Semel & Wiig, 1982) were administered to students prior to and at the conclusion of the intervention, and after a further 12 weeks. Data analysis focused upon improvement in students' coding performance following the intervention.

The results indicated that strategy training assisted the students in the respective groups to improve and maintain their processing performance following instruction. That is, the simltaneous group improved on the simultaneous tasks but not on the sequential or planning tasks; the sequential group improved their performance on sequential, but not on the simultaneous or planning tasks; and the two control groups showed no improvement on the coding or planning measures.

A secondary objective of the study was to examine transfer of learning to language processing and production. In brief, the results of the analyses showed that the sequential training group made significant gains on language processing during the intervention and consolidated this improvement during the follow-up phase. The simultaneous, stimulation, and control groups generally showed little change in performance across the period of the study.

Analysis of individual student data attempted to identify why some children showed greater improvement than others. This examination revealed that 9 of the 10 children in each of the experimental groups improved their performance on the relevant coding measure, and it appeared that the lower ability students showed greater improvement than their higher ability peers. This trend did not appear to extend to the language measures.

Laboratory Versus Real-Life Problems

The second study had three aims: (a) to replicate the effect of the PBI process using the same sequence as applied in the first study; (b) to examine differences across students with varying abilities; and (c) to examine the effect of different training materials used in conjunction with PBI. Students in this study were of similar age and ability to those in the earlier study; all attended special classes in one of four large high schools, different from those in study 1.

Following pretesting, students were assigned to either the high or the low sequential processor group on the basis of their serial processing competence. Students were then assigned to experimental pairs by their regular teacher and these pairs were then randomly assigned to one of three groups. One group received instruction using training materials similar to those used in other *laboratory* studies; a second used tasks related to *real-life* or day-to-day activities; and, the third received no intervention. Therefore, students were assigned to six groups, crossing training task with ability (Ashman, 1986b).

Both project teachers worked with all experimental group students. For the first half of the intervention, one teacher worked with the laboratory materials while the other used the real-life task. At the midway point, this arrangement was reversed, thus minimizing the confounding effect of teachers upon treatments. Lessons plans, similar to those used in the first study were developed, and observations and tape recorded and written records of sessions were undertaken to monitor consistency.

The success of the intervention was evaluated by comparing pre- and posttest performances of the students on the processing and achievement tests. Students (low and high ability combined) who received training using the real-life activities outperformed the laboratory group and continued to improve into the follow-up period. This suggested that the more broadly based training may have encouraged students to use their skills away from the training context, and thus, obtain experience that might promote the unassisted use of serial processing strategies. In contrast, the students using laboratory materials improved up to the posttest session, and maintained their standard at the follow-up session.

To determine whether improvement was dependent upon the initial processing competence, data were analyzed according to the high or low serial processing conditions. The results showed that the low-ability students in the training groups made substantial performance gains while not exceeding the scores of their high-ability peers. Differences between the task conditions (laboratory versus real-life) were not found. Similar results were reported by Petersen and Swing (1983). In the present study, it appeared that the high-ability students may not have been as highly motivated to achieve as the low-ability classmates, perhaps due to the hypothetical nature of the training materials.

In this investigation, the transfer of learning to achievement tests was also examined. Only one significant result was found, for arithmetic. This Kaufman Assessment Battery for Children (K-ABC) achievement test is predominartly a mental arithmetic task and it could be expected that the development and use of serial strategies would enhance recall.

Discussion

Generally speaking, the purpose of the studies reported here was the development of an instructional model that provides a systematic educational approach suitable for use with mildly intellectually disabled students. The results of interventions up to this point have shown general improvement by the students involved in both their attitude toward learning and their performance. Moreover, the studies have led to optimism concerning the value of a unified assessment-instructional approach for enhancing processing competence, one that is concerned with the *whole* process rather than elements (Borkowski & Büchel, 1983).

What are the future directions? The ultimate goal of PBI is application within the classroom, managed by the regular classroom teacher. The current series of studies has moved in that direction. This requires consideration of process versus skill training, and in one study the efficacy of process/skill training has been examined. Moreover, it is recognized that the dynamics within the laboratory and the classroom are quite different, and that changes in the PBI procedures will be required to allow for interactions with class-size groups of students. However, the essential assessment and instruction components of PBI should remain constant (Conway, 1985).

In conclusion, PBI appears to offer a valid extension of assessment into the area of instruction and intervention. Although it is recognized that considerable examination of, and refinement to, the procedures is still required, the changes in student behavior and performance indicates that there is much to be gained. Moreover, PBI offers much to the classroom teacher in terms of philosophy, attitude, and methods, and seems to be appropriate for teachers working in resource and regular classroom contexts. Of course, the final test of the efficacy and success of Process-Based Instruction will be its acceptance and use by classroom teachers. For further information relating to the development and practical application of PBI, see Ashman and Conway (1989).

References

Anderson, J. R., Greeno, J. G., Kline, P. J., & Neves, D. M. (1981). Acquisition of problem solving skills. In J. R. Anderson (Ed.), *Cognitive skills and their acquisition*. Hillsdale, NJ: Erlbaum.

Ashman, A. F. (1978). *Relationship between planning and simultaneous-successive processing*. Unpublished doctoral dissertation, University of Alberta, Edmonton, Canada.

Ashman, A. F. (1985). Process-based interventions for retarded students. *Mental Retardation and Learning Disability Bulletin*, *13*, 62–74.

Ashman, A. F. (1986a). Aeronautical decision making. *SAFE*, *3*, 1–8.

Ashman, A. F. (1986b). *Cognitive training with mildly intellectually handicapped adolescents* (Report to the Australian Research Grants Scheme). Newcastle, NSW: Department of Education, University of Newcastle.

Ashman, A. F., & Conway, R. N. F. (1989). *Cognitive strategies for special education*. London: Routledge.

Belmont, J. M., & Mitchell, D. W. (1987). The general strategies hypothesis as applied to cognitive theory in mental retardation. *Intelligence*, *11*, 91–105.

Berger, R. M., Guilford, J. P., & Christensen, P. R. (1957). A factor-analytic study of planning abilities. *Psychological Monographs: General and Applied*, *71*, (6, Whole No. 435).
Borkowski, J. G., & Büchel, F. P. (1983). Learning and memory strategies in the mentally retarded. In M. Pressley & J. R. Levin (Eds.), *Cognitive strategy research: psychological foundations* (pp. 103–128). New York: Springer-Verlag.
Borkowski, J. G., & Cavanaugh, J. C. (1979). Maintenance and generalization of strategies by the retarded. In N. R. Ellis (Ed.), *Handbook of mental deficiency, psychological theory, and research* (pp. 569–617). Hillsdale, NJ: Erlbaum.
Brown, A. L. (1974). The role of strategic behavior in retardate memory. In N. R. Ellis (Ed.), *International review of research in mental retardation* (Vol. 7, pp. 55–111). New York: Academic Press.
Brown, A. L., & Campione, J. C. (1986). Psychological theory and the study of learning disabilities. *American Psychologist*, *41*, 1059–1068.
Conway, R. N. F. (1985). *Remediation using the information-integration model.* Paper presented at the annual meeting of the American Educational Research Association, Chicago, II.
Das, J. P., Kirby, J. R., & Jarman, R. F. (1979). *Simultaneous and successive cognitive processes*. New York: Academic Press.
Feuerstein, R., Rand, Y., Hoffman, M. B., & Miller, R. (1980). *Instrumental enrichment: An intervention for cognitive modifiability*. Baltimore: University Park Press.
Federicksen, N. (1984). Implications of cognitive theory for instruction in problem solving. *Review of Educational Research*, *54*, 363–407.
Hayes-Roth, B. & Hayes-Roth, F. (1979). A cognitive model of planning. *Cognitive Science*, *3*, 275–310.
Kaufman, A. S. (1984). K-ABC and controversy. *Journal of Special Education*, *19*, 409–444.
Kaufman, A. S., & Kaufman, N. L. (1983). *Kaufman assessment battery for children: Interpretative manual*. Circle Pines, MN: American Guidance Service.
Kirby, J. R., & Ashman, A. F. (1984). Planning skills and mathematics achievement. *Journal of Psychoeducational Assessment*, *2*, 9–22.
Kops, C., & Belmont, I. (1985). Planning and organizing skills of poor school achievers. *Journal of Learning Disabilities*, *18*, 8–14.
Kramer, J. J., & Engle, R. W. (1981). Training awareness of strategic behavior in combination with strategy training: Effect on children's memory performance. *Journal of Experimental Child Psychology*, *32*, 513–530.
Luria, A. R. (1973). *The working brain*. Harmondsworth: Penguin.
Manzo, A. V. (1968). *Improvement of reading comprehension through reciprocal questioning*. Unpublished doctoral dissertation, Syracuse University, New York.
Marsh, G. E., Price, B. J., & Smith, T. E. C. (1983). *Teaching mildly handicapped children: Methods and materials*. St Louis: C. V. Mosby.
Miller, G. A., Galanter, E., & Pribram, K. H. (1960). *Plans and the structure of behavior*. New York: Holt.
Osguthorpe, R. T., & Scruggs, T. E. (1986). Special education students as tutors: A review and analysis. *RASE*, *7*, 15–26.
Palincsar, A. S., & Brown, A. L. (1984). Reciprocal teaching of comprehension-fostering and monitoring activities. *Cognition and Instruction*, *1*, 117–175.

Petersen, P. L., & Swing, S. R. (1983). Problems in classroom implementation of cognitive strategy instruction. In M. Pressley & J. R. Levin (Eds.), *Cognitive strategy research: Educational applications* (pp. 267–287). New York: Springer-Verlag.

Rand, Y., Tannenbaum, A. J., & Feuerstein, R. (1979). Effects of instrumental enrichment on the psychoeducational development of low-functioning adolescents. *Journal of Educational Psychology*, *71*, 751–763.

Schofield, N. J., & Ashman, A. F. (1987). The cognitive processing of gifted, high average, and low average ability students. *British Journal of Educational Psychology*, *57*, 9–20.

Semel, E. M., & Wiig, E. H. (1982). *Clinical evaluation of language functions: Diagnostic battery examiner's manual*. Columbus, OH: Merrill.

Siegler, R. S. (1976). Three aspects of cognitive development. *Cognitive Psychology*, *8*, 481–520.

Simon, H. A. (1978). Information-processing theory of human problem solving. In W. K. Estes (Ed.), *Handbook of learning and cognitive processes (Vol. 5—Human information processing)*. Hillsdale, NJ: Erlbaum.

Simon, H. A. (1980). Problem solving and education. In D. T. Tuma & R. Reif (Eds.), *Problem solving and education: Issues in teaching and research*. Hillsdale, NJ: Erlbaum.

Smith, P. K., & Dutton, S. (1979). Play and training in direct and innovative problem solving. *Child Development*, *50*, 830–836.

Spitz, H. H., Minsky, S. K., & Bessellieu, C. L. (1985). Influences of planning time and first-move strategy on Tower of Hanoi problem solving performance of mentally retarded young adults and nonretarded children. *American Journal of Mental Deficiency*, *90*, 46–56.

Sternberg, R. J. (1980). Sketch of a componential subtheory of human intelligence. *Behavior and Brain Sciences*, *3*, 573–614.

Tharp, R. G., & Gallimore, R. (1985). The logical status of metacognitive training. *Journal of Abnormal Child Psychology*, *13*, 455–466.

Turner, L. A., & Bray, N. W. (1985). Spontaneous rehearsal by mildly mentally retarded children and adolescents. *American Journal of Mental Deficiency*, *90*, 57–63.

Part 4
Case Studies of Interactive Assessment

One way to learn the specific aspects and applications of a method—whether of assessment, psychotherapy, highway paving, or cake baking—is to examine individual cases in substantial detail. In this section we present two intensive case studies derived from quite different theoretical perspectives. In presenting these the editors want to emphasize that they are selective rather than representative. That is to say, a clinical method depends to some extent on the individual preferences, skills, and experience of its practitioners as well as on their theoretical orientations. Other practitioners, even under the same set of theory, might do things differently. In addition, these two cases represent only two of several possible theoretical orientations.

Kaniel and Tzuriel in Chapter 17 demonstrate the application of a "mediated learning" approach to the assessment and treatment of persons with a major psychiatric disorder. Their method is derived from Feuerstein's theory of structural cognitive modifiability and mediated learning experience, and their assessment tools are those of the Learning Potential Assessment Device. Their chapter extends both the theoretical and the applied aspects of Feuerstein's system, and provides a demonstration of the dual role of interactive assessment as a clinical tool and as a research tool.

Chapter 18 by Paour and Soavi represents an approach that is not yet widely familiar among English-speaking psychologists and educators. Called "operatory learning," their method is essentially neo-Piagetian. These authors base their work on the observation that deficient performance often reflects a fixation in cognitive development at the preoperatory level. They demonstrate that this particular fixation may be characterized as failure to have acquired the "pairing relation," i.e., the concept that two or more events may be related to each other in more-or-less arbitrary ways. When their training overcomes that specific deficiency, greater cognitive, intellectual, and learning potential is revealed.

17
Mediated Learning Experience Approach in the Assessment and Treatment of Borderline Psychotic Adolescents

Shlomo Kaniel and David Tzuriel

The development of diagnostic and therapeutic approaches during the last decade has been accompanied by an increasing awareness of the important effects of cognitive factors and social milieu on the formation of mental structures and behavior patterns (Maultsby, 1984; Meichenbaum, 1974, 1977).

Novel approaches to the treatment of persons with psychopathological conditions have emphasized the role of the social milieu in rehabilitation, especially of those with borderline psychotic conditions. One of the main problems in the treatment of these persons is finding an optimal balance between ensuring a protective environment and allowing exposure to the stresses and conflicts of normal life conditions. The mediated learning experience (MLE) treatment presented in this chapter is an effort to address that optimal balance, as well as other issues concerning assessment and treatment.

The MLE theory (Feuerstein & Rand, 1974; Feuerstein, Rand, Hoffman, & Miller, 1980) is based on an "active modificational" approach (Feuerstein, 1970), which has generated three applicative systems: (a) the dynamic assessment of individual learning potential, whose major objective is the evaluation of cognitive modifiability above and beyond a person's manifest level of functioning; (b) a cognitive education program known as Instrumental Enrichment (IE), and the conceptualization of interactive processes that lead to the increase of cognitive modifiability; and (c) establishment of a situation in which the modifiability assessed through dynamic assessment and enhanced by IE and MLE will become reinforced by an environment in which modifiability is a major need for survival.

In the first part of the chapter the theoretical assumptions of the MLE approach are presented. In the second part, there is a discussion of the MLE theory and its derivative systems: the Learning Potential Assessment Device (LPAD; Feuerstein, Rand, & Hoffman, 1979), the Instrumental Enrichment Program, and modification of environment (Feuerstein et al., 1980). In the last part, we present a case study of an adolescent diagnosed as psychotic, who was given a "dynamic" assessment and then was treated for several years using the MLE approach.

Theoretical Assumptions of the MLE Approach

The clinical procedures using the MLE approach in treatment of mentally retarded or mentally disturbed adolescents are based upon several assumptions of the theory of structural cognitive modifiability (SCM; Feuerstein et al., 1980). The same theoretical principles that guide the treatment of persons whose main problems are cognitive also guide the treatment of those whose main problems are emotional. From this point of view, a person is perceived as a whole and not fragmented artificially into cognitive and emotional components. In fact, in many cases it is difficult, if not impossible, to make a distinction between these two areas of human functioning. The theoretical principles of SCM allow enough flexibility to adjust both mediational (cognitive) processes and environmental conditions to each person's specific requirements.

According to the first assumption, the human organism is conceived of as an open system given to continuous changes. Thus, an observed low level of functioning is not accepted as a fixed ceiling for one's capacity, nor perceived as a predictor of one's social and/or occupational adjustment in the future. Low-functioning persons, as well as their parents and teachers, are encouraged to set long- and short-term goals and expectations for adequate integration in society.

The second assumption of the theory of SCM is that retarded performance is reversible (Filler, Robinson, Smith, Vincent-Smith, Bricker, & Bricker, 1975). Redevelopment of low-performing individuals may occur through helping persons to acquire efficient learning strategies, working habits, thinking skills, and behavior patterns (Feuerstein et al., 1980). In fact, reversibility of low functioning may occur spontaneously given proper change in life circumstances, as shown by studies on early experiential deprivation (Clarke & Clarke, 1976; Skeels, 1966; Skodak, 1968).

The third assumption is related to the distinction between distal and proximal etiologies. Distal etiology refers to those determinants that do not lead directly and invariably to certain specific outcomes, but rather have a trigger effect. Examples of distal factors are genetic factors, organic deficiencies, a history of stimulus deprivation, a family's impoverished language, and emotional disturbance of children and/or parents. Proximal etiology, on the other hand, is composed of those determinants that, when triggered by a distal factor, lead directly and invariably to specific cognitive outcomes. When, for certain reasons, the distal determinants do not succeed in triggering the proximal determinant, or are prevented from doing so, the expected end product may not necessarily appear. The most important proximal factor is the mediated learning experience (Feuerstein et al., 1980). Because of its importance, the MLE concept is discussed later in detail.

The fourth assumption of the MLE approach refers to a synchronized integrated treatment of various areas of functioning (cognitive, social, personal). Due to the complexity of the human organism, it is assumed that treatment of psychotic adolescents is most efficient within an ecological framework in which all aspects of human functioning are taken care of. At different phases of the treatment process, emphasis can change from one area to another according to the individual's current needs and therapeutic goals. It is also our assumption that changes in one area of functioning are transferred to other areas. Example: Focused intervention in the cognitive area is transferred by a diffusion process to the social functioning and/or emotional aspects that were not directly treated. A detailed description of the mediated learning experience theory is given in several papers (Feuerstein, 1977; Feuerstein & Rand, 1974; Jensen, Feuerstein, Rand, Kaniel, & Tzuriel, 1986; Tzuriel & Haywood, Chapter 1 this volume). Because of space limitations readers are referred to those sources. It is important to emphasize that because MLE is, by definition, an environmental variable, the deficits produced by its absence or insufficiency may be more readily reversible than they might be if these were "constitutional" deficits. According to MLE theory, no limits are set for the mediational process; neither are critical periods implied for development. Although early childhood can be considered an optimal period for MLE, a great deal can be achieved at later stages of development by providing adequate MLE.

The MLE theory serves as a basis for three main applicative systems: the Learning Potential Assessment Device (LPAD), the Instrumental Enrichment Program (IEP), and the shaping of the environment. All three systems are based on the same theoretical principles and are used integratively in treatment of low-functioning and/or emotionally disturbed individuals. They are presented here briefly.

The Learning Potential Assessment Device

LPAD, developed by Feuerstein et al. (1979), is the most well-developed of the dynamic assessment procedures. The main objective of the LPAD is to assess the cognitive modifiability of individuals, to identify those factors that bring about poor performance, and to assess the nature and amount of mediation required to change that performance. The whole assessment process involves teaching of prerequisite cognitive functions, work habits, rules, principles, and operations. Clients are first taught to solve a given problem using a cognitive principle, operation, or strategy such as classification, transformation, or systematic search. Then, they are given progressively new and complex problems that constitute variations on the initial task.

The LPAD is characterized by four changes or shifts that distinguish it from normative, static tests: (a) a shift from product to process orientation; (b) a modification of test structure; (c) a change of the test situation, especially of the examiner-client relationship; and (d) a shift in the interpretation of results. Detailed accounts have been given elsewhere (Feuerstein et al., 1979; Feuerstein, Haywood, Rand, Hoffman, & Jensen, 1986; Feuerstein & Shalom, 1967; Rand & Kaniel, 1987; Tzuriel & Feuerstein, this volume; Tzuriel & Haywood, Chapter 1 this volume).

Of most interest within the context of a therapeutic approach is the shift in the examiner-client relationship. The examiner is actively involved in the teaching-testing process by providing feedback on success and failure, and attaching meaning to certain behavior. The examiner focuses on efficient and inefficient modes of functioning, interprets results, and arouses attention and challenge. The examiner's care goes beyond the assessment objectives and carries with it therapeutic elements. It is no wonder that for many individuals the LPAD situation constitutes a turning point in their history of failure, passivity, apathy, frustration, and bitterness. Two points should be noted regarding the LPAD administration. First, the motivational change that occurs is not sufficient to make the client's problem solving behavior successful and efficient. Continual feedback transcending the immediate task should be provided using a variety of communicational modalities. Second, the LPAD process can be a starting point for a long-range process in the treatment of borderline psychotic adults. The line between assessment and therapy becomes blurred as the examiner moves within the testing situation to a therapeutic situation. In some cases the LPAD becomes a "springboard" to a cognitive therapeutic approach. Although one cannot expect truly structural changes within an assessment situation, even with dynamic assessment, it is possible to derive an indication of what future changes may be possible, and of what will be required to achieve those changes.

The Instrumental Enrichment Program

The IEP (Feuerstein et al., 1980) was designed mainly to modify those intellective functions that are conceived to be responsible for ineffective thinking, learning, and performance. The IEP is a way of providing the MLE that might have been deficient during earlier stages of development. The major goal of the IEP is to enhance the cognitive modifiability of the individual. This goal is broken down into six subgoals: (a) correction of deficient cognitive functions; (b) teaching of sepcific concepts, operations, and vocabulary required by the IEP; (c) development of an intrinsic need for adequate cognitive functioning and spontaneous use of operational thinking by production of crystallized schemas and habits; (d) production of insight and understanding of one's own thought processes; (e) production of task-intrinsic motivation, reinforced by attaching meaning to operations and content in a broader social context; and (f) change in the manner of viewing oneself from a passive recipient of information to an active generator of information.

The IEP consists of a set of content-controlled "instruments" (curriculum units or groups of lessons) containing paper and pencil exercises. The program is usually integrated into a shcool curriculum, spread over 2 to 3 years (400 hours) with a minimum of three sessions per week. The attainment of all the subgoals depends largely on the interaction among the three elements of student, teacher, and instruments. There is no doubt that among all the components, the teacher's contributions are of greatest importance, especially in attaining subgoals b and d. In general, each instrument is focused on a small set of cognitive functions, and the redevelopment of dysfunctional areas, while incorporating others in a more diffused way. The exercises are designed to capture the interest of the students and enhance task-intrinsic motivation by being graded in difficulty and balanced with respect to required effort and challenge. The repetition that is often used aims at achieving crystallization and automatization of schemas by varying types of exercises (applications) while holding constant the underlying principle.

Systematic research carried out recently has shown success of the program as assessed by tests of intelligence and personality-motivational measures (Burden, 1987; Feuerstein, Rand, Hoffman, & Miller, 1979; Rand, Tannenbaum, & Feuerstein, 1979; Raziel, 1981; Redfield, 1984; Sar-Shalom, 1978; Savell, Twohig, & Rachford, 1986; Thickpenny, 1982; Tzuriel & Alfassi, 1987; Walker & Meier, 1982).

Although the main goal of the IEP is to enhance cognitive modifiability, it can have a great effect on the affective and behavioral areas of functioning. This approach is very similar to principles of the cognitive therapy paradigm (Maulstby, 1984; Meichenbaum, 1974, 1977; Meichenbaum & Asarnow, 1979). Although the principles are similar, the philosophical foundations, specific concepts, procedures, and techniques are different. Our basic assumption, verified by clinical experience, is that changes in cognitive structures are transferred by a diffusion process to the affective and behavioral areas. In other words, the affective and behavioral changes are inherent in the structural changes that have taken place.

Shaping of the Environment

An integrative component of the MLE approach in treatment of mentally disturbed or mentally retarded persons is shaping of the environment. According to this approach, exceptional children should be placed in a normal educational environment where they can be confronted with daily life problems. The conventional procedures of placing such persons in special settings (e.g., mental hospitals, institutions for the mentally retarded, special education schools) are frequently explained by the need to protect them from society's pressures as well as to protect society from their "bizarre," antisocial, or aggressive behavior. Cut off from normal peer models for imitation, the developing individuals are "channeled" to identify with an imitate peer models who suffer the same or other difficulties. Thus, living in special settings prevents these persons from returning to normal ways of behavior. Following this shaping of the environment approach, Feuerstein and Krasilowsky (1972) integrated 25 severely disturbed adolescents into a group of normally functioning adolescents. The criteria for placement of the disturbed adolescents were: total or functional illiteracy, low intelligence (40 to 75 IQ), primary emotional disturbance, and severe behavior disorders. About 20% of these adolescents were considered borderline or psychotic. They had been either hospitalized or seriously considered for hospitalization. Others had been rejected from normal or special school systems because of the severity of their dysfunctional behavior.

Four major intervention principles were applied in the treatment of these exceptional adolescents who were integrated within the normal group structure: unconditional acceptance, reduction of anxiety, induced regression, and planned and controlled relations with peers.

1. The unconditional acceptance provided the individual, and the group feelings of belonging, regardless of behavior, were essential in order to establish the basic trust of adolescents. In practical terms this meant that no adolescent was ever rejected because of either behavior problems or signs of maladjustment. Even when behavior was considered dangerous in the immediate environment, everything was done to avoid rejection.
2. Anxiety had been generated by repeated failures and by feelings of incompetence in meeting age-specific academic and social functioning. Because the major source of frustration lay in the area of learning, it was important that schooling be presented to them in a more successful way. Accordingly, the adolescents were placed in two special classes that were organized around a great variety of nonacademic activities. The high level of tolerance displayed by the teachers allowed for spontaneous expressive behavior in class. In this way, the children openly expressed their need to devalue the area of performance that was the cause of their anxiety. Much of the early time at school was spent outside of the classroom on long and instructive talks. At the same time, major steps were taken to develop school functioning through individualized tutoring given by their group workers.

3. Induced regression (Alpert, 1975) helped these children to indulge in infantile, need-fulfilling behavior, especially in their relations with caring adults and peers. Many of these children had learned to control their behavior by confrontation with social reality. Unfortunately, this was achieved only by means of total blockage of their intellectual and social capacities. There was no ability to discriminate between areas of desirable activity and activity leading to rejection and punishment. Induced regression enabled those unfulfilled needs to be met and decreased the resistance to modification.
4. Planned and controlled relations with a normal peer group constituted the most essential principle of the treatment. The major theoretical assumptions underlying this principle are as follows: Adolescence is characterized by resistance to influence from the adult world, attempts to separate from previous attachments, and, at the same time, a great need to "belong." The peer group is the most important and potent medium for creating new identities, thus helping adolescents to solve the conflict between their tendency to be independent and the need to "belong." Because the ability of adults to socialize adolescents by transmitting attitudes, values, and motives is limited, it is essential to use the peer group as the main transmitter of values, as well as the principal means of modifying and shaping behavior. These theoretical assumptions are true for the great majority of normal adolescents and even more for disturbed adolescents. Following the principle of controlled relations with normal peers, the disturbed adolescents lived in close relationship with "normal" adolescents. Both groups met on the grounds, in the dining room, and in various group activities. They were able to associate as individuals. They could make friends or come into conflict with one another. In order to control behavior and to make use of these interactions, the group was provided with a relatively large number of workers (four group workers to 25 adolescents). These adults spent their time exclusively with the clients, so that they could intervene at the right moment, help with inevitable distress situations, or mediate the social meaning of daily events.

The results of Feuerstein and Krasilowsky's (1972) study showed a dramatic change in the treatment group, manifested by the absolute disappearance of delinquent behavior, as well as higher achievement in academic, social, and occupational areas as compared to their initial level of functioning. All of the adolescents entered military service. (Service in the Israel Defense Force is seen in Israel as an external objective criterion of adequate development and is crucial for social integration.) This clearly demonstrated the enormous degree of reversibility that one can expect. The capacity of the majority of the children to function very close to normal was shown by the fact that they were accepted by their normal peer groups, their own families, and society at large, whereas in the past they had been rejected. It seems that life within the group can be viewed as the basis of a "corrective emotional experience" whose effects are felt both in the adaptational capacities and in the emotional makeup of the children (Alpert, 1975).

The importance of peers has also been emphasized by Filler et al. (1975) in a comprehensive study on classification of children. Their first recommendation was that public school systems as a whole must be encouraged to develop programs for all children, even the most severely handicapped, within the domain of regular schools.

In the following section we describe the dynamic assessment and MLE-based treatment of a borderline psychotic, low-functioning adolescent. We emphasize that there have not been, as yet, any systematic experiments to study the MLE integrative approach with its implications for cognitive and emotional areas.

Case Report

History and Previous Testing

Peter was born 24 years earlier in Europe to survivors of the Holocaust. When Peter was 9, his parents immigrated to Israel and established themselves occupationally and economically. The father works as a merchant and the mother as a teacher. Both have an academic education. Peter is the firstborn and has two sisters and one brother. His first sister was born 3 years after Peter. Until Peter was 3 years old, the parents did not report any special behavior, though they recognized that Peter was not relaxed. He cried easily in response to little frustrations, such as losing a toy. He did not like physical touch and avoided interactions with strangers. Peter began kindergarten at the age of 3 at that time the teacher helped the parents to realize that Peter was an exceptional child. The kindergarten teacher told the parents that Peter sat alone, engaging in solitary "intelligent" activities for a long time. Any attempt to disengage him resulted in crying and deep anger. It seemed as if he were running from reality into inner worlds. His language was adequate but it was difficult for him to understand the relations between sentences or between the ideas he was expressing. At the age of 6, Peter was referred for diagnosis to a clinic where he was observed and tested by a few professionals. The reason for referral was "atypical behavior." One psychiatrist labeled him as "moderate autistic," and another's diagnosis was "schizophrenic reaction of childhood." On the Peabody Picture Vocabulary Test his IQ was 63. The psychiatrist reported that "this score is minimal and is not really indicative of the child's potential." Peter was at that time distractible, anxious, and not truly attending to the test instructions and content.

After receiving treatment by traditional supportive psychotherapy, pharmacotherapy, and placement in a special education school, a reevaluation was carried out when he was 9 years old. According to the report at that time, Peter had attended a special school for children with emotional behavior problems for the preceding 3 years. This had been recommended because his atypical behavior prevented him from participating in a regular class. During this period his behavior was characterized by many of the pathognomonic features of schizophrenic children, such as limited speech, almost no contact with people, hand fluttering, jumping, and confusion of reality with fantasy. He was viewed as a symbiotic, dependent child with an inadequate self-concept and poor differentiation of self from the external environment. There was also evidence of anxiety and a need for immediate impulse gratification due to low frustration tolerance.

When Peter and his parents came to Israel, he was placed in a regular school in a special education class. Three years later, at the age of 12, he went back to Europe for reevaluation at his parents' initiative. On the WISC-R, he attained a Verbal IQ of 79, a Performance IQ of 90, and a Full Scale IQ of 83. Great variability among the subscales was also reported (e.g., Information, 4; Object Assembly, 12). Academically, Peter functioned at about the early fourth grade (3 years behind his chronological age). The psychologist who tested Peter referred to the discrepancies in subtests by commenting, "There is a sufficient variability to suggest uneven intellectual development and greater potential." Behaviorally, Peter was attentive, with a tendency to become overexcited, which once resulted in a short outburst of aggression. In general, his behavior was appropriate, though somewhat immature. It is important to note that there was no comment in the report about schizophrenic or psychotic behavior. It seems reasonable to assume that the fact that Peter studied in a regular school, observing and modeling his normal peers, might be the reason for moderation of his psychotic behavior.

Dynamic Assessment by the LPAD

When Peter was 13 years old, his parents referred him for LPAD assessment and reevaluation. During testing he gave the impression of a highly motivated young adolescent, cooperative and attentive. Peter had well-developed moral standards, though on a conventional level. He complained about his friends' unjust behavior toward others, their messiness and untidiness, and claimed that their behavior was responsible for his social isolation. At home, he was given almost no opportunities for independence. His relationships with his two younger sisters and brother were strained. He interfered with their games and drove away their friends, usually by screaming and singing aloud so as to embarrass them.

In general, the LPAD results indicated an initial adequate ability to form abstractions and draw inferences. He showed analytic and synthetic capacities and succeeded in learning to formulate rules and derive predictions about possible solutions to problems. His long-term memory, as well as his span of working memory, were efficient. He was able to relate to several sources of information simultaneously, transfer two-dimensional forms into three dimensions and verbally anticipate the correct solutions. There were some difficulties in spatial orientation and in coding and decoding of visual stimuli. On the affective level, whenever he failed, even when he made a minor mistake, he showed a tendency for regression by withdrawing from interaction with the examiner. Many times, when encountering pressure, he would escape by asking to go to the toilet. His passivity was expressed in a minimal investment of mental effort when coping with problems. His passive tendency had apparently developed as a result of a long history of failures. This tendency was probably strengthened by his long tenure in special education settings, where ineffective study habits had been accepted. The dynamic assessment process, however, served as a turning point by providing Peter with opportunities to overcome some barriers that hindered his learning. For example, one of Peter's difficulties was in following a sequence of instructions, but when the examiner focused his attention on registering the input, Peter could follow the instructions systematically. Sometimes, when asked about a specific topic Peter responded without distinguishing among parts of the answer, bringing up everything he knew and not really giving a clear answer. He had a tendency to change his train of thought or mental set in the middle. For example, when he was working on oral multiplication, which he answered correctly, he suddenly switched to subtraction. When he received proper mediation he manifested a great change in his performance.

It should be noted again that the learning situation of the LPAD is characterized by (a) good rapport and intensive interaction with the mediator, (b) exertion of optimal pressure for progress and rewarding of efforts, a combination of mediation of feelings of competence and an active-modifying approach, (c) the lack of time limits, and (d) gradual progression of task difficulty.

At this point the differences between the static-conventional tests given to Peter previously and the dynamic testing process were striking. In contrast to the static testing, the LPAD permitted the setting of different goals and different means of intervention. The static diagnosis and the consequent labeling (process) set low goals for Peter. He was placed in a special education class, labeled as an autistic child, and expected to continue his life in a very protected institutional environment. The LPAD, on the other hand, revealed Peter's high learning potential, which in turn led to much more optimistic goals: regular education and regular environment. The active modificational approach, combined with the LPAD results, provided Peter, his parents, and his helping environment (therapist, teachers, social worker) with the power and motivation to cope with the long duration of the treatment. Furthermore, with the static diagnosis there is difficulty in pointing out the means and processes of intervention. Its static characteristics make it quite hard to reveal the problems in the cognitive and emotional processes of the examinee. The dynamic interaction methods of the LPAD, on the other hand, allowed us both to reveal the deficient cognitive functions and affective-motivational aspects, and also to suggest specific methods of intervention.

The most important conclusions derived from the LPAD, in regard to Peter's treatment, were the following:

1. It was important to emphasize the input phase and make sure that information would be registered.
2. Helpers should mediate to Peter the specific inadequacies of his communication system: he cannot be understood when he changes his responses in the middle of a thought.
3. One should help Peter understand how to organize and plan his communication according to his listener's perspective; in other words, to develop less egocentric styles.

These techniques were applied successfully in the assessment, and therefore could be transferred to the treatment phase. It must be emphasized again that the dynamic assessment and the intervention that follows are not two separate phases; rather, they are a long process, with each part complementing the other. In the next section we present Peter's treatment as deduced and continued from the dynamic-interactive assessment process.

The Treatment

The treatment objectives were centered around four areas: (a) social learning, (b) family relationships, (c) cognitive functions, and (d) academic achievement. In order to facilitate attainment of these objectives, a treatment program was designed that included the following components: (a) individual psychotherapy sessions, combined with individual lessons of Instrumental Enrichment; (b) counseling parents with the goals of fostering Peter's independence and finding a balance between optimistic expectations and realistic limitations; and (c) placement in a normal educational environment and counseling of teachers and staff, using the treatment principles already mentioned. This assistance included preparation for the next day's lessons in order to achieve immediate successes. During vacations attempts were also made to close the gaps in academic achievements.

Individual Sessions

In his first assessment session, Peter came early and spoke of various subjects, jumping from one topic to another. His everyday knowledge was vast, containing news and facts absorbed from the media of radio, television, and newspapers. This knowledge reflected his alertness, curiosity, and interest in the world around him. He also demonstrated suspiciousness as reflected by his perception of many objects in the room as dangerous to health (e.g., orange juice, sandwiches). He constantly blamed his parents and the examiner for his condition, and demanded that his file in the clinic be burned. Peter showed a high level of anxiety and would hold the examiner's hand with excitement. The assessment sessions gradually changed in the direction of including more psychotherapeutic elements.

Simultaneous with the psychotherapeutic sessions, Instrumental Enrichment lessons were given. This was in accord with the MLE approach in which cognitive and emotional elements should be treated integratively, thus allowing a change in one area to be diffused to the other. For example, on the Organization of Dots, usually the first instrument taught in IE, the learner is given visual models (i.e., squares and triangles) and is required to find the shapes in a cloud of dots and draw them. This task requires definition of a problem, planning, systematic exploration of alternatives, and control of impulsivity. Difficulties on this task are not only used to correct cognitive impairments but are also "bridged" to daily life situations. During the treatment sessions the therapist and Peter discussed Peter's cognitive deficiencies in relation to behavioral and emotional difficulties, such as defining a social problem, exploration of reasons and causal factors, planning behavioral steps, and controlling impulsive reactions.

As a result of the assessment process it was decided to focus mainly on two phases of the mental process: input and output. This included, for example, systematic gathering of information (input), simultaneous consideration of multiple sources of information (input), adjusting responses to external demands (output), and using nonegocentric communication. The repetitive nature of the tasks reinforces crystallization of the acquired skills and enhancement of efficiency. The necessity to plan ahead in Organization of Dots, together with "bridging" to real-life situations, helped Peter to understand the importance of planning and organizing the expression of his ideas so that they could be conveyed to others and understood by them. One of the techniques used was to allow Peter to speak on any subject and even to jump from one topic to another, but only on condition that he state beforehand that he was going to speak on another topic. He was required to give reasons for illogical statements. Sometimes the therapist pretended he did not understand Peter's ideas in order to elicit more reasonable and accurate answers. Due to the very good rapport established between the psychologist and Peter, the demands, some of which could be considered strict, were accepted with almost no resistance. The acceptance of the demands might also be explained by Peter's need to structure his environment.

Another technique used with Peter was role playing. This could take place only in the third year of treatment, because one of Peter's main difficulties was in imagining himself in different positions. In role playing, several social skills were learned, such as opening a discussion with a new friend, making eye contact in conversations, initiating a talk with a girl, and adjusting his steps while walking with another person. The role playing was not restricted to the therapy room, but also took place in vivo: in streets, shops, and buses. Although these sessions were very successful, Peter insisted on stopping them. This was probably because these experiences touched too closely on his main problems and caused a high degree of anxiety.

Many sessions were focused on daily life experiences, with the purpose of leading Peter to insight about the relation between his behavior and its consequences. He was encouraged to develop an internal locus of control and causality by reasoning, hypothesizing, and drawing conclusions. The topics used in these cognitive interventions were brought up by Peter himself. For example, Peter accused one of his past psychologists of being a liar because he placed Peter in a special education setting, and therefore, prevented him from making progress. This topic was used as a lever to compare Peter's actual functioning in school to his performance during the LPAD diagnostic sessions. The comparison was based on facts such as grades, teachers' perceptions, examiners' remarks, and changes in performance and in level of efficiency. This cognitive analysis helped Peter to differentiate between ability and achievement and to gain insight into the possible reasons for the gap between them, and to construct reality in a novel way.

In the first 5 years, treatment was concentrated mainly around IE and academic studies. Meetings were not held intensively, but took place only when Peter had vacations from his boarding school. Overall, there were about 10 to 15 meetings per year, approximately one a month. These sessions also served as therapeutic dialogues on various topics (anxiety, aggression to parents, sexual problems). In the last 3 years of treatment, the content of the sessions was chosen mainly by Peter, and no IE was given.

Some of the sessions were focused on the importance of attending the boarding school as a means for social development. The discussions were around such issues as helping roommates, teasing and insulting, loneliness, and relationships with girls. MLE principles were used to organize Peter's experience and suggest alternative solutions. Usually,

Peter was encouraged to arrive at solutions; however, when no solution was achieved, suggestions were offered and independent choice was encouraged.

In his third year in the boarding school, Peter had a traumatic sexual experience when a friend induced him to masturbate in the shower. He could not discuss this event and became very upset, excited, and aggressive to the point of almost striking the therapist. This behavior was extraordinary, especially in view of Peter's generally polite, controlled, and cooperative behavior. The sexual topic was raised several times in later sessions and discussed more openly, with fewer and fewer episodes of suppression and acting-out.

Other topics raised during treatment were related to vocational aspirations. When therapy was started, Peter demonstrated unrealistically high aspirations, as expressed in his wishes to be a physician, a lawyer, or an airplane pilot. No attempt was made to lower his aspirations or directly confront him with the gap between his level of functioning and the required demands of each profession. The requirements were analyzed with him objectively. As time passed, his ambitions became more realistic and directed toward the completion of matriculation examinations and finding a job suitable for a high school graduate.

One of the most promising changes that had taken place was Peter's attitude toward serving in the army. It should be emphasized that in Israeli society service in the army, which is obligatory, serves as a strong integrative factor and is taken into account later in job applications. At the start of the interventions, Peter expressed his wish to return to his native European country and did not want to consider any idea of army service. It seemed that he interpreted the source of his problems as immigration to Israel. He believed that returning to Europe would give him the opportunity for a fresh start. Today Peter understands the significance of army service for his vocational future and social integration. He has also developed identification with the country, as indicated by his wish to build his life in Israel and serve in the army.

Peter made much progress regarding his independence. He resisted any help while entering the army and requested that he serve far from his home. He comes home every 2 weeks and the conflicts with his parents about his independence have almost disappeared. It seems that he has reached a balance between dependency and autonomy.

Counseling Parents

Parallel to the therapeutic sessions, there were about five or six sessions each year with Peter's parents. The parents were very devoted and strongly believed in the MLE approach. A central idea in counseling the parents was their progress and development together with Peter's development. Because it was very important for them to protect their son from the external world, it was recommended that they permit Peter to cope by himself with challenges and to develop his independence as he matured, just as any other child would. These sessions, therefore, were focused on strengthening the parents' belief in Peter and understanding that his difficulties were part of growing up. Guidance was also given on how to neutralize the fighting between Peter and siblings and prevent him from embarrassing them and turning their friends away from the house. Much counseling time was invested in strengthening the parents' belief that life with regular children in a boarding school would be very beneficial to Peter's growing independence and social mainstreaming. When Peter was on school vacations, his parents were asked to allow him to travel, go shopping, and plan his activities alone. They were also counseled not to comment on mistakes and to reward independent attempts at mastery. Overall, during an 8-year period they had 15 to 17 hours of counseling. During this period, they slowly modified their overprotective behavior as evidenced by the decrease of the frequency of their visits to the boarding school. The mother became increasingly able to ignore behavior that previously had bothered her. Peter was allowed to open a bank account, and no attempt was made to ask what he was doing with the money. He was no longer required to tell exactly where and when he was going out or when he was coming back.

Learning in a Normal Educational Environment

At the start of treatment, immediately after the dynamic assessment sessions, Peter was referred to a regular boarding school for children whose background could be described as culturally disadvantaged. Before the start of the program a staff meeting was arranged to report the LPAD results and recommendations. The main objective that was set for the staff was to help Peter increase his social adjustment. This would be carried out by living with normal peers who would give him honest feedback on his behavior, as well as provide him with models for imitation. The secondary objective was to close the gaps in academic studies. These goals were facilitated by placing Peter in a class, one grade below his age, and helping him with individual lessons after school. The staff preparation made Peter's entrance into the school smoother.

No problems appeared in the first month. In the second month there was a trend toward regression, as reflected by Peter's tendency to stay in his room most of the day and to act aggressively toward peers as if he were under attack. In the third month an urgent call from school conveyed the information that Peter was fighting with everyone who even hinted at an insult. In a staff meeting with the therapist this behavior was explained as a necessary, though painful, process, and that in the future he might try to find a balance. The principle of induced regression (see above) was applied here in that Peter was permitted to be aggressive. The assumption was that this regression would release Peter from his emotional inhibition and meet his unfulfilled needs, thus decreasing resistance to modification. The principle of unconditioned acceptance was also applied in that the staff enabled Peter to remain in school despite his aggression, and directed him gradually to obey the rules of school.

A social worker of the boarding school, working together with the therapist, was asked to discuss the aggressive incidents with Peter in order to find appropriate ways of reacting. Her work was continued later in the therapeutic sessions during his vacations. There was a need to focus on simple behavior, such as what to do when friends tease and how to approach a teacher to ask for a higher grade on a test. His behavior in these areas was extreme, leading to negative responses. As time passed, his behavior became more balanced and stabilized, for example, from greeting the same person 20 times a day to more socially acceptable modes of interaction. This change occurred in response to well-intentioned remarks and reactions by the staff and peers. This again emphasized the importance of living in a normal educational environment.

After a while Peter was accepted by his peers. He was even elected to one of the class committees, and the teasing stopped. He also succeeded in his studies, which permitted his transfer after 2 years to a similar boarding school that had a higher academic level. This school had various programs at different academic levels, including programs leading to matriculation examinations.

When Peter changed schools, the same stages of treatment were repeated: instruction to the staff at the beginning of the year; crisis after 3 months; further instruction to the staff; individual help in academic areas; and therapeutic sessions during vacations. In these 2 years (3rd and 4th of intervention) the progress was slow. This can be attributed to the fact that in this school the pupils were not tolerant and gave Peter a hard time by insulting and rejecting him. There were several attempts to speak with his classmates in order to change their attitude and behavior, but without much success. After 2 years at the second school, the time came for Peter's induction into the army. We had to convince the army to postpone Peter's induction in order to permit him an additional 2 years of academic studies and more progress in social areas. It was easy to convince the army but not Peter and his parents. Peter would have preferred anything to returning to boarding school life. It was necessary to devote several sessions to the issue as well as to request the intervention of Prof. Reuven Feuerstein, whom Peter accepted as an authority figure. Peter and his parents were finally convinced that he should continue for an additional 2 years in a boarding school of the same type as that in which he was previouly enrolled. In these 2 years Peter made very great progress, both socially and academically, and even completed two final examinations. Because Peter was 2 years older than his classmates, an age gap that disturbed him very much, he was given responsibilities for younger students in lower grades, such as waking them up in the morning and escorting them on trips. Peter showed devotion to these tasks and received much appreciation. During the summer vacation he worked as a messenger boy and file clerk in various offices. He earned money and learned to handle it, including opening a bank account and using a checkbook.

Peter was drafted into the army 6 years ago within the framework of a special army program, with easier basic training, but afterward he continued in a regular army course. He served first as a cleaner and later as an assistant supplies manager. Later, Peter lived on an army base and enjoyed his independence. In reports received from his superiors, it has been noted that Peter functions with high devotion and adequate adjustment to his work, and that there is almost no difference between him and other military personnel. His superiors were very satisfied with his service and gave him very good references upon his discharge. During his service, Peter was also involved in two main activities: evening studies for final exams in math, history, and geography, and lessons for his driving license.

Discussion

The treatment according to the MLE approach was characterized by the following:

1. The use of a dynamic-interactive assessment approach made possible the validation of optimistic objectives in cognitive, academic, and emotional areas. The assessment was contered on specific social learning tasks, cognitive functions, and academic achievement. By avoiding labeling, we were able more accurately to perceive specific difficulties and to set optimal expectations.
2. Individual treatment sessions were used for IE, general academic studies, and psychotherapy. The bridging between areas also facilitated transfer from one area to another and enabled more efficient thinking processes and an optimal balance between cognitive and emotional areas. All these components are perceived integratively as part of the MLE approach, and facilitated Peter's modifiability.
3. In accordance with the principles of the Treatment Group technique (Feuerstein & Krasilowsky, 1972), the following four principles were applied in Peter's treatment: (a) unconditional acceptance; (b) reduction of anxiety; (c) induced regression; and (d) planned and controlled relationships with normal peers.
4. In an ecological integrative approach, all factors surrounding the child were taken into account: normal educational environment,

psychotherapy, counseling parents and teachers, and academic tutoring. All these combined factors permitted significant modification as well as a balance between optimal protection and remaining in normal life conditions.

There was some evidence of successful treatment. If Peter had not come to us, but instead had remained in his former school and been treated according to previous diagnoses, we would have expected certain patterns of behavior and experience. Peter would have continued his studies in a special education school. He would have regressed in his social behavior. He would have lived in his closed world with total dependence on his parents. He probably would have developed more serious symptoms of psychiatric disorders, even psychosis, that would have required hospitalization. The treatment Peter did receive totally changed his path of development. He finished high school, was accepted into army service, and he successfully completed his army duty. His social adjustment has been much improved. He is now able to communicate with people and conduct his daily life independently. There is more than a hope that in the future Peter will be able to cope with challenges as they arise. He still needs counseling and assistance, but they are becoming less important. It is hard to designate Peter's vocational objectives, but there is no doubt that he can function at a higher level than he is at now.

It can be concluded that only dynamic-interactive assessment, especially in the form of the LPAD, could set such optimistic goals and give such specific objectives and means to achieve them. The success of the treatment, which was continued straight from the LPAD integrated by one person, affords great hope in modifying and helping borderline psychotic adolescents.

Acknowledgment. The client in this case study was treated by the first author, who was supervised by Professor Reuven Feuerstein.

References

Alpert, A. (1975). A special therapeutic technique for certain development disorders in prelatency children. *Amercian Journal of Orthopsychiatry*, *27*, 256–270.

Burden, R. (1987). Feuerstein's Instrumental Enrichment Program: Important issues in research and evaluation. *European Journal of Psychology of Education*, *2*, 3–16.

Clarke, A. M., & Clarke, A. D. (1976). *Early experience, myth and evidence*. London: Open Books.

Feuerstein, R. (1970). A dynamic approach to the causation, prevention and alleviation of retarded performance. In H. C. Haywood (Ed.), *Social-cultural aspects of mental retardation* (pp. 341–377). New York: Appleton Century Crofts.

Feuerstein, R. (1977). Mediated learning experience: A theoretical basis for cognitive modifiability during adolescence. In P. Mittler (Ed.), *Research to practice in mental retardation. Volume 2: Education and training*. Baltimore: University Park Press.

Feuerstein, R., Haywood, H. C., Rand, Y., Hoffman, M. B., & Jensen, M. (1986). *Examiner manual for the Learning Potential Assessment Device*. Jerusalem: Hadassah-WIZO-Canada Research Institute.

Feuerstein, R., & Krasilowsky, D. (1972). Interventional strategies for the significant modification of cognitive functioning in the disadvantaged adolescent. *Journal of the American Academy of Child Psychiatry*, *11*, 572–582.

Feuerstein, R., & Rand, Y. (1974). Mediated learning experience: An outline of the proximal etiology for differential development of cognitive functions. *International Understanding* (Issue edited by L. G. Fein entitled *Cultural Differences in the Development of Cognitive Processes*), *9–10*, 7–37.

Feuerstein, R., Rand, Y., Hoffman, M. B., Hoffman, M., & Miller, R. (1979). Cognitive modifiability in retarded adolescents: effects of Instrumental Enrichment. *American Journal of Mental Deficiency*, *83*, 539–550.

Feuerstein, R., Rand, Y., & Hoffman, M. B. (1979). *The dynamic assessment of retarded performance: The Learning Potential Assessment Device: theory, instruments, and techniques*. Glenview, IL: Scott, Foresman.

Feuerstein, R., Rand, Y., Hoffman, M. B., & Miller, R. (1980). *Instrumental Enrichment: An intervention program for cognitive modifiability*. Glenview, IL: Scott, Foresman.

Feuerstein, R., & Shalom, H. (1967). Methods of assessing the educational level of socially and culturally disadvantaged children. *Megamot*, *15*, 177–187. (In Hebrew)

Filler, J. W., Robinson, C. C., Smith, R. A., Vincent-Smith, L. J., Bricker, D. D., & Bricker, W. A. (1975). Mental retardation. In N. Hobbs (Ed.), *Issues in the classification of children* (Vol. 1, pp. 194–238). San Francisco: Jossey Bass.

Jensen, M., Feuerstein, R., Rand, Y., Kaniel, S., & Tzuriel, D. (1986). Cultrual difference and cultural deprivation: A theoretical framework for differential intervention. In R. M. Gupta & P. Coxhead (Eds.), *Cultural diversity and learning efficiency*. London: Macmillan.

Maultsby, M. C. Jr. (1984). *Rational behavior therapy*. Englewood Cliffs, NJ: Prentice-Hall.

Meichenbaum, D. (1974). Self-instructional training: A cognitive prosthesis for the aged. *Human Development*, *17*, 273–280.

Meichenbaum, D. (1977). *Cognitive behavior modification*. New York: Plenum.

Meichenbaum, D., & Asarnow, J. (1979). Cognitive-behavior modification and metacognition development. In P. C. Kendall & S. D. Hollon (Eds.), *Cognitive behavioral interventions: theory, research, and procedures* (pp. 225–282). New York: Academic Press.

Rand, Y., & Kaniel, S. (1987). Group administration of the LPAD. In C. Lidz (Ed.), *Dynamic assessment* (pp. 196–214). New York: Guilford.

Rand, Y., Tannenbaum, A., & Feuerstein, R. (1979). Effects of instrumental enrichment on the psychoeducational development of low-functioning adolescents. *Journal of Educational Psychology*, *71*, 751–763.

Raziel, S. (1981). *Effects of mediated learning experience on cognitive modifiability, locus of control and self esteem.* Unpublished master's thesis, Bar Ilan University, Israel. (In Hebrew).

Redfield, D. (1984, April). Application of instrumental enrichment to college students. Paper presented at the annual meeting of the American Educational Research Association, New Orleans.

Sar-Shalom, Y. (1978). *The efficiency of the Instrumental Enrichment program for cognitive and didactic modification of seminar students.* Unpublished MA Thesis, Bar Ilan University, Israel (In Hebrew).

Savell, J. M., Twohig, P. T., & Rachford, D. L. (1986). Empirical status of Feuerstein's "Instrumental Enrichment" technique as a method of teaching thinking skills. *Review of Educational Research*, *56*, 381–409.

Skeels, H. M. (1966). Adult status of children with contrasting early life experience. *Monographs of the Society for Research in Child Development*, *31*, 3–18.

Skodak, M. (1968). Adult status of individuals who experienced early intervention. In B. W. Richards (Ed.), *Proceedings of the First Congress of the International Association for the Scientific Study of Mental Deficiency*. Reigate (Surrey), UK: Michael Jackson.

Thickpenny, J. P. (1982). *Teaching thinking skills to deaf adolescents: The implementation and evaluation of Feuerstein's Instrumental Enrichment.* Unpublished master's thesis, University of Auckland, New Zealand.

Tzuriel, D., & Alfassi, M. (1987, March). *Cognitive and motivational changes as a function of Instrumental Enrichment and initial cognitive modifiability.* Paper presented at the 21st Convention of the Israeli Psychological Association, Tel Aviv.

Walker, S., & Meier, J. (1982). *Instrumental Enrichment Program*. New York: Office of Educational Evaluation, New York City Publich Schools.

18
A Case Study in the Induction of Logic Structures

JEAN-LOUIS PAOUR and GUYLAINE SOAVI

Our purpose in this chapter is to illustrate the method of "induction of logic structures" by intensive study of a single case. This method is both assessment and treatment. The assessment aspect reflects the notion that one way to learn about any phenomenon is to change it deliberately and under specifiable conditions, and to observe its characteristics under the changed conditions. Such a method seems particularly well suited to the examination of *processes* of thought and the development of those processes. We have taken this case from one of the studies presented in Chapter 5 by Paour in this volume. The philosophy, theoretical structure, and detailed procedures used in the method of induction of logic structures are described in that chapter and thus are not repeated here.

The Basic Study

Goals and Design

We have conducted 12 experiments in the current series of studies of induction of logic structures, and have selected this one for presentation in detail for three principal reasons: (a) it is recent; (b) its 2-year duration permits a detailed description of the cognitive changes that occurred, giving us some confidence in the results; (c) it illustrates what we have found to be a powerful training procedure for inducing concrete logic structures in mentally retarded persons who may be fixated at a preoperatory level of the development of reasoning.

This study was designed initially as a test of our analysis of the conceptual and functional aspects of cognitive fixation at a given preoperatory level. In addition, this case helped us to refine our description of how induced operatory thought can be functionally integrated into the problem-solving repertoire.

Subjects were 22 mentally retarded children with the following characteristics: Mean age, 128 months (SD = 16 months); mean mental age 77 months (SD = 13 months); mean IQ 57 (SD = 7 points). Selection criteria were (a) IQ less than 68 on a standard individual intelligence test such as the Stanford-Binet, and (b) inability or great difficulty in inferring "arbitrary" contextual relations (i.e., relations that exist by definition rather than by natural dependency) between objects in paired relationships. All attended the same special school for mildly and moderately retarded children and adolescents, a non-mainstreamed school that served about 90 children. In the mornings, these children received academic instruction adjusted individually to their achievement levels. In the afternoons they had "free choice" activities such as sports, dance, handicrafts, and dramatic expression. The sample of 22 was divided into 11 who received the special training and 11 "control" children.

Each of the 11 training group children received 24 individual training sessions spread over two consecutive academic years (Table 18.1). The content of the training exercises was predesigned, but their presentation was abjusted to the individual developmental levels and requirements of the children. Thus, in the course of intervention, parallel forms of some exercises, as well as an adaptation of the original training situation (described below), were created. During training sessions, the subjects' actions, as well as their verbalizations, were systematically recorded. Subjective indications of their response to the tasks, such as attention, interest, or pleasure, were noted. These records enabled us to follow the progress of the children through training sessions and posttests in a longitudinal manner.

Each of the 11 control children received an equal number of sesions in the same type of setting: an isolated room, sessions of about 40 minutes' duration, with one-to-one interaction, and participation with their consent. During these sessions, the control children either read or listened to stories, depending on their ability, and discussed the stories.

TABLE 18.1. Schedule of the study.

Time	Event
October–December, 1982	Pretest
January–March, 1983	Training sessions 1 to 6
March–April, 1983	Training sessions 7 to 12
June, 1983	Posttest 1.1
July–September, 1983	School vacation
October–November, 1983	Posttest 1.2
November, 1983–February, 1984	Training sessions 13 to 18
April–June, 1984	Training sessions 19 to 24
June, 1984	Posttest 2.1
July–September, 1984	School vacation
October–November, 1984	Posttest 2.2
June, 1986	Delayed posttest

Training and control sessions were conducted alternately by two advanced graduate students in developmental psychology.

The Training

In accordance with our hypothesis concerning fixation at the preoperatory level (see Chapter 5 by Paour, in this volume), we devised a training program directed toward three hierarchical goals: (a) to stimulate *comparison* of objects both before and after their transformation, (b) to induce *representation* of differences in terms of relational ties from which regularities can be inferred and rules can be abstracted, and (c) to induce the ability to *coordinate* these relational rules into a global system of transformation. The following is a brief description of the training situation (Paour, 1975, 1980, 1985; Soavi, 1986).

The materials consist of a "transformation box" (see Figure 5.2) and groups of several kinds of objects that can be transformed on different criteria. The transformation box has four compartments, each arranged as follows:

Subject side. This side has two openings: one on the top through which objects are inserted, and one on the bottom from which the objects that have been substituted by the examiner are taken out.

Examiner side. This side has two separate levels: the top level, where objects that have been inserted remain, and the lower level, where the examiner can substitute objects through an opening (to be taken out on the other side by the subject).

During training, one can use from two to four compartments, depending on the particular study. The compartments that are not being used are covered by a piece of cardboard. Both the subject and the examiner have their own identical supply of objects. For each compartment used, there is a rule governing the correspondence between objects introduced by the subjects (into the top level) and objects substituted by the examiner (into the bottom level): thus, the transformation occurs regularly and predictably from top to bottom of any given compartment. The difficulty of the exercise depends on (a) the number of compartments in use at once, (b) the kind of rules for substitutions, (c) the nature of the objects, (d) the transformed properties, and (e) the kind of coordinations required.

Each training session follows the same sequence.

1. The examiner asks the subject to describe the objects, gives guidance in this task as needed, and then asks for a free grouping of the objects.
2. Free activity: Each "play" consists of the subject's putting into the top part of the box any one of 12 objects, using any one of the available compartments.
3. First general verbalization: "What does the box do?"

4. Guided activity: 12 more objects freely placed. Depending on the functional level previously observed, the examiner gives help by one or another of the following: (a) calling attention to the unused compartments; (b) focusing attention on the object that has been introduced; (c) focusing attention on the object that has been retrieved; (d) asking, after retrieval of an object, what has happened; (e) asking the subject to predict what is going to happen; (f) asking the subject to use the previously abstracted rules to predict what is going to happen.
5. Second general verbalization: "What does the box do?" When an answer is not clear, a specific question is asked about the function of each compartment that is used.
6. Anticipation test: Subjects are asked to anticipate the result of proposed transformations (i.e., the objects are not actually "transformed"). These are of five kinds: (a) direct (anticipation of the result); (b) reciprocal (specification of the object that would have to be introduced in order to produce a given "transformed" object); (c) generalization to objects that are only slightly different from the objects actually used; (d) generalization to quite different and even incongruent objects; (e) for each of the compartments actually used, invitation of the subject to comment on the transformations that are possible or impossible.
7. Coordination of the transformation rules: (only in the last two steps, described later).

The intervention protocol consists of five hierarchical steps. Steps I to III are directed to the subject's achievement of goals a and b, while steps IV and V are directed to goal c (see Figure 5.2):

I. Be aware of the substitutions and abstract the differences as consequences of an arbitrary relation that ties "introduced" objects (put by subject into the top of the box) to "transformed" ones (put by the examiner into the bottom of the box).
II. Be able to specify the properties that have been transformed and those that have not been transformed.
III. Be able to abstract relative transformations (by degree, as opposed to the absolutes used in steps I and II).
IV. Be able to reach the logical identification of a target object by additive coordination of absolute transformation rules.
V. Be able to reach the logical identification of a target object by compensatory coordination of relative transformation rules.

Anne at the Beginning of the Training

Anne was chosen from the 11 training group subjects because she was representative of the group in terms of the amount of training completed and of her total cognitive progress. She held exactly the median position at the last posttest. Further, her case is specifically instructive because of the great difficulty she encountered at the beginning of training. Anne's case allows us to understand, far better than would faster subjects who show little difficulty, the mechanism of developmental fixation and the ways in which the intervention might have worked.

Anne is an attractive, pleasant, native French girl who was, at pretest, 10 years and 3 months old. Five years earlier she had been removed from her family following a catastrophic parental crisis, and had been placed in a total-care residential institution. She had joined the special school 2 years before pretest, following total failure in a regular first-grade class.

Anne's attitudes and behavior were characteristic of her situation. She was a very affectionate child who regularly sought contact with adults, around whom she adopted infantile behavior in order to elicit mothering. By contrast, she was aggressive and frequently quarrelsome with her peers. In the initial contacts (pretesting and first training sessions) she exhibited instability and extreme difficulty in concentration (looking all around, not listening to the examiner, talking constantly but without continuity). It was necessary to encourage her and to direct her attention to the tasks. Her explanations were quite confused and her graphic and motor representations very imprecise. She could not read, and had just barely begun to discriminate certain syllables; in arithmetic, she could only add two-digit numbers, without carrying.

The results of the pretesting suggested mild mental retardation. On the New Metric Test of Intelligence (Zazzo, Gilly, & Verba-Rad, 1966), Anne obtained a mental age of 6 years and an IQ of 58. Tests of conservation of number confirmed this retardation: Anne was totally nonconserving according to tests that are passed by the majority of children at 7 to 8 years (conserving the number of tokens when their spatial alignment is changed, conserving the number of beads when they are poured from one container to another).

The First Six Sessions: Deficient Information Seeking and Inability to Abstract a Paired Relation

The first six training sessions provide an example of fixation. In fact, despite help and practice, Anne was not successful in establishing a relationship between the object placed into the box and the one retrieved from it. Analysis of her difficulty permitted us to separate the cognitive aspects from the functional aspects in the etiology of her fixation.

The Cognitive Obstacle

A cognitive obstacle to Anne's ability to solve these transformation problems became apparent during the "guided activity" phase. In fact, in her most highly developed responses to the question that immediately followed each trial ("What happened?"), Anne mentioned only the two objects, the one introduced into the top of the box and the one retrieved from the bottom: "You gave me a big card; the other one was little." "You gave me a closed one; the other one was open." Clearly, Anne gave evidence by her qualification of the objects (big–little, closed–open) that she had perceived the relevant differences. In spite of this, neither relation was connected explicitly by an abstraction that permitted her to go back and forth between them. She merely described, in a quite mechanical way, the beginning and final states of the objects rather than any relational qualities. Even when she would give a description that seemed relatively abstract (the name of the object not being mentioned), e.g., "You gave me a closed one, I [put in] an open one," she did not connect the two conditions. Even so, these were the *most* elaborated responses. More typically, Anne would refer only to the retrieved object ("You gave me a long fish," "She gave a broken spoon"), without ever referring to the relevant difference.

Her verbal responses to the second general question (task 5: "What does the box do?") permit us to interpret more clearly what she said immediately after the trial. These responses were totally centered on the act and/or the states: "to put," "she gave some things," "You put some toys, sometimes the same, sometimes not the same," "Me this, you that" (designating two objects), "She put in some blues and some reds." These responses are characteristic of a lower level of understanding than the concept of paired relations. At that level, the two elements, (the causal context of effective actions, and temporal contiguity) are distinctly perceived, but the *paired relation* as such is not abstracted inasmuch as the elements to be paired are not understood as dependent on some arbitrary relation (i.e., pairing on such dimensions as relative size, color, or position).

We learned from her responses to task 6 (anticipation) that Anne's responses reflected a *conceptual order* barrier, i.e., a problem of cognitive level, rather than any difficulty of verbal expression. In fact, she failed 57% of the total number of anticipations, and 70% when one excludes from the total those that related to nontransformation. Further, she considered as acceptable some transformations that were actually impossible given the rules of the task. Finally, her identification of the nontransforming compartments was not always either correct or well established. At the end of sessions 3 and 4, for example, she attributed changes to the nontransforming compartment.

Deficient Functioning

The first six sessions made it clear that Anne was not functioning very effectively in this situation. Although on the whole her ineffectiveness was commensurate with her developmental level, she seemed to us to exhibit a further dificiency in her functioning. At the beginning of the intervention Anne's behavior did not seem to correspond to her ability. Then, given guidance, and without our observing any general developmental progress, the discrepancy was progressively reduced.

The description of the objects (task 1) offers a prime example of deficient functioning. In the first sessions, Anne did not spontaneously identify the qualities and characteristics of the objects when we asked her to describe the materials. In fact, without exhausting the types of objects, she designated several individual objects simply by naming: "There are spoons, pencils, and squares, . . ." "A pack of cigarettes, envelopes, boxes, that's umbrellas." This poor level of spontaneous description seems to be related to a general *outer-directedness* in cognitive functioning (Zigler, 1972): Anne had difficulty sustaining attention, moved around, looked from side to side, and tried to start discursive conversations.

Although she did not improve her response when we asked her to give a better description of a specific object, she did give a more complete description when we isolated a pair of the same objects that differed only on a single criterion; e.g., "A pencil, it's broken, that one, it's not broken." Even if it is not a question of comparison (because, as in the transformation exercises, she did not *compare* the objects), the help afforded by their proximity improved her verbalization and therefore apparently the quality of the information available for reflection. Her arranging of the objects confirmed that she discriminated their qualities: for example, in the second session she made separate piles of objects that were strictly identical (according to their nature, and in two sizes).

For a long time, such progress remained dependent on the help of the examiner. Up to and including the fifth session, her spontaneous descriptions were as impoverished as the initial ones. From the sixth session on she gave richer descriptions *spontaneously*: ". . . red fish and blue fish, big ones and little ones." Anne still was not comparing the objects, but she did adopt a prerequisite attitude by describing more completely the stock of objects and by identifying them by the dimensions on which they differed. This new exigency marked a breakthrough, after the fifth session, into the phase of spontaneous activity. Anne then verbalized spontaneously on every trial, and continued to do so throughout the intervention.

Here we are referring to *attitude*, because from the sixth session on Anne spontaneously applied a level of description that *corresponded to her cognitive developmental level*. This attitude was shown to be stable, inasmuch as the examiner did not have to intervene any further in the task of description: we could no longer refer to any apparent separation between her ability to abstract differences—and then later to abstract their properties—and her spontaneous description of the objects. This attitude came to be generalized to other situations. In fact, during the posttest, like the majority of the other training group subjects but contrary to the control subjects, Anne had a tendency to describe spontaneously the material presented to her according to the same requirement. On the Tower of Hanoi problem, for example, she described the arrangement exhaustively. She counted the pencils that served as the shaft, announced their color, pointed at and counted the disks and called out each by a different qualifier and even specified the color of the stand in which the pencils were set. This attitude transferred as well to scholastic learning, as shown by the teachers' reports that they had observed it independently. The attitude appeared significant to the extent that it affected directly the quality of information input and retention.

The initial deficient functioning was revealed further by progressive improvement in the area of planning of actions. During the first three sessions, Anne had a tendency to concentrate on the same compartment for long periods. In the first session, she put her first eight objects into the same compartment; in the second, she put six consecutive objects into the same compartment and did the same thing in the guided phase in spite of the examiner's indicating the presence of the other one. This behavior was repeated in the third session, but disappeared for good thereafter. Thus, even though she did not place all 12 objects of one trial into a single compartment, as we have observed in Haitian children from extremely deprived sociocultural conditions (Robeants, 1987), Anne certainly had an initial tendency not to explore the full range of the materials available to her.

The choice of the object to be introduced was similarly not very well controlled. We observed, for example, up to the sixth session, some sequences in which Anne reintroduced, as many as four or five times, the object that she had just retrieved. At this level, however, we could hardly expect progress, inasmuch as the concept of paired relations was not yet present even in rudimentary form.

Finally, in the fifth session, progress toward control over her actions was revealed by guessing: "I bet it's the same." Even though this confident expression did not concern the outcome of a transformation, it nevertheless revealed a quite relevant awareness of the problem: to predict what was going to come out of the box. We would expect that this representation would lead her to seek out rules that would allow her to predict effectively.

At the end of the first six training sessions it appeared clear that Anne had not attained a developmental level corresponding to the abstracting of paired relations (Orsini-Bouichou, 1975; Wallon, 1942). The obstacle that she encountered was quite clearly a cognitive one: it corresponded to the inability to relate the elements of a pair in an abstract way. This inability resisted the help offered by the materials and by the examiner's guidance, because her functional progress was not accompanied by conceptual progress. The observation of this resistance permitted us to understand that the inability to relate two objects abstractly could be responsible for a durable fixation at the preoperatory level.

Sessions 7 to 12: The Progressive Abstraction of Transformation Rules, and More Efficient Functioning

Two out of the other 10 training group subjects showed the same difficulties. We had to devise for them an adaptation of the original training situation in order to foster the understanding of an abstract relation between the "introduced" and the "retrieved" objects.

Adaptation of the Task

The Apparatus

The apparatus consists of three wooden U-shaped pieces. There is a vertical slit on each side through which one pulls a long strip of paper. On the paper strip are glued pictures of four transformation steps of an object or animal (for example, a fish becoming larger). Because the strip is pulled through slits in the wooden pieces, only one picture at a time is exposed.

Each session includes the transformation of three different properties. Each exercise is presented twice: the first time without stopping, and the second time with a stop after each step in the transformation. After the continuous presentation, the examiner asks, "Tell me what you saw, what happened." After presentation of each picture in the discontinuous series the examiner asks, "Remember how it was before? What happened?" Following both presentations, the examiner says, "Explain to me what you saw. What happened there?"

After this adapted presentation, pictures (not on a paper strip) that correspond to the extreme values of those from the paper strip are used in the regular transformation box procedure.

First Statements of an Abstract Paired Relation

Anne was given this adapted presentation, called "movie," in the seventh and eighth sessions. We were able to see that the new cognitive attitudes described earlier had been clear forerunners of a sudden appearance of new abilities.

As early as the first continuous presentation, Anne was able to label the four transformation steps as "big, little, medium, medium." After the first discontinuous presentation, *and for the first time*, she stated a relation among the stimuli: "It is the same ducks, but their shapes change, medium, big." In the second exercise of this same session she applied the concept of *becoming* in characterizing the transformation: "It *gets* little, medium, big, and tall."

To our surprise, she even referred spontaneously to an unchanged property: "It's the shapes that change, but the color is the same." Further, she inhibited the earlier impulse to name the object in her general description of what happened in this "exhibit," as she said.

The Progressive and Simultaneous Construction of More Abstract Properties and More General Relations

By examining Anne's performance in sessions 7 to 12, we can gain a detailed description of the progressive building of a more general conditional relation based on the progressive abstraction of simple object properties.

This cognitive progress took the form of a decontextualization of the rules that Anne had given in the first and second verbalization tasks (3 and 5). The progressive nature of this change was suggested by the lability and insecurity of the emerging new abilities. The steps were:

1. The names of the objects disappeared in the general statement by the ninth session: "It is not the same; I put a yellow and you put a red." But Anne still felt the need for an example, because she followed that observation with the comment, "If I put a yellow marble, you put a red marble."
2. This former need disappeared with the 10th session in the first verbalization: "I give you a short one and you give me a long one." Here only the values of the transformed property were mentioned, without the names of the objects.
3. Totally abstract properties were referred to in the second verbalization of this same session: "This one changes the shape, the colors they are not changed (pointing to compartment #1), this one changes the color, it does not change the shape (compartment #2), it was the same color and the same shape, they are alike."
4. The nontransformed values and properties were also referred to spontaneously from this 10th session on.

This progressive change was reflected as well in Anne's initial description, in which she referred to all the values in a coordinated way: "Red and yellow beads, and red and yellow pieces of chalk," "long and short and red and blue fishes." It was shown as well in the optional free-arrangement task, in which the values (colors, sizes) rather than merely the kinds of objects constituted the grouping principles (e.g., *red* beads and pieces of chalk, *yellow* beads and pieces of chalk).

Anne's 90% success rate in the anticipation tasks (excluding the nontransformation rule) indicates that she had abstracted actual and general rules of transformation. Applying the rules of this activity, she firmly rejected impossible transformations, and consistently identified each transformation with its appropriate compartment (e.g., #1 transformed color, #2 shape). Even so, her statements after each trial remained much less abstract than her answers to the general questions. Even in the 12th session she began by describing the initial object, then described the retrieved object, and only then the relation between the two. This demonstrated her persistent reliance on verbal description of the objects in order to abstract the transformed properties.

Growth of the Functional Cognitive Aspects of Action Mastery

In the meantime, Anne experienced a steady growth of action mastery. This was reflected primarily in her choice of compartments and of objects to be transformed, which became an efficient way of discovering the transformation rules.

In the seventh session, Anne adopted a systematic method of exploring compartments by alternating her plays across available compartments. When three compartments were open, she extended her alternating strategy, going invariably from left to right.

Her choices of objects to be transformed also reflected some relatively efficient strategies. First, she introduced all the different kinds of objects. Second, she introduced them in such a way that the reciprocal transformations were explored (e.g., large-to-small as well as small-to-large). Third, when double transformation rules were in play, Anne's choices seemed to represent an effort to achieve constancy of a property. These strategies were neither systematic nor durable in the course of intervention, apparently because they rapidly became unnecessary as her mastery of the task increased. Across sessions, she reduced the number of trials to criterion in the free-activity part, until by the 10th session she needed no more than six trials to discover the transformation rules. She no longer needed to try out the bidirectionality of each transformation rule or to find out exactly what happened to each kind of object or to each transformed property. In the 12th session, after only six trials she was able to infer the set of rules and their effects on new and different objects in the anticipation test. A clear indication of her new planning mastery was her firm refusal to continue in the guided phase, arguing that she had "already discovered what the box does."

At the same time, we observed a growing need for precision in labeling the different properties. She revealed this new cognitive attitude in her spontaneous descriptions, naming all the different kinds of objects and all the properties by which they differed. This attitude was apparent also in her attempts, sometimes clumsy, to use different words to qualify all of the steps in the transformation process revealed in the "movie" apparatus, such as "little, medium, *big* and *tall*" in the seventh session. Another example was her need to describe spontaneously the invariant values or properties associated with the transformation compartments.

All of these new manifestations of ability had to have been based in changes in her cognitive development. Their application suggests that new and efficient cognitive habits had been established and that she had internalized a more pressing need for precision in gathering and giving information. These changes were reflected in her general behavior: Anne became much less distractible, more intrinsically interested in the tasks, more invested in the preparation of the materials, and she seemed to enjoy the challenge of discovering the rules governing the transformation activity.

In evaluating Anne's cognitive progress, it is important to observe that the examiner never gave answers, nor precisely named objects, values, or properties. These specifications were elicited from Anne and were ultimately consequences of her own reflection. There are no magic tricks in the transformation box. Its arbitrary relationships, psychopedagogical devices, problems, and the examiner's guidance were directed toward changing Anne into a more active and effective information processor. The examiner guided, but Anne discovered the rules, the properties, the values, and Anne applied them more and more systematically to new cases.

Following the 12 sessions of the first year, Anne had clearly progressed to a significantly higher mode of thought (level IIb; see Chapter 5 by Paour, in this volume). The training had helped to free her from the functional difficulties she had endured for many years.

First Posttest: Functional Progress but Conceptual Fixation

There were two progress probes during the first year of this case study: the first just after the period of training at the end of the academic year (June), and the second at the beginning of the next academic year (October, same year). These probes revealed significant progress in functioning, as shown on the Tower of Hanoi problem, but only a slight gain on Raven's Standard Progressive Matrices and the Piagetian tasks.

Improvement in Cognitive Functioning

Anne's performance on the Tower of Hanoi problem (Borys, Spitz, & Dorans, 1982) showed clearly that she had improved in cognitive functioning during her training (see Chapter 5 by Paour, in this volume, for discussion of the choice of this task as a criterion). Before training, Anne was unable to complete the problem, even with two disks, earning zero points out of a possible 10. Like the majority of the other subjects in the two groups, she did not apply the rules and did not construct her tower on the correct "target."

Her initial performance on the posttest looked very much like that of her pretest trials. In trials 1 and 3 she placed the small disk on the target base, then made a "large-on-small" error (trial 1) and constructed the tower on the wrong base (trial 3). In spite of this poor beginning, she learned rapidly how to manage the small disk, and in trials 2, 4, and 5 she succeeded with no errors and the minimal number of moves. Two observations support the conclusion that her success in this task was related to some kind of general comprehension: (a) she was directly successful in the first two trials of the second placement task; (b) she was able to anticipate the correct placement of the small disk on five anticipatory questions (i.e., trials on which the task was not actually performed).

Her enhanced cognitive efficiency was demonstrated most clearly on the three-disk tasks. In fact, Anne failed only on the first trial of each of the two placements. Moreover, she stopped herself as soon as she perceived that the initial placement was wrong. This attitude on her part suggests that she was capable of constructing a clear and appropriate representation of the task, and also that she was able to control her behavior in accordance with that representation. The increased precision that appeared during training was apparent in her ability to describe verbally and without error the sequence of movements necessary to relocate the tower; however, Anne did not abstract the general rule for using three disks, i.e., that one must put the small disk on the target. In this task she failed all five of the anticipations required.

Anne's 8-point score was superior to that of all but one of the subjects in the control group (see Table 5.12). By comparison with the data of Byrnes and Spitz (1977), Anne's score on these tasks was superior both to the mean score of their retarded adolescents and to that of nonretarded children of Anne's mental age. Because the training was not specifically addressed to this task, and the performance of the control group demonstrates that mere repetition of the test is not sufficient to bring about performance changes, we can conclude that the training itself led to Anne's significant improvement in problem solving.

Continuing Fixation at Preoperatory Level in Conservation Tasks

Raven's Standard Progressive Matrices was used as a criterion of generalization of the cognitive processes observed during the training phase. Solution of the matrix problems requires abstraction of arbitrary relations, as does the training task, but the form of the problems, the stimuli, and the kind of relations that one must abstract are all very different from those in the transformation box situation, i.e., the training task.

One can see in Anne's performance on the Progressive Matrices (Tables 18.2 and 18.3) both the extent and the limits of her transfer of training (first two columns in Table 18.2). She earned credit for 12 of the 24 items of the A and B sets, as opposed to 8 at pretest, reflecting her progress during training. Even so, she still gave wrong answers, in set A

TABLE 18.2. Anne's responses to Sets A, B, and C of Raven's Standard Progressive Matrices, by item and date of test.[a]

Item	11/82	6/83	6/84	10/84	6/86
A1	+	+	+	+	+
A2	6/+	+	+	+	+
A3	+	+	+	+	+
A4	1/+	+	+	+	+
A5	2/+	+	+	+	+
A6	4	+	+	+	+
A7	4	+	+	4/+	2/+
A8	6	6/+	+	+	1
A9	4	5	+	+	+
A10	+	6	+	+	+
A11	3	6	6	6	6
A12	6	6	1	6	6
B1	4	+	+	+	+
B2	5	+	+	+	3
B3	2	+	+	+	+
B4	5	+	6/+	+	+
B5	6	5	2	+	+
B6	5	2/4	2/+	+	2
B7	1	3/1	4	3	1
B8	3	4	+	+	+
B9	+	1	+	+	1
B10	+	2	+	+	+
B11	2	3	+	3/4	+
B12	6	2	+	+	2
C1			+	2/+	+
C2			+	3	+
C3			4	2/+	+
C4			+	+	4
C5			8	1	4
C6			6	+	5
C7			+	6	6
C8			8	+	+
C9			+	3	+
C10			8	7	+
C11			8	4	+
C12			8	7	4

[a] Numbers indicate incorrect responses; + indicates correct response. Example: 6/+ indicates that Anne's initial response to this item was incorrect, and then she corrected it spontaneously.

TABLE 18.3. Anne's scores, and mean scores of trained and control subjects, on Sets A and B[a], Raven's Standard Progressive Matrices, by date of testing.

	Date of testing				
Subject(s)	11/82	6/83	6/84	10/84	6/86
Anne	8	12	20	20	16
Trained	8.09	14.09	16.88	19.55	
	(3.01)[b]	(3.27)	(3.50)	(2.90)	
Control	8.27	9.72	10.18	9.90	
	(2.50)	(2.40)	(2.70)	(2.50)	

[a] Because of their low scores on Set B, control group children were not given Set C; thus, scores entered here are the sum of scores on Sets A and B.

[b] Parenthetical entries are standard deviations.

as well as in set B, when required to coordinate two relations simultaneously, that is, when she had to keep in mind and apply relations governing two or more dimensions. At this time, she had not yet been exposed to exercises that required the *coordination* of transformation rules. These results are generally in agreement with our description of cognitive level IIb as demonstrated in her training.

The conservation tests supported this interpretation. In fact, this new ability to relate pairs of elements permitted her to resist perceptual conflict (number versus length) in a situation that she had failed at pretest, the one in which two aligned groups are composed of objects of quite different size (small and large beads). Even though Anne succeeded in recognizing the constancy of number when the objects had already been placed in end-to-end correspondence on the table, she was no longer successful in this task when, as in the pouring out of the beads, the end-to-end correspondence had to be constructed mentally. Thus, the validity of the progress that she had apparently made during training was confirmed both by her successes and by her failures.

Mastery of a Skillful Problem Solving Style and the Ability to Coordinate Transformation Rules

The 12 sessions of the second year were devoted to abstraction, and subsequently coordination, of relative transformation rules by unidirectional steps. Anne was able to do only 20 of the 24 exercises that we had designed originally.

Mastering Relative Transformation Rules

Sessions 13 to 16 were devoted to exercises that were comparable in difficulty to those presented at the end of the first year, except that in one of the compartments they required a double transformation. Following the long summer break, it seemed wise to review the exercises that had been mastered previously in order to consolidate what she had already learned. In view of the results, it turned out that it had been unnecessary to go back over exercises that seemed not to present any particular problem.

Anne showed that she could still be quite effective: she explored the compartments from left to right in two successive passes, and continued to describe the properties that were not transformed, which sometimes led her to mention some properties not brought up during the session and even some that had never before been used in the training. Even so, she was moving progressively during these four sessions into the habit of mentioning the transformed property immediately after each trial without first describing the two objects.

Sessions 17 to 19 were devoted to exercises in which we introduced two additional problems: (a) relative transformations, and (b) simultaneous use of four compartments (rather than three). Introduction of relativity of the transformations led Anne to return temporarily to previously discarded behavior: (a) in the first pass of any compartment, she again described both the introduced and the retrieved objects in detail, without giving any general rule, whereas in the second pass, by contrast, she followed that description with a general rule, e.g., "bigger size"; (b) her general rule included some examples, which had not been observed in any of the previous sessions (13 to 16).

This temporary regression diminished from the first to the third of these exercises. Thus, in session 19, Anne did not give the names of the objects after each trial ("thickness has changed, it is bigger, the head has not changed"), nor did she give any example in her general verbalization ("that changes the head, it is lowered a little; it changes thickness, gets a little smaller; the head comes back up; it changes thickness to bigger, the heads do not change"). Anne did not yet know how to express the relativity of the transformation economically, but described it according to the property accompanying the meaning of the transformation. Only in the later sessions would she use a single verb to qualify this type of transformation: "the thickness gets less, the size gets bigger, the size gets smaller." She was, however, not to reach the stage of freedom from the transformed properties in which a single precise verb-adjective combination would evoke the transformation in play, such as "gets smaller, gets lighter."[1]

Anne continued to explore the four compartments systematically and to memorize the placement of each transformation without error. Finally,

[1] Translator's note: In the original, the reference was to "a single precise verb." In French, that is possible: "*elle diminue*, *elle éclaircit*," but in the simple English that a person such as Anne would use, two words, a verb and an adjective, are required: "it *gets smaller*, it *gets lighter*."

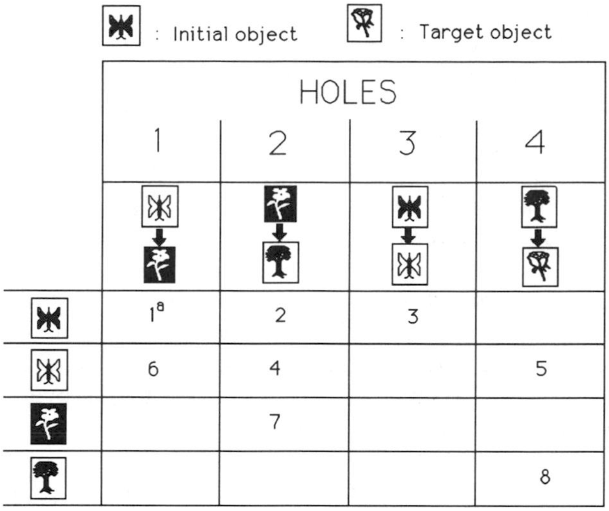

General rule:

"Me I put a red butterfly you a yellow butterfly (shows H3) / I put the butterfly here (H1) and you gave me back a yellow flower which I put in here (H2) in order to get the tree / here (H4) I must get the red flower because there is just one hole left.

[a]Numbers refer to successive introductions

FIGURE 18.1. Activity chart, session 21, showing Anne's use of coordination of transformation rules.

her rate of success in the anticipation phase attests to her ability to anticipate the consequences of a relative transformation in both directions, including both new and incongruous objects.

The Ability to Coordinate Transformation Rules and Evidence of a Skillful Problem Solving Style

The final sessions were addressed to coordination of transformation rules (i.e., to use two or more dimensions simultaneously). Session 21 illustrates Anne's functional efficiency toward the end of the training.

Figure 18.1 shows the activity chart and the final general rule guiding Anne's actions. In this exercise the coordination phase was not preceded by exploration; instead, she had to discover the function of each compartment with respect to the target object (in this case, a rose). This kind of problem is particularly useful for observing planning behavior.

In the first pass, transformation of the initial red butterfly, Anne looked for the function of each compartment by moving systematically from left to right. In the second pass, she no longer proceeded in this exploratory way, but escaped the compartment 3 where she had just transformed the butterfly. In the final pass, she put the tree directly in the correct hole. It would be difficult to perform any better!

This high degree of control suggested a perfect representation of the task and of her action in it. She clearly understood the requisite logical and temporal relations related to her general rule: "and," "in order to," "I must have," "because." She also demonstrated a certain precision of vocabulary, awareness of sequences, and the expression of a feeling of logical necessity.

In session 23 we observed perfect representation and control: "If I put the little white fish here it gives me back a long one but of the same color, and then we put it here and it becomes fat, and then here and it is red." In these final sessions in which it was necessary to discover the rules before advancing to the coordination phase, Anne made only one pass per compartment and immediately enunciated the transformation rule.

In the last session Anne was given an exercise that required her to compensate for the effect of the transformation rules in order to obtain the desired object. In fact, the rules were associated in such a way that the subject had to be willing temporarily to abandon the objective on one dimension in order to be able to transform on the other: two compartments had a diminishing effect, the one reducing thickness and the other the inclination of the head, whereas the third simultaneously increased both thickness and inclination. Following the "discovery of rules" phase, Anne was asked to transform a moderately thick duck whose head was lowered into a thinner duck with its head raised. She began by only reducing thickness. Then, after having observed that it would be necessary to use the "double transformation" compartment, she proceeded to raise the head to the required position while simultaneously increasing the thickness of the picture. Finally, she reduced the thickness to that required, observing, "Here, I got it!" Anne then succeeded on the two other exercises in the minimal number of plays.

Anne at the Two Posttests and at Follow-Up

Two planned posttests, one in June (second year) and the other from October to November (second year), completed the experiment. In anticipation of writing this report, we conducted a follow-up in June 1986 as a final posttest.

Accession to a Concrete Operatory Level of Thought

Each posttest consisted of five Piagetian conservation tests for establishing the stage of concrete operations.

At the initial posttest, Anne was shown to be conserving totally in the two tests of conservation of number (lining up tokens and pouring out beads). In all the situations presented, conservation as well as non-conservation, she gave correct answers based on the arguments of identity or compensation, and similarly refuted the counterarguments of the experimenter. She expressed such a feeling for evidence in the test of pouring out of beads that we were surprised to find her not conserving in the test of conservation of mass.

At the next posttest, Anne was shown to be totally conserving on all five tests. On each of these tests, and especially on the last two (area and weight-volume dissociation) that comprise numerous and diverse transformations, she gave evidence of her understanding of constant properties. On the test of area, for example, she used the three arguments of conservation and spontaneously offered other transformations that do not affect the constancy of the relevant properties. On all these tests, she described as well some other transformations that would affect constant properties. On the test of dissociation, at the first weighing in which there was a difference in weight between the two stimuli (same diameter and same height), she showed only a brief hesitation. Then before their immersion she declared that the weight of the stimuli did not affect the height of the water. Very quickly, she stated to the experimenter that "I am right, and the weight does nothing," "the size is important, the height also, if you put two little ones it will be equal to one big one." Moreover, on the standard test of conservation of volume she gave only correctly argued conservation responses, whatever the material of the stimuli to be immersed (plastic, wax, or Lego blocks).

Table 5.7 of Chapter 5 shows that at the end of the intervention Anne had quite clearly surpassed the subjects of the control group, of whom only two had attained the operatory level on the test of placement of tokens. On the basis of conservation tests, we can state confidently that the intervention radically modified Anne's way of thinking. Together with six other subjects in the training group, she had fully acceded to concrete operatory thought.

Mental Age Gains

The developmental gains shown on the conservation tests were supplemented by improvement on the New Metric Test of Intelligence (NMTI) and on Raven's Progressive Matrices. Generalization of her improvements to these tasks suggested that Anne had functionally integrated her cognitive gains.

On the NMTI, just as on the conservation tests, Anne's performance was clearly different from that of the control subjects, whereas her progress fit perfectly with that of the training group. Table 18.4 shows also that her IQ gain was maintained, because at the final posttest her

TABLE 18.4. Mental age (months) and IQ (New Metric Test of Intelligence) of Anne, trained subjects, and control subjects, by testing date.

	Mental Age					IQ				
	Anne	Trained		Control		Anne	Trained		Control	
Test date		M	SD	M	SD		M	SD	M	SD
11/82	72	78	6	76	11	55	58	6	56	9
6/84	96	99	19	80	16	64	63	5	53	10
6/86	114					65				

score was almost identical (65) to that obtained 2 years earlier, at initial posttest (64).

The progress that Anne made on the Progressive Matrices (Tables 18.2 and 18.3) reflects a generalization of her ability to coordinate relations that appeared progressively in the course of the second year of training. Here as well, Anne's progress from beginning to end of the intervention was clearly superior to that of the control group. Nevertheless, this test revealed some limitations on her progress. First, from pretest to last posttest Anne consistently failed designs A11 and A12. Second, even on the posttest of October 1984, when Anne's score was highest, the cognitive requirements of the problems interfered with the coordination of relations as they appear in the C series. Finally, her score on the final posttest (June 1986) was lower than that on the two immediately preceding tests (June 1984 and October 1984), but was still higher than that of the pretest (November 1982).

Cognitive Functioning Style

On the two 1986 posttests, Anne solved immediately the two-disk problem of the Tower of Hanoi. When tested the following June, she did not immediately succeed in anticipating the three-disk placements in the course of the first three trials. On the first trial she placed the small disk on the wrong base, and stopped herself immediately. She then constructed the tower on the wrong base on the second trial, and succeeded on the third trial but in nine rather than seven plays. She improved her performance on the second placement, although on the first trial, even though she was on her way to finishing the problem successfully, she constructed it on the wrong base, probably because she was disturbed by the preceding problem. Her difficulty in anticipating, especially on the three-disk placements, was apparent in her total failure to anticipate the placement of the small disk. But in the course of the four-disk trials, she did succeed in constructing an accurate representation. On none of the six trials of the first problem did she succeed in the minimal number of placements, 15. In the second problem, she succeeded on the last two trials following four transfers that were correct but too long. It is important to note that all of her four-disk anticipations were correct!

This progressive understanding was confirmed by the October posttest. In fact, Anne succeeded right away in virtually all of the two-, three-, and four-disk placements (exceeding the minimal number of placements on only the first trial of the second three-disk problem), and she correctly anticipated the placement of the small disk on all the transfers. However, Anne was to fail on five-disk problems: in spite of her wish to persist, she did not master the placements and stopped at a point when she was only rarely reaching her objective.

Comparison with the control group shows Anne's progress dramatically. On the October posttest, 8 of the 11 control subjects had a score of 0 on the three-disk problems, whereas the two others obtained 7 and 8 points. In the training group, seven of the nine subjects earned at least 8 points. Although the majority of the control subjects showed absolutely no progress on this test, Anne became capable of solving problems whose solution required efficient cognitive functioning, most notably the four-disk problems. The June 1986 (final) posttest showed that Anne had not lost any of her effectiveness in this task, although she still was not able to solve the five-disk problems.

Conclusions

The case of Anne has served to demonstrate our method of induction of logic structures. Her progress, which was not unique, is clarified by that of the training group subjects and contrasted with that of the control subjects. The duration of the observations, as well as the description of the difficulties that she overcame, has led us at the end of this chapter to think that the induction of the *concept of paired relations*, then that of *general rules of dependence*, and finally that of their coordination, are the basis of a profound change. Both the nature of the intervention and our analysis of the posttest data assure us that this change was authentic, durable, and generalizable. Anne's gains, as well as those of the other experimental subjects, support the method of *induction of logic structures* as a means of assessment of cognitive potential.

But can we say that Anne is more *intelligent* today than she was before the training? Such a question is difficult, even redoubtable (Spitz, 1986). It seems to us, moreover, that it is easier to answer this question at the individual level than at the general level of the educability of intelligence. What is more, the answer must depend upon the criteria that one holds for intellectual growth and upon the instrumentation of those criteria.

First, Anne is certainly more competent in the sense that her post-training level of reasoning was quite superior to her pretraining level. In fact, the distal posttest confirmed the overall stability of the operatory behavior sequences within the group of conservation tests. Her representation of objects and cognitive problems was shown to be at once both more complex and much closer to what one would expect to find in the day-to-day logical functioning of any normal adult. The difference between Anne's functioning and "normal" functioning has been reduced. Today, she is distinguished only by a quantitative difference, i.e., by degree, and not by a radical qualitative difference as was the case prior to training.

From this latter point of view, we can state that Anne is unquestionably *more intelligent than the subjects in the control group* and that she will retain this superiority so long as the control subjects do not reach the concrete operatory level. Moreover, we have observed a relative concordance between her mental age in June 1986 and the developmental age that one could infer from the conservation tests. Although Anne's IQ remains in the mildly mentally retarded range, we can point out that she has continued to achieve some *acquisitions* (i.e., examples of structural cognitive growth) at a rate that is superior to that of the control subjects.

The Progressive Matrices and the Tower of Hanoi tests show that Anne has functionally integrated the new cognitive tools and systems that the training has helped her to construct. We can therefore state with certainty that she is more intelligent than the control subjects in the sense that *she knows how to process information and resolve problems* better than they do.

The relationships between operatory thought and academic and vocational learning are not well understood. It is, however, reasonable to think that if attainment of the concrete operatory level does not always constitute a necessary condition for fundamental academic learning, it certainly constitutes a facilitating condition. Anne's scholastic evolution supports this point of view: with five other subjects from the training group (but none from the control group) she was placed in September 1985 in a specialized education class. These are classes that are integrated into schools that offer basic academic instruction combined with prevocational training. We do not mean to attribute this academic advance to the cognitive training alone; nevertheless, we do want to point out that in view of her academic progress her teachers have judged her to be able to follow a more demanding curriculum than she had had before training.

This institutional change is a two-edged sword. Having changed her academic foundation, Anne is confronted with new requirements and is encountering new problems. According to her school report of June 1987, she does not seem to have surmounted the new problems fully. In fact, her teachers have pointed out some difficulties that, every allowance being made, correspond to those that she showed initially. From this latter aspect, it is clear that *Anne is not fundamentally more intelligent*. Her intellectual "dynamic" has not been radically turned around. She has not spontaneously acceded to the next higher level of reasoning (preformal), and the reports of her teachers and the deterioration of her Progressive Matrices scores leaves one suspecting that her functioning is still deficient in this task. If the acquired cognitive changes are shown to be stable, it would seem more difficult to produce long-term modifications in individual functional modalities. Labile by their nature, and especially in mentally retarded persons, such functioning needs to be continually supported.

Our training does not have the scope of a general program of cognitive education. Its force and perhaps its limitations derive from its focus on well-specified developmental objectives and the application of strict principles of intervention. A program of cognitive education must certainly take into account many other aspects and components of cognitive functioning. One can, however, offer the hypothesis that the induced acquisition of concrete operatory structures constitutes a facilitating condition, truly amplifying the effectiveness of other intervention strategies that might be more focused on functioning.

This kind of cognitive intervention and its ultimate generalizations to other stages of development can therefore constitute one element and one referent for any general program of cognitive education.

Acknowledgments. This study constitutes the experimental phase of the second author's doctoral dissertation, done at the University of Provence. This chapter was translated from the original French by H. Carl Haywood.

References

Borys, S. V., Spitz, H. H., & Dorans, B. A. (1982). Tower of Hanoi performance of retarded young adults and nonretarded children as a function of solution length and goal state. *Journal of Experimental Child Psychology*, *33*, 87–110.

Byrnes, M. M., & Spitz, H. H. (1977). Performance of retarded adolescents and nonretarded children on the Tower of Hanoi problem. *American Journal of Mental Deficiency*, *81*, 561–569.

Orsini-Bouichou, F. (1975). *Régularités dans les organisations spontanées chez l'enfant et genèse des comportements cognitifs* [Regularities in children's spontaneous organizations and the origins of cognitive behavior]. Unpublished doctoral dissertation, Université René Descartes, Paris.

Paour, J.-L. (1975). Effet d'un entraînement cognitif sur la compréhension et la production d'énoncés passifs chez des enfants déficients mentaux [Effect of cognitive training on the understanding and production of passive statements in mentally retarded children]. *Etudes de Linguistique Appliquée*, *20*, 88–110.

Paour, J.-L. (1980). *Construction et fonctionnement des structures opératoires concrètes chez l'enfant débile mental: Apport des expériences d'apprentissage et d'induction opératoires* [Construction and functioning of concrete operatory structures in the mentally retarded child: Support from experiments in operatory induction and learning]. Unpublished doctoral dissertation, Université de Provence, Aix-en-Provence.

Paour, J.-L. (1985). De l'induction des structures logiques à la modification du fonctionnement [From the induction of logic structures to the modification of functioning]. *Revue Suisse de Psychologie*, *44*(3), 135–147.

Robeants, M.-J. (1987). *Etude du développement et du fonctionnement cognitif d'enfants Haïtiens* [A study of the cognitive functioning of Haitian children]. Unpublished doctoral dissertation, Université de Provence, Aix-en-Provence.

Soavi, G. (1986). *Une analyse du fonctionnement cognitif chez l'enfant retardé mental à propos de la genèse observée et provoquée de la relation de couple* [An analysis of cognitive functioning in mentally retarded children according to the observed and induced genesis of the pairing relation]. Unpublished doctoral dissertation, Université de Provence, Aix-en-Provence.

Spitz, H. H. (1986). *The raising of intelligence: A selected history of attempts to raise retarded intelligence*. Hillsdale, NJ: Erlbaum.

Wallon, H. (1942). *L'évolution psychologique de l'enfant* [The psychological development of the child]. Paris: Armand Colin.

Zazzo, R., Gilly, M., & Verba-Rad, M. (1966). *Nouvelle Echelle Métrique de l'Intelligence* [New Metric Scale of Intelligence]. Paris: Armand Colin.

Zigler, E. (1969). Developmental versus difference theories of mental retardation and the problem of motivation. *American Journal of Mental Deficiency*, *73*, 536–556.

Zigler, E. (1972). Rigidity in the retarded: A reexamination. In E. Trapp & P. Himelstein (Eds.), *Readings in the exceptional child: Research and theory* (2nd ed., pp. 141–162). New York: Appleton-Century-Crofts.

Part 5
Public Policy Issues in Psychoeducational Assessment

Few educational issues have stirred up as much activity in the public policy realm in recent years as has the question of the use of standardized, normative intelligence tests to determine educational placement, especially placement of children from minority ethnic groups. The policy issues are multifaceted and extraordinarily complex, with theoretical, psychometric, sociopolitical, and legal aspects. Solutions that have been suggested have not always been based on the most careful reflection because the debates have been especially passionate. At the same time, it is useful to recognize that intelligence testing is a singularly powerful achievement of psychology. For limited purposes, intelligence tests do their job well. The urgent question today is whether or not that is a job that still needs to be done in the same way as in the past.

In Chapter 19, Utley, Haywood, and Masters outline the major arguments against the continued use of standardized, normative intelligence tests for educational placement, examine the available empirical evidence on those arguments, and present the need for alternative assessment approaches. Finding the weight of evidence to be against some of the most familiar arguments (e.g., that intelligence tests themselves are "biased" against minority children, and that the tests have differential predictive validity), they make a different case for the need for alternative methods of assessment.

The *Larry P.* and PASE cases have become famous in the literature of psychoeducational assessment, as well as in that of case law. Litigation has been focused on the issue of whether or not standardized intelligence testing is inherently discriminatory when used for educational placement. In Chapter 20, Elliott, both a psychologist and a legal scholar, examines these issues from a combined psychological and legal perspective. His analysis of the testimony in these famous court cases suggests both the passion with which the litigation has been pursued and the obvious fact that something is wrong in the way educational placement decisions are made.

19
Policy Implications of Psychological Assessment of Minority Children

Cheryl A. Utley, H. Carl Haywood, and John C. Masters

The insistent demand for "nondiscriminatory" testing procedures in psychoeducational assessment, especially of children from minority groups, has had a substantial base in case law (e.g., Larry P. v. Wilson Riles, 1979; Mattie T. et al., v. Charles E. Holladay et al., 1979; see also Elliott, Chapter 20 in this volume) as well as federal legislation (e.g., Title VI of the Civil Rights Act of 1964; Section 504 of the Vocational Rehabilitation Act of 1973; Education of All Handicapped Children Act of 1975). Professional organizations, such as the American Psychological Association, the American Educational Research Association, and the National Council on Measurement in Education, have adopted policy statements addressed to the possibility of bias in mental tests. Innovative assessment practices with minority children have been developed in efforts to minimize the discrepancy in intelligence test scores between minority and majority children and to prevent inappropriate or disproportionate assignment of minority children, relative to majority children, to special education classes (Jones, 1976, 1988; Sewell, 1987). These concerns constitute issues in psychometrics and educational practice, but they also constitute public policy issues.

A major criticism regarding the use of standardized intelligence tests is that they may be culturally biased against poor, minority children as compared to majority children, because of differences in culture, language, values, and experiential background, and therefore may not be appropriate tools with which to assess the intelligence of minority children. Psychologists and other social scientists have sought alternative psychoeducational assessment procedures designed to minimize the discrepancy between test performance and ability that many think they have observed in both minority and majority children. In this chapter we review the psychometric and educational issues relevant to psychoeducational assessment with particular emphasis on minority children, examine alternative psychoeducational assessment procedures, and discuss issues of public policy in this domain.

Psychometric Issues

Persistent minority-majority differences in intelligence test scores have been the topic of intense debate among educators, social scientists, and behavior geneticists. Black and Hispanic children characteristically score significantly below the mean value for majority children on normative, nationally standardized intelligence tests. This basic datum is clear and undisputed. The question is whether or not differences in IQ (the manifest variable; the score on a test of intelligence) reflect differences in intelligence itself (the latent, unobservable variable that is assumed to be measured by intelligence tests). The observed race differences in IQ have frequently been attributed to the technical and scientific inadequacy of these tests: test bias and the validation procedures used in the construction and standardization of intelligence tests.

Test bias refers to the presence of "systematic errors of measurement as opposed to chance or random, patternless errors" (Reynolds & Brown, 1984). Conceptually, the study of test bias has been concerned with the measurement of average test scores and the extent to which obtained measurements systematically overestimate (or underestimate) the true (error-free) scores for members of one group relative to members of another group. From this perspective, the concept of test bias is viewed as a set of statistical properties that are divorced from subjective value judgments, legal mandates, and ethical issues of fairness and unfairness (Jensen, 1980).

A basic assumption of the psychometric perspective is that intelligence is normally distributed in the population and that intelligence test scores are distributed according to a Gaussian or bell-shaped curve (Haywood, 1974; Wyne & O'Connor, 1979). Because the means of the distributions of IQ for minority and majority children differ by approximately 15 points or one standard deviation, the proportion of individuals in one group who fall in the upper and lower ranges of the distribution of the other group can be calculated and compared. The proportion of minority children with IQs below 70 (and who are thus psychometrically eligible for a diagnosis of mental retardation) is approximately six times greater than the proportion of majority children who score in that range. By contrast, approximately 16% of majority children have IQs above 115, but only about 3% of minority children have scores in that range.

The arguments against the use of standardized intelligence tests with minority children have centered around claims of test bias from a variety of sources (Bond, 1982; Laosa, 1977; Oakland & Parmelee, 1985). Reynolds and Brown (1984) have summarized the potential sources of test bias as follows:

1. *Inappropriate content.* Minority children have not had the same exposure to material in the test questions or other stimulus materials as have majority children. The tests are geared primarily toward white middle-class environments, vocabulary, and values.
2. *Inappropriate standardization samples.* Ethnic minorities are inadequately represented in standardization samples used in the collection of normative data. Williams (Wright & Isenstein, 1977) has criticized the WISC-R (Wechsler, 1974) normative sample for including black subjects only in proportion to the United States total population. Out of 2,200 children in the WISC-R standardization sample, 330 were members of ethnic minorities. Williams contended that such a small absolute number had little effect on the norms of the test. In earlier years, it was not unusual for standardization samples to be all white (e.g., the 1937 Binet and 1949 WISC).
3. *Examiner and language bias.* Because most psychologists are white and speak only standard English, they may intimidate minority subjects. They are also unable to communicate adequately with minority children—for example, they may be insensitive to ethnic pronunciations of words on the tests. Lower scores for minority persons, then, may reflect this intimidation and difficulty in the communication process, rather than lower ability.
4. *Inequitable social consequences.* As a result of bias in educational and psychological tests, minority group members, already at a disadvantage in the educational and vocational markets because of past discrimination, and thought as a result of their test scores to be unable to learn, are disproportionately relegated to dead-end tracks. Labeling effects also fall in this category.
5. *Measurement of different constructs.* Related to item 1 above, this position asserts that the tests measure different attributes when used with children from other than the white middle-class culture on which the tests are largely based, and thus do not measure validly the intelligence of minority group members.
6. *Differential predictive validity.* Although tests may predict accurately a variety of outcomes for white middle-class children, they do not predict successfully any relevant behavior for minority group members. Further, there are objections to the use of the standard criteria against which tests are validated with minority cultural groups. That is, scholastic or academic attainment levels in white middle-class schools are themselves considered by many black psychologists to be biased as criteria (Reynolds, 1982, pp. 179–180).

Most of the assertions of inappropriateness of standardized intelligence tests for minority children are linked to these aspects of psychometric validity: (a) content validity, (b) predictive or criterion validity, and (c) construct validity.

Content Validity

Content validity is the determination of item parameters, such as item difficulty, item discrimination, item characteristic curves, and their use in item selection, modification, and scoring (Ironson & Sebkovial, 1979; Johnson, 1980). Most of the empirical evidence regarding possible bias in content validity has centered on item difficulty. Item difficulty may be due to the degree of cultural specificity in the individual items on the test, factual content of the items, and/or familiarity with the informational content of items. Research is directed by the question: To what extent are the items on standardized intelligence tests relatively more difficult for minority children than for majority children? To determine whether or not there are differences between groups, the rank order of item difficulties (percent passing each item) and the magnitude of the Item × Group interaction are calculated. Comparisons of the performance levels of black and white persons on standardized intelligence tests have shown that the order of item difficulty is similar for both groups. In addition, the cross-racial correlations of item difficulties for standardized intelligence tests have been very high (e.g., .98 for Raven's Progressive Matrices and the Stanford-Binet, .96 for the WISC). The hypothesis of test bias as related to item difficulty in content validity for different cultural groups has not been empirically supported.

Predictive Validity

Another aspect of validation that would reflect test bias is the degree to which intelligence test scores differentially predict the academic performances of minority and majority persons. To determine whether intelligence tests have equivalent predictive validity for minority and majority children the essential question is: Do similar test scores predict the same level of success for members of different population subgroups? Two types of studies have been conducted in order to examine differential predictive validity: (a) correlations between the tests and the criterion measures, often referred to as investigations of differential validity; and (b) regression equations, referred to as investigations of differential prediction (Linn, 1982).

Differential validity studies have been conducted to determine whether IQ predicts equally well across different population subgroups such criterion variables as scores on standardized tests of school achievement or school grades. Correlation coefficients ranging from .50 to .70 for both minority and majority groups have been reported between standardized intelligence tests, such as the WISC, WISC-R, and Stanford-Binet (Form L-M), and scores on standardized school achievement tests, such as the California Achievement Test, Wide Range Achievement Test, Metropolitan Achievement Tests, Stanford Achievement Tests, and

California Test of Mental Maturity (Sattler, 1974, 1988). When teacher-assigned grades are the criterion, substantially lower correlations are found for minority than for majority children (Goldman & Hartig, 1976; Messé, Crano, Messé, & Rice, 1979).

Differential prediction is determined by calculating the coefficient of correlation between the test and some criterion and then by calculating a linear regression equation (Cleary, Humphreys, Kendrick, & Wesman, 1975). Differential prediction studies are thus designed to examine the variability of observed criterion scores around their predicted values, intercepts, and slopes for two different groups. In psychometric terms, the principal question is: Do the regression lines have the same criterion scores, the same intercepts, and the same slopes? Differences in criterion scores indicate that predictions can be made with greater accuracy for individuals in one group than for individuals in another group. Differences in intercept suggest that the average score on the criterion is higher for members of one group than for members of the other group. Differences in slope suggest that the predicted criterion scores are more unstable (i.e., change more rapidly) for members of one group than for members of the other group.

Test bias in predictive validity studies is "determined by the direction and the magnitude of the differences between predicted and observed criterion scores for members of a given group. . . ." (Wigdor & Garner, 1982, p. 76). Underprediction occurs when members of one group do not perform as well on the actual criterion. On the other hand, overprediction occurs when members of one group tend to perform better on the criterion. Thus, the regression lines in the predicted equation for two groups may yield biased predictions that are either against members of one group or in favor of members of the other group.

Investigations of differential prediction have been conducted with minority and majority elementary and secondary school children. The question has been whether intelligence tests are biased against minority children such that the IQs derived from them underestimate the academic abilities of these children. There is little evidence that standardized intelligence tests such as the WISC-R predict academic performance differently for minority groups than for majority groups (Oakland & Parmelee, 1985; Reschly & Sabers, 1979; Reynolds, 1982; Reynolds & Gutkin, 1980; Travers, 1982).

Construct Validity

Construct validation involves inferences about what psychological attributes underlie test performance. According to Wigdor and Garner (1982, p. 61), the focus of construct validation in testing is to identify "the characteristics of ability by establishing a relationship between a measurement procedure (e.g., a test) and an unobserved underlying trait," such as intelligence or scholastic performance. A common statistical method employed is factor analysis, a correlation technique designed to investigate patterns of interrelationships of performance among individuals (Johnson, 1980).

With regard to construct validation, test bias would exist, "when a test is shown to measure different hypothetical traits (psychological constructs) for one group than another or to measure the same trait but with differing degrees of accuracy" (Reynolds & Brown, 1984, p. 26). Conversely, tests would be considered "nonbiased" when similar factor structures are found for minority groups and majority groups. Should the factor structure of standardized intelligence tests for minority children vary substantially from that of the standardization sample of these tests, the construct validity would be questionable. Factor analytic studies suggest that the overall factor structure of the WISC-R for minority children is highly comparable to that for majority children (Gutkin & Reynolds, 1980; McShane & Cook, 1985; Reschly, 1978, 1980; Sandoval, 1982; Sattler, 1988). Findings do not support the notion that the WISC-R measures different attributes in minority children and majority children.

Among theories specifically related to minority children, the psychometric perspective does not refute claims of test bias. The empirical evidence herein reviewed does not support allegations that differences in test scores between minority and majority children are due to (a) the relative difficulty of the item content, (b) an underestimation of the abilities of minority children, and (c) the measurement of different attributes for different minority groups. This explanation of individual differences in intelligence between minority and majority children has been extensively criticized because it excludes any considerations that pertain to the ethical issues of fairness and unfairness and the educational consequences resulting from the use of test scores as criteria for testing and evaluating minority and majority children.

Educational Issues

Standardized intelligence tests play a central role in the classification and subsequent placement of minority and majority children into different types of educational programs. The pedagogical principle underlying the placement of children into homogeneous groups is that instruction can be accomplished most effectively if children are grouped on the basis of real or perceived ability (Resnick, 1979). The provision of instruction tailored to each child's learning aptitude has resulted in the emergence of three types of educational programs: (a) regular or "mainstream," (b) compensatory education, and (c) special education (Anderson, 1982).

The regular education program includes the vast majority of children, those whose intelligence quotients (IQs) are within two standard deviations of the population mean on standardized intelligence tests, and who have no significant sensory impairment, emotional disturbance, or learning disability. Compensatory education programs are designed for low-achieving children who are enrolled in regular education programs but who, supposedly because of unfavorable environmental circumstances such as poverty, need additional individualized instruction in the basic skills (e.g., reading, spelling, and arithmetic) (Haywood, 1982). Special education programs are designed for children diagnosed as gifted, sensory handicapped, multiply handicapped, mentally retarded, learning disabled, or behavior-disordered (Kirk & Gallagher, 1989). Educators in general seem to believe that special education programs for sensory handicapped children are justified and effective. On the other hand, the practice of assigning children to special education programs based on ability grouping has not seemed to improve student achievement (Slavin, 1987) or to have closed the gap in performance levels on standardized intelligence tests among minority and majority children (Ogbu, 1978).

Disparities continue to exist in the achievement levels of minority and majority children in the regular education program. Data assembled as a part of the National Assessment of Educational Progress indicate that reading test scores of black children were 15% lower than those of white children at age 9, 23% lower at age 13, and 27% lower at age 17 (Children's Defense Fund, 1985). These achievement data are consistent with comparisons of scores on intelligence tests. For example, Coleman, Campbell, Hobson, McPortland, Mood, Weinfeld, & York (1966) compared several minority groups (African-American, Mexican-American, Puerto Rican, and Native American) from a national sample of 3rd, 6th, 9th, and 12th grades on tests of verbal and nonverbal ability, reading comprehension, mathematics, and general information. Differences in test scores of one standard deviation were found between minority and majority children on every test at all four grades. With respect to intelligence tests, Jensen (1985), among many others, has reported that the average IQ of minority children, in particular black children, is 85, approximately one standard deviation below the average score for white children. Such differences persist, whether one uses verbal or nonverbal tests, relatively culturally rich or "culture-fair" tests, or whether one assesses intelligence or school achievement.

Current testing practices have also influenced the development and evaluation of compensatory education programs. The educational objectives of these programs have been guided by one principal question: To what extent have compensatory education programs facilitated the academic and intellectual growth of minority children as compared to majority children so as to minimize differences between these groups of children? Evaluative reports on the effectiveness of compensatory education programs have shown student gains in the academic achievement levels of minority children relative to majority children (Darlington, 1986; Haywood, 1982). For example, in a National Institute of Education study, first-grade students showed average gains of 12 months in reading and 11 months in math and third-grade students gained 8 months in reading and 12 months in math during a 7-month compensatory education program (reported by Haywood, 1982). Significant gains in IQ have also been associated with compensatory education, but follow-up studies have indicated that such gains have not been sustained over the early years of elementary school experience (Consortium for Longitudinal Studies, 1983; Ogbu, 1978).

Minority children are statistically overrepresented in EMR ("educable," i.e., mildly, mentally retarded) classes relative to their numbers in the population (Chinn & Hughes, 1987; Finn, 1982; Manni, Winikur, & Keller, 1984; Tucker, 1980). For example, in California, Hispanic children constitute 15.22% of public school children, but make up 28.34% of the EMR enrollment (California State Department of Education, 1970). Prasse and Reschly (1986) observed that black children are "placed in programs for the mildly retarded at a rate that significantly exceeded a comparison to the percentage of black children in the school base population, and that rate was excessive when contrasted with the placement of white children in the same program for the mildly retarded" (p. 334). Finn (1982) cited some interesting demographic trends reported in a data base assembled by the Office of Civil Rights (1978):

1. The average percentage of minority children in EMR classes exceeds the average percentage of majority children in such classes in every state except four: Iowa, New Hampshire, Vermont, and West Virginia.
2. The highest EMR placement rates for minority children are in the southern states, followed by the northeastern and midwestern states.

Concerns have been raised that the more frequent classification of minority children as EMR may reflect the use of special education classes for these children as a "dumping ground," that is, as a means of excluding minority children from regular education classes (Dunn, 1968; Heller, Holtzman, & Messick, 1982). The assignment to EMR classes is often tantamount to a "sentence" for the duration of a minority child's school experience. Once assigned to EMR classes a child is unlikely to return to a regular education track. For example, in one epidemiological study of mental retardation in Riverside, California, it was reported that "only 19% of the children placed in special education were returned to the regular classroom. Twenty-three percent dropped out of school, 46% were eventually excluded from school or were placed in other programs and institutions, and 11% aged out of the program" (Mercer, 1979a, p. 2).

There is significant controversy over the extent to which standardized intelligence and achievement tests are used in the identification-assessment-placement process of minority and majority children into special education programs. Strickland and Turnbull (1990) argued that no single procedure should be used as the sole criterion for determining placement into special education. The assessment process requires the integration of test results with information obtained from multiple sources, such as adaptive behavior scores, language samples, teacher reports, and interviews. It has been noted, however, that the decisions made by both psychologists and teachers rely on test scores as primary criteria for placement (Matuszek & Oakland, 1979). A consistent finding by Poland, Ysseldyke, Thurlow, & Mirkin (1979) and Ysseldyke, Algozzine, Regan, & McGue (1979) is that achievement test scores represent the single most important source of data for evaluating the performance of students. Bickel (1982, p. 197) further noted that the use of intelligence test scores, coupled with achievement tests, in placement decisions involves a process in which poor achievement "nominates" a student for referral and the IQ "anoints" him or her into a particular classification. Despite the fact that multifactored assessment procedures are required for placement into special education classes, standardized intelligence and achievement test scores continue to play a persuasive role in the classification process.

Standardized intelligence tests are the mechanisms by which children are placed into different academic environments, where the distribution of educational resources, hence the quality of instruction, may vary substantially. Because special and low-ability classes frequently emphasize social adjustment and vocational training rather than the acquisition of academic knowledge and proficiencies, minority children placed into these classes fall farther and farther behind children in the regular classes on standardized tests of academic achievement. In EMR classes, instructional practices are often based on a "watered-down" curriculum in which there is little emphasis on the development of academic knowledge. Consequently, EMR children have been shown to progress more academically in regular classes than in segregated, self-contained classes.

Overall, studies of the effectiveness of academic instruction have shown that specific features of instructional programs may be of greater relevance to improved achievement than is the type of administrative arrangement, e.g., self-contained or resource room, in which EMR children have been placed (Corman & Gottlieb, 1978; Jenkins & Mayhall, 1976). For example, the direct instruction of basic skills, the use of informal assessment techniques, and the implementation of behavior management programs are features of effective instructional programs that have been successful in teaching poor and minority children enrolled in regular education programs, compensatory programs, and self-contained and resource classrooms (Brookover & Lezotte, 1979; Rosenshine & Berliner, 1978). In addition, programs that emphasize the acquisition of problem solving processes and use of rehearsal strategies have improved the cognitive functioning of EMR children (Feuerstein, Rand, Hoffman, & Miller, 1980).

A very important issue that must be resolved in the psychoeducational assessment of minority and majority children is the utility of standardized assessment, particularly intelligence test scores, in the development of effective educational programs. Although standardized intelligence test scores are used for purposes of classification and diagnosis, they are not prescriptive. Standardized intelligence tests are not used to identify a child's functional needs (e.g., cognitive processing, adaptive motivation), to recognize obstacles that may or may not interfere with their learning ability, and to develop instructional practices designed to minimize the discrepancy between learning performance and learning potential. In the case of minority children, Heller et al. (1982) remarked that

> the predictive power of IQ does not necessarily make it a good measure of mental processes: different processes may underlie the same IQ scores for different groups of children, and different types of remediation may be necessary in cases of poor performance. For example, it has been frequently argued that levels of motivation and effort of minority students are systematically different from those of white students. Similarly, language factors undoubtedly affect performance more for some groups than others. IQ tests administered entirely in English to students for whom English is a second language are an extreme case in point. Because of these and a host of other factors, there is no way to directly infer the source of a child's difficulty from incorrectly answered test items, nor does a test score or a profile of subscores provide the kinds of information needed to design an individualized curriculum for a child in academic difficulty. (p. 19)

Therefore, it is imperative that teachers and school psychologists demonstrate that the use of standardized intelligence tests in instructional programming for EMR students leads to effective instructional practices for minority children and that these practices help students with learning difficulties to overcome learning obstacles and improve their academic performance.

Alternative Psychological Assessment Procedures

In spite of the lack of evidence supporting allegations of test bias and differential measurement and prediction when standardized intelligence tests are used with minority and majority children, the routine use of such tests as the principal criterion for such educational decisions as special class placement, particularly for minority children, has been prohibited. There is evidence, however, suggesting that both psychologists and teachers rely solely or heavily on intelligence tests for the classification of children into special programs and these tests have limited usefulness in designing educational programs.

The weight of the evidence on test bias is now on the opposite side; that is, that "bias" in tests cannot account for ethnic group differences in IQ. Further, it appears to be unlikely that standardized intelligence tests predict academic learning criteria differentially for minority and majority persons. Even though they cannot be associated with either test bias or differential prediction, IQ differences persist and in fact are quite consistent across studies by different investigators. One solution to that problems would be to assume that the tests "discriminate against" minority persons, and then to discount the scores. To adopt such a solution would mean adding some constant to the IQs of minority persons in order to produce a mean IQ for each ethnic group that would be equivalent to the mean IQ in the population as a whole. The logic of that solution would require that the IQs of majority persons be reduced by some constant, on the assumption that the tests had overestimated their intelligence, and in order also to produce a group mean IQ equivalent to that of the population as a whole. The result of that solution would be to "declassify" some number of minority children from special education programs. That result would deny them special educational services. It would free them from the disadvantage of being thought less able than majority children, but by "declassifying" them it would also make them ineligible for special help in cases of particular educational need.

Another approach would be to assume that minority children rather often have special educational needs, but that those needs do not necessarily reflect low ability. It is quite possible that there are circumstances, often associated with minority, immigrant, or socioeconomic status, that result in need for a different kind of educational assistance than one sees in majority children. Such needs might be related to "transculturality" (changing cultures), language difference, and inadequate transfer of their culture from one generation to the next, as well as reduced opportunities to learn from participation in the normal institutions of a society (Feuerstein & Rand, 1974; Haywood, 1988). Such conditions could mask or limit their access to their own intelligence, without destroying intelligence itself (Haywood & Switzky, 1986a, 1986b). To the extent that that is true, the assessment task is to design and use tests that can reveal the processes by which children perceive, think, and learn, identify deficient processes, estimate the kinds and amounts of intervention required to overcome the deficits, and prescribe educational treatments. Such an approach would not be based on an assumption that whole ethnic groups are less intelligent than are others, but would recognize the correlation between ethnicity and social advantage/disadvantage and would help to provide special educational services to children who need them rather than denying those services because of some presumed "discrimination." Indeed, we would argue that it is greatly more discriminatory to deny needed services than to identify individual children as persons who have special education needs—provided that identification of their needs leads to their getting more adequate education!

Thus, there is a growing and widespread need to develop alternative procedures that can address the educational issues that, in turn, affect the academic progress of minority children in regular education classes. The following alternative procedures have been developed for the explicit purpose of eradicating issues of bias in assessment of minority children: (a) culture-fair or culture-reduced tests, (b) adaptive behavior, and (c) dynamic assessment.

Culture-Fair Tests

Culture-fair and culture-reduced tests have been constructed to eliminate the inherent bias in standardized intelligence tests and to minimize the effects of cultural differences in test performance. Such tests depart from traditional tests in several important ways. First, unlike standardized intelligence tests, culture-fair tests are not timed; if necessary, the directions can be given orally or in pantomime. Second, draw-a-person tests, which measure body concept and differentiation, have been used as culture-fair indices of intellectual ability (e.g., Goodenough Harris Draw-A-Person Test). Third, tests that require nonverbal responses rather than verbal ones may be more appropriate for children whose language or dialect is different from the language presented in standardized tests (e.g., Raven's Progressive Matrices, Cattell Culture Fair Intelligence Test).

Culture-fair tests have been criticized as being, nevertheless, "culture-bound" and not truly culture-free. Cohen (1969) has argued that

> nonverbal tests concentrate on the ability to reason "logically." . . . It is the very nature of these logical sequences that the most culture-bound aspects of the middle-class, "analytic" way of thinking are carried. Even more critical than either the quantitative or qualitative information components of such tests are the analytic mode of abstraction and the field-articulation requirements they embody. (p. 828)

The general consensus by researchers concerning the utility of culture-fair tests as alternative measures to standardized tests is that they do not eliminate cultural differences in test performance (Bond, 1982).

Adaptive Behavior

The concept of adaptive behavior plays a significant role in the diagnosis and classification of persons with mental retardation. According to Grossman (1977, 1983), the definition of mental retardation includes the measurement of intelligence and adaptive behavior. Adaptive behavior is viewed as "the effectiveness or degree with which individuals meet the standards of personal independence and social responsibility expected of their age and cultural group . . ." (p. 157). For school-age children, an important index of adaptive behavior is performance on standardized intelligence and/or achievement tests. Grossman (1983) has held that the skills required for adaptation during childhood and early adolescence involve complex learning processes. This involves the process by which knowledge is acquired and retained as a function of the experiences of the individual. Difficulties in learning are usually manifested in the academic situation, but in the evaluation of adaptive behavior, attention should focus not only on the basic academic skills and their use, but also on skills essential in coping with the environment, including concepts of time and money, self-directed behavior, social responsiveness, and interactive skills. (p. 26).

A more specific concern directly related to the classification of minority children as EMR is the application of the dual-criterion standard, i.e., the inclusion of adaptive behavior scores in conjunction with standardized intelligence test scores in the assessment process. Minority children with low intelligence test scores and adequate adaptive behavior scores would not be eligible for placement into such classes. In such cases, the number of children, in particular minority children, classified as EMR would be reduced as compared to the numbers of children who would be classified on the basis of IQ alone.

Generally, two types of studies have been done to examine the effects of applying the dual-criterion standard in the diagnosis of mild mental retardation. In the first type of study, interest has been focused on the effects of applying the adaptive behavior criterion in addition to an IQ-less-than-70 criterion. For example, Mercer (1973) demonstrated that the application of the dual-criterion standard and a lower IQ cutoff score reduced the prevalence rates for black students from 44.9 to 4.1 per 1,000 students, and for Mexican-American students from 149.0 to 60.0 per 1,000 students. Similarly, Heflinger, Cook, and Thackrey (1987) found prevalence rates to be less than 0.5% when using the dual-criterion system.

The second type of study has been focused on the declassification of students who had already been labeled mentally retarded on the basis of the single (IQ) criterion. Mascari and Forgnone (1982) reported a declassification rate of 45% of Florida students when the dual criterion was applied. Childs (1982) showed a declassification rate of 45% in Texas. Collectively, both types of studies have shown that the inclusion of adaptive behavior measures along with IQs in the diagnosis of mild mental retardation reduces markedly the number of students eligible for special education services.

The System of Multicultural Pluralistic Assessment (SOMPA)

This comprehensive assessment instrument consists of a variety of measures designed to assess the achievement levels of children from culturally diverse backgrounds and to influence classification and placement decisions of school-age mentally retarded children (Kazimour & Reschly, 1981; Mercer, 1973, 1979a,b). Standardization is based upon a stratified sample of 2,100 children varying in sociocultural group (anglo, black, & Hispanic), socioeconomic status (SES), age, and gender.

Unlike traditional assessment approaches, the SOMPA integrates three conceptual models and evaluates the performance of children from each of the following perspectives: (a) medical, (b) social system, and (c) pluralistic. In the medical model, "biological anomalies, disease processes, sensory or motor impairments, or other pathological conditions in the organism," (Mercer, 1979a, p. 42) are evaluated. In addition to the acquisition of medical information, the sociocultural characteristics of the individual are an integral part of the evaluation process. Sociocultural characteristics may be associated with certain pathological conditions. For example, social, cultural, and economic factors contribute to brain disorders of prenatal and perinatal origin which in turn affect the cognitive development of children during their elementary school years (Avery, 1985). Instruments in the medical model include health history inventories, weight and height, visual and auditory screening tests, visual-motor tasks, and perceptual-motor tests.

The social system model is concerned with "the social organizations within which the child is living and the child's role performance within those organizations" (Mercer, 1979a, p. 46). Normal behavior is defined according to the role performance and expectations of other group members. By contrast, abnormal or deviant behavior occurs when group expectations are not met. The extent to which children use their adaptive behavior and coping skills to adjust to the social environment is important in making the distinction between "pseudo-retardation" and "quasi-retardation." Pseudo-retardation is defined by low IQ that may be the result of extraneous factors such as unfamiliarity with test situations, anxiety in test situations, or the lack of exposure to test questions. Quasi–mental retardation, on the other hand, is characterized by low IQ but adaptive behavior scores that are in the normal range. Instruments embracing this model are the Adaptive Behavior Inventory for Children (ABIC, Mercer, 1979a), a measure of social role performance across the domains of family, community, peer group, nonacademic school, earner consumer, and self-maintenance from the perspective of the primary caretaker or parent, and the WISC-R, a measure of achievement and school functioning level.

The pluralistic component of the SOMPA defines normality/abnormality according to the sociocultural backgrounds of children. The philosophical assumptions underlying this model are that: (a) tests measure a child's innate ability as well as his/her differential exposure to certain sociocultural and physical environments; (b) children from similar sociocultural backgrounds have approximately the same opportunities to learn test content, have the same motivation, and test-taking experiences; and, (c) children from different sociocultural backgrounds have average "learning potential" or intellectual abilities and that differences in test scores result from differences in reinforcement in behavior, test-taking experiences, and exposure to learned material on various tests (Mercer, 1979a). Instruments include four sociocultural scales (Family Size, Family Structure, SES, and Urban Acculturation) designed to provide information about the extent to which the sociocultural backgrounds of children differ from the dominant American culture.

Dynamic Assessment

Dynamic assessment refers to a method of psychological assessment that departs substantially from standardized intelligence testing in several fundamental ways, as summarized in Table 19.1. A philosophical assumption of this approach is that ability consists of a finite number of identifiable processes of thought, perception, learning, and problem solving, referred to as cognitive functions, which are "compounds of native ability, attitudes, work habits, learning history, motives, and strategies" (Feuerstein, Rand, & Hoffman, 1979). These cognitive functions are developed through mediated learning experiences and transmitted by child-rearing agents, parents, grandparents, and teachers (Feuerstein & Rand, 1974; Haywood & Wachs, 1981). Relative ineffectiveness at learning is due to inadequate mediated learning experiences, resulting in inadequate development of cognitive functions at the input, elaboration, and output phases of information processing (Feuerstein, et al., 1979; Jensen & Feuerstein, 1987). Although the method of dynamic assessment can be

TABLE 19.1. Differential characteristics of normative and dynamic assessment.

	Methods of assessment	
Dimensions	Normative	Dynamic
Goals	Classification, prediction	Identification of cognitive processes; Estimation of learning potential; Prescriptive
Method of administration	Standard/No help; Control of distal stimulus	Dynamic (teaching); Control of proximal stimulus
What is assessed	Achievement	Learning in new tasks
Assumptions	Equal opportunity to learn, past predicts future	Learning and generalization of principles indicate potential
Comparison	Subject with norms	Subject with self over time and across domains

Note. From "Dynamic Assessment: Issues, Research, and Applications" by H. C. Haywood and J. D. Bransford, March 1984, paper presented at the XVII Gatlinburg Conference on Research in Mental Retardation, Gatlinburg: TN. Copyright 1984 by Haywood and Bransford. Reprinted by permission.

applied to the examination of most psychological processes, it has been used to assess cognitive functions, and in particular, "learning potential" (Feuerstein et al., 1979).

Psychologists have recognized that there is a difference between performance on standardized intelligence tests and learning potential. The measurement of potentiality in intellectual development is rooted in the theory of cognitive modifiability and conceptually defined as the "zone of proximal development" (Arbitman-Smith, Haywood, & Bransford, 1984; Brown & Ferrara, 1985; Budoff & Hamilton, 1976; Campione, Brown, & Bryant, 1985; Feuerstein et al., 1979; Minick, 1987; Vygotsky, 1978). This is "the distance between the actual developmental level as determined by independent problem solving and the level of potential development as determined through teaching under adult guidance or in collaboration with more capable peers" (Vygotsky, 1978, pp. 85–86). This approach assumes that "for everybody there is a discrepancy between performance and potential, that the discrepancy is explainable in part by relatively ineffective cognitive processes, and that the acquisition of such processes can reduce the discrepancy" (Haywood, 1984).

"Dynamic" refers to the fact that in this method of assessment the examiner, instead of remaining studiedly neutral and objective, actually teaches systematic cognitive operations. This approach relies on a test-teach-test procedure with process-oriented tests designed to show how much a person's performance can be improved when generalized cognitive principles of thought and understanding are taught during the psychological assessment sessions. The traditional one-session testing situation (e.g., standardized intelligence test) is replaced by a three-step procedure (pretest, training for teaching, posttest) (Budoff, 1975; Budoff & Corman, 1973)

The essence of this method is to invoke the scientific principle of "strong inference," i.e., to disprove all available alternative explanations of poor learning and problem solving performance before inferring that poor performance is due to an incapacity to learn. The examiner recognizes that learning and problem solving often depend upon some prior knowledge, and that failure on a problem solving task may result from a lack of essential information, or from inadequate development of essential strategies and processes of learning, as well as a lack of capacity to learn or to comprehend a solution. Children do not get low ability estimates for not having had the opportunities to learn the appropriate cognitive strategies for success on standardized measures of intelligence. For example, it is commonly observed that the intelligence test scores of EMR children, particularly minority children diagnosed as EMR, are depressed because of impulsive responding, i.e., they give answers to test questions before they have considered the questions carefully and analytically. The application of dynamic assessment principles would involve teaching them to slow down and to think about test questions analytically so as to bring about changes in their test scores. Such teaching during the assessment process usually results in substantially higher performance levels on standardized intelligence tests for low-achieving children (Budoff, 1975), and reveals sources of low performance other than low ability itself.

Dynamic assessment would be interesting, but of limited utility, if it were used merely to "correct" misclassification based on standardized intelligence tests. Many culturally different persons, even though not validly classifiable as mentally retarded, slow learning, or learning disabled, do have need of special educational services, special teaching approaches, and modifications to their educational programs if they are to learn effectively in schools that are geared to the dominant culture. Indeed, precisely because of the circumstances that yield cultural difference, many minority children may have undeveloped learning potential resulting from inadequate opportunities to acquire essential cognitive processes, information, and skills (Feuerstein et al., 1979). It would be a mistake simply to take them out of inappropriate classifications and then to assume that the problem is solved. We need to have assessment instruments and procedures that can help psychologists and educators to go beyond the classification questions and to prescribe and deliver the special help that many such children need in order to become effective learners.

Dynamic assessment appears to offer solutions to several problems encountered by minority children in tesk-taking situations. As Haywood (1988) observed,

> A more appropriate approach is to give them new learning tasks that have not been encountered before, observe their learning processes, teach them some principles of learning and problem solving, observe how readily they learn given teaching, and then require them to apply the principles to the solution of new problems. In other words, the best predictor of learning is learning, not knowledge that one presumes to have accumulated in situations that examiners do not know and could not control . . . one searches for maximal rather than typical performance, for cognitive processes rather than products of presumed prior opportunities to learn, for the amount of teaching needed to achieve certain levels and types of learning rather than the success/failure ratios, and for specific process deficiencies (and the means for their correction) that underlie previous learning failure, rather than merely for evidence that certain content areas have not been mastered. (p. 44)

Such changes in assessment procedures are sufficiently radical to qualify them as issues of public policy.

Policy Implications

It is common policy in the American educational system to use psychoeducational assessments as evaluation and assignment mechanisms. The evaluation component is intended to identify or diagnose aspects of performance, achievement, or ability that may not be effectively addressed in the typical classroom or by typical teaching methods and materials. The assignment component is prescriptive: based upon some criterion (e.g., a range of test scores) and the availability of services, the assessment will lead to a student's assignment to a special classroom, program, or school that is designed to provide learning and instruction that will be more effective for that student.

The general policy of using psychoeducational assessment in this fashion becomes a policy *issue* when there is concern about its validity, effectiveness, and fairness. This is certainly the case with respect to psychoeducational assessment of children and assignment to special learning environments. The basic issue is whether assessment devices and techniques are equally valid for minority and majority groups if there are differences in the average scores for these groups and thus in the likelihood that children from one group will be assigned to special learning environments. The effectiveness of these learning environments for the education of children assigned to them is a separate issue. It is yet another totally separate issue whether a student's right to the "least restrictive environment" (that is compatible with that student's individual welfare and development) is fulfilled or denied by assignment to a special learning environment on the basis of a psychoeducational assessment, or whether such assignment or classification stigmatizes children. And it is a totally separate issue whether the particular skills and knowledge conveyed in such special environments represent the imposition of the majority culture on minority populations, thus infringing upon their heritage and group identity. Although all of these issues are individual and separate from one another, they are nevertheless worthy of consideration together because they have a common link: psychoeducational assessment is likely to be the conduit into classification and assignment to special learning environments.

We have reviewed the literature regarding the validity of psychoeducational assessment for minority and majority populations and concluded that the tests that have been studied are valid for the assessment of minority as well as majority persons. We suggest, then, that the flaw in the policy of assessing children in the schools using the instruments most commonly employed does not derive from the differential validity (or invalidity) of the tests themselves. Nevertheless, the uses to which valid instruments are put, and the decisions and actions that are undertaken on the basis of scores derived from those instruments, are additional facets of the overall policy of classification and assignment that may be flawed in ways that undermine the utility, effectiveness, or fairness of the policy for certain groups of persons, such as minorities.

It is not within the scope of this chapter to ponder the pros and cons of special learning environments, such as EMR classrooms, in terms of stigmatization, their effectiveness, or whether it makes sense that children from minority and majority groups should be referred to them in representative proportions. If one assumes that they are not stigmatizing, that they are effective (in producing better life outcomes for children properly referred to them than would be achieved without such referral), and that the assessment instruments used for such assignments are appropriate for that purpose, then any greater representation of a minority group would simply indicate that the sorts of preparedness to learn that children from that group bring to the school context call for a different type of learning environment if the purpose of schooling is to be accomplished as effectively as it is by the regular classroom track for persons from other groups who bring a different (not better, nor worse) preparedness into the educational system. To the extent that these assumptions are incorrect, the policy of tracking children into special learning environments may be questioned, again even if the assessment mechanism appears to be valid.

One final caveat should be noted. Our review suggests that psychoeducational assessment instruments on which minority and majority groups score differently are valid according to a variety of criteria that are relevant to the tests' theoretical underpinnings. It might be said that such instruments actually have several kinds of validity, one of which is validity with respect to the use to which the test is put. Tests that yield an intelligence quotient might possess strong validity in terms of being able to predict aspects of performance and achievement that can be linked to the concept of intelligence, but at the same time they might have poor validity in predicting responsiveness to a particular educational regimen that adapts teaching to meet certain needs. Put differently, a test that is used to assess how well or how rapidly a child learns may not predict how that child might best be taught. For such a purpose the best assessment might be one that targets how a child learns so that instruction may be tailored either to the child's manner of learning or toward changing how the child learns. In short, there is validity-for-a-given-purpose, and an instrument that is valid for one purpose (e.g., predicting correlates of intelligence) may not be valid for another (prescribing the best sort of educational experience).

We have intended to show here that (a) standardized intelligence tests are not reasonably called upon to do jobs that we now see as important; (b) ethnic minorities may be especially subject to erroneous decisions and placements based upon standardized intelligence tests, not because of test bias or poor predictability but because ethnically and culturally different persons might often have need of different educational approaches that are not identified by standardized normative tests; (c) these are legitimate public policy issues; and (d) dynamic assessment has the potential to be an important adjunct to standardized intelligence tests, especially for use with ethnic minorities and other persons who are socially different, such as handicapped persons, culturally different persons, and persons whose primary language is other than that of their dominant culture.

To capitalize on the potential of dynamic assessment for addressing these policy issues, certain regulations, expectations, and beliefs that are already in place will have to be changed. Prominent among those is the concept of intelligence itself as a characteristic whose measurement can and should be used to predict performance in a wide variety of future learning contexts. Such a concept might very possibly have outlived its usefulness. Indeed, prediction of academic performance should probably not be a major goal of psychoeducational assessment. Second, classification as a major goal in psychoeducational assessment should probably be abandoned in favor of an approach based more firmly on recognition of huge individual differences across persons. Third, in the practice of school psychology it will be necessary to abandon the expectation that assessment of learning aptitudes, problems, and prescriptions can be done in 60 minutes! Finally, since dynamic assessment of learning potential yields information about adequate or inadequate development of specific cognitive processes, teaching will have to be adjusted to include stimulation of acquisition and elaboration of important cognitive processes rather than being focused principally on accumulation of information and skill.

References

Anderson, B. (1982). Test use today in elementary and secondary schools. In A. K. Wigdor & W. R. Garner (Eds.), *Ability testing: Uses, consequences, and controversies (Part 2). Report of the Committee on Ability Testing, National Research Council* (pp. 232–285). Washington, DC: National Academy Press.

Arbitman-Smith, R., Haywood, H. C., & Bransford, J. D. (1984). Assessing cognitive change. In P. H. Brooks, R. D. Sperber, & C. McCauley (Eds.), *Learning and cognition in the mentally retarded* (pp. 433–471). Hillsdale, NJ: Erlbaum.

Avery, G. (1985). Effects of social, cultural, and economic factors on brain development. In J. M. Freeman (Ed.), *Prenatal and perinatal factors associated with brain disorders* (pp. 163–176). Bethesda, MD: National Institutes of Health.

Bickel, W. E. (1982). Classifying mentally retarded students: A review of placement practices in special education. In K. A. Heller, W. H. Holtzman, & S. Messick (Eds.), *Placing children in special education: A strategy for equity* (pp. 182–229). Washington, DC: National Academy Press.

Bond, L. (1982). The IQ controversy and academic performance. In S. Turner (Ed.), *Behavior modification in black populations: Psycho-social issues and empirical findings* (pp. 95–120). New York: Plenum Press.

Brookover, W. B., & Lezotte, L. W. (1979). *Changes in school characteristics coincident with changes in student achievement.* East Lansing, MI: Michigan State University, College of Urban Development (ERIC Document Reproduction Service No. ED 182 465).

Brown, A. L., & Ferrara, R. A. (1985). Diagnosing zones of proximal development. In J. Wertsch (Ed.), *Culture, communication, and cognition: Vygotskian perspectives* (pp. 273–305). New York: Cambridge University Press.

Budoff, M. (1975). *Learning potential among educable retarded pupils.* Technical report, grant No. RO1 MH 18553-03. Washington, DC: National Institute of Mental Health.

Budoff, M., & Corman, L. (1973). *The effectiveness of a group training procedure on the Raven learning potential measure with children of diverse racial and socioeconomic backgrounds.* RIEP Print #58. Cambridge, MA: Research Institute for Educational Problems.

Budoff, M., & Hamilton, J. (1976). Optimizing test performance of the moderately and severely mentally retarded. *American Journal of Mental Deficiency, 81*, 49–57.

California State Department of Education (1970). *Placement of underachieving minority group children in special education classess for the educable mentally retarded.* Sacramento: California State Department of Education.

Campione, J. C., Brown, A. L., & Bryant, N. R. (1985). Individual differences in learning and memory. In R. J. Sternberg (Ed.), *Human abilities: An information processing approach* (pp. 103–126). New York: Freeman Press.

Children's Defense Fund (1985). *An analysis of the President's FY 1986 budget and children.* Washington, DC: Children's Defense Fund.

Childs, R. E. (1982). A study of the adaptive behavior of retarded children and the resultant effects of this use in the diagnosis of mental retardation. *Education and Training of the Mentally Retarded, 17*, 109–113.

Chinn, P. C., & Hughes, S. (1987). Representation of minority students in special education classes. *Remedial and Special Education, 8*(4), 41–46.

Cleary, T. A., Humphreys, L. G., Kendrick, S. A., & Wesman, A. (1975). Educational uses of tests with disadvantaged students. *American Psychologist, 30*, 15–41.

Cohen, R. A. (1969). Conceptual styles, culture conflict, and nonverbal tests of intelligence. *American Anthropologist, 71*, 828–856.

Coleman, J. S., Campbell, E. Q., Hobson, C. J., McPortland, J., Mood, A. M., Weinfeld, F. D., & York, R. L. (1966). *Equality of educational opportunity.* Washington, DC: U.S. Government Printing Office.

Consortium for Longitudinal Studies. (1983). *As the twig is bent . . . lasting effects of preschool programs.* Hillsdale, NJ: Erlbaum.

Corman, L., & Gottlieb, J. (1978). Mainstreaming mentally retarded children: A review of research. In N. R. Ellis (Ed.), *International review of research in mental retardation* (Vol. 9, pp. 251–275). New York: Academic Press.

Darlington, R. B. (1986). Long-term effects of preschool programs. In U. Neisser (Ed.), *The school achievement of minority children: New perspectives* (pp. 159–189). Hillsdale, NJ: Erlbaum.

Dunn, L. M. (1968). Special education for the mildly retarded—is much of it justifiable? *Exceptional Children, 35*(1), 5–22.

Education of All Handicapped Children Act of 1975, Sec. 121 a. 5, 20 U.S.C. Sec. 1401 (1977).

Feuerstein, R., Haywood, H. C., Rand, Y., Hoffman, M. B., & Jensen, M. (1986). *Examiner manual for the Learning Potential Assessment Device.* Jerusalem: Hadassah-WIZO-Canada Research Institute.

Feuerstein, R., & Rand, Y. (1974). Mediated learning experiences: An outline of proximal etiology for differential development of cognitive functions. *International Understanding*, *9–10*, 7–37.

Feuerstein, R., Rand, Y., & Hoffman, M. B. (1979). *The dynamic assessment of retarded performers: The Learning Potential Assessment Device, theory, instruments, and techniques*. Baltimore: University Park Press.

Feuerstein, R., Rand, Y., Hoffman, M. B., & Miller, R. (1980). *Instrumental Enrichment*. Baltimore: University Park Press.

Finn, J. D. (1982). Patterns in special education placement as revealed by the OCR surveys. In K. A. Heller, W. H. Holtzman, & S. Messick (Eds.), *Placing children in special education: A strategy for equity* (pp. 322–381). Washington, DC: National Academy Press.

Goldman, R. D., & Hartig, L. K. (1976). The WISC-R may not be a valid predictor of school performance for primary-grade minority children. *American Journal of Mental Deficiency*, *80*(6), 583–587.

Grossman, H. J. (Ed.) (1977). *Manual on terminology and classification in mental retardation*. Washington, DC: American Association on Mental Deficiency.

Grossman, H. J. (Ed.) (1983). *Classification in mental retardation*. Washington, DC: American Association on Mental Retardation.

Gutkin, T. B., & Reynolds, C. R. (1980). Factorial similarity of the WISC-R for Anglos and Chicanos referred for psychological services. *Journal of School Psychology*, *18*(1), 34–39.

Haywood, H. C. (1974). Distribution of intelligence. *Encyclopedia Britannica* (15th Ed.), 672–677.

Haywood, H. C. (1982). Compensatory education. *Peabody Journal of Education*, *59*, 272–300.

Haywood, H. C. (1984, October). *Alternative approaches to psychoeducational assessment of minority children*. Paper presented at the Association for Public Policy Analysis and Management Research Conference, New Orleans.

Haywood, H. C. (1988). Dynamic assessment: The Learning Potential Assessment Device. In R. Jones (Ed.), *Pschoeducational assessment of minority group children: A casebook* (pp. 39–63). Berkeley, CA: Cobb & Henry.

Haywood, H. C., & Bransford, J. D. (1984, March). *Dynamic assessment: Issues, research, and applications*. Introductory paper for a symposium on Dynamic Assessment given at the XVII Gatlinburg Conference on Research in Mental Retardation, Gatlinburg, TN.

Haywood, H. C., & Switzky, H. N. (1986a). The malleability of intelligence: Cognitive processes as a function of polygenic-experiential interaction. *School Psychology Review*, *15*, 245–255.

Haywood, H. C., & Switzky, H. N. (1986b). Transactionalism and cognitive processes: Reply to Reynolds and Gresham. *School Psychology Review*, *15*, 264–267.

Haywood, H. G., & Wachs, T. D. (1981). Intelligence, cognition, and individual differences. In M. J. Begab, H. C. Haywood, & H. L. Garber (Eds.), *Psychosocial influences in retarded performance. Vol. 1. Issues and theories in development* (pp. 95–126). Baltimore: University Park Press.

Heflinger, C. A., Cook, V., & Thackrey, M. (1987). Identification of mental retardation by the System of Multicultural Pluralistic Assessment: Nondiscriminatory or nonexistent? *Journal of School Psychology*, *25*, 121–127.

Heller, K. A., Holtzman, W. H., & Messick, S. (1982). *Placing children in special education: A strategy for equity*. Washington, DC: National Academy Press.

Ironson, G. H., & Sebkovial, N. J. (1979). A comparison of several methods for assessing item bias. *Journal of Educational Measurement*, *16*, 209–225.

Jenkins, R. H., & Mayhall, W. F. (1976). Development and evaluation of a resource teacher program. *Exceptional Children*, *43*, 21–29.

Jensen, A. R. (1980). *Bias in mental testing*. New York: Free Press.

Jensen, A. R. (1985). The nature of black-white differences on various psychometric tests. *Behavioral and Brain Sciences*, *8*(1), 359–368.

Jensen, M. R., & Feuerstein, R. (1987). The Learning Potential Assessment Device: From philosophy of practice. In C. S. Lidz (Ed.), *Dynamic assessment: An interactional approach to evaluating learning potential* (pp. 379–402). New York: Guilford.

Johnson, S. T. (1980). Major issues in measurement today: Their implications for black Americans. *Journal of Negro Education*, *49*(3), 253–262.

Jones, R. L. (1976). *Mainstreaming and the minority child*. Reston, VA: The Council for Exceptional Children.

Jones, R. L. (1988). *Psychoeducational assessment of minority group children: A casebook*. Berkelely, CA: Cobb & Henry.

Kazimour, K. K., & Reschly, D. J. (1981). Investigation of the norms and concurrent validity for Adaptive Behavior Inventory for Children (ABIC). *American Journal of Mental Deficiency*, *85*(5), 512–520.

Kirk, S. A., & Gallagher, J. J. (1989). *Educating exceptional children*. Boston, MA: Houghton Mifflin.

Laosa, L. M. (1977). Nonbiased assessment of children's abilities: Historical antecedents and current issues. In T. Oakland (Ed.), *Psychological and educational assessment of minority children* (pp. 1–20). New York: Brunner/Mazel.

Larry P. v. Wilson Riles (1979). 495 F. Supp. 926 (N. D. Cal. 1979) No. 80.4027. (9th Cir., Jan, 1980).

Linn, R. (1982). Ability testing: Individual differences, prediction, and differential prediction. In A. K. Wigdor & W. R. Garner (Eds.), *Ability testing: Uses, consequences, and controversies (Part 2). Report to the Committee on Ability Testing, National Research Council* (pp. 335–388). Washington, DC: National Academy Press.

Manni, J. L., Winikur, D. W., Keller, M. R. (1984). *Intelligence, mental retardation, and the culturally different child*. Springfield, IL: Charles C Thomas.

Mascari, B. G., & Forgnone, C. (1982). A follow-up study of EMR students four years after dismissal from the program. *Education and Training of the Mentally Retarded*, *17*, 288–292.

Mattie, T., et al. v. Holladay, et al. (1979). DC-75-31-S (N.D. Miss. 1979).

Matuszek, P., & Oakland, T. (1979). Factors influencing teacher's and psychologists' recommendations regarding special class placement. *Journal of School Psychology*, *17*, 116–125.

McShane, D., & Cook, V. (1985). Transcultural intellectual assessment. In B. B. Wolman (Ed.), *Handbook of intelligence: Theories, measurement, and applications* (pp. 737–785). New York: Wiley.

Mercer, J. R. (1973). *Labeling the mentally retarded: Clinical and social system perspectives on mental retardation*. Berkeley, CA: University of California Press.

Mercer, J. R. (1979a). *System of Multicultural Pluralistic Assessment Technical Manual*. New York: Psychological Corporation.
Mercer, J. R. (1979b). In defense of racially and culturally nondiscriminatory assessment. *School Psychology Digest*, *8*, 89–115.
Messé, L. A., Crano, W. D., Messé, S. R., & Rice, W. (1979). Evaluation of the predictive validity of tests of mental ability for classroom performance in elementary grades. *Journal of Educational Psychology*, *71*, 233–241.
Minick, N. (1987). Implications of Vygotsky's theories for dynamic assessment. In C. S. Lidz (Ed.), *Dynamic assessment: An interactional approach to evaluating learning potential* (pp. 116–140). New York: Guilford.
Oakland, T., & Parmelee, R. (1985). Mental measurement of minority-group children. In B. B. Wolman (Ed.), *Handbook of intelligence: Theories, measurement, and applications* (pp. 699–736). New York: Wiley.
Office of Civil Rights (1978). *Elementary and secondary civil rights survey. Sample selection*. Washington, DC: U.S. Department of Health, Education, & Welfare.
Ogbu, J. U. (1978). *Minority education and caste: The American system in cross-cultural perspective*. New York: Academic Press.
Poland, S., Ysseldyke, J., Thurlow, M., & Mirkin, P. (1979). *Current assessment and decision making in school settings as reported by Directors of Special Education* (Research Report No. 14). Minneapolis, MN: University of Minnesota, Institute for Research on Learning Disabilities.
Prasse, D. P., & Reschly, D. J. (1986). Larry P.: A case of segregation, testing or program efficacy. *Exceptional Children*, *52*(4), 333–346.
Reschly, D. J. (1978). WISC-R factor structure among Anglos, blacks, Chicanos, and Native American Papagos. *Journal of Consulting and Clinical Psychology*, *46*, 417–422.
Reschly, D. J. (1980). *Nonbiased assessment*. Unpublished manuscript. lowa State University, Department of Psychology, Ames, lowa.
Reschly, D. J., & Sabers, D. L. (1979). Analyses of test bias in four groups with regression definition. *Journal of Educational Measurement*, *16*(1), 1–9.
Resnick, L. B. (1979). The future of IQ testing in education. *Intelligence*, *3*, 241–253.
Reynolds, C. R. (1982). The problem of bias in psychological assessment. In C. R. Reynolds & T. B. Gutkin (Eds.), *The handbook of school psychology*. New York: Wiley.
Reynolds, C. R., & Brown, R. T. (1984). *Perspectives on bias in mental testing*. New York: Plenum Press.
Reynolds, C. R., & Gutkin, T. B. (1980). A regression analysis of test bias on the WISC-R for Anglos and Chicanos referred for psychological services. *Journal of Abnormal Child Psychology*, *8*(2), 237–243.
Rosenshine, B. V., & Berliner, D. C. (1978). Academic engaged time. *British Journal of Teacher Education*, *4*, 3–16.
Sandoval, J. (1982). The WISC-R factoral validity for minority groups and Spearman's hypothesis. *Journal of School Psychology*, *20*(3), 198–204.
Sattler, J. M. (1974). *Assessment of children's intelligence*. Philadelphia: W. B. Saunders.
Sattler, J. M. (1988). *Assessment of children*. San Diego, CA: Jerome M. Sattler.
Section 504 of the Vocational Rehabilitation Act of 1973, 29 U.S.C. §794. Regulations at 45 C.F.R. §84 (1977).

Sewell, T. (1987). Dynamic assessment as a nondiscriminatory procedure. In C. S. Lidz (Ed.), *Dynamic assessment: An interactional approach to evaluating learning potential* (pp. 426–443). New York: Guilford.

Slavin, R. E. (1987). Ability grouping and student achievement in elementary schools. A best-evidence synthesis. *Review of Educational Research*, *57*(3), 293–336.

Strickland, B. B., & Turnbull, A. P. (1990). *Developing and implementing individualized education programs*. Columbus, OH: Merrill.

Title VI of the Civil Rights Act of 1964m 42 U.S.C. Sec. 2000d. Regulations at 45 C.F.R. Sec. 121 (1977).

Travers, J. R. (1982). Testing in educational placement: Issues and evidence. In K. A. Heller, W. H. Holtzman, & S. Messick, (Eds.), *Placing children in special education: A strategy for equity* (pp. 230–261). Washington, DC: National Academy Press.

Tucker, J. A. (1980). Ethnic proportions in classes for the learning disabled: Issues in nonbiased assessment. *Journal of Special Education*, *14*(1), 93–105.

Vygotsky, L. (1978). *Mind in society: The development of higher psychological processes*. New York: Cambridge University Press.

Wechsler, D. (1974). *Wechsler Intelligence Scale for Children—Revised*. Cleveland, OH: Psychological Corporation.

Wigdor, A. K., & Garner, W. R. (1982). *Ability testing: Uses, consequences, and controversies (Parts 1 and 2)*. Report of the Committee on Ability Testing, National Research Council. Washington, DC: National Academy Press.

Wright, B. J., & Isenstein, V. R. (1977). *Psychological tests and minorities*. Rockville, MD: NIMH, DHEW Publication No. (ADM) 78–482.

Wyne, M. D., & O'Connor, P. D. (1979). *Exceptional children: A developmental view*. Lexington, MA: D.C. Heath.

Ysseldyke, J., Algozzine, R., Regan, R., & McGue, M. (1979). *The influence of test scores and naturally occurring pupil characteristics on psychoeducational decision making with children* (Research Report No. 14). Minneapolis: University of Minnesota, Institute for Research on Learning Disabilities.

20
Larry P., PASE, and Social Science in the Courtroom: The Science and Politics of Identifying and Educating Very Slow Learners

ROGERS ELLIOTT

It is a durable and well-nigh universal finding in the field of ability testing that there is a difference between the average performance of American blacks and whites amounting to about a standard deviation and existing at every age examined, from preschool onward (Coleman, et al., 1966; Hall & Kaye, 1980; Jensen, 1980; Oakland, 1978; Reschly & Sabers, 1979; Reynolds, 1983; Loehlin, Lindzey, & Spuhler, 1975). To illustrate, Figure 20.1, taken from the judicial opinion in the trial under discussion, *Larry P. v. Wilson Riles* (1979) shows the distribution of WISC-R scores for three ethnic groups in California a decade ago. Differences of like magnitude exist for school and college grades, selection and employment tests, and their criteria (see, e.g., Jensen, 1980; Klitgaard, 1985; Wigdor and Garner, 1982).

One implication of the distribution shown in Figure 20.1 is that, if an IQ level is established below which a child is eligible for (and hence more likely to be placed in) a special class for educable mentally retarded (EMR) children, disproportionate numbers of black and Hispanic children will be in such classrooms. More generally, ability tests used for selection will serve to exclude Chicanos and, especially, blacks, from schools and jobs.

Not surprisingly, blacks have attacked such tests as biased and discriminatory, and in the case of IQ tests used in special education placement, black psychologists organized a nationwide attack, beginning about 1969:

> The Association of Black Psychologists fully supports those parents who have chosen to defend their rights by refusing to allow their children and themselves to be subjected to achievement, intelligence, aptitude, and performance tests which have been and are being used to A. Label Black people as uneducable. B. Place Black children in "special" classes and schools. C. Perpetuate inferior education in Blacks. D. Assign Black children to educational tracks. E. Deny Black students

*Much of the material in this chapter was originally published in *Litigating Intelligence* (Auburn House, Dover, MA, an imprint of Greenwood Publishing Group, Inc., 1987); used with permission.

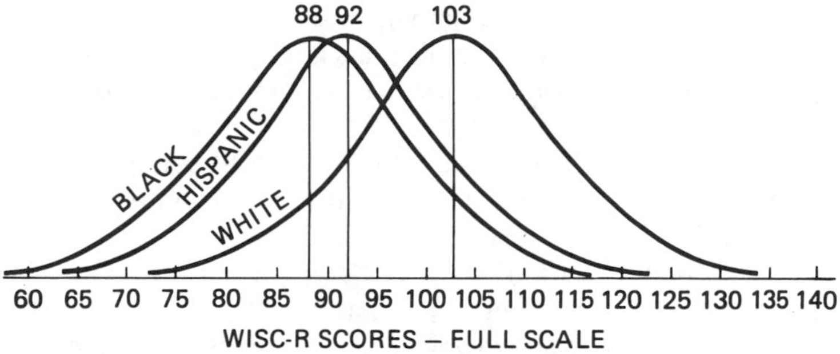

FIGURE 20.1 The distribution of WISC-R raw scores for three ethnic groups in California in 1979. From the judicial opinion in the trial of *Larry P. v. Wilson Riles*, 1979, 343 F. Supp. 306 (1972); 495 F. Supp. 926 (1979).

higher educational opportunities. F. Destroy positive growth and development of Black people. (Williams, 1970).

Black professionals in San Francisco challenged that city's use of IQ tests in placement. They located six black children who had been placed in EMR classes and whose IQs were near the top of the range then in use for placement. The children had had histories of repeating early grades and of very low achievement. Black psychologists retested the children in very nonstandard ways, producing IQs nearly 20 points higher than had been found earlier, and with this as background, brought suit.

The result was *Larry P.*, in which individual IQ tests[1] were banned by Federal District Judge Robert F. Peckham for use in placing black children into EMR classes in California. The specific complaints were that the six black children in San Francisco had had irreparable harm done to their educational careers by being inappropriately and pejoratively labeled and stigmatized by being placed into "deadend" (Judge Peckham's word) EMR classes, primarily because of scores obtained on IQ tests said to be racially and culturally biased against blacks. Plaintiffs sought and finally got relief in the form of a test ban and a quota controlling the proportion of black EMR placement at the level of black representation in the school population.

No one disputed the fact that black children were represented in EMR classes at over twice their proportion in the general school population. But all of the chief terms of the pleadings, and some questions implied by them, were hotly disputed at the trial: for example, the meanings of "culture," test bias, intelligence, mental retardation, and stigma; the nature of EMR education; the role of expectation in education; and the power of the schools to repair academic deficits. The case was, as

[1] The Wechsler Intelligence Scales for Children (WISC and WISC-R), the Stanford-Binet Intelligence Test (S-B), and the Leiter International Performance Scale.

much as anything else, a debate among psychologists and lawyers about the scientific status of tests of intellectual ability, and about the social and political implications of what such tests had to say about race and disadvantage.

Judge Peckham affirmed nearly all of the plaintiffs' contentions, finding that standardized IQ tests were biased against blacks and played a critical role in the decision to place children into EMR classes; that EMR classes constituted very bad education, being rather a burden than a benefit; that "intelligence" means something innate; that a fair test of intelligence must yield equal scores for two racial groups unless they are different genetically, which they are not; that bias in an intelligence test is therefore manifested by group differences in scores on it; that *socioeconomic* differences are not sufficient to account for the black-white differences in "intelligence," though *sociocultural* differences are sufficient to account for differences in scores on IQ tests; and that the average black deficit in school-related abilities can probably be repaired by appropriate educational interventions.

A comparison case (*PASE* (Parents in Action on Special Education) *v. Hannon*, 1980), with the same complaints, and featuring several of the same plaintiffs' witnesses, was filed in Chicago in 1975, and was tried in 1980. Here, Judge John Grady of the United States District Court found that the tests (save for a total of eight items) were not biased or discriminatory, that socioeconomic differences *were* sufficient to account for black-white differences in IQ, and that cultural differences were of little or no effect.

A social science consensus exists about many of the disputed issues, and it existed at the time of the trials. By consensus, I mean agreement among psychologists most experienced and most expert according to the standards of their peers (e.g., Cronbach, 1984; Humphreys, 1979; Hunter, Schmidt & Rauschenberger, 1984; Linn, 1982; Sattler, 1982; Scarr, 1981; Thorndike & Hagen, 1977; Vernon, 1979); I do not mean lack of controversy. According to this consensus, there is a general mental ability usually called intelligence and represented by verbal facility; problem solving ability; logical and quantitative reasoning; facility in learning, discriminating, and generalizing; and facility in forming concepts and applying them in novel situations. Measures of mental ability are fairly good predictors of academic success and most job performance, and as good for blacks as for whites. The black-white difference appears early in development, certainly by age 4, prior to schooling, and it persists.

There is less consensus about the sources of intelligence in nature and nurture, though some degree of heritability in the range of .2 to .8 is almost universally assumed. There is very little consensus about the degree (if any) to which population gene frequencies account for the measured black-white difference. There is also little consensus among experts about the plasticity of mental ability, and the power of known educational methods to alter it. Finally, few agree, because few if any really know, about how best to educate children who are slow learners either generally or in particular areas—how best to deal, in short, with the mildly retarded or learning disabled (and in the case of the latter, even how to diagnose it).

The two cases considered here would have been interesting to social scientists even had they both come out alike. Had the *Larry P.* opinion prevailed, for example, we would have the interesting case of the failure of expert consensus in a venerable area of psychological research to prevail in the political arena. Had the consensus prevailed, as in *PASE*, we might have learned less about science and politics even as we were encouraged more by the persuasive power of the data. But the opposed opinions invite scrutiny, so as to discover what might be behind the difference, and to begin to see what strategies or tactics might improve the weight of good, and make clear the deficiencies of bad, social science evidence in the courtroom setting.

Before considering some of the less substantive, but nonetheless influential contextual differences between the two lawsuits, several influential witnesses ought to be identified. Three testified in both trials: Leon Kamin of Princeton, well known for his work establishing the eugenic, racist, and hereditarian predilections of several early developers of ability tests, and his strong environmentalist position on the provenance of IQ; George Albee of the University of Vermont, also highly environmentalist and testifying on mental retardation; and Gloria Powell of UCLA, a black pediatrician and frequent witness on cultural bias in the assessment of mental retardation. Three others are named more than once in this chapter: Jane Mercer, a sociologist from the University of California, Riverside, who developed a well-known scale of adaptive behavior and is a proponent of the view that tests and schools provide only a limited assessment of intelligence (*Larry P.*); Asa Hilliard of Georgia State University, then as now a highly visible critic of standardized ability and achievement tests (*Larry P.*); and Robert Williams of Washington University, Hilliard's counterpart in *PASE* and a founder of the Association of Black Psychologists, whose views were quoted above.

Differences in Context

There were a series of factors surrounding the trials that had less to do with social science evidence and its effects than with law and politics. They had to do with vagaries of context: the winds of political pressure, the personalities of such major participants as judges and lead attorneys, the choice of tactics in case presentations, and so on. Here are some of them that may have affected the different outcomes in these cases, and may therefore make hazardous any attribution to the role of social science as the basis for outcome.

1. *Larry P.* was filed and initially argued during the heat of the desegregation controversy in San Francisco in 1971 and 1972, and sympathy for black causes was arguably greater at that time and that place than in Chicago in 1980.

   The decade of the 1970s had begun with great successes in the cause of black civil rights. It had become clear at least since the Moynihan (1965) and Coleman et al. (1966) reports that simple desegregation would not go far to improve the distressed conditions of most American blacks. The Supreme Court, in *Griggs v. Duke Power Co.* (1971), had in effect approved the stringent views about appropriate uses of ability tests prevailing in the Equal Employment Opportunity Commission (EEOC), and it endorsed the view that disparate impact alone built at least a strong presumption of discrimination. In *Keyes v. School District No. 1* (1972), it went far in opening the door to suits for affirmative action to integrate schools by proportionality. And the impetus for mainstreaming, seen in such famous cases as *Hobson v. Hansen* (1967), *Mills v. Board of Education* (1971) and *PARC v. Pennsylvania* (1971), and represented in psychology by Dunn (1968) and Hobbs (1975), was running at full tide.

   As the decade wore on, the limits of mainstreaming mentally retarded children, of busing, and of integration itself became clearer. The Supreme Court gave less and less deference to the EEOC in cases concerning disparate impact and test validity (see Lerner, 1978), and it slowed the momentum of affirmative action in school integration in *Pasadena Board of Education v. Spangler* (1976) and *Milliken v. Bradley* (1974). Reviewers like St. John (1975) and Stephan (1978) questioned the value of integration in helping black children, and scholars—e.g. Gottlieb (1981); MacMillan and his colleagues (MacMillan, Jones, & Meyers, 1976; Meyers, MacMillan, Yoshida, 1980)—reviewing the effect of mainstreaming on EMR children, found little, if any, effect on their achievement and mixed effect on self-concept.

   By 1980, the mood was different. The city of Chicago was nearing the end of a decade of negotiation with the government (the issue never got to trial) concerning integration, but by 1980 there were far fewer white students (28%, including large numbers of students not eligible for busing in the earliest grades) to integrate with than there had been in 1970. Also, the Chicago Board of Education (CBE) had revised its procedures to be the very model (at least on the books) of careful and legally mandated assessment of the handicapped, including the mentally handicapped.
2. In *Larry P.*, the state began by entertaining the notion of genetic difference as a cause of racial IQ difference. They eventually dis-

avowed this defense, in favor of an "agnostic" position, but its odor permeated the trial. In PASE, there was never any question of using such a defense, and the name of Arthur Jensen (the chief modern expositor of the genetic difference hypothesis) was scarcely heard in the land.

3. Chicago was, as noted, a predominantly black school district. Two important conditions ensued: First, because the district was 60% black in school population, the degree of disproportionate enrollment of black children into EMR classes was limited—it was 80%, but that is not much compared with the factor-of-two rates of disproportion in California. Second, school officials who were black testified for the defense in *PASE*, and some 40 black psychologists used the challenged tests; it was clear that they found the tests useful in assessing black children. In California, the defense was carried primarily by white bureaucrats and experts.
4. The sides were more evenly matched in *PASE* than in *Larry P.* The defense in *Larry P.*, a Leviathan of a case, was carried essentially by one lawyer, with little help, against a platoon of very competent public interest and private *pro bono* lawyers and their assistants. In *PASE*, the Board of Education assigned three lawyers, with their assistants, to the case, and the case was smaller in scope and complexity. Conversely, the plaintiffs' team in *PASE* was less cohesive and less coherent in attack.
5. The judges were different, both in temper and in history. Peckham is well known to be a liberal judge. It is not conceivable, with the choice he was given, between finding test bias or genetic inferiority of blacks, that he would have decided for the latter.

   Judge Grady was skeptical in general, and of the plaintiffs' claims in particular. He simply dismissed the notion of cultural difference-not-deficit offered to him. He was quite familiar with the deprivations of much of black life in Chicago, and their effects, and castigated both sides for pussyfooting around these conditions and effects.

   Judge Peckham had also presided over two cases directly relevant to the issue of *Larry P.* One was *Diana v. State Board of Education* (1970), which was resolved by various consent decrees, including an explicit quota controlling the number of Chicano children placed in EMR classes. The other was the preliminary injunction phase of *Larry P.* itself, in which Judge Peckham had found as an undisputed fact that IQ tests were culturally biased, and which had resulted in a ban of IQ tests for use in placing black children in EMR classes. The judge, in short, had ample precedent for his final decision in his own earlier ones, and would, like most of us, have been predisposed to cognitive consistency. Judge Grady had no such history of prior commitment on the issues.

These differences in judicial temper and style will appear several times in the discussion to follow. They may not have been critical to the differences in trial outcome, but I cannot say that there is any factor that outweighs their importance.

6. The cases in *PASE* were briefer, and the two sides less intransigently unaccommodating, than in *Larry P.* There were not the same extended discussions of stigma and self-concept, or of mainstreaming and its effects, or of the inadequacies of EMR education. In *PASE*, EMR classrooms were granted, even by plaintiff witnesses, to be appropriate for many EMR pupils; in *Larry P.*, they were scorned by plaintiffs for use by *any* pupil. In *Larry P.*, black witnesses had no use for tests, and no stake in the state school bureaucracy; in *PASE*, one of the chief black plaintiffs' witnesses had a senior position on the Chicago Board of Education (and two of his subordinates testified for the defense). In contrast to the nonstandard and unprofessional testing done by black psychologists in *Larry P.*, the retesting of plaintiff children in *PASE* was done by an experienced black school psychologist using standard procedures, an expert who found the WISC-R useful despite its putative bias. The flow of examination in *PASE* was less often disrupted by objections than in *Larry P.*
7. Both sides in *PASE* had the materials of *Larry P.* The *PASE* defense had more to learn from the mistakes of its counterpart in *Larry P.* than the plaintiffs did. Most especially, the defense learned to stress three arguments either not made or not prevailing in *Larry P.*: the socioeconomic status (SES) basis of black deficit; the relevance of tests for schools, even though both tests and schools might be in some sense biased; and internal evidence against test bias. These constitute the substantive issues to which we now turn.

Differences in Evidence and Argument

The trials differed primarily in defense strategies, and chief differences were (a) the heavy emphasis in *PASE* on a socioeconomic argument to account for black deficits; (b) the view that schools do represent the dominant white culture, just as the tests do, and that the tests have criterion validity *because* they are culturally loaded; and (c) considerable evidence, given very short shrift in *Larry P.*, of the lack of any internal evidence of test bias.

Note that the question of a separate black culture pervades the other issues. At one limit, a translated IQ text might be considered unfair if used, say, on native Africans, even if it predicted performance in Western schools, because both school and test might be inappropriate institutions in an alien culture. That is, it might truly be the case that persons in such a culture display social and physical problem solving skills in ways far more independent of test performance than would be the case in American society.

Indeed, Judge Peckham accepted the notion of a separate American black culture that "translates the phenomena of intelligence into skills and knowledge untested by standardized intelligence tests" (*Larry P. v. Wilson Riles*, 1979, p. 960) (495 F. Supp. 960). Such a view transforms what appears to be a deficit into something more neutral, just a difference. It also carries the implication, realized to a degree in the case of bilingual and bicultural programs, that there ought to be a separate curriculum for a separate culture.

It is difficult, however, to imagine what schools would teach to various ethnic groups in place of the reading comprehension and quantitative reasoning skills that are the primary locus of deficit. In the case of American blacks, there is virtually no native language and little ancestral culture around which to build a curriculum. Critics of the schools' education of blacks characteristically fail to suggest an appropriate pedagogy that would not also help all pupils.

Two things are true: American blacks have unique shared history and experiences, the stuff of ethnicity; and American blacks are part of the American culture. If the uniqueness and difference are emphasized, then the importance of other artifacts and institutions of mainstream culture, like tests and schools, can be minimized. But if the similarity and belongingness of blacks to the wider culture is emphasized, then the intellectual deficits are serious. In both the present cases, explanation of black intellectual deficits in the same terms that would account for white deficits threatens cultural-difference arguments.

Plaintiffs in *PASE*, following the successful line in *Larry P.*, attacked the notion that poverty and its nutrition and health correlates could account for much, if any, of the black IQ deficit. That is about as far as defendants in *Larry P.* took the SES argument; indeed, they criticized the evidence for environmental effects from cross-race adoption or intervention studies. But in *PASE*, defendants were able to show associations between "poverty pockets" in the city of Chicago and the presence of federal compensatory education programs (Head Start, Title I), as well as the rate of EMR placement. Furthermore, in Chicago a black middle class existed in numbers sufficient to show a low rate of EMR placement where it was concentrated.

Moreover, in *PASE* it was defendants, not plaintiffs, who introduced the Scarr and Weinberg (1976) adoption studies, and the effects of interventions to show how improved home and school conditions were associated with higher black IQs. (The same studies in *Larry P.* were used by plaintiffs to show the effects of acculturation into the "Anglocentric" world.)

The reception of the evidence of Gloria Powell, the black pediatrician who appeared for plaintiffs in both cases, is instructive. She gave ample testimony about the effects of mother-child "synchrony" and verbal interaction upon child IQ, and even brought up the effects of maternal education and intelligence on children. (These were the strongest effects on IQs of 4-year-olds in the Broman, Nichols, & Kennedy, 1975, study, on which she relied heavily.) But she stoutly refused to relate the fact that black mothers on average had less education or provided poorer verbal models than white mothers to their children's deficits in school-related abilities. Judge Peckham never pressed this inconsistency, but Judge Grady did, and Powell simply would not budge from her view that the deficit in IQ could be caused only by test bias against black culture.

The most dramatic evidence used by defendants in *PASE* was the thesis of Nichols (1970/1971) which showed virtually no difference in IQ between black or white samples matched in SES. In *Larry P.*, conversely, several defense experts testified to the common finding that the black deficit is large even in samples matched in SES, and plaintiffs' attorneys quite deliberately evoked and emphasized such testimony, because it took away the SES explanation of race difference and left the judge with the choice of finding either test bias or genetic inferiority.

The defense in *PASE* hammered home the point that IQ tests did help to predict school performance. They welcomed the plaintiffs' view that ability tests, school grades, and achievement tests were all part of the same culture, and virtually invited the plaintiffs to attack the criterion—i.e., the schools. In *Larry P.*, Jane Mercer had done that, and Judge Peckham saw that equalizing minority scores on intelligence tests "raises difficult questions regarding which skills are appropriate for our schools and society" (*Larry P. v. Wilson Riles*, 1979, p. 955). In *PASE*, Robert Williams suggested adding various minority studies units to curricula but had little else to offer. The defense simply granted that schoolchildren in Chicago were not being trained for life in (at various times) Greece, China, Tasmania, or (in Judge Grady's final comparison) "another planet." Grady did not appear to feel it was his place to establish curricula, or to pronounce the standard curricula biased against blacks, or even to suggest that it might be changed.

And where in *Larry P.* there was some persuasive evidence that IQ tests predicted black grades less well than white grades, (as well as evidence that tests predicted equally well), evidence in *PASE*, provided by plaintiffs themselves, indicated that the prediction of achievement scores for low-achieving blacks in Chicago was quite strong (correlations of about .50), even though smaller than that for low-achieving whites (correlations about .60) perhaps because the variance of black scores was smaller. Moreover, the Gordon and Rudert (1979) review, demonstrating strong and roughly equal criterion validity in both groups, was by that time available to Judge Grady (and his decision shows that he read it). Thus was criterion validity for the Chicago curriculum established.

Finally, internal validity was established by reference to work, chiefly by Gordon and Rudert (1979) but including studies by Miele (1979) and Nichols (1970/1971), that demonstrated no race-by-item interaction in IQ test items, even while showing large race differences on virtually all items. It is clear from his opinion, in which he actually quotes from their paper (*PASE v. Hannon*, 1980, p. 880) F., that Judge Grady was impressed with the arguments of Gordon and Rudert against the "cultural diffusion" hypothesis. This hypothesis states, roughly, that the reason blacks do less well than whites on virtually every item is that there is a black-white cultural barrier across which all items of information from the Anglocentric culture pass with nearly uniform delay. This view requires that such tests as block design or Raven's matrices be as culturally "loaded" as tests of vocabulary and information. Such a view is regarded as inplausible by Gordon and Rudert, among others, and Judge Grady, following his survey of several hundred items, obviously did not believe it either.

No factor, of course, stands alone. Judge Grady was interested in the tests at a far more microanalytic level than Judge Peckham, and he was, therefore, fascinated by testimony at the item or subtest level, starting with the very first witness, Leon Kamin. By the end of the trial he was not satisfied that he had been given good evidence on the race-by-item issue, and called for papers on the subject, which he quite evidently read, along with the tests. This is a case of preestablished intellectual style forcing, and not merely hearing, the evidence.

The cases differed on two final points, both having to do with defining intelligence. First, Judge Peckham, repeating Judge Wright's error in *Hobson v. Hansen* (1967), accepted the plaintiffs' view that an unbiased intelligence test must measure innate potential. That was Jane Mercer's point (Mercer, 1979) in adjusting WISC-R scores for sociocultural variables, so that a disadvantaged black child with an IQ of 85 might be said to have a "true" IQ of 100. This view comports, of course, with the notion that the tests are biased against blacks because they do not truly capture some aspects of black intelligence. The reading in *PASE* was that intelligence was *developed* intellectual abilities, primarily related to schooling and validated, as we have seen, by scholastic achievement.

The second aspect of how the two cases differed radically in conceiving intelligence was the scope of its definition. Plaintiffs in *Larry P.* adopted a capacious view of intelligence as being successful adaptation to several environments, of which school was merely one. Even with respect to school, it was not simply academic performance that measured adaptation, it was also success in the role of student, including deportment, participation in music, art, and so on. Thus, grades were better measures of adaptation than achievement tests, and adaptive behavior in the home and community was as good as scholastic intellectual performance in indexing intelligence.

These views, by making schooling in academic subjects just one of several life roles, and school just another 6-hour environment, minimize the importance of the life of the intellect. They also emphasize a conception of intelligence as talent broadly conceived, in the manner of Gardner (1983) and Guilford (1967), a view that emphasizes several talents (e.g., music, dance) that may have little to do with scholastic performance.

In *PASE*, however, Judge Grady pressed hard on the significance of nonintellectual adaptive behavior for intelligence. George Albee had testified that knowing how to get along with others, knowing the rules of baseball and basketball, and knowing how to get around in the city were characteristic of adaptive behavior, hence of intelligence. Grady asked him what he made of good scholars who were not good on the playground, and vice versa. Were mastering arithmetic and getting along with others to be considered the same thing? Albee answered that intelligence is usually considered to be made up of several abilities, and is not just the cognitive ability tested by IQ tests. The judge finally said,

> I don't think anybody today, at least, would say that it is. I just want to steer us away from any false issue here. I don't think anyone in saying that an IQ test measures the entire spectrum of human achievement or human capacity. I think what we are concerned with is, does it do anything worthwhile? There is no point in talking about apples and oranges if that is what we are talking about. (Record of trial, p. 159)

Because it was granted that the IQ test was used primarily to assess scholastic ability, the defense had little more to do than to establish that it predicted achievement in both racial groups about equally well, which, with allowance for the greater range restriction among blacks, it did.

Effects of These Cases[2]

The real-world net effects of these cases on the cognitive abilities and school retention of what were once known as mildly retarded children (65

---

[2] The data here are chiefly the result of several interviews done in late 1984 in California, with Fred Hansen and Ken Bill of the Department of Education; Alice Bryant, Psychological Services, Los Angeles Unified School District; Curtis Cooper, Special Education Services, San Francisco Unified School District; John Kingsbury and his staff, Special Education, Alum Rock Unified School District; Gorden Gareth, Special Education, San Jose Unified School District. In addition, I have relied on an article by Cordes (1986) and discussions in 1988 and 1989 with James Colwell, a school psychologist in the San Francisco district. For information on Chicago, there is an APA *Monitor* article (Cordes, 1983), and I have talked with Sharon Weitzman, a lawyer who directs Designs for Change, a research and advocacy group overseeing the mandated change, in special education assessment in Chicago; and with various officials of the Chicago Board of Education.

to 80 IQ range) are, of course, not yet well known, as we are too close to the decisions. But something is already known about the shifting of numbers and programs, and the changes in modes of assessment.

In California (as of 1984) there were 12,000 to 13,000 EMR children, down from the 1968–69 high of 58,000. This is a prevalence rate below what is often accepted for the more serious, biologically involved category of trainable mentally retarded (TMR). Indeed, my recent informal survey of state and local special education officials indicated a continuation of the process that began about the time that *Larry P.* was first filed: the qualitative change in the EMR population from the generally normal very slow learner (the normal tail of a normal distribution) toward the more serious impairment characteristic of the TMR child (see, e.g., MacMillan & Borthwick, 1980). Simultaneously, the declassified EMR children have returned to regular classes or to other special education categories, chiefly learning disabled (LD), an umbrella category that now includes about half of all special education placements. In it may be found children with brain injuries, hyperactive children, children with special perceptual or reading deficits, children with emotional disorders, severe underachievers, and, increasingly, slow learners of IQ levels that are in the 65 to 80 range (see, e.g., Campione, Brown, & Ferrara, 1982; Shepard, Smith, & Vojir, 1983).

Table 20.1 shows the recent prevalence in Los Angeles for various ethnic groups in EMR, TMR, developmentally handicapped and LD categories. Note that the prevalence rates for EMR are very low: about 0.3% for whites, Hispanics, and American Indians and about twice that for blacks, who are also overrepresented in the largest category, LD. Note also that the segregated classroom is quite common for LD students, and this is true not only for Los Angeles but for other cities I visited. In San Francisco, blacks made up 22% of the public school population, 46% of the population of special day classes, and 54% of the clientele of resource specialist programs, which are typically for LD students. In Alum Rock, a part of the San Jose district, the number of special day classes had not decreased since 1969, but instead of having 21 EMR classes of about 11 children each, there were now some 4 EMR classes, about 17 primarily LD classes, and 2 diagnostic classes. Clearly, a switch to LD status by no means guaranteed either mainstreamed or racially integrated status. For the state as a whole, blacks made up 9% of the school population and 15% of the EMR and TMR total in 1984. Because TMR rates are usually *not* disproportionate, the black EMR proportion is still probably close to twice the school population proportion.

Many, perhaps half, of all children removed from EMR classes in California *have* been placed in regular classrooms, which means that they have been returned to the very environments they had failed in initially. The court order requires all returned students to get some transitional help. But since the early 1970s, thousands of children have never been

TABLE 20.1. Ethnic compostion of certain special education programs, 1983–84 school year, Los Angeles Unified School District.[a]

Program		Asian	Ethnic groups Hispanic	Black	White	Total
EMR:	NO.	64	889	842	360	2,178
	%[c]	2.93	40.82	38.66	16.53	100
	RATE[d]	0.15	0.32	0.73	0.31	0.39
TMR:	NO.	68	826	392	368	1,661
	%	4.09	49.72	23.60	22.15	100
	RATE	0.16	0.29	0.34	0.32	0.29
DH:	NO.	38	338	165	212	763
	%	4.98	44.30	21.62	27.78	100
	RATE	0.09	0.12	0.14	0.18	0.14
LD:	NO[b]	294	8,358	6,577	5,416	20,774
	%	1.42	40.23	31.65	26.07	100
	RATE	0.69	2.98	5.68	4.69	3.74
District population		42,114	280,106	115,642	115,269	554,848
	%	7.59	50.48	20.84	20.77	99.9

Note: EMR, educable retarded; TMR, trainable mentally retarded; DH, developmentally handicapped; LD, learning disabled.

[a] American Indians, Filipinos, and "others" are not shown. Their numbers are included in the totals, but are very small.

[b] About 800 pupils receiving Designated Instructional Services. About 7,000 pupils in Special Day Classes. About 13,000 pupils in Resource Specialist Program.

[c] The percentage of the category represented by members of each ethnic group.

[d] The percentage of each ethnic group in this category.

placed in EMR who would have been so placed before that time. Some of these children get assistance as LD students, but many do not, because the criterion for eligibility as LD is to be achieving significantly below ability, and very slow learners are often achieving close to their limited ability.

The LD category, being a large catchall, is a wonderful locus of ambiguities where monetary constraints, conceptual fuzziness, human need, and politics all meet. California has a cap of 10% of the population to be funded as handicapped. In San Francisco, they simply exceed the limit and rely on state tolerance. Alum Rock is in a consortium with other districts so that if one district is under quota, another may go over. Definitionally, the state requires that there be a severe discrepancy between intellectual ability and achievement in one or more of the areas specified in Section 56337(a) of the Education Code, which include listening, reading, writing, and math skills. Severe discrepancy is indexed as any discrepancy in the two relevant (standardized) scores that is 1.5 times the standand deviation of the population of such difference scores. "But if standardized tests are considered to be invalid for a specific pupil, the discrepancy shall be measured by alternative means" (Los Angeles Unified School District Student Guidance Services Division, 1984). Because the tests may be considered invalid for most minority children, and because the alternative means of assessing ability include adaptive behavior scales, like the Adaptive Behavior Inventory for Children (ABIC) (Mercer, 1979), known to be only slightly correlated with intelligence tests, it is nearly always possible to find the "hook" that will make a child eligible for service. There is some test shopping, too, so that if a discrepancy doesn't appear on the Wide Rang Achievement Tests (WRAT), for instance, it might on the Woodcock-Johnson.

Still, one effect of cutting down the EMR category has been to cast many children adrift in the mainstream with little or no special help. (At the very least, the much-maligned EMR classroom is small, and easy to compete in.) The effect is mitigated to a degree by the presence of compensatory education programs in areas of high rate of school failure, but the special education professionals I have talked with say that dropping out of school after repeated failure is an increasing problem with these once-EMR-eligible very slow learners. Even the EMR vocational programs in high schools have declined in number, along with the EMR population itself. One goal of the plaintiffs was to get an education that was better than the "survival skills" that are the focus of EMR curricula. Fewer EMR children are learning survival skills, but there has been no comparable increase in the quality of education for slow learners.

The requirement to answer to a court has made school boards and school psychologists very shy about recommending any minority child for EMR placement. The moratorium on tests began 4 years before the final *Larry P.* decision, by way of preliminary injunction, and psychologists could see the quota coming, as it had come already for Hispanic children in the *Diana* settlement of 1970. Defense Exhibit 1 in the trial was a file of letters written in 1976 from school boards lamenting the loss of a useful instrument (the IQ test), and relating tales of Hispanic parents who fought to have their children placed or re-placed into quota-controlled EMR classrooms so they could find a place where they would not fail. As we have seen, disproportionate black placement has persisted, despite the burdens of justification it imposes, and it would seem to be a function neither of tests nor of any current racism. EMR quotas for Hispanics are easier to keep to, as there are alternative programs, (e.g., bilingual programs) for Hispanic children not available to blacks.

The system for assessing possible EMR children at present in California is a charade. An IQ test may be used with a child referred for assessment; however, if it then appears that the child might be placed in EMR, everyone must behave as if no test had been given. But the fact that no score is given by the psychologist in the placement conference is a tip-off about its nature. If the tests are physically taken out of the hands of psychologists, as it appeared to me had happened in San Jose and San Francisco (there were stacks of discarded WISC-R kits piled into storage cabinets), then the psychologists are perforce to be left to other devices, and that is exactly what has happened.

By 1986, at least one school psychologist complained to the Office of Civil Rights that the San Francisco Unified School District had resorted to unnormed and unvalidated assessment methods (Landers, 1986), thus turning the tables on the plaintiffs, who had made the same claim about IQ tests. The complaint was true, and the Office of Civil Rights did, in fact, forbid the use of one of the items. As of 1989, when I last conducted interviews in the city, school psychologists were using bits and pieces of various tests, and of course these ad hoc combinations had neither the norms nor the reliability and validity data customarily required of tests. A group of staff psychologists had also appealed the use of such unprofessional methods to the American Psychological Association in 1984 and 1985 and, for their pains, were accused of disloyalty by the functionary then in charge of special education (Landers, 1986).

In Chicago, the ban on tests is even more thoroughgoing than it is in California—tests can't be used for *any* special education category.[3] For although defendants in *PASE* won at court, they lost by virtue of a consent decree in the large, 10-year-old desegregation negotiation that required them not to permit discrimination in *any* kind of classroom. A plan developed as a result of the decree obliges the Board of Education to desegregate EMR classes and not to use IQ tests for anyone; and to provide transition help for children put back into regular classes. About 2,000 black children, of the 10,000 in EMR classrooms, have been placed into regular classes, most with a pull-out-for-special-help resource option. The rate of EMR placement for black children in Chicago is still very high, at about 2.5%, more than three times the rate in California. An advocacy group, Designs for Change, monitors the Chicago Board of Education's compliance. The Designs for Change spokesperson told me that many children have dropped out of school, and that the board has not increased the size of its LD staff to accommodate this increased demand for services occasioned by reassessment. With straitened finances, and the redeployment of its psychologists to the reassessment job, the

[3] One strategy of the plaintiffs' advocates appears to have been to insist that new tests be developed and validated specifically for diagnosing EMR status. This is an extremely difficult task. The Chicago Board of Education showing that some of their tests discriminated between EMR and "transition" students was objected to on the grounds that the proscribed IQ tests had been used to set up such groups in the first place. If no valid test could be developed, then adaptive behavior scales could be the main basis of reassessment, and their use is well known (Reschly, 1981) to make a majority of children who are eligible for EMR on an IQ basis ineligible on the adaptive behavior basis. Such an effect had occurred in Champaign, Illinois, with the use of Mercer's (1979) SOMPA system. Ironically, her system could not be employed in Chicago, though she was a consultant there, because it involves one of the forbidden tests, the WISC-R (see Cordes, 1983, for a discussion).

board has a backlog of demand for special education services, particularly from Hispanics, who are underrepresented (as in California) in almost every category.[4]

In addition to the unencouraging results of regular classroom placement, the plaintiffs' advocates in Chicago are unhappy with the new methods of assessment. The Board of Education is careful to say that, although its psychologists use tests whose outcome *could* be reported in specific numbers, they are in fact used for the psychological observation of individual performance—just, as it were, a sort of standardized observational technique. It is hard to read through this heavily legalized message, but it sounds as if they are testing without (overtly) scoring: Given the constraints of the consent decree, it is hard to imagine what else they could do because scores would create norms, which would then manifest a race difference. Thus, both the Draw-a-Man and the Kohs Block Design tests are used, but no score is reported; the psychologists do not have to write anything down. No labels are applied; rather, a narrative record is provided.

Because quotas prevent disproportionate placement of minorities into EMR in California, the inevitable increase in subjectivity and discretion of assessors that occurs in the absence of norms will simply add noise to the decision-making process. In Chicago, where there are no quotas, per se, the plaintiffs' advocates are very suspicious of the great fluidity and discretion in the assessment process. Because they feel that the "overplacement" of blacks arose in part from abuse of discretion, they are not happy with the increase in mystery that has replaced reliance on well-known objective tests. The executive director of designs for Change said she would actually prefer a rule—e.g., no placement unless the pupil scores less than two standard deviations below the norm on a standard test like the Iowa Test of Basic Skills. Note, however, that such reliance, although more objective, is unlikely to remove the racial disproportion: the tests of mental ability on which blacks score a standard deviation below whites include school achievement tests. Use of such a rule would therefore not really meet the objections of the black professionals, quoted early in this chapter, who included achievement tests among their targets.[5]

---

[4] It is thought that the availability of English as a Second Language programs "hides" many Hispanic children who might otherwise be served in LD or EMR programs, both in Chicago and in California. Thus, for example, the establishment of a strong bilingual program in Illinois in the mid-1970s was accompanied by a decrease in Hispanic EMR placement rate. It went from 2.0% to 1.2% from 1973–74 to 1975–76. One result was the modification of the complaint to exclude Hispanics from the plaintiff class in *PASE*.

The use of achievement tests will do most of what the use of IQ tests would do, with the single exception of the unique use for which Binet developed the test in the first place: to help school officials decide why a child is failing. If such a child performs well on an IQ test, then one looks for motivational and emotional difficulties; if not, then one might consider special, slowed-down instruction.

In California, the broad conception of intelligence urged on the court by plaintiffs has won wide official acceptance in the districts I looked at. Thus, among the mimeographed materials I received in San Francisco, in addition to explications of Feuerstein's (1979) dynamic assessment method, were a précis of Gardner's (1983) *Frames of Mind* and literature on Guilford's (1967) structure-of-intellect model. These views permit a definition of giftedness, for example, that is the counterpart of any definition of retardation stressing adaptive behavior; that is, classes for the gifted can, by selecting students gifted in art, music, and dance, mitigate the ethnic disproportions that sole reliance on IQ would produce.

It is possible, of course, that schools should encourage a wider variety of skills than they have traditionally. Their custodial role in the care and development of the whole child is receiving ever-greater attention and support in an economy that takes larger proportions of parents out of the home. The same economy, however, rewards intellectual development. With limited resources, the tensions created by the contending views of intelligence and the appropriate goals for schools will be severe. The politics of race has heightened this tension, and current demands that

[5] I spoke with a black professional in pupil services in Chicago, who would I am sure not want to be named. The phone interview was as clear an example of the problems associated with the attempts to settle complex social problems adversarially as I have come across. She wanted me to put in writing exactly what I wanted from them, because she had learned long since that casual conversations with Designs for Change tended to end in court. She said Designs for Change will not be satisfied with any assessment method that does not result in removing over 60% of the black children from EMR—that is, achieves the prevalence rate promoted by Mercer in her testimony in *Larry P.* The Iowa Test for Basic Skills will not do this, and, of course, it has not be validated for the purpose of identifying black EMR children (indeed, what has?).

The use of adaptive behavior scales, would probably result in greater removal of EMR children, but, says my informant, the school personnel hear more complaints from parents who want to keep their children in EMR than from those who want them out.

The two sides in this dispute simply will not communicate except through lawyers; there is no trust whatever that I can discern. It may be all right for hostile parties to impoverish their communication by reliance on lawyers, provided they can cut their ties. But both the parties in Chicago are concerned for the educational problems of children, problems that will not go away.

schools not only do more but do it better will strain them ever more. Let us turn explicitly, then, to the policy implications of these decisions.

Policy Implications of These Cases

It cannot be said that all of the changes just reviewed were the result of judicial decision. There were strong movements in the early 1970s in the California legislature to achieve mainstreaming and reduce disproportion in EMR; Congress passed the Education for All Handicapped Act in 1975; the Chicago Board of Education modernized its assessment procedures throughout the 1970s. Courts affected the political process and were affected by it. Mainstreaming was an idea of great political force, and probably would have prevailed in any case. Disproportionate representation in low tracks had been the subject of frequent litigation. So the political involvement in these lawsuits was of a piece with these movements: to achieve more equal status for blacks, and to mainstream the mildly handicapped in order to reduce the stigma and, perhaps, the educational burden of EMR placement.

But the attack on the most venerable of tests of mental ability, the individual intelligence tests, was new (Bersoff, 1981), and that was an exercise in black pride, an effort to explain the large difference in performance (because it was clear, after all, that the tests were not the cause of disproportionate placement) that has continued to exist without tests as much as it did before the ban; both trials established that there were racially disproportionate achievement rates prior to any IQ testing. If there were any winners in *Larry P.* it was the black professionals who found the plaintiffs and brought the suit that declared one famous set of measures of black deficit invalid. But the other targets, the achievement tests, are too close to the curriculum. To attack tests of arithmetic and language skills, however much they correlate with IQ tests, is to attack a vital institution of Western industrialized culture, the school itself.

For special education, the negative results are reduced precision and objectivity of assessment, reduced precision of placement, reduced morale of and faith in the professionals charged with assessment, some downgrading of the once-central importance of developing intellectual skills, and reduced services for slow-learning, non-LD children in the 65 to 80 range. The positive results are broader and newer kinds of assessment (if there is time for the breadth, and norms for the novel tests) and some fresh thinking about programs for children having difficulty in school.

There is a limit on the effect courts and legislatures can have upon education, if by that we mean the development of intellectual skills and not just changes in special education categories or in racial composition of schools and faculties. For example, Wrubel (1979) studied the impact of court directives on schools (including the directives arising out of the *Larry P.* preliminary injunctions), and found very little impact. Kirp, Kuriloff, & Buss, et al. (1975) studied compliance with two famous cases concerning education of the retarded, *PARC* and *Mills*, and with the California legislative changes of the early 1970s. They concluded that in no case did much basic change occur in the educational systems, and what little change did occur came only after enormous and sustained effort.

In particular, courts and legislatures cannot make group and individual differences disappear; neither can they develop the cognitive abilities of children. Students need instruction suited to their current skills, and the slower or further behind they are when they first appear in schools, the more, and more intensive, instruction they need. As highly experienced observers have noted (Bereiter, 1985; Resnick, 1979), though the law may call for sundry labels like LD, EMR, and CD (culturally disadvantaged), children differently labeled often have a similar deficit, which requires a similar remedy (e.g., intensive instruction in reading and other basic skills).

What is needed, then, is more teaching, which means more teachers and smaller student-to-teacher ratios. As long as budgets are tight, such classes are likely to occur only for special education categories, and the assessment and decision-making apparatus—tests and the like—is going to continue to be needed. But if we ever came to appreciate the real return on good early education, in the sense that Berrueta-Clement, Schweinhart, Barnett, Epstein, and Weikart (1984) have shown for preschool programs, then, as Resnick (1979) has pointed out, classes will be small enough to preclude much of the need for classification and testing; the behavior of the pupil and the experience of the teacher will be all that are necessary to guide instruction.

More intensive, low-ratio teaching will also ameliorate a serious problem with mainstreaming. Mainstreaming implies large variability of academic and social behavior in a classroom. Such variability makes it hard for teaching, and there is a point beyond which teachers (and many parents) will not tolerate the effect on the class of laggard intellectual performance or disruption.

Until such changes in staffing are made, we need some improvement in the classification scheme. Most importantly, we need either (a) a program for non-LD children in the 65 to 80 IQ range in which classes are smaller than average (I assume many self-contained LD classes serve this purpose, but, as we have seen, there are tight budgetary caps on funding the LD category); or (b) better assistance to such mainstreamed children even though they do not qualify as LD. That is, resource or "pull-out" programs should be for *any* student in need, and not just a certain category of student.

As long as testing is to continue, professionals ought to be allowed to use whatever instruments they find useful, including WISC-Rs and

Standford-Binets. The irony in California is that blacks are "protected" from EMR placement by quota (or, if the quota is not kept, by the burden of explanation and the threat of lawsuit borne by the school boards), but within the black population so protected, pupils are denied the advantage of being assessed and classified by useful instruments (the IQ tests). One possible effect of leaving assessment to teacher judgment can be seen in the recent report of a controlled study of an early, highly structured educational intervention for very poor "high-risk" black children in North Carolina (Ramey & Haskins, 1981). The first cohorts of their day-care intervention group and the controls are now in public schools. Although the day-care group had averge IQs at age 5, they were almost uniformly grouped into the lowest academic groups by their teachers when they entered public school. Ramey and Haskins state:

> We have also come to suspect that the process of schooling is very different for high-risk children and other children attending the public schools. Teachers tend to relegate high-risk children to the lowest academic group, although such placement does not always correspond with the intellectual ability of all these children as measured by standarized tests. (p. 109)

Perhaps one small change would solve several problems, and that would be to stop referring to intelligence tests as such and to start calling them tests of developed scholastic ability, or school functioning level, or the like. Such a name change would remove some of the onus of low scores. It is fairly evident that the public attributes something more innate, general, and permanent to "intelligence" than do professionals in the consensus, who regard it as referring to current performance.

As to the black-white differences, a policy recommendation is difficult, because it requires patience. Twenty-five years ago Moynihan (1965) wrote a policy planning document on the Negro family, outlining what he termed "the tangle of pathology" of much of black life: broken homes, illegitimacy, unemployment, welfare, school achievement deficits, and drug use. The report shocked many readers, and angered several civil rights advocates for seeming to blame the victim, much as tests are attacked for the bad news they bring. Moynihan's view was that family cohesiveness was the chief, perhaps the only guarantee against pathology of such scope and dimension, and that the main support for families would be better employment opportunities for black males. The relatively superior school performance of the children of poor immigrant Jewish, Chinese, and Japanese families was, to him, evidence of the power of family cohesiveness sustained by the employment and industry of male heads of household.

A generation later, life for blacks has become better for a few, and worse for many (Wilson, 1978). It is no longer true, for example, that only a third of black children live in households of which a single mother is the head. Today, over half of all black children are in that circumstance, even though the status of the relatively small black middle-class has improved substantially.

This chapter does not address job-training and employment strategies, although we may note that effective ones have not been created on a large scale. Given this situation, what, in addition to more intensive regular teaching, might be done to reduce the black intellectual deficit? The literature supports the use of preschool interventions in which deliberate practice in cognitive skills is given, and, in some cases, child-training advice is given to mothers.

There have been three recent reviews of two decades of research on such preschool interventions (Berrueta-Clement et al., 1984; Lazar & Darlington, 1982; Ramey, Bryant, & Suarez, 1985). In his commentary at the end of the Lazar and Darlington monograph, Ramey sums up in part as follows:

> The major finding is that children from preschool programs were less likely to repeat a grade or be placed in special education classes than were their controls. . . .
>
> For the 1976 consortium follow-up data there are not significant differences in IQ between program and control groups and the evidence concerning achievement test data is not very convincing of substantial program effects. . . .
>
> In fact, the mean IQ performance at follow-up for the children from the four projects having more nearly randomized designs is approximately one standard deviation below the national average, for both program and control children. . . .
>
> It is my opinion that given the complex and little-understood forces operating to sustain lower intellectual performance among this society's lower socio-economic groups—including limited economic opportunities, racial and social discrimination, and genetic limitations, to mention just a few—we are unlikely to witness full realization of human potential through limited educational experiments. Therefore, the expectations of success from such efforts must be constrained by experience. . . .(Ramey, in Lazar & Darlington, 1982, pp. 147–149)

Ramey's own project, the Carolina Abecedarian Project, is a strong, well-reported model (Ramey & Haskins, 1981). Low-income black children were enrolled by random assignment as infants, at 3 months of age, or were left to their normal home circumstances, with the provision of the social work, medical, and nutritional supplementary services common to both groups. The day-care program was a cognitively and socially oriented program emphasizing language, with a child-to-staff ratio varying from 3:1 to 5:1. Children attended 6 to 8 hours per day, 5 days a week, 50 weeks a year, until entry into public kindergarten. The IQ differences (Stanford-Binet) were about 9, 15, and 12 points at 2, 3, and 4 years, respectively; and at 5 years, children in the experimental group a mean IQ of 98 on the Wechsler Preschool and Primary Scale of

Intelligence (WPPSI), with the figure for the control group being 91. These differences do not match the enormous effects reported for the Milwaukee project (Garber & Heber, 1981), but they are well described and fully reported.

The Abecedarian Project is not cheap, and its effects are modest. The project assesses home environmental and psychosocial factors, which yield equally low scores for both groups in comparison to middle-class homes, so that even the experimental children are still spending most of their time in an intellectual and motivational context unlikely either to amplify preschool efforts or to facilitate later school achievement. The alternatives to such projects are weaker interventions, like Head Start, or a long wait before the black middle-class becomes larger and, where it exists, more firmly established.

I think it will be true for the foreseeable future that school-based improvements in the intellectual repertoires of poor black children will be counteracted by effects of home and neighborhood. A great social shift is needed to change those important environments. Even with goodwill and determined effort, however, any such shift will take generations. This picture may be minimally satisfying to those who take the long view or who distrust the process and consequences of more rapid social shifts. Persons most hurt by present circumstances, however, are least likely to indulge in statesmanlike delay of gratification. Present circumstances make unlikely in the near term any large expenditures either for preschool and school enrichment programs for the poor, or any new policies designed to strengthen the black middle class.

In the meantime, some black advocates will continue to deny that anything is wrong, except with the tests, with the grading system and achievement tests that constitute the criteria, and with the schools. They will continue to believe that if only teachers had higher expectations of black children, or if only they taught, in some never-specified way, *correctly*, then the black-white gap would close.

Let me end this section by adverting to a conflict in Minneapolis. The school board there, under Superintendent Richard Green, has adopted a policy of "promotional gates," according to which students must pass "benchmark" tests, given at the end of kindergarten, second, fifth, seventh, and ninth grades, in order to move up to the next grade.

The test involved at the kindergarten level is like any readiness test: recognizing letters, colors, and numbers, understanding simple concepts, ordering simple numerals, and the like. In the 1984 spring testing, some 300 kindergarten children were not promoted, and they were disproportionately minority children, particularly blacks. (Kenneth Rustad, of the Department of Guidance and Assessment Services, sent me ethnic data. Passing rates for blacks were about 74% in 1984 and 1985, compared with white rates of 94%, for a difference, given normality, just slightly smaller than one standard deviation.)

A few black parents wanted to protest such disproportionate failure to be promoted to regular first-grade classes but were dissuaded from doing so. The president of the Minneapolis Urban League noted that there had been warnings for 2 years of such "gates," and considerable contact with parents about pupil progress: "Parents began to realize that this was also a quiet indictment of them, of how they had done in preparing the child in the previous five years" (*New York Times*, September 16, 1984, p. 10).

This news item is a poignant illustration of the dilemmas of policy. Black children are on average underprepared before they arrive at school, and school does not repair this relative deficit. Blaming families who are transmitting their own relative lack of experience with middle-class intellectual skills does not seem any more useful than blaming schools, or going to court to forbid the use of the test or of the "gates" policy that precludes social promotion. All that exist are a few options with modest potential for amelioration: preschool programs, family support systems of the kind discussed by Zigler and Seitz (1982), remedial work after school or during summers (one sixth of the failing kindergarten children passed their test after going to summer school), and more intensive work during regular classes.

The costs of these programs is high, and the results will come but gradually. Impatience will be a constant temptation, both for taxpayers and civil rights advocates. One of the common effects of injunctions and court orders is to stimulate anger and resistance, as we have seen most plainly in the history of court-ordered busing, often to the detriment, and with the resegregation of, the schools. It is more difficult (at least for this observer) to see how the present lawsuits did anything good for black children than it is to see harm. Apart from cases of blatant discrimination and well-substantiated harm, courts will (I think) do themselves and the rest of society a service by staying out of the school business.

There is indeed a national crisis in education, especially in the development of useful intellectual and other skills among disadvantaged minority children (Elliott, 1988; Humphreys, 1988; Levin, 1985). What is needed is thoughtful leadership, a willingness to spend large sums of money, and a widespread constituency of support that sees that resources devoted today are an enormously cost-effective and humane investment. What is not needed are poor policy decisions coming out of a forum very ill-equipped to decide them. With that, we turn to our final section, on the use of social science in the adversarial system of the courts.

The Adversary System as a Way of Finding Facts

Wolf (1981) and Rossell (1980) have contributed thoughtful analyses of the role of social science in school equity and integration cases, and nothing in the present analysis of these two lawsuits would lead one to a brighter conclusion than theirs about the capacity of the court system to make intelligent use of social science.

Social science data are rarely conclusive, so that they are uncommonly arguable (particularly in a forum given uncommonly to argument). They confirm enough of common sense to be easily dismissed as *only* common sense. And their data, unlike those of physics or chemistry, are sufficiently accessible to laymen—that is, so close, incremental, and supplementary to ordinary knowledge—that it is easy for laymen to distort their meaning or dismiss their value. Everyone is a bit of a psychologist in a way that not everyone is a bit of a chemist. One of the most influential bodies of social science data, on jury size, for example, was dismissed by Justice Lewis Powell as "numerology" (*Ballew v. Georgia*, 1978). The result is that the value of even the best social science data may be hard to discern in relatively neutral settings. But in settings where adversaries are seeking not truth but victory, then what modest value social science data have can easily be wholly nullified.

The fact that a consensus on some matters exists in social science (as I claim exists concerning test bias and race) does not mean that it will be noncontroversial. Kamin, in his *PASE* testimony (Record of Trial 107–108), compared the controversy over test bias with the disagreement among psychiatrists concerning the insanity of some defendant, and said that the disagreement in each case implied shaky evidence. His argument exemplified two faults. First, Kamin compared applications of general principles to particular cases in a field marked by ambiguities of definition and diagnosis, with evidence about a set of general principles in a field where definitions of prediction, criterion, and bias are readily operationalized and amenable to sophisticated analysis. In a less partisan climate he would have been less likely (I hope) to have done so. Second, he takes the sheer fact of controversy, regardless of the merits of the two sides, as precluding the possibility of consensus. Evolution is a still controversial theory, and well-credentialed experts can be found to argue against it; nonetheless, a consensus exists among well-qualified experts.

The problem in court is that if there are two marginally qualified experts against the scientific consensus and 200 well-qualified experts in it, the court will hear two on each side. And if one side represents popular myth (e.g., "of course tests are biased against blacks—they've had little chance to learn what is tested"), then the odds against the scientific consensus get longer. Unfortunately, the most valuable consensus, in the sense of providing useful information, is precisely the one that contradicts the popular myth.

Even where the subject of expert testimony is hard science, the court is a less than ideal way of finding the truth of some matter. The adversarial procedure means that one position is presented at a time, without answer, comment, or discussion, sometimes (as in *Larry P.*) for weeks. Cross-examination of the experts on one side is done not by peer experts but by a lawyer whose skill in the subject is a hastily acquired patchwork, and whose skill in cross-examination will vary enormously with the luck of the draw and the money available. Even direct testimony may be poorly evoked, or weakened by procedures that control admissibility of evidence and trial conduct. Jerome Sattler, a defense expert on intellectual assessment of children, was interrupted some 20 times in the first half hour of his testimony in a clear effort to disrupt the continuity of presentation of evidence of criterion validity of IQ tests, evidence that was potentially very damaging to the plaintiffs' case in *Larry P.* In a scientific forum that would not happen.

Thus, Judge Peckham heard over 2 months of plaintiffs' witnesses relentlessly building their case before the other side called a witness. It is possible that really brilliant cross-examination might have blunted the effect, but fact-finding should not have to depend on so thin a reed. Fundamental terms like culture, intelligence, bias, or retardation never got defined clearly; concepts like correlation, or the effect of restriction of range on correlation, never were adequately understood by the judges. Judge Grady, during closing arguments, asked "What's the correlation between an IQ of 60 and GPA?" (closing arguments, p. 134). The defense attorney, with unusual courage, said, "With all due respect, Judge, that is a nonsensical question." It is not customary for attorneys to tell judges that they are either stupid or missing the point, however. In the scientific forum, of course, the bracing effect of pointing out error is uninhibited by the presence of robed authority.

One very significant difference in these two trials was in the willingness of the judges to accept a broad range of social science data. Judge Peckham, as was noted, was faced with the choice of finding either test bias or racial genetic difference as the cause of IQ differences, neither side having made much of a case for SES or home-environment causation. Had he accepted the general evidence of test validity and nonbias at all levels of education, especially in predicting standard achievement scores, he could scarcely have found much if any bias at the levels at issue in the trial. So he adopted the strategy of other governmental agencies (like the EEOC)—confronting test differences that threaten opportunities for minorities. He particularized the validation requirements so much (he insisted on evidence of prediction of teacher grades rather than achievement test scores, for young, low-achieving, black children of California) that the large quantity of data available generally on the prediction of black school achievement became almost irrelevant, even though the great weight of the evidence before and since the trial denies the plaintiffs' view.

Judge Grady, on the other hand, was asking about bias at the item level from the first day of the trial, and he ended by pleading with both sides to give him any and everything they had on race difference in item-passing rates. Furthermore, he accepted scholarly articles, supplied to him at the end of the trial, on general issues of race bias in prediction and as well as on internal analyses. The defense had printed a booklet of excerpts from testing experts on criterion validity and other matters, and to this was added papers by Jensen (1976), Miele (1979), and the thesis of Nichols (1970/1971). It seems clear that these papers, along with that by Gordon and Rudert (1979) were influential on the decision.[6]

For a judge to call for papers that had never been testified to and subjected to cross-examination is unusual. But Judge Grady's style was to be very open to information, and to ask many pressing questions, to both sides, though more to plaintiffs than to defendants. Thus, he wanted to know why, if environment is the key to IQ scores, similarly situated children score differently; why black children in the same school environment with whites do not catch up;[7] why, if the IQ test is of the same culture as the school and its tests, the correlation between the two measures is only .4; why, given that low correlation, anyone would think the IQ useful; if knowing English grammar was part of middle-class culture and what middle-class culture was; what witnesses meant when they talked about "early stimulation"; whether a sample was representative; how the plaintiffs would validate a test for use with EMR children (to their claim that IQ tests were not validated for such use, he asked how could they know what it [validation] wasn't if they couldn't tell him what it was?); and so on.

Science is, among other things, skepticism of attitude. Some judges appear to be more tough-minded (like Judge Grady) than others (like Judge Peckham), but whether trials like these draw such judges is a matter of chance. It is not foreseeable that judges will be systematically trained to think routinely in terms of base rates and control groups, to check representativeness, to insist on data rather than anecdotes, and so on. There is little enough of that even among social scientists, and we

---

[6] It is ironic that Judge Grady has been more severely castigated (see, e.g., Bersoff, 1981) for his armchair analysis of item bias than has Judge Peckham for his wrong view of what test bias is. There are, I think, two reasons for this. First, the *PASE* decision only hints, in citing Gordon and Rudert (1979), that social science literature might be involved. No other papers are cited, though it is clear that the judge read several. Second, in finding eight items that ought not be used for blacks, Judge Grady said, "I believe the following items are either racially biased *or so subject to suspicion of bias* that they should not be used" (PASE v. Hannon, 1980, p. 875, emphasis supplied). One may recognize suspiciousness without claiming to substitute subjective judgment for empirical analysis.

---

[7] Kamin's answer was that the schools failed black children. The judge asked how he knew that. Kamin said it must be so, or else the black children would have caught up.

cannot expect that judges, to say nothing of juries, will save social science either from the inadequacies of the adversarial system, or from those of its "experts" for whom politics may mean more than science.

Indeed, one egregious flaw in the adversarial system is its use of experts. There are two major problems. First, "experts" has a much broader meaning in the court than in the judgment of peers. Thus, the two chief critics of intelligence tests from the point of view of black culture, Asa Hilliard (in *Larry P.*) and Robert Williams (in *PASE*) had expert status in the area of test bias in court by virtue of being both psychologists and black, but they have little or none among psychologists who specialize in testing. They lack the training and the scholarship to qualify as scientific experts in that field.

Some of what they had to say was the stuff of everyday discourse—beliefs and anecdotes, unchecked by reported fact—about the Afrocentricity of American black culture; the ease of repairing the school achievement deficit in children (Hilliard said there were data, never presented, to show 3 years' gain in only 32 hours of remedial training); the power of teacher expectancy (Williams related a story of a Florida teacher who, mistaking high locker numbers for IQ scores, expected so much from her class that they did very well); and the invalidity of the WISC (for Hilliard, doing well was a matter of having an obsessive-compulsive personality, and one could, if of sufficient reputation, make up a test like the WISC in one's living room). Sometimes the two witnesses simply had facts wrong: Williams, for example, claimed that scholastic ability tests usually underpredicted black scholastic performance; that there is test bias against Asians (apparently, he did not realize how well they perform); that Galton invented the normal curve; and that Binet used an 80% to 90% passing criterion to accept items for a particular age group.

Various plaintiffs' experts ignored or did not know that there was little or no effect of race or dialect of examiner on IQ scores of blacks; that the Rosenthal-Jacobsen (1968) study did not report a change in teacher behavior, and was in several respects inadequate; that the Coleman report did not show improved black performance from placing formerly segregated blacks into mainly white classrooms, and so on.

Without an unusually knowledgeable lawyer, or a format in which other experts can challenge mistakes, qualify generalities, or expose half-truths, these misstatements simply pass into the record for later reflection by the judge. Judge Peckham, a believer, swallowed the testimony of Hilliard and Powell pretty much whole. Judge Grady, a skeptic, dismissed most of what Williams and later, Powell, had to say.[8]

The second difficulty with using experts adversarially is captured by Cronbach's (1975, p. 12) epigrammatic statement: "There is a fundamental difference between the style of the advocate . . . and the style of the scholar. An advocate tries to score every point, including those he knows he deserves to lose." Attorneys do not hire experts whose testimony will not help them, and they tempt even those qualified experts who agree with them to say both more, by way of certainty and conclusion, and less, by way of limitation and qualification, than they would do in the company of knowledgeable and critical peers. The theory appears to be that the several partial truths encouraged by zealous adversarial combat will add up to the whole truth. That might be the case if there were a critical discourse among the experts to bring out the weaknesses of each position, but there is no provision for such a colloquy in court.

The best example of the expert-as-partisan in these lawsuits is probably Kamin, a man whose knowledge of the intelligence test literature is detailed and encyclopedic (e.g., 1974) but whose selection of data to make the environmentalist argument, even outside the courtroom, has been frequently criticized (Fulker, 1975; Loehlin et al, 1975; Scarr, 1976).

Kamin discussed the history of testing at both trials. At the first, *Larry P.*, he had the following to say when asked why sex differences and race differences had been dealt with differently in test construction (Record of Trial):

> Let me answer in the following way: I am struck at the discrepancy in the treatment of the sex difference versus the treatment of the race difference and the treatment of the social class difference for that matter.
>
> I can see no scientific ground why one should eliminate questions which appear to show that one sex is doing better than the other and not eliminate questions which appear to show that one social class is doing better than another or that one race is doing better than the other.
>
> It seems to me this has to reflect the preconceptions of the people who are making up these tests. . . .
>
> Evidently, when they found the items discriminated between blacks and whites or between upper- and lower-class people, judging from the quotations which I have earlier cited, I would imagine that the test makers felt that these differences simply validated the test as a test of intelligence; after all, Terman had predicted

---

[8] As his opinion (PASE v. Hannon, 1980, p. 836 and Footnote 3) shows, Judge Grady was quite unimpressed by some of the experts:

> In some instances, I am satisfied that the opinions expressed are more the result of doctrinaire commitment to a preconceived idea than they are the result of scientific inquiry . . . I have not disregarded the expert testimony in this case, but neither do I feel bound by it. The factual determinations to be made are well within the capability of any competent trier of fact.

At one point in the trial (Record of Trial, p. 1558) the plaintiffs' attorney objected to a defense witness answering a question about the cultural bias of intelligence tests on the ground that the witness, a school official, was not a qualified psychologist. Judge Grady overruled, saying, "The fact that someone wears a hat that says 'psychologist' should not overly impress anyone who has sat through two weeks of this trial."

> before any data was available that tests would show that blacks are less intelligent than whites.
>
> So I would imagine he would not be particularly upset or alarmed and certainly not surprised if he found these items, indeed, did discriminate between the two races (pp. 875–876).

Of course, the great distinction between the sex and race cases here is that, on average, there are no, or only slight, differences in the school performances of the sexes (or, for that matter, in almost any cognitive ability, spatial reasoning perhaps expected—see Maccoby and Jacklin, 1974), in great contrast to those of the two races in question, or of different social classes. Even if Terman and Merrill (1937, p. 34) had not made it clear that sex differences were not large or numerous, McNemar's (1942) work would show it. At trial, both Lloyd Humphreys of the University of Illinois and Leo Munday of the test department of Houghton Mifflin testified that the sex differences that existed favored one sex or another about equally, as Terman and Merrill had said. There are, in fact, tests of mental ability (e.g., the Raven's matrices; Thurstone's primary abilities) whose items have not been edited for sex differences, that produce equal scores for the sexes (see Jensen's 1980 review). Because there was a large pool of items on which the sexes were close, those evoking large differences could be rejected. For race differences, there were very few items that did *not* produce significant differences, and rejecting those that did, therefore, would leave very little to make up a test with.

By 1980, when he appeared again as witness in *PASE*, Kamin gave substantially the same testimony, though he said he had by that time seen Jensen's book on bias (Jensen, 1980, of which Kamin was a reviewer), and he had the opportunity to see the paper by Gordon and Rudert (1979), calling his *Larry P.* testimony "disingenuous." Judge Peckham had been impressed with Kamin's testimony, citing it favorably, and ignoring the contrary testimony of Humphreys and Munday. Judge Grady, however, dismissed Kamin's testimony with a quotation from Gordon and Rudert (1979). It is possible that the judges' preestablished opinions and intellectual styles, or their early established theories of the cases, and the selective assessment of evidence that would have followed, led them to their different conclusions. For anyone interested in good social science having its day in court, that is cold comfort.

What can be done? Courts are a part of the political process, and, like legislatures, are affected by political movements. If dominant political forces concur in the belief that ability tests are unfair to blacks, then so much the worse for the tests. But in cases like these, judges are making complex social policy decisions alone. Most other political decision makers can get some help obtaining and evaluating evidence on complex issues. The Congress has staffs and research organizations, and the president can have advisors as nonpartisan as he would like. But for lawsuits like these, even if panels of qualified experts could be convened to observe and to critique the evidence given in them, the critiques could rarely be reported in a way that would affect a judge; judges are not supposed to look at evidence that is not before the court.

The courts are not just occasionally inhospitable to facts, they sometimes reject them outright. Judge Roth, presiding over the remedy hearings in *Bradley v. Milliken* (1971) refused to take testimony on the possibility and size of the "white flight" that might ensue from his huge school-integration order (Wolf, 1981). And if the Constitution said what he said it said, he was right; if departure from proportionality of race in schools is fundamentally wrong, then it is irrelevant that there might be costs associated with achieving it: *fiat justitia ruat coelum*. As one of *PASE* plaintiffs' attorneys said in her closing argument, "The only other explanation [of black disproportion in EMR] other than a problem with the evaluation and placement would be that black children are intellectually inferior to white children. We think that explanation is contrary to the Constitution and all the federal statutes" (Closing arguments, p. 70). And, as noted, Judge Peckham's softer rejection of evidence for IQ-achievement validities was a similar political proscription of data.

The point here is not that courts are necessarily worse than legislatures. If the citizens of a democracy want to protect their myths or their special interests, then we must not be surprised to see legislatures and courts act to do that. In some respects we may even prefer courts for these functions. We generally attribute greater wisdom to them than to legislatures, even though the latter have greater resources, perhaps because we need to feel that a decision we can do little about, because its source cannot be called to account, is a better one.

Psychologists, knowing some myths not to be true, will need to find a way to educate judges and legislators. To improve expert testimony, they should see, first, that cases are ably defended. That means lots of money and, in complex cases like these, several good attorneys coherently led and ably advised by good consultants. A team like that will go some ways toward showing up the inadequacies of nonexpert "experts"; and it can spend the time needed to effect clarity of the presentation of its case.

Second, no expert should mislead by commission or omission. The best way to inhibit resort to half-truth or outright error is probably to report it as quickly as possible both to professional peers and to the public. Many inexpert "experts" will not care much—the constituency for Hilliard and Williams was not psychometricians, but blacks—but other, better qualified psychologists might be concerned to be widely known as partisan in the use of data. Even here, of course, the more partisan the psychologist, the less likely he or she will be affected by the opinion of other, usually more prudent peers.

Beyond all that, citizens, including judges, are educated by the cumulative force of data. It is vastly easier to argue in 1988 that ability tests used for employment or scholastic selection and placement are equally valid for blacks and whites than it was in 1975, when many of these cases were begun or in progress (see, e.g., Heller, Holtzman, & Messick, 1982; Hunter, Schmidt, & Rauschenberger, 1984; Manning & Jackson, 1984; Sattler, 1982; Wigdor & Garner, 1982). The message, again, is that patience is what is required, along with fidelity to the scientific canon that forbids misrepresentation. Patience is a scarce resource in a world that cannot take its issues back to the lab or seminar, but must decide them when they are brought. Scientists, however, need not live by the rules of that world, anymore than that world needs to live by the rules of scientific procedure.

References

Ballew v. Georgia. (1978). 435 U.S. 223.

Bereiter, C. (1985). The changing face of educational disadvantagement. *Phi Delta Kappan*, *66*, 538–541.

Berrueta-Clement, J. R., Schweinhart, L. J., Barnett, W. S., Epstein, A. S., & Weikart, D. P. (1984). Changed lives: The effects of the Perry Preschool Program on youths through age 19. *Monographs of the High/Scope Educational Research Foundation*, No. 8.

Bersoff, D. N. (1981). Testing and the law. *American Psychologist*, *36*, 1047–1056.

Bradley v. Milliken. (1971). 338 F. Supp. 582.

Broman, S. H., Nichols, P. L., & Kennedy, W. A. (1975). *Preschool IQ: Prenatal and early developmental correlates*. Hillsdale, NJ: Erlbaum.

Campione, A. C., Brown, A. L., & Ferrara, R. A. (1982). Mental retardation and intelligence. In R. J. Sternberg (Ed.), *Handbook of human intelligence* (pp. 392–490). New York: Cambridge.

Coleman, J. S., Campbell, E. Q., Hobson, C. J., McPortland, J., Mood, A. M., Weinfeld, F. D., & York, R. L. (1966). *Equality of educational opportunity*. Washington, DC: U.S. Office of Education, U.S. Government Printing Office, OE 38001.

Cordes, C. (March, 1983). Chicago school reassessment renews debate on role of tests. *APA Monitor*, *14*, No. 3, 14–15.

Cordes, C. (April, 1986). Assessment in San Francisco. *APA Monitor*, *17*, No. 4, 16–17.

Cronbach, L. J. (1975). Five decades of public controversy over mental testing. *American Psychologist*, *30*, 1–13.

Cronbach, L. J. (1984). *Essentials of psychological testing*. New York: Harper & Row.

Diana v. State Board of Education. (1970). C-70-37 RFP N. D. Cal.

Dunn, L. M. (1968). Special education for the mildly retarded—is much of it justifiable? *Exceptional Children*, *35*, 5–22.

Elliott, R. (1988). Tests, abilities, race, and conflict. *Intelligence*, *12*, 333–350.

Feuerstein, R. (1979). *The dynamic assessment of retarded persons*. Baltimore: University Park Press.

Fulker, D. W. (1975). Review of *The science and politics of IQ* by L. J. Kamin. *American Journal of Psychology*, *88*, 505–519.

Garber, H. L., & Heber, R. (1981). The efficacy of early intervention with family rehabilitation. In M. J. Begab, H. C. Haywood, & H. L. Garber (Eds.), *Psychosocial influences in retarded performance* (Vol. 2). Baltimore: University Park Press.

Gardner, H. (1983). *Frames of mind*. New York: Basic Books.

Gordon, R. A., & Rudert, E. E. (1979). Bad news concerning IQ tests. *Sociology of Education*, *52*, 174–190.

Gottlieb, J. (1981). Mainstreaming: Fulfilling the promise? *American Journal of Mental Deficiency*, *86*, 115–126.

Griggs v. Duke Power Co. (1971). 401 U.S. 424.

Guilford, J. P. (1967). *The nature of human intelligence*. New York: McGraw-Hill.

Hall, V. C., & Kaye, D. B. (1980). Early patterns of cognitive development. *Monographs of the Society for Research in Child Development*, *45*, Serial No. 184.

Heller, K. A., Holtzman, W. H., & Messick, S. (Eds.) (1982). *Placing children in special education: A strategy for equity*. Washington, DC: National Academy Press.

Hobbs, N. (Ed.) (1975). *Issues in the classification of children*. San Francisco: Jossey-Bass.

Hobson v. Hansen. (1967). 269 F. Supp. 401.

Humphreys, L. G. (1979). The construct of general intelligence. *Intelligence*, *3*, 105–120.

Humphreys, L. G. (1988). Trends in levels of academic achievement of blacks and other minorities. *Intelligence*, *12*, 231–260.

Hunter, J. E., Schmidt, F. L., & Rauschenberger, J. (1984). Methodological, statistical, and ethical issues in the study of bias in psychological tests. In C. R. Reynolds & R. T. Brown (Eds.), *Perspectives on bias in mental testing*. New York: Plenum.

Jensen, A. R. (1976). Test bias and construct validity. *Phi Delta Kappan*, *58*, 340–346.

Jensen, A. R. (1980). *Bias in mental testing*. New York: Free Press.

Kamin, L. J. (1974). *The science and politics of I.Q.* Potomac, MD: Lawrence Erlbaum.

Keyes v. School District No. 1. (1972). 313 F. Supp. 67.

Kirp, D. L., Kuriloff, P. J., & Buss, W. G. (1975). Legal mandates and organizational change. In N. Hobbs (Ed.), *Issues in the classification of children* (Vol. 2). San Francisco: Jossey-Bass.

Klitgaard, R. (1985). *Choosing elites*. New York: Basic Books.

Landers, S. (1986, December). *APA Monitor*, p. 18.

Larry P. v. Wilson Riles (1979). 343 F. Supp. 306 (1972). 495 F. Supp. 926 (N. D. Cal. 1979).

Lazar, I. & Darlington, R. (1982). Lasting effects of early education. A report from the consortium for longitudinal studies. *Monographs of the Society for Research in Child Development*, *47*, Serial No. 192.

Lerner, B. (1978). The Supreme Court and the APA, ERA, NCME test standards: past references and future possibilities. *American Psychologist*, *33*, 915–919.

Levin, H. M. (1985). The educationally disadvantaged: A national crisis. *The State Youth Initiatives Project Working Paper 6*, 1985. Public/Private Ventures, 399 Market St., Philadelphia.

Linn, R. (1982). Ability testing: Individual differences, prediction, and differential prediction. In A. K. Wigdor & W. R. Garner (Eds.), *Ability testing: Uses, consequences, and controversies*. Washington, DC: National Academy Press.

Loehlin, J. C., Lindzey, G., & Spuhler, J. N. (1975). *Race differences in intelligence*. San Francisco: Freeman.

Los Angeles Unified School District Student Guidance Services Division. (1984, January 6). Bulletin No. 36.

Maccoby, E. A., & Jacklin, C. N. (1974). *The psychology of sex differences*, Stanford, CA: Stanford University Press.

MacMillan, D. L., & Borthwick, S. (1980). The new educable mentally retarded: Can they be mainstreamed? *Mental Retardation*, *18*, 155–158.

MacMillan, D. L., Jones, R. L., & Meyers, C. E. (1976). Mainstreaming the mildly retarded: Some questions, cautions, and guidelines. *Mental Retardation*, *14*, 3–10.

Manning, W. H., & Jackson, R. T. (1984). College entrance examinations. In C. R. Reynolds & R. T. Brown (Eds.), *Perspectives on bias in mental testing*. New York: Plenum.

McNemar, Q. (1942). *The revision of the Stanford-Binet Scale*. Boston: Houghton Mifflin.

Mercer, J. (1979). *System of multicultural pluralistic assessment*. New York: Psychological Corporation.

Meyers, C. E., MacMillan, D. L., & Yoshida, R. K. (1980). Regular class education of EMR students, from efficacy to mainstreaming. In J. Gottlieb (Ed.), *Perspectives on handicapping conditions*. Baltimore: University Park Press.

Miele, F. (1979). Cultural bias in the WISC. *Intelligence*, *3*, 149–164.

Milliken v. Bradley. (1974). 418 U.S. 717.

Mills v. Board of Education. (1971). 348 F. Supp. 866.

Moynihan, D. P. (1965). *The Negro family: The case for national action*. Washington, DC: U.S. Government Printing Office.

Nichols, P. L. (1971). The effects of heredity and environment on intelligence test performance in 4 and 7 year white and Negro sibling pairs. Doctoral dissertation, University of Minnesota, 1970). *Dissertation Abstracts International*, *32*, 101B–102B. (University Microfilms No. 71-18, 874).

Oakland, T. (1978). Predictive validity of readiness tests for middle and lower socioeconomic status Anglo, black and Mexican American children. *Journal of Educational Psychology*, *70*, 574–582.

PARC v. Pennsylvania. (1971). 343 F. Supp. 179.

Pasadena Board of Education v. Spangler. (1976). 427 U.S. 424.

PASE v. Hannon. (1980). 506 F. Supp. 831.

Ramey, C. T., Bryant, D. M., & Suarez, T. M. (1985). Preschool compensatory education and the modifiability of intelligence: A critical review. In D. Ditterman (Ed.), *Current topics in intelligence* (pp. 247–296). Norwood, NJ: Ablex.

Ramey, C. T., & Haskins, R. (1981). The causes and treatment of school failure: Insights from the Carolina Abecedarian Project. In M. J. Begab, H. C. Haywood, & H. L. Garber (Eds.), *Psychosocial influences in retarded performance* (Vol. 2). Baltimore: University Park Press.

Reschly, D. J. (1981). Evaluation of the effects of SOMPA measures on classification of students as mildly mentally retarded. *American Journal of Mental Deficiency*, *86*, 16–20.

Reschly, D. J., & Sabers, D. L. (1979). Analysis of test bias in four groups with the regression definition. *Journal of Educational Measurement*, *16*, 1–9.

Resnick, L. B. (1979). The future of IQ testing in education. *Intelligence*, *3*, 241–253.

Reynolds, C. R. (1983). Regression analysis of race and sex bias in seven preschool tests. *Journal of Psychoeducational Assessment*, *1*, 169–178.

Rosenthal, R., & Jacobson, L. (1968). *Pygmalion in the classroom*. New York: Holt, Rinehart and Winston.

Rossell, C. H. (1980). Social science research in educational equity cases: A critical review. *Review of Research in Education*, *8*, 237–295.

Sattler, J. (1982). *Assessment of children's intelligence and special abilities* (2nd Ed.). Boston: Allyn & Bacon.

Scarr, S. (1976). Review of *The science and politics of IQ*. by L. J. Kamin. *Contemporary Psychology*, *21*, 98–99.

Scarr, S. (1981). *Race, social class, and individual differences in IQ*. Hillsdale, NJ: Erlbaum.

Scarr, S., & Weinberg, R. A. (1976). IQ test performance of black children adopted by white families. *American Psychologist*, *31*, 726–739.

Shepard, L. A., Smith, M. L., & Vojir, C. P. (1983). Characteristics of pupils identified as learning disabled. *American Educational Research Journal*, *20*, 309–331.

Stephan, W. (1978). School desegregation: An evaluation of predictions made in *Brown v. Board of Education*. *Psychological Bulletin*, *85*, 217–238.

St. John, N. (1975). *Desegregation outcomes for children*. New York: Wiley.

Terman, L. M., & Merrill, M. A. (1937). *Measuring intelligence*. Cambridge, MA: Houghton Mifflin.

Thorndike, R. L., & Hagen, E. P. (1977). *Measurement and evaluation in psychology and education* (4th ed.). New York: Wiley.

Vernon, P. E. (1979). *Intelligence: Heredity and environment*. San Francisco: Freeman.

Wigdor, A. K., & Garner, W. R. (1982). *Ability testing: Uses, consequences, and controversies*. Washington, DC: National Academy Press.

Williams, R. L. (1970). Black pride, academic relevance, and individual achievement. *Counseling Psychologist*, *2*, 18–22. (Paper presented at the meeting of the American Psychological Association, Honolulu, Hawaii, September, 1972.)

Wilson, W. J. (1978). *The declining significance of race: Blacks and changing American institutions*. Chicago: University of Chicago Press.

Wolf, E. P. (1981). *Trial and error*. Detroit: Wayne State University Press.

Wrubel, P. (1979). *An assessment of the impact of the courts on local school boards*. Stanford, CA: Institute for Research on Educational Finance and Governance.

Zigler, E., & Seitz, V. (1982). Social policy and intelligence. In R. J. Sternberg (Ed.), *Handbook of human intelligence* (pp. 586–641). New York: Cambridge.

The Status and Future of Interactive Assessment

H. Carl Haywood and David Tzuriel

This volume begins with the notion that there is a need to reexamine the whole enterprise of psychoeducational assessment, and perhaps to supplement our traditional psychometric approaches and tools with new ones addressed to different goals. Different authors present different views of the nature and extent of the problems. Their criticism varies in emphasis, including problems of classroom education, problems with psychometric models and properties, problems of social integration and social justice, and even legal problems. There is the further notion that changes in theoretical concepts of the nature, development, and modifiability of human ability should be followed by conceptually consistent changes in the goals and methods of assessing ability. These are formidable challenges. It is unlikely that the very few chapters in this book have responded completely and satisfactorily to these challenges.

Several "interactive" approaches to psychoeducational assessment are proposed, each following from its own conceptual scheme regarding both the nature of ability and the goals of assessment. This diversity of approach introduces two sources of danger. The first is the temptation to believe that the success of any one set of methods of interactive assessment demonstrates the validity of the generic notion of interactive assessment. In our opinion, it would be wiser to interpret such successes as indicating the possibility of development and application of alternatives to standardized, normative assessment. Further, each technical approach is a derivative of its own conceptual system; therefore, the demonstrated success of any one approach should be seen as strengthening its underlying conceptual system. The second source of danger is the opposite: the temptation to believe that the lack of demonstrated success of any one method constitutes evidence against the validity of the generic notion itself. Failure of any one of these approaches could mean any of the following: (a) that the method had not been adequately operationalized; (b) that the method, but not its conceptual base, is deficient; (c) that the conceptual base, but not the method itself, is deficient; or (d) that the subject sample was inappropriate.

Of course, a theory or a method that has too many built-in excuses for failure has little value. After examining the chapters in this volume, it seems to the editors that there is much work to be done before the broad approach of interactive assessment can be either validated or discredited as a whole.

First, all of the theoretical systems reported here need to be extended, strengthened, and stated more clearly in ways that lead to the possibility of testable hypotheses, and "tightened" in the sense of leading to a smaller number of applications. For example, interactive assessment adherents should decide whether they believe in a small number of widely generalizable cognitive processes that are essential to learning and performance in extremely diverse contexts, or whether, on the other hand, performance depends upon more "domain-specific" processes. Feuerstein's theory of structural cognitive modifiability and mediated learning experience is by far the most complex and comprehensive of these theories, and that may constitute one of its problems: it explains too much, with interdependent parts of the theory. It is also the least empirically derived and supported. Paour's concepts of fixation, chronic deficient performance, the importance of the "pairing relation," and operatory learning all appear to be empirically derived, but their application my be more limited (to mentally retarded or chronically underfunctioning persons—the populations sampled in that group's research). The Lerntest approach rests perhaps on the least complex theoretical system—both a virtue and a potential deficiency. Das's essentially neuropsychological approach may be too limited in its choice of functions to emphasize, although its principal parts have clearly been derived empirically; that is, it might explain too little.

Second, empirical research in this field has not been blessed either with great breadth or with great volume. An example is the critical issue of domain independence versus domain specificity. Advocates of the "independence" position so far have been content merely to assert, without supporting evidence, that a small number of basic cognitive processes underlies perception, thinking, learning, and problem solving across a broad spectrum of content and contexts. Advocates of the "specificity" hypothesis have done research, failed to find great generalizability of training in specific cognitive operations, and have concluded prematurely that there is no generalizability. A more appropriate question would be: what does one have to do, with what subjects, over what period of time, to produce wide content/context generalizability of trained cognitive operations? Evaluative research has been perhaps too narrow. There have been several demonstrations that the teaching that occurs in interactive assessment leads to higher levels of postteaching performance than is true of subjects who did not receive teaching. That seems to lead only to the conclusion that people can learn from teaching! Studies of the longer term validity of interpretations derived from interactive assessment have been few and far between.

Third, there is still great conflict within the psychometric establishment regarding the necessity to establish the metric properties of interactive assessment. One example is the question of test reliability. Clearly, traditional test-retest reliability is not a useful concept when the method of testing includes interposed teaching—that is, when one sets out deliberately to change the phenomenon that is being assessed. It is, however, quite sensible to insist upon established test-retest reliability of the same instruments when they are given without interposed teaching or feedback. Another aspect of reliability, interjudge reliability of inferences derived from interactive assessment, is also critical. Some research suggests that it is possible to make quite gross judgments reliably, and that reliability of diagnostic inferences becomes less and less adequate the more one tries to make fine, detailed inferences. This whole topic demands additional research. Finally, the issue of validity is extremely challenging. It is difficult to agree upon external criteria of validity, especially when the major goal of assessment is not to predict future performance (without specific intervention) but rather to specify what is needed in order to defeat such predictions based upon standardized, normative assessment. In the grossest sense, it will be necessary to specify essential treatments (such as educational programs) differentially on the basis of interactive assessment, then actually deliver those programs, and then assess the subjects' differential progress as a function of their initial interactive assessment performance.

Fourth, it is undeniably true that all interactive methods require more skill and greater investment of time from examiners, and a willingness on the part of subjects also to invest more time and effort in assessment. In some of these systems, an investment of 10 or more houre is normal. Many school psychologists are accustomed to having only from 1 to 3 hours to spend with each subject. School officials will surely ask why they should invest in methods that require several times as many hours from the psychologists as do present methods. The answer, of course, lies in what one derives from the assessment. If it can be done quickly, but without useful results, it might be less economical than spending more time and deriving useful information. The challenge, then, is to be certain that the information derived is worth the investment required to get it, and that the information is then used in such a way as to result in educational (or other) benefit for the subjects.

In spite of such large and difficult problems, interactive approaches to psychoeducational assessment appear to offer useful and even rich alternatives to standardized, normative assessment. Their clinical utility, as demonstrated in the case studies presented here, is convincing. These approaches appear to offer the possibility of more adequate assessment of handicapped persons (e.g., mentally retarded, sensory impaired, emotionally disturbed persons) and persons with learning disabilities, than do standardized, normative tests. They appear also to offer the possibility of some solution to "nondiscriminatory" assessment and educational programming for persons in minority ethnic groups and those in "transcultural" status: immigrants and those with language differences.

The richness of interactive approaches has just begun to be explored and exploited. The editors and the contributors hope that this volume will lead to greater exploration and greater exploitation.

Author Index

Page numbers in italics indicate entries in references sections.

Subject Index